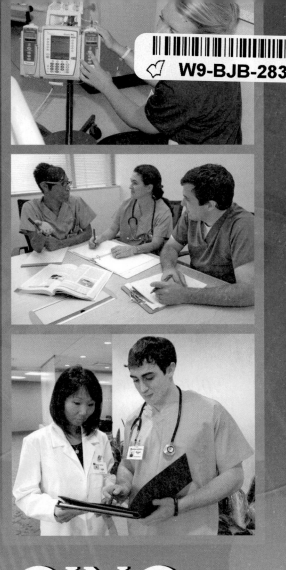

LEADING
and MANAGING
in NURSING
Revised Reprint

FIFTH EDITION

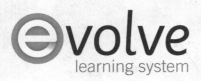
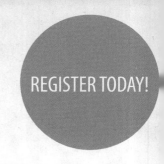

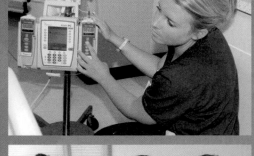

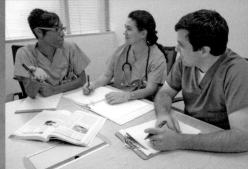

Patricia S. Yoder-Wise

Texas Tech University Health
   Sciences Center
Lubbock, Texas
Texas Woman's University-Houston
Houston, Texas

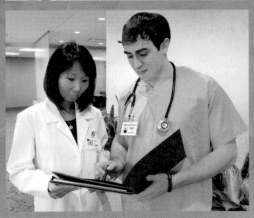

LEADING and MANAGING in NURSING Revised Reprint

FIFTH EDITION

ELSEVIER
MOSBY

3251 Riverport Lane
St. Louis, Missouri 63043

LEADING AND MANAGING IN NURSING, FIFTH EDITION, Revised Reprint   ISBN: 978-0-323-24183-0

Notices

Knowledge and best practice in this field are constantly changing. As new research and experience broaden our understanding, changes in research methods, professional practices, or medical treatment may become necessary.

Practitioners and researchers must always rely on their own experience and knowledge in evaluating and using any information, methods, compounds, or experiments described herein. In using such information or methods they should be mindful of their own safety and the safety of others, including parties for whom they have a professional responsibility.

With respect to any drug or pharmaceutical products identified, readers are advised to check the most current information provided (i) on procedures featured or (ii) by the manufacturer of each product to be administered, to verify the recommended dose or formula, the method and duration of administration, and contraindications. It is the responsibility of practitioners, relying on their own experience and knowledge of their patients, to make diagnoses, to determine dosages and the best treatment for each individual patient, and to take all appropriate safety precautions.

To the fullest extent of the law, neither the Publisher nor the authors, contributors, or editors, assume any liability for any injury and/or damage to persons or property as a matter of products liability, negligence or otherwise, or from any use or operation of any methods, products, instructions, or ideas contained in the material herein.

Library of Congress Cataloging-in-Publication Data (in PHL)

Leading and managing in nursing / [edited by] Patricia S. Yoder-Wise.—5th ed.
    p. ; cm.
Includes bibliographical references and index.
ISBN 978-0-323-24183-0 (pbk.)
1. Nursing services—Administration. 2. Leadership. I. Yoder-Wise, Patricia S., 1941-
[DNLM: 1. Nurse Administrators—organization & administration. 2. Leadership. WY 105 L4325 2011]
RT89.L43 2011
362.17′3—dc22

                                                                          2010025915

Acquisitions Editor: Nancy O'Brien
Associate Developmental Editor: Angela Perdue
Publishing Services Manager: Deborah L. Vogel
Senior Project Manager: Jodi M. Willard
Design Direction: Teresa McBryan

Printed in United States of America

Last digit is the print number: 9   8   7   6   5   4   3   2   1

This book is dedicated to the families and friends who supported all of us who created it, to the faculty who use this book to develop tomorrow's emerging leaders and managers, and to the learners who have the vision and insight to grasp today's reality and mold it into the future of dynamic nursing leadership. Special recognition goes to Anne Mitchell and Vickilyn Galle for their leadership in safe patient care. You are our heroes!!

Lead on! ¡Adelante!

CONTRIBUTORS

Michael R. Bleich, PhD, RN, NEA-BC, FAAN
Dean and Carol A. Lindeman Distinguished Professor of
    Nursing
School of Nursing
Oregon Health and Science University
Portland, Oregon
Chapter 1: Leading, Managing, and Following

Mary Ellen Clyne, MSN, RN, NEA-BC
Executive Director
Clara Maass Medical Center
Belleville, New Jersey
*Chapter 16: Strategic Planning, Goal-Setting, and
    Marketing*

Mary Ann T. Donohue, PhD, RN, APN, NEA-BC
Vice President of Clinical Care Services
Jersey Shore University Medical Center
Neptune, New Jersey
Chapter 17: Leading Change

Karen A. Esquibel, PhD, RN
Assistant Professor
Texas Tech University Health Sciences Center
Anita Thigpen Perry School of Nursing
Lubbock, Texas
Chapter 9: Cultural Diversity in Health Care

Michael L. Evans, PhD, RN, NEA-BC, FACHE, FAAN
Dean and Professor
Goldfarb School of Nursing at Barnes-Jewish College
St. Louis, Missouri
Chapter 3: Developing the Role of Leader

Victoria N. Folse, PhD, APN, PMHCNS-BC, LCPC
Director and Associate Professor, School of Nursing
Illinois Wesleyan University
Bloomington, Illinois
Chapter 20: Managing Quality and Risk
Chapter 23: Conflict: The Cutting Edge of Change

Denise K. Gormley, PhD, RN
Assistant Professor and Director, Graduate Programs in
    Systems-Focused Nursing
University of Cincinnati, Academic Health Center,
    College of Nursing
Cincinnati, Ohio
Chapter 19: Collective Action

Ginny Wacker Guido, JD, MSN, RN, FAAN
Regional Director for Nursing and Assistant Dean
Washington State University Vancouver
Vancouver, Washington
Chapter 5: Legal and Ethical Issues

Debra Hagler, PhD, RN, ACNS-BC, CNE, ANEF
Clinical Professor and Coordinator for Teaching
    Excellence
Arizona State University
College of Nursing & Health Innovation
Phoenix, Arizona
Chapter 29: Managing Your Career

Catherine A. Hill, MSN, RN, CS
Director of Quality
Texas Health Resources
Dallas, Texas
Chapter 28: Self-Management: Stress and Time

Cheri Hunt, MHA, RN, NEA-BC
Vice President for Nursing/Chief Nursing Officer
The Children's Mercy Hospital
Kansas City, Missouri
*Chapter 11: Caring, Communicating, and Managing with
    Technology*

Karen Kelly, EdD, RN, NEA-BC
Associate Professor
Southern Illinois University Edwardsville
Edwardsville, Illinois
Chapter 10: Power, Politics, and Influence

Karren Kowalski, PhD, RN, NEA-BC, FAAN
Professor
Texas Tech University Health Sciences Center
Anita Thigpen Perry School of Nursing
Lubbock, Texas;
Grant/Project Director
Colorado Center for Nursing Excellence
Denver, Colorado
Chapter 18: Building Teams Through Communication and
    Partnerships
Chapter 24: Managing Personal/Personnel Problems

Mary E. Mancini, PhD, RN, NE-BC, FAHA, FAAN
Professor and Associate Dean
The University of Texas—Arlington
College of Nursing
Arlington, Texas
Chapter 7: Healthcare Organizations
Chapter 8: Understanding and Designing Organizational
    Structures

Dorothy A. Otto, EdD, MSN, RN, ANEF
Associate Professor
University of Texas Health Science Center
School of Nursing
Houston, Texas
Chapter 9: Cultural Diversity in Health Care

Janis B. Smith, RN, DNP
Director, Clinical Information Systems
The Children's Mercy Hospital
Kansas City, Missouri
Chapter 11: Caring, Communicating, and Managing with
    Technology

Susan Sportsman, PhD, RN
Dean, College of Health Sciences and Human Services
Midwestern State University
Wichita Falls, Texas
Chapter 13: Care Delivery Strategies
Chapter 14: Staffing and Scheduling

Trudi B. Stafford, PhD, RN
Vice President and Chief Nursing Officer
Baylor All Saints Medical Center
Fort Worth, Texas
Chapter 12: Managing Costs and Budgets

Angela L. Stalbaum, MSN, RN, NE-BC
Chief Nursing Officer
Seton Family of Hospitals—Seton Medical Center Austin
Austin, Texas
Chapter 4: Developing the Role of Manager

Diane M. Twedell, DNP, RN, CENP
Nurse Administrator
Mayo Clinic
Rochester, Minnesota
Chapter 15: Selecting, Developing, and Evaluating Staff
Chapter 27: Role Transition

Ana M. Valadez, RN, EdD, NEA-BC, FAAN
Professor Emerita
Anita Thigpen School of Nursing
Texas Tech University Health Sciences Center
Lubbock, Texas
Chapter 4: Developing the Role of Manager

Rose Aguilar Welch, EdD, RN
Professor of Nursing
California State University, Dominguez Hills
Carson, California
Chapter 6: Making Decisions and Solving Problems

Crystal J. Wilkinson, MSN, RN, CNS-CH, CPHQ
Assistant Professor
Texas Tech University Health Sciences Center
Lubbock, Texas
Chapter 25: Workplace Violence and Incivility

Patricia S. Yoder-Wise, RN, EdD, NEA-BC, ANEF,
FAAN
Texas Tech University Health Sciences Center
Lubbock, Texas
Texas Woman's University-Houston
Houston, Texas
Chapter 2: Patient Safety
Chapter 26: Delegation: An Art of Professional Practice
Chapter 30: Thriving for the Future

Margarete Lieb Zalon, PhD, RN, ACNS-BC, FAAN
Professor
Department of Nursing
University of Scranton
Scranton, Pennsylvania
Chapter 21: Translating Research into Practice
Chapter 22: Consumer Relationships

EVOLVE RESOURCES

Instructor's Manual and PowerPoint Slides
Barbara D. Powe, PhD, RN
Director, Cancer Communication Science
American Cancer Society
Atlanta, Georgia

Test Bank
Joyce Engel, PhD, RN, BEd, MEd
Associate Professor
Department of Nursing
Brock University
St. Catharines, Ontario

PHOTOGRAPHY

Dennis Scanio
Florissant, Missouri

Peer review is a critical aspect of most publications. Peers tell us what is strong and what is missing. They direct the content of a publication from their area of knowledge and experience. These individuals provide insightful comments and suggestions to hone the information presented in a text or article, and we are indebted to them. The end result of their efforts, as in any peer review process, is a stronger presentation of information for the readership. We are grateful to the masked reviewers of this publication. Thank you!

Martha C. Baker, PhD, RN, CNE, ACWS-BC
Director of BSN Program/Professor of Nursing
St. John's College of Nursing
Southwest Baptist University
Springfield, Missouri

Kathleen Becker, RN, BSN, MSN, MEd
Professor of Nursing
St. Louis Community College
St. Louis, Missouri

Jacqueline Rosenjack Burchum, DNSC, FNP-BC, CNE
Associate Professor
College of Nursing
University of Tennessee Health Science Center
Memphis, Tennessee

Beth-Anne M. Christopher, MS, RN
Instructor
Adult Health and Gerontological Nursing
Rush University College of Nursing
Chicago, Illinois

Tammy S. Czyzewski, BA, BSN, MS, RN-BC, NEA-BC
Assistant Professor of Nursing
Sinclair Community College
Dayton, Ohio

Victoria Todd Durkee, PhD, APRN
Associate Professor
Nursing Department
University of Louisiana at Monroe
Monroe, Louisiana

Donna Egnatios, RN, MSN, CCM, NEA-BC
Nurse Manager—Home Health
Scottsdale Health Care
Scottsdale, Arizona

Mary L. Fisher, PhD, RN, CNE, BC
Professor of Nursing/Associate Vice Chancellor for Academic Affairs/Associate Dean of the Faculties
Academic Affairs
Indiana University/Purdue University
Indianapolis, Indiana

Shirley Garick, PhD, MSN, RN
Professor of Nursing
Department of Nursing
Texas A & M University—Texarkana
Texarkana, Texas

Judith A. Gentry, APRN, MSN, OCN, CNE
Assistant Professor of Clinical Nursing
School of Nursing
Louisiana State University Health Sciences Center
New Orleans, Louisiana

Earl Goldberg, EdD, APRN, BC
Associate Professor
Nursing and Health Sciences
Lasalle University
Philadelphia, Pennsylvania

Nancy C. Grove, PhD, RN, BSN, MEd, MSN
Adjunct Associate Professor
School of Nursing
University of Pittsburgh
Pittsburgh, Pennsylvania

Bonnie L. Kirkpatrick, RN, MS, CNS, CNL
Clinical Instructor
School of Nursing
Ohio State University College of Nursing
Columbus, Ohio

Patricia A. La Brosse, APRN-BC
Psychiatric/Mental Health
Clinical Nurse Specialist
Nursing Services
University Medical Center
Lafayette, Louisiana

Dimitra Loukissa, PhD, RN
Associate Professor
School of Nursing
North Park University
Chicago, Illinois

Dorothea E. McDowell, PhD, RN
Professor of Nursing
Nursing Department
Salisbury University
Salisbury, Maryland

Lynn A. Menzel, RN, MA
Case Manager
Case Management
Martin Memorial Medical Center
Stuart, Florida

Denise Top Rhine, RN, MEd, CEN
Professor of Nursing
Nursing Department
Oakton Community College
Des Plaines, Illinois

Jack E. Rydell, RN, MS
Assistant Professor
Nursing Department
Concordia College
Moorhead, Minnesota

Gail Scoates, RN, MS
Adjunct Faculty
School of Nursing
Illinois Wesleyan University
Bloomington, Illinois

Christina Leibold Sieloff, PhD, RN
Associate Professor
College of Nursing
Montana State University
Bozeman, Montana

Jaynelle F. Stichler, DNSc, RN, EDAL, FACHE, FAAN
Professor and Concentration Chair—Leadership in
    Healthcare Systems
School of Nursing
San Diego State University
San Diego, California

Mary Pat Szutenbach, PhD, RN, CNS
Assistant Professor
School of Nursing
Regis University
Denver, Colorado

Karen S. Ward, PhD, RN, COI
School of Nursing
Middle Tennessee State University
Murfreesboro, Tennessee

Constance Woulard, RN, MSN
Associate Chief Nurse
Extended Care Rehab
Grand Canyon University
Des Moines, Iowa

ACKNOWLEDGMENTS

This fifth edition of *Leading and Managing in Nursing* revised reprint, reminds me of the numerous people over the years who have continued to build on what the first edition presented. From edition one, where I heavily relied on the U.S. Postal Service, FedEx, Kinko's, and an Internet service provider, to today where everything was completed electronically, we have increased the intensity of information about leading and managing to respond to the increased intensity of need for such information.

The first edition was conceived at a meeting in New Orleans. Darlene Como, then with Mosby, and I sat hunched over a table identifying chapters and content and then prospective authors. This textbook revolutionized how texts addressed leading and managing content. Previously, texts about managing consisted primarily of words and a few graphs and charts. The introduction of color, stories, exercises, photographs of nurses in situations where leading and managing are expected, a research and/or literature perspective, and boxes of information changed the face of texts devoted to helping students learn about leading and managing. The title was chosen carefully: ending the words in "-ing" was designed to show a dynamic process important to nursing. Although the text has increased in size, the first edition had large white spaces for margins in which the exercises and key words appeared. In later editions, these spaces were replaced with more content to accommodate the increased amount of information about leading and managing. The workbook was first a separate publication, then it was incorporated into the text, and now it is online. This flow represents the movement of nursing education across the country from tear-out pages to electronic access. This evolution of content and design was made possible by each of the authors and editors from the first edition through to the fifth.

Special acknowledgment goes to the team at Elsevier—the "behind the scenes" people who turn Word documents into a graphically appealing and colorful presentation. To our editor, Nancy O'Brien; to our developmental editor, Angela Perdue; to our editorial assistant, Kevin Clear; and to our project manager, Jodi Willard: THANKS!

To the authors who made this edition possible: thank you for helping the next generation of nurses be well prepared to enter the profession of nursing and to exercise both leadership and management in responsible and artistic ways. To the faculty who have used this textbook and provided feedback, we listened and, as with the reviewers, incorporated suggestions as needed.

Most of all, for me personally, I have to thank my husband and best friend, Robert Thomas Wise. He has lived through five editions of this text and knows by now that when the deadlines tighten, his humor and creativity need to increase. And they do! His willingness to take on more of the things that might be deemed mutual tasks is a small example of his ongoing support. You are the best!

As has been true since the beginning of *Leading and Managing in Nursing* revised reprint, we who created and revised this edition learned more about a particular area and the impact of each area on the whole of leadership and management. Our learning reflects the condition of nursing today: there is no room for stagnation on any topic. The context in which nurses lead and manage is constantly changing—so the key to success is to learn continuously. Keep learning, keep caring, and maintain our passion for nursing and the patients we serve. That message, if nothing else, must be instilled in our leaders of tomorrow.

Lead on! ¡Adelante!

Patricia S. Yoder-Wise
RN, EdD, NEA-BC, ANEF, FAAN
Texas Tech University Health Sciences Center
Lubbock, Texas

Leading and managing are two essential expectations of all professional nurses and are more important than ever in today's rapidly changing healthcare system. To lead and manage successfully, nurses must possess not only knowledge and skills but also a caring and compassionate attitude. After all, leading and managing are both about people.

Volumes of information on leadership and management principles can be found in nursing, healthcare administration, business, and general literature. The numerous journals in each of these fields offer research and opinion articles focused on improving leaders' and managers' abilities. The first four editions of this text demonstrated that learners, faculty, and registered nurses in practice found that a text that synthesized applicable knowledge and related it to contemporary practice was useful. Whereas clinical nursing textbooks offer exercises and assignments designed to provide opportunities for learners to apply theory to patients, nursing leadership and management textbooks traditionally offered limited opportunities of this type. We changed that tradition in 1995 by incorporating application exercises within the text and a workbook section for learners. With the third edition, we changed that tradition yet again by linking this text to a website where case studies exemplify a chapter's point and provide even more recent references. The fourth edition again broke a new pathway for learning, providing a web-based course available through Evolve. Now, we've added the workbook to the website so students can readily access those activities that faculty suggest. In addition, the fourth edition adds to critical content areas—patient safety and workplace violence. Patient safety was added because of the critical importance it has in the way leaders and managers must make decisions. Protecting the patient is an obligation of all who engage in patient care. Workplace violence was added because of its prevalence in the workplace and its threat to patient safety, personnel safety, retention, and recruitment.

This book results from our continued strong belief in the need for a text that focuses in a distinctive way on the nursing leadership and management issues of today and tomorrow. We continue to find that we are not alone in this belief. Before the first edition, Mosby, primarily through the efforts of Darlene Como, solicited faculty members' and administrators' ideas to determine what they thought professional nurses most needed to know about leading and managing and what type of text would best help them obtain the necessary knowledge and skills. Their comprehensive list of suggestions remains relevant in this edition. This edition incorporates reviewers from both service and education to be sure that the text conveys important and timely information to users as they focus on the critical roles of leading, managing, and following. Additionally, we took seriously the various comments by faculty and learners offered as I met them in person or heard from them by email.

CONCEPT AND PRACTICE COMBINED

Innovative in both content and presentation, *Leading and Managing in Nursing* revised reprint merges theory, research, and practical application in key leadership and management areas. Our overriding concern in this edition remains to create a text that, while well grounded in theory and concept, presents the content in a way that is real. Wherever possible, we use real-world examples from the continuum of today's healthcare settings to illustrate the concepts. Because each chapter contributor focuses on synthesizing the assigned content, you will find no lengthy quotations in these chapters. We have made every effort to make the content as engaging, inviting, and interesting as possible. Reflecting our view of the real world of nursing leadership and management today, the following themes pervade the text:

- Every role within nursing has the basic concern for safe, effective care for the people we exist for—our clients and patients.

- The focus of health care is shifting from the hospital to the community.
- Healthcare consumers and the healthcare workforce are becoming increasingly culturally diverse.
- Today virtually every professional nurse leads, manages, and follows, regardless of title or position.
- Consumer relationships play a central role in the delivery of nursing and health care.
- Communication, collaboration, team-building, and other interpersonal skills form the foundation of effective nursing leadership and management.
- Change continues at a rapid pace in health care and society in general.
- Movement toward evidence-based practice is long overdue.
- An anticipation of healthcare delivery over the next several years will rely on the above themes for nurses.

DIVERSITY OF PERSPECTIVES

Contributors are recruited from diverse settings, roles, and geographic areas, enabling them to offer a broad perspective on the critical elements of nursing leadership and management roles. To help bridge the gap often found between nursing education and nursing practice, some contributors were recruited from academia and others from practice settings. This blend not only contributes to the richness of this text but also conveys a sense of oneness in nursing. The historical "gap" between education and service must become a sense of a continuum and not a chasm.

AUDIENCE

This book is designed for undergraduate learners in nursing leadership and management courses, including those in BSN-completion courses and second-degree programs. In addition, we know that nurses in practice, who had not anticipated formal leadership and management roles in their careers, use this text to capitalize on their own real-life experiences as a way to develop greater understanding about leading and managing and the important role of following. Because today's learners are more visually oriented than past learners, we have incorporated illustrations, boxes, and a functional full-color design to stimulate

interest and maximize learning. In addition, numerous examples and The Challenge in each chapter remain to provide relevance to the real world of nursing.

ORGANIZATION

We have organized this text around issues that are key to the success of professional nurses in today's constantly changing healthcare environment.

First, it is important to understand the core concepts of leading and managing and how the theories and foci differ from each other. For example, headship (holding a formal position or title) does not always mean that person is demonstrating leadership. Next, nurses should understand key concepts as they relate to leading and managing. You will find key organizational information that ranges from our chief concern of patient safety to a basic understanding about the types of organizations delivering care to the changing demands for quality, technology, and cost-effectiveness. Consumer relationships influence how to deliver care and relationships with staff. Cultural diversity does not focus so much on understanding diversities of patients (appropriate for clinical textbooks) as it does on understanding and valuing diversities in employees (critical to leading and managing) and the influence of diverse staff on diversities of patients. The text then transitions from the critical elements of teams and how they interact to accomplish work to the individual expectations and influences we must have throughout our careers.

Because repetition plays a crucial role in how well learners learn and retain new content, some topics appear in more than one chapter and in more than one section. For example, prior editions addressed disruptive behavior, although it was not called that. Several of the chapters in this current edition address the issue of disruption in the workplace. The issue of workplace disruptions or violence are so prevalent in today's healthcare world that we have devoted a chapter to the issue to pull several key points together. We have also made an effort to express a variety of different views on some topics, as is true in the real world of nursing. This diversity of views in the real world presents a constant challenge to leaders and managers, who address the critical tasks of creating positive workplaces so that those who provide direct care thrive and continuously improve the patient experience.

DESIGN

The functional full-color design, still distinctive to this text, is used to emphasize and identify the text's many teaching/learning strategies, which are featured to enhance learning. Full-color photographs not only add visual interest but also provide visual reinforcement of concepts, such as body language and the changes occurring in contemporary healthcare settings. Figures elucidate and depict concepts and activities described in the text graphically.

TEACHING/LEARNING STRATEGIES

The numerous teaching/learning strategies featured in this text are designed both to stimulate learners' interest and to provide constant reinforcement throughout the learning process. In addition, the visually appealing, full-color design itself serves a learning purpose. Color is used consistently throughout the text to help the reader identify the various chapter elements described in the following sections.

CHAPTER OPENER ELEMENTS

- The introductory paragraph briefly describes the purpose and scope of the chapter.
- Objectives articulate the chapter's learning goals, typically at the application level or higher.
- The Challenge presents a contemporary nurse's real-world concern related to the chapter's focus.

ELEMENTS WITHIN THE CHAPTERS

Glossary Terms appear in color type in each chapter. Definitions appear in the Glossary at the end of the text.

Exercises stimulate learners to think critically about how to apply chapter content to the workplace and other real-world situations. They provide experiential reinforcement of key leading and managing skills. Exercises are highlighted within a full-color box and

are numbered sequentially within each chapter to facilitate using them as assignments or activities.

Research Perspectives and *Literature Perspectives* illustrate the relevance and applicability of current scholarship to practice. Perspectives always appear in boxes with a "book" icon in the upper left corner.

Theory Boxes provide a brief description of relevant theory and key concepts.

Numbered boxes contain lists, tools such as forms and work sheets, and other information relevant to chapter content that learners will find useful and interesting.

END OF CHAPTER ELEMENTS

The Solution provides an effective method to handle the real-life situations set forth in *The Challenge*.

The Evidence contains one example of evidence related to the chapter's content or it contains a summary of what the literature shows to be evidence related to the topic.

Need to Know Now summarizes the most critical key points for new graduates in preparation for their transition to the workforce.

Chapter Checklists summarize key concepts from the chapter in both paragraph and itemized list form.

Tips offer practical guidelines for learners to follow in applying some aspect of the information presented in each chapter.

References and *Suggested Readings* provide the learner with a list of key sources for further reading on topics found in the chapter.

OTHER TEACHING/ LEARNING STRATEGIES

The *Glossary* contains a comprehensive list of definitions of all boldfaced terms used in the chapters.

COMPLETE TEACHING AND LEARNING PACKAGE

In addition to the text *Leading and Managing in Nursing*, Instructor Resources are provided online through Evolve (http://evolve.elsevier.com/Yoder-Wise/). These resources are designed to help instructors present the material in this text and include the following assets:

- **UPDATED!** PowerPoint Slides for each chapter with lecture notes where applicable (over 600 slides total)
- **UPDATED!** ExamView Test Bank with over 750 multiple-choice questions.

  Rationales are based on AONE Competencies and the most recent ANA Scope and Standards for Nurse Administrators. Answers are also provided.
- **UPDATED!** Instructor's Manual
  - Chapter Objectives
  - Chapter Outline
  - Terms to Know
  - Teaching Suggestions
  - Instructions for Text Chapter Exercises
  - Skills Checklist

  - Discussion/Essay Questions
  - Experiential Exercises and Learning Activities
  - Suggested Guest Speakers
- **UPDATED!** Application Activities and Answers
- **UPDATED!** Case Studies for each chapter
- **NEW!** Sample Exercise Answers
- **UPDATED!** Image Collection (over 50 images)
- **UPDATED!** Online Course with twenty-eight modules presented in a consistent organizational structure, including features such as an overview, critical questions, objectives, reading assignments, learning activities, and case studies.

Student Resources can also be found online through Evolve (http://evolve.elsevier.com/Yoder-Wise/). These resources provide students with additional tools for learning and include the following assets:

- Sample Résumés
- WebLinks

LEARNER'S GUIDE

As a professional nurse in today's changing healthcare system, you will need strong leadership and management skills more than ever, regardless of your specific role. You will also need to be an independent, dependable follower. The fifth edition of *Leading and Managing in Nursing* not only provides the conceptual knowledge you will need but also offers practical strategies to help you hone the various skills so vital to your success as a leader and manager.

Because repetition is a key strategy in learning and retaining new information, you will find many topics discussed in more than one chapter. In addition, as in the real world of nursing, you will often find several different views expressed on a single topic. This repetition reinforces ideas and illustrates how one concept has multiple applications. Rather than referring you to another portion of the text, the key information is provided within the specific chapter, but perhaps in less depth. Because leading and managing are skills that require specific situation considerations, you can see why such a diversity of views exists.

To help you make the most of your learning experience, try the following strategy. Read the opening paragraph of each chapter. This preview should create a context for your reading. The objectives suggest what your accomplishments should be by the time you conclude the chapter. Look at the end of the chapter for the checklist of the key big points. *The Challenge* allows you to "hear" a real-life situation and always poses the question, "What do you think you would do if you were this nurse?" (*The Solution,* at the end of the chapter, examines what one individual did in this situation and again asks you to think about how that fits for you and why.) The Introduction and subsequent content, like any text, provide critical information. For some learners, it is useful to skim those headings and the box content to gain an overall sense of the concepts inherent in the chapter. For others, reading and reflecting from the beginning of the chapter to the end might be useful. The material in boxes (boxes, tables, Research Perspectives, Literature Perspectives, and Theory Boxes) is designed to augment understanding of the content in the text narrative. The Evidence at the end of the chapters highlights what we know in at least one case about the topic. The checklist at the end of each chapter highlights the key points the chapter presented, and tips illustrate ways to apply the content just studied. After you complete each chapter, stop and think about what the chapter conveyed. What does it mean for you as a leader, follower, and manager? How do the chapter's content and your interaction with it relate to the other chapters you have already completed? How might you briefly synthesize the content for a non-nurse friend? Reading the chapter, restating its key points in your own words, and completing the text exercises and online activities will go far to help you make the content truly your own.

We think you will find leading and managing to be an exciting, challenging field of study, and we have made every attempt to reflect that belief in the design and approach of this edition.

LEARNING AIDS

The fifth edition of *Leading and Managing in Nursing* continues to incorporate important tools to help you learn about leading and managing and apply your new knowledge to the real world. The next few pages graphically point out how to use these study aids to your best advantage.

The vivid full-color chapter opener *photographs* and other photographs throughout the text help convey each chapter's key message while providing a glimpse into the real world of leading and managing in nursing.

The *introductory paragraph* tells you what you can expect to find in the chapter. To help set the stage for your study of the chapter, read it first and then summarize in your own words what you expect to gain from the chapter.

The list of *Objectives* helps you focus on the key information you should be able to apply after having studied the chapter.

In *The Challenge*, practicing nurse leaders/managers offer their real-world views of a concern related to the chapter. Has a nurse you know had similar or dissimilar challenges?

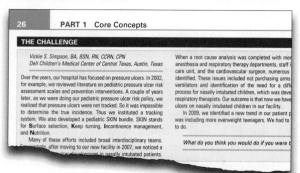

Most chapters contain at least one *Research Perspective* or *Literature Perspective* box that you can identify by the "book" icon in the upper left corner. These boxes summarize articles of interest and point out their relevance and applicability to practice. Check the journal that the article came from to find a list of indexing terms to help you locate additional and even more recent articles on the same topic.

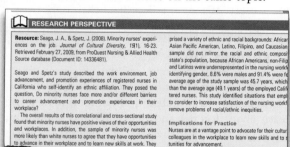

Most chapters contain a *Theory Box* to highlight and summarize pertinent theoretical concepts.

THEORY BOX		
Theories for Planned Change		
KEY CONTRIBUTORS	**KEY IDEA**	**APPLICATION TO PRACTICE**
Six Phases of Planned Change* Havelock (1973) is credited with this planned change model.	Change can be planned, implemented, and evaluated in six sequential stages. The model is advocated for the development of effective change agents and used as a rational problem-solving process. The six stages are as follows: 1. Building a relationship 2. Diagnosing the problem 3. Acquiring relevant resources 4. Choosing the solution 5. Gaining acceptance 6. Stabilizing the innovation and generating self-renewal	Useful for low-, low-complex change.
Seven Phases of Planned Change† Lippitt, Watson, and Westley ...ted with this	Change can be planned, implemented, and evaluated in seven sequential phases. Ongoing sensitivity to forces in the change process is essential. The seven phases are as follows: 1. The client system becomes aware of the need for change. ...ship is developed between the client system and	Useful for low-, low-complex change.

Every chapter contains numbered *Exercises* that challenge you to think critically about concepts in the text and apply them to real-life situations.

Key terms appear in boldface type throughout the chapter. (A list of all key terms used in the chapter appears at the end of the chapter and the Glossary at the end of the text contains a list of their definitions.)

The *boxes* in every chapter highlight key information such as lists and contain forms, worksheets, and self-assessments to help reinforce chapter content.

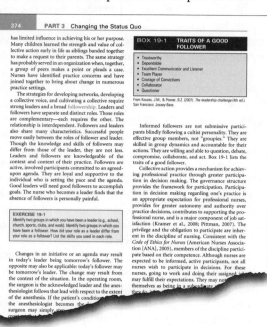

The *tables* that appear throughout the text provide convenient capsules of information for your reference.

TABLE 17-2	SELF-ASSESSMENT: HOW RECEPTIVE ARE YOU TO CHANGE AND INNOVATION?		
Read the following items. Circle the answer that most closely matches your attitude toward creating and accepting new or different ways.			
1. I enjoy learning about new ideas and approaches.		Yes	Depends
2. Once I learn about a new idea or approach, I begin to try it right away.		Yes	Depends
3. I like to discuss different ways of accomplishing a goal or end result.		Yes	Depends
4. I continually seek better ways to improve what I do.		Yes	Depends
5. I commonly recognize improved ways of doing things.		Yes	Depends
6. I talk over my ideas for change with my peers.		Yes	Depends
7. I communicate my ideas for change with my manager.		Yes	Depends
8. I discuss my ideas for change with my family.		Yes	Depends
9. I volunteer to be at meetings when changes are being discussed.		Yes	Depends
10. I encourage others to try new ideas and approaches.		Yes	Depends

If you answered "yes" to 8 to 10 of the items, you are probably receptive to creating and experiencing new and different ways of doing things. If you answered "yes" to 5 to 10 of the items, you are probably conditionally based on the fit of the change with your preferred ... of doing things. If you answered "no" to 4 to 10 of the items, you are probably not receptive, at least initially, to new ways... "yes," "no," and "depends" an approximately equal number of times, you are probably ... situations.

The numerous full-color *illustrations* visually reinforce key concepts.

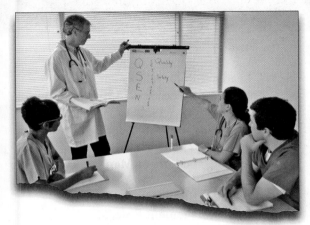

Each chapter ends with these features:

The Solution provides an effective method to handle the situation presented in the Challenge.

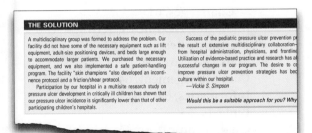

THE SOLUTION

A multidisciplinary group was formed to address the problem. Our facility did not have some of the necessary equipment such as lift equipment, adult-size positioning devices, and beds large enough to accommodate larger patients. We purchased the necessary equipment, and we also implemented a safe patient-handling program. The facility "skin champions "also developed an incontinence protocol and a friction/shear protocol.

Participation by our hospital in a multisite research study on pressure ulcer development in critically ill children has shown that our pressure ulcer incidence is significantly lower than that of other participating children's hospitals.

Success of the pediatric pressure ulcer prevention p[...] the result of extensive multidisciplinary collaboration[...] from hospital administration, physicians, and frontline[...] Utilization of evidence-based practice and research has a[...] successful changes in our program. The desire to c[...] improve pressure ulcer prevention strategies has bec[...] culture within our hospital.

—Vickie S. Simpson

Would this be a suitable approach for you? Why[...]

The Evidence identifies at least one piece of evidence by citing an article, or it identifies a list of evidence-based/best practices about the chapter.

THE EVIDENCE

A strong correlation has been established between nurse practice environments and patient outcomes. Aiken et al. (2008) added to an established program of research and analyzed data from 10,184 nurses and 232,342 surgical patients in 168 Pennsylvania hospitals to determine the effects of nurse practice environments on nurse and patient outcomes. Outcomes included nurse job satisfaction, burnout, intent to leave, and reports of quality of care including mortal-

ity and failure to rescue pati[...] study reinforces findings fr[...] of 94 research studies exam[...] nurse staffing to patient outc[...] Agency of Healthcare Resea[...] published in 2007 by Kane [...] Kane et al. showed that [...] was associated with redu[...] reduced failure to rescue, [...]

Need to Know Now is designed to summarize what the authors think is expected of most new graduates in their first professional positions.

The *Chapter Checklist* provides a quick summary of key points in the chapter. To help you keep in mind the broad themes of the chapter, read it immediately *before* you start reading the chapter. Reading it afterwards highlights the key big points.

The *Tips* offer guidelines to follow for each chapter before applying the information presented in the chapter.

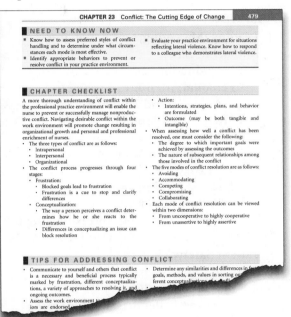

CHAPTER 23 Conflict: The Cutting Edge of Change | **479**

NEED TO KNOW NOW

- Know how to assess preferred styles of conflict handling and to determine under what circumstances each mode is most effective.
- Identify appropriate behaviors to prevent or resolve conflict in your practice environment.
- Evaluate your practice environment for situations reflecting lateral violence. Know how to respond to a colleague who demonstrates lateral violence.

CHAPTER CHECKLIST

A more thorough understanding of conflict within the professional practice environment will enable the nurse to prevent or successfully manage nonproductive conflict. Navigating desirable conflict within the work environment will promote change resulting in organizational growth and personal and professional enrichment of nurses.
- The three types of conflict are as follows:
  - Intrapersonal
  - Interpersonal
  - Organizational
- The conflict process progresses through four stages:
  - Frustration:
    - Blocked goals lead to frustration
    - Frustration is a cue to stop and clarify differences
  - Conceptualization:
    - The way a person perceives a conflict determines how he or she reacts to the frustration
    - Differences in conceptualizing an issue can block resolution

- Action:
  - Intentions, strategies, plans, and behavior are formulated
  - Outcome (may be both tangible and intangible)
- When assessing how well a conflict has been resolved, one must consider the following:
  - The degree to which important goals were achieved by assessing the outcomes
  - The nature of subsequent relationships among those involved in the conflict
- The five modes of conflict resolution are as follows:
  - Avoiding
  - Accommodating
  - Competing
  - Compromising
  - Collaborating
- Each mode of conflict resolution can be viewed within two dimensions:
  - From uncooperative to highly cooperative
  - From unassertive to highly assertive

TIPS FOR ADDRESSING CONFLICT

- Communicate to yourself and others that conflict is a necessary and beneficial process typically marked by frustration, different conceptualizations, a variety of approaches to resolving it, and ongoing outcomes.
- Assess the work environment t[...] iors are endorsed [...]
- Determine any similarities and differences in f[...] goals, methods, and values in sorting ou[...] ferent conceptualizations of a c[...]

The *Glossary* at the end of the text lists in alphabetical order all the terms that are boldfaced in the text.

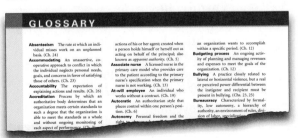

GLOSSARY

Absenteeism The rate at which an individual misses work on an unplanned basis. (Ch. 24)

Accommodating An unassertive, cooperative approach to conflict in which the individual neglects personal needs, goals, and concerns in favor of satisfying those of others. (Ch. 23)

Accountability The expectation of explaining actions and results. (Ch. 26)

Accreditation Process by which an authoritative body determines that an organization meets certain standards to such a degree that the organization is able to meet the standards as a whole and without ongoing monitoring of each aspect of performance. (Ch. [...]

actions of his or her agent; created when a person holds himself or herself out as acting on behalf of the principal; also known as *apparent authority*. (Ch. 5)

Associate nurse A licensed nurse in the primary care model who provides care to the patient according to the primary nurse's specification when the primary nurse is not working. (Ch. 13)

At-will employee An individual who works without a contract. (Ch. 19)

Autocratic An authoritarian style that places control within one person's position. (Ch. 6)

Autonomy Personal freedom and the right to [...]

an organization wants to accomplish within a specific period. (Ch. 12)

Budgeting process An ongoing activity of planning and managing revenues and expenses to meet the goals of the organization. (Ch. 12)

Bullying A practice closely related to lateral or horizontal violence, but a real or perceived power differential between the instigator and recipient must be present in bullying. (Chs. 23, 25)

Bureaucracy Characterized by formality, low autonomy, a hierarchy of authority, an environment of rules, division of labor, specialization [...]

Each of these sections is designed to help learners transfer the words of the text into a personal understanding about what leading, managing, and following mean. Achieving success in those roles helps nurses to be effective team members and to contribute to positive patient care outcomes.

CONTENTS

PART 2   MANAGING RESOURCES

PART 3   CHANGING THE STATUS QUO

PART 4   INTERPERSONAL AND PERSONAL SKILLS

PART 1

Core Concepts

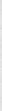

Leading, Managing, and Following

Michael R. Bleich

Leading, managing, and following are integral to professional nursing practice. Engaging in constructive behaviors associated with these concepts influences patient care and organizational outcomes, regardless of position title. By examining self-motivation and confidence in relation to power, authority, influence, decision making, conflict, and change, the professional nurse is enabled to lead, manage, and follow with meaning and purpose.

OBJECTIVES

- Relate leadership and other organizational theories to behaviors that serve as important functions of professional nursing.
- Link self-knowledge and emotional intelligence to the constructive use of power, influence, and authority needed for professional practice.
- Develop strength in optimizing one's personal attributes to effectively lead, manage, and follow.
- Apply organizational strategies to improve interprofessional collaboration and care delivery in complex clinical settings.
- Improve decision making as a leader, manager, or follower by enlarging the view of the patient to include the social network and organizational outcomes.

TERMS TO KNOW

complexity theory	management	tacit knowledge
emotional intelligence	management theory	values
followership	motivation	vision
leadership	process of care	
Magnet™ recognition	social networking	

THE CHALLENGE

Ruby R. Jason, MSN, RN, NEA-BC
Division Director, Women and Children's Division,
*   Doernbecher Children's Hospital*
Oregon Health & Science University, Portland, Oregon

In accepting a formal leadership position as an emergency department (ED) director, I was the fourth "formal" director in 3 years in
a unionized 32-bed inner-city ED. The attitude of "management"
versus "staff" was evident within the informal leadership structure
in which power and authority rested with a group of senior nurses
with over 10 years of service. I noted that formal policies and procedures did not reflect actual practices; specifically, the patient flow
process depended entirely on the senior "charge" nurse's style

and preferences; no one challenged his or her "authority," including
the physicians. Instead, staff adapted to whoever was in charge,
causing daily variability in patient flow. The time between the
patient arriving in the ED and being evaluated and treated by an ED
physician was controlled by the charge nurse—one assigned
patients chronologically, another by chart review, and another by
acuity. On my first day, one of the most senior members of the staff
informed me, "We were here before you, and we will be here long
after you are gone." The implication was that my formal authority
was something they neither respected nor accepted.

What do you think you would do if you were this nurse?

INTRODUCTION

The nursing profession constitutes the backbone of
the healthcare system both in numbers and in its span
of influence across the clinical spectrum. Bearing the
responsibility of keeping patients safe requires vigilance, acute observation, knowledge of care delivery
processes, and a willingness to act—to engage with
patients, families, and other nurses; health disciplines;
and agencies. This willingness and the way one
engages in these actions constitute leading, managing,
and following (Meyer & Lavin, 2005).

As important as it is to ensure that patients have
safe passage through the health system maze, nursing
functions performed beyond the bedside also incorporate nursing knowledge and values. For instance,
nurses develop evidence-driven clinical protocols,
design care delivery systems through initiatives
such as Transforming Care at the Bedside (TCAB)
(Chaboyer et al., 2009), and adapt to ever-changing
shifts in human resources. Nurses influence policy
leading to health reform and lead social change
movements. These activities expand the depth and
breadth of nursing work, demanding even more
sophisticated knowledge of ways to lead, manage,
and follow.

At the heart of patient safety, care delivery design,
policy development, and point-of-care clinical performance is a central tenet: the nurse must bridge
critical thinking with critical action in complex
healthcare settings to achieve positive patient and

organizational outcomes. This decision making is
not isolated but, instead, is done with others to collectively influence constructive change. Decision
making and the corresponding actions taken are
core work performed in engagement with others. This
core work demands that nurses be leaders, managers,
and followers at the point-of-care, unit, institutional,
and even societal levels.

Too often, nurses new to the profession believe
their ability to perform clinical procedures is what
makes them appear professional to those receiving
care, to their peers, or to the public. They may believe
that leadership is left to those holding management
positions or that following means blindly adhering to
the direction of others. These nurses fail to realize that
their professional nursing image and success depend
equally on the poise and influence they demonstrate
in decision making and in engaging with others,
which requires effective leading, managing, and following behaviors. These behaviors are the first lens
through which patients, families, supervisors, and
other professionals view them and gain confidence in
their abilities.

The way nurses lead, manage, and follow has
changed over time. Formerly, nurses took direction
from physicians or senior nurses, such as "head" or
"charge" nurses. These roles still exist today, but the
expectation has shifted from top-down order giving
with an expectation of unquestioning following to a
model in which shared decision making with collaborative action is the norm. Knowledge expansion and

the array of treatment interventions available to patients have grown beyond what a command and control model can accommodate in traditional hierarchically led organizations. This is because patient acuity requires immediate and autonomous responses separate from those that can be preassigned. Health care is now delivered in a collaborative and, most often, an interprofessional manner, with select roles (e.g., charge nurses) serving as an information and care coordination conduit. New roles have emerged, such as the clinical nurse leader (CNL) (Porter-O'Grady, Clark, & Wiggins, 2010). The CNL is a systems navigator and bedside-focused care coordinator educated to deliver care and intercede with care delivery processes to ensure clinical and organizational outcomes. And, as technology is increasingly available in all clinical settings, knowledge management, decision-support, and social networking tools can be used to expand beyond tradition-bound organizations, linking professionals to solve complex care and health systems problems (Cross & Parker, 2004). Social networking, as used here, relates to webs of relationships supported by technology to rapidly transmit and receive information.

The study of leadership and organizational behavior has never been more important to patients who face making complex health decisions or to the nursing discipline in an era of major health reform. Each nurse—from point-of-care nurses to those in expanded roles—is held accountable to make the best use of scarce nursing resources. Professional nurses are expected to meet the organizational mission and goals, avert medical errors, achieve patient satisfaction, and ensure positive patient outcomes. In addition, organizations expect nurses to contain costs when delivering patient care, contribute to quality improvement and change initiatives, and interact with other healthcare team members to resolve clinical and organizational problems. These expectations mean that each nurse must be effective in leading, managing, and following.

In this chapter and in Chapters 3 and 4, various perspectives of the concepts of leading (leadership), managing (management), and following (followership) are presented. These concepts are integrated, meaning that nurses can lead, manage, and follow concurrently. Leading, managing, and following are not role-bound concepts—the nurse leads, manages,

and follows within any nursing role. This chapter highlights the distinctiveness of each concept separately for ease of understanding the differences, beginning with operational definitions.

Leadership is the process of *engaged decision making* linked with *actions taken* in the face of complex, unchartered, or perilous circumstances present in clinical situations for which *no standardized solution exists*. In exercising leadership, the leader assesses the context surrounding the situation, creates and adapts strategies based on scientific evidence and tacit knowledge, and guides others to broad-based outcomes that, at a minimum, alleviate risk and harm. Effective nurse leaders approach decision making and action setting by communicating direction, using principles to guide the process, and projecting an air of self-assurance. These traits evoke security in those associated with the task at hand, which, in turn, fosters reasonable risk taking.

Nurse leaders can be found at all levels, from practitioners who are novice to expert, in all personality types, and without regard to gender, ethnicity, or age. In fact, leadership is enacted by a willingness to identify and act on complex problems in an ethical manner. Ethical leadership is not coercive or manipulative of others; the leader informs others of the goal to be attained so solutions can be co-created in the best manner to serve clinical and organizational needs. Leadership can be misused when coercive relationships form, information is withheld, and the true goals are withheld.

Management is an engaged process of guiding others through a *set of derived practices and procedures* that are evidence-based and known to satisfy *preestablished outcomes* based on repeated clinical situations. In this chapter, management does not refer to persons holding top positions of authority (e.g., nurse director, chief nursing officer). Management-based decisions and actions may be routine in frequency and low in complexity; however, they increasingly are highly complex and require sophisticated skills and abilities. For example, pain management requires knowledge of the derivative causes of the pain and knowledge of a set of interventional choices applied to the situation at hand and can require simple to complex actions. The challenge of management is to maintain enthusiasm for followers who can become bored or fatigued with tasks that require vigilance but are sustained and repeated and yet are essential for clinical care.

Management differs from leadership in that the behaviors and activities required occur in clinical situations that are less ambiguous; the outcomes are known and a sequence of actions is prescribed, either in writing or through historical practices that are embedded in the organization's culture.

Followership is engaging with others who are leading or managing by contributing to problem identification, completing tasks, and providing feedback for evaluation. Followers provide a *complementary set of healthy and assertive actions* to support the leader (who is forging into unknown, complex problem solving) or the manager (who is directing and coordinating predetermined actions to achieve outcomes). Dynamic interplay exists between and among individuals when leading, managing, and following—and this interplay defines, in part, a culture that contributes to patient, family, and healthcare team achievement. The nurse as follower promotes clinical and organizational outcomes by practicing acquiescence to individuals leading or managing the team over certain tasks, such as direction setting, politicking, pacesetting, or planning. Followership is not passive direction taking but, rather, behaviors that model collaboration, influence, and action with the leader or manager. Followers are as individualistic as leaders (Kellerman, 2012).

The collective behaviors that reflect leading, managing, and following enhance one another. All interdisciplinary healthcare providers, including professional nurses, experience situations each day in which they must lead, manage, and follow. Some formal positions, such as charge nurse or nurse manager, require an advanced set of leading and managing know-how to establish organizational goals and objectives, oversee human resources, provide staff with performance feedback, facilitate change, and manage conflict to meet patient care and organizational requirements. In other positions, the nursing role itself demands shifting among leading, managing, and following, almost on a moment-by-moment basis. For instance, nurses lead, manage, and follow in daily clinical practice through assignment making, patient and family problem solving, discharge planning, patient education, and coaching and mentoring staff.

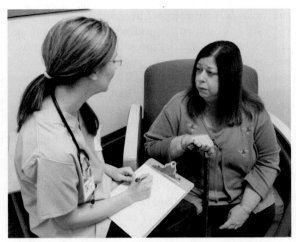

Being empathetic and showing sensitivity to the experiences of others help nurse leaders develop their emotional intelligence.

EXERCISE 1-1

Using the definitions of leadership, management, and followership, imagine that you are faced with a critically ill patient whose family members are spread throughout the country. Some family members are holding vigil at the patient's side, whereas others are calling the patient care unit incessantly, taking time away from other patient care responsibilities. You recognize the family's care and concern, yet you want to move from a reactive stance to a proactive position. How would you engage in solving this problem in a leader role? A manager role? A follower role? In which role would you be most comfortable? Least comfortable? Which role would lead to the best outcomes?

PERSONAL ATTRIBUTES NEEDED TO LEAD, MANAGE, AND FOLLOW

Leading, managing, and following require different skills from those associated with the technical skills-based aspects of nursing. Goleman (2000) and others refer to emotional intelligence—possessing social skills, interpersonal competence, psychological maturity, and emotional awareness that help people harmonize to increase their value in the workplace. Nurses have countless interactions within the course of a workday. In each interaction, nurses can hone their ability to lead, manage, or follow as an emotionally intelligent practitioner within five domains. The domains address:

- Deepening self-awareness (stepping outside oneself to envision the context of what is happening, while recognizing and owning feelings associated with an event)
- Managing emotions (owning feelings such as fear, anxiety, anger, and sadness and acting on these feelings in a healthy manner; avoiding passive-aggressive and victim responses)
- Motivating oneself (focusing on a goal, often with delayed gratification, such that emotional self-control is achieved and impulses are stifled)
- Being empathetic (valuing differences in perspective and showing sensitivity to the experiences of others in ways that demonstrate an ability to reveal another's perspective on a situation)
- Handling relationships (exhibiting social appropriateness, expanding social networks, and using social skills to help others manage emotions)

Emotionally intelligent nurses are credible as leaders, managers, and followers because they possess awareness of patient, family, and organizational needs, have the ability to collaborate, show insight into others, and commit to self-growth. When coupled with performing clinical tasks and critical thinking, the emotionally intelligent nurse demonstrates expanded capabilities. The synergy associated with credibility and capability fuse to become markers of professional

nursing. Without self-reflective skills, growth in emotional intelligence is stymied, work becomes routinized, and a nurse can experience a lack of synchrony with others. Box 1-1 is a composite of the attributes that add to the credibility and capability of nurses to lead, manage, and follow.

EXERCISE 1-2

Referring back to Exercise 1-1, how would a nurse with highly developed emotional intelligence lead, manage, or follow in reference to problem solving? What kind of social networking skills would be needed for goal attainment? Emotional intelligence is developed through insight into one's self. Develop a journal or create a feedback circle with other emotionally intelligent colleagues to promote self-awareness about biases, framing complex problems and promoting contextual awareness—seeing a problem through the lens of others. Prepare a sociogram—a list of key relationships to determine balance, perspective, and opportunities for social network expansion. Using these tools, create a personal recipe for enhancing your own emotional intelligence.

THEORY DEVELOPMENT IN LEADING, MANAGING, AND FOLLOWING

Theory has several important functions for the nursing profession. First, theory can help address important questions for which answers are needed. Second, theory (and the expanding array of research methods available to researchers) adds to evidence-based care and management practices (Melnyk & Fineout-Overholt, 2011). Third, theory directs and sharpens the ability to predict or guide clinical and organizational problem solving and outcomes. Nurses often have less exposure to organizational theories than to clinical theories. Leadership, management, and organizational theories are still evolving as the complexity of healthcare organizations grow and the variables that influence care delivery increase and become more apparent. Unfortunately, a single universal theory to guide all organizational and human interactions does not exist. Theory can also guide the thinking about the complexity found in health care today by exploring various elements such as workforce supply, the demand for care, economics, the work environment, and the interrelationships among them.

BOX 1-1	**ATTRIBUTES OF LEADERS AND MANAGERS**

- Use focused energy and stamina to accomplish a vision.
- Use critical-thinking skills in decision making.
- Trust personal intuition and then back up intuition with facts.
- Accept responsibility willingly and follow up on the consequences of actions taken.
- Identify the needs of others.
- Deal with people skillfully: coach, communicate, counsel.
- Demonstrate ease in standard/boundary setting.
- Examine multiple options to accomplish the objective at hand flexibly.
- Are trustworthy and handle information from various sources with respect for the source.
- Motivate others assertively toward the objective at hand.
- Demonstrate competence or are capable of rapid learning in the arena in which change is desired.

Theory development associated with leading, managing, and following concepts has been a process of testing, discarding, expanding, creating, and applying. These theories overlap. Terms such as *leadership theory, transformational leadership, servant leadership, management theory,* and *motivational theory* and even attempts at *followership theories* are interrelated and cannot be categorized in any mutually exclusive manner. Developing theories for leading, managing, and following is a complicated task. Furthermore, the theories that leaders, managers, and followers use are drawn from yet another set of theories, many addressed in this book. These include change theory, conflict theory, economic theory, clinical theories, individual and group interaction theories, communication and social networking theories, and many more.

The Theory Box in this chapter is organized as an overview to highlight two sets of theoretical work that are commonly referenced: leadership theories (including management and followership concepts) and motivational theories (because of the magnitude of research that explored human behavior and reward structures). As more disciplines have embraced leadership and management theory development, other theories have grown increasingly rich and multidimensional. The complex factors associated with clinical care and organizational functioning explain why no single theory fully addresses the totality of leading, managing, and following. (See the Literature Perspective at the right and the Theory Box on pp. 9-11.)

The development of leadership, motivation, and management theory rapidly evolved at the beginning of the twentieth century when people moved in masses to industries that were aimed at mass production. As the population shifted from agricultural communities to urban manufacturing environments, the factors that promoted efficient production were studied. Leadership theory grew by examining the influence of charismatic leaders on the workforce, followed by the uncovering of the motivational factors that supported worker job satisfaction and, later, the environmental determinants that contributed to or deterred workers from achieving production quotas. (Note that the theories developed in manufacturing industries were then applied to other non-manufacturing settings.)

Leadership theory developed as a system of knowledge to extrapolate the traits and behaviors of leaders who were considered successful at influencing situations, people, and events to attain organizational goals, especially productivity. Leadership theory was first studied by sociologists and psychologists. It is readily apparent today that leadership is a process of engaging with others, and therefore motivational theories naturally overlapped with leadership theory. Motivational theories were attempts to explain how non-management workers sustained behaviors to

LITERATURE PERSPECTIVE

Resource: Kerfoot, K.M. (2009). Leadership: Social identity and guiding from within. *Dermatology Nursing, 21*(1), 45-47.

Kerfoot presents a concise and concentrated history of leadership as a concept, shifting from command-and-control modes in which inheritance played a role (as in Royalty) to military power–based leadership; the next era notes the leader as celebrity, reflected through hierarchical structures and endowed with information.

Generational differences have formed new models of leadership as a construct. Contingency theory shifts to a relationship-oriented view of what is needed to effect change. Today, Kerfoot suggests, an important consideration is the social identity of the group in relationship to its leaders. New research from organizational psychology suggests that the best leaders come from within a group—and that groups are best led from within. She reflects on the body of science that suggests that leaders who are separate from the group or hold different social identities lead from the outside rather than from the inside. Identifying the many types of social identities within healthcare organizations, she explains why nurse leaders reflect the differing expectations of the groups they lead—and so appear different.

Implications for Practice
It is important, Kerfoot suggests, to assess the social identity of the group that one expects to lead and to determine where gaps exist. If the social identity of the group is mismatched with the individual who wants to lead, then building on common values and experiences is an important first step. Also, engaging others from within the group and co-leading is an additional practice strategy. When leading in a situation in which there is a social identity gap, identifying the group's needs and functions and setting priorities for change will facilitate organizational success. Ultimately, the creation of a shared vision is needed for sustained leadership-followership success.

THEORY BOX

Leadership Theories

THEORY/CONTRIBUTOR	KEY IDEA	APPLICATION TO PRACTICE
Trait Theories Trait theories were first studied from 1900 to 1950. These theories are sometimes referred to as the *Great Man* theory, from Aristotle's philosophy extolling the virtue of being "born" with leadership traits. Stogdill (1948) is usually credited as the pioneer in this school of thought.	Leaders have a certain set of physical and emotional characteristics that are crucial for inspiring others toward a common goal. Some theorists believe that traits are innate and cannot be learned; others believe that leadership traits can be developed in each individual.	Self-awareness of traits is useful in self-development (e.g., developing assertiveness) and in seeking employment that matches traits (drive, motivation, integrity, confidence, cognitive ability, and task knowledge).
Style Theories Sometimes referred to as *group and exchange* theories of leadership, style theories were derived in the mid-1950s because of the limitations of trait theory. The key contributors to this renowned research were Shartle (1956), Stogdill (1963), and Likert (1987).	Style theories focus on what leaders do in relational and contextual terms. The achievement of satisfactory performance measures requires supervisors to pursue effective relationships with their subordinates while comprehending the factors in the work environment that influence outcomes.	To understand "style," leaders need to obtain feedback from followers, superiors, and peers, such as through the Managerial Grid Instrument developed by Blake and Mouton (1985). Employee-centered leaders tend to be the leaders most able to achieve effective work environments and productivity.
Situational-Contingency Theories The situational-contingency theorists emerged in the 1960s and early 1970s to mid-1970s. These theorists believed that leadership effectiveness depends on the relationship among (1) the leader's task at hand, (2) his or her interpersonal skills, and (3) the favorableness of the work situation. Examples of theory development with this expanded perspective include Fiedler's (1967) Contingency Model, Vroom and Yetton's (1973) Normative Decision-Making Model, and House and Mitchell's (1974) Path-Goal theory.	Three factors are critical: (1) the degree of trust and respect between leaders and followers, (2) the task structure denoting the clarity of goals and the complexity of problems faced, and (3) the position power in terms of where the leader was able to reward followers and exert influence. Consequently, leaders were viewed as able to adapt their style according to the presenting situation. The Vroom-Yetton model was a problem-solving approach to leadership. Path-Goal theory recognized two contingent variables: (1) the personal characteristics of followers and (2) environmental demands. On the basis of these factors, the leader sets forth clear expectations, eliminates obstacles to goal achievements, motivates and rewards staff, and increases opportunities for follower satisfaction based on effective job performance.	The most important implications for leaders are that these theories consider the challenge of a situation and encourage an adaptive leadership style to complement the issue being faced. In other words, nurses must assess each situation and determine appropriate action based on the people involved.

Continued

THEORY BOX—cont'd

Leadership Theories

THEORY/CONTRIBUTOR	KEY IDEA	APPLICATION TO PRACTICE
Transformational Theories Transformational theories arose late in the past millennium when globalization and other factors caused organizations to fundamentally re-establish themselves. Many of these attempts were failures, but great attention was given to those leaders who effectively transformed structures, human resources, and profitability balanced with quality. Bass (1990), Bennis and Nanus (2007), and Tichy and Devanna (1997) are commonly associated with the study of transformational theory.	Transformational leadership refers to a process whereby the leader attends to the needs and motives of followers so that the interaction raises each to high levels of motivation and morality. The leader is a role model who inspires followers through displayed optimism, provides intellectual stimulation, and encourages follower creativity.	Transformed organizations are responsive to customer needs, are morally and ethically intact, promote employee development, and encourage self-management. Nurse leaders with transformational characteristics experiment with systems redesign, empower staff, create enthusiasm for practice, and promote scholarship of practice at the patient-side.
Hierarchy of Needs Maslow is credited with developing a theory of motivation, first published in 1943.	People are motivated by a hierarchy of human needs, beginning with physiologic needs and then progressing to safety, social, esteem, and self-actualizing needs. In this theory, when the need for food, water, air, and other life-sustaining elements is met, the human spirit reaches out to achieve affiliation with others, which promotes the development of self-esteem, competence, achievement, and creativity. Lower-level needs will always drive behavior before higher-level needs will be addressed.	When this theory is applied to staff, leaders must be aware that the need for safety and security will override the opportunity to be creative and inventive, such as in promoting job change.
Two-Factor Theory Herzberg (1991) is credited with developing a two-factor theory of motivation, first published in 1968.	Hygiene factors, such as working conditions, salary, status, and security, motivate workers by meeting safety and security needs and avoiding job dissatisfaction. Motivator factors, such as achievement, recognition, and the satisfaction of the work itself, promote job enrichment by creating job satisfaction.	Organizations need both hygiene and motivator factors to recruit and retain staff. Hygiene factors do not create job satisfaction; they simply must be in place for work to be accomplished. If not, these factors will only serve to dissatisfy staff. Transformational leaders use motivator factors liberally to inspire work performance.

THEORY BOX—cont'd

Leadership Theories

THEORY/CONTRIBUTOR	KEY IDEA	APPLICATION TO PRACTICE
Expectancy Theory Vroom (1994) is credited with developing the expectancy theory of motivation.	Individuals' perceived needs influence their behavior. In the work setting, this motivated behavior is increased if a person perceives a positive relationship between effort and performance. Motivated behavior is further increased if a positive relationship exists between good performance and outcomes or rewards, particularly when these are valued.	Expectancy is the perceived probability of satisfying a particular need based on experience. Therefore, nurses in leadership roles need to provide specific feedback about positive performance.
OB Modification Luthans (2008) is credited with establishing the foundation for Organizational Behavior Modification (OB Mod), based on Skinner's work on operant conditioning.	OB Mod is an operant approach to organizational behavior. OB Mod Performance Analysis follows a three-step *ABC* Model: *A*, antecedent analysis of clear expectations and baseline data collection; *B*, behavioral analysis and determination; and *C*, consequence analysis, including reinforcement strategies.	The leader uses positive reinforcement to motivate followers to repeat constructive behaviors in the workplace. Negative events that de-motivate staff are negatively reinforced, and the staff is motivated to avoid certain situations that cause discomfort. Extinction is the purposeful non-reinforcement (ignoring) of negative behaviors. Punishment is used sparingly because the results are unpredictable in supporting the desired behavioral outcome.

accomplish goals or how leaders and corresponding environmental factors influenced worker productivity. Motivational theories were developed primarily by psychologists. Note that these early theoretical developments were *role-based* and *hierarchical* in reference to the way organizations were driven by top-down supervisor-subordinate relationships, which was the predominant model in place at the time.

Management theory comprised the body of knowledge that describes how managers should conduct themselves to keep an organization operating effectively. Management theory encompassed variables such as how work is organized, planning is accomplished, change is managed, and production quotas are determined. Because of the diverse nature of activities that contribute to management theory development, representatives from a broad range of disciplines, including managers, psychologists, sociologists, and anthropologists, have contributed to its development.

Again, leadership, motivational, management, and other related organizational theories overlap, although they are often presented as distinctive, depending on the discipline of the theorist. Regardless, each area of theory development continues to evolve, incorporating new knowledge about organizational culture, structure and function, motivation, learning and development, team functioning, and other contemporary factors, such as globalization, diversity, generational differences, and gender equity.

THE PROMISE OF COMPLEXITY THEORY

Too often, theories are believed to have been developed in the distant past. However, new theories are continually being created, tested, and put into practice—a function carried out by nurse scientists and others. Complexity theory has emerged from the work of physical sciences and, more recently, social sciences. It is addressed here because healthcare organizations and nursing curricula are embracing complexity science as a new way of viewing both clinical and organizational issues that have not responded to traditional science, or top-down hierarchies.

Classic science developed theory on assumptions concerning the examination of the "parts" of the patient and the division of organizational tasks to understand the "whole." Complexity science promotes the idea that the world is full of systems that interact and adapt through relationships. The interactions may appear to be random, rather than controlled, and decisions emerge that make sense through the interactions. Stated another way, professional nurses are being responsive to patient and family dynamics, disease interactions, non-hierarchical communications and decision making, and the identification of new patterns of human responses through the use of complexity science. Complexity science, therefore, expands the repertoire of nursing interventions beyond cause-and-effect predictive strategies and expands the repertoire of nursing actions to include strategies that are multidimensional.

In complexity theory, traditional organizational hierarchy plays a less significant role as the "keeper of high-level knowledge." It is replaced with decision making distributed among the human assets within an organization without regard to hierarchy. Leaders and managers who use complexity science approaches spend less time trying to control the future and more time influencing, innovating, and responding to the many factors that influence health care. In complexity science, every voice counts, and every encounter between and among patients and staff may add to effective decision making because decisions and actions taken are co-created by all.

In reference to leadership, management, and followership, how do these definitions differ using complexity science principles?

Leadership was presented as dealing with the unknown, formulating solutions in reaction to complex presenting circumstances. The definition suggests that responding to and drawing on human resources is important when navigating unknown circumstances, and complexity science supports the idea that overprescribing solutions to complex problems fails to yield the best solution. Leadership, then, does not require hypervigilant control over events but, rather, an engaged interaction with the event and people who are part of it.

The earlier definition of management potentially has less of a role in complexity sciences. The nature of organizations requires that certain processes be put into place and standardized. When problems are of a routine nature, they can often be solved using linear step-by-step prescriptive models. Complexity science does not attempt to replace decisions that can be standardized through cause-and-effect science but, rather, is extended to complement situations in which this approach is not ideal. Nevertheless, analyzing patterns, examining relationships, and being open to complexity approaches if causal strategies are not effective is a fit with complexity science (Meleis, 2011).

Followership is a central tenet of complexity sciences. No longer is the follower a passive participant but, rather, a central player in the networks that command a full expression of ideas, stories, and lessons learned. As stated earlier, the follower acquiesces to the leader at times. In complexity science, the leader is not hierarchically related to the follower. Rather, each individual brings to the problem-solving network and the particular patient/family encounter the capacity to lead, manage, and follow. It is the flow among and between these roles in which individuals in formal positions foster an environment that empowers, encourages risk taking, and diminishes fear and organizational silence on matters that are critical to patient and organizational outcomes. (See the Research Perspective on p. 13.)

Marion and Uhl-Bien (2001) identify five ways in which complexity science encourages individuals to lead, manage, and follow. Those who use complexity principles:

Develop Networks. A network is any related group with common involvement in an area of focus or concern. Social networks are found within organizations but also beyond organizational boundaries.

RESEARCH PERSPECTIVE

Resource: Chen, C., Wang, S., Chang, W., & Hu, C. (2008). The effect of leader-member exchange, trust, supervisor support on organizational citizenship behavior in nurses. *Journal of Nursing Research: JNR, 16*(4), 321-327.

The authors acknowledge that leadership is a social exchange process, enhanced by trust between the leader and member in exchanges that take place. Further, they recognize that there are organizational "citizenship" behaviors that foster a positive working climate. This research brings together the variables of the quality of working relationships between leaders and followers, which they reference with the term *member,* with the organizational work climate itself, which they describe as *organizational citizenship behavior.* This research adds to research that has been conducted in corporate but non-healthcare settings. The central importance of nursing in the healthcare workforce justified the focus on nurses for a target group, and the research was conducted using a convenience sample in three medical centers in three regional hospitals. The sample included 14 head nurse and 200 nurse dyads with a response rate of 71.4%. Measurement was conducted using various instruments that determined the quality of leader-member exchanges, organizational citizenship behavior, supervision support, and trust in the head nurse from the staff nurse perspective.

Implications for Practice

The results document that the quality of relationships that exist in leader-follower roles (in this case, the formal role of head nurse with his or her related staff nurses) creates trust in the leader. Not all leader-follower relationships are the same; those with more access to the leader create more intense opportunities for feedback and support, rewards, and favorable assignments. This finding suggests that leader and followers must mutually engage with each other to ensure balance in ongoing relationships. The leader-member relationships are of higher quality; in these relationships, it is more likely that a sense of community will exist in which the members feel engaged as citizens of the work group and the organization. The culture of the organization is influenced by the willingness of the community members to engage in reciprocal support, going above and beyond the call of duty—beyond a sense of doing just what is obligatory. In summary, leader and follower relationships are important to nurture, and when these relationships are nurtured, trust between the leader and follower develops. Trust is an essential ingredient for creating a sense of community in which its members support and balance each other through the complexity of nursing work.

For example, a nursing program is not considered a part of the hospital or agency setting where clinical experiences take place; however, common interests (supply and preparation of a qualified workforce and demand for clinical services) make this network critically important for both organizations.

Encourage Non-hierarchical, "Bottom-Up" Interaction Among Workers. As noted earlier, those who lead, manage, and follow are not considered to be within the traditional hierarchy. Shared governance is an example of decision making in which staff at any level in the hierarchy is engaged in shaping policy and practices that affect patient care. In this model, each nurse is a valued human resource, with rich perspective, and a potential voice to shape direction.

Become a Leadership "Tag". The term *tag* references the philosophic, patient-centered, and values-driven characteristics that give an organization its personality, sometimes called *attractors* or *hallmarks of culture,* similar to values. Although the performance of procedures and functions may be similar in clinical settings, the intangible "caring" attractor can drive organizational performance in a manner that exemplifies caring, whereas another organization focuses on cost-efficiencies. The term *tag* refers to these distinctions.

Focus on Emergence. The concept of emergence addresses how individuals in positions of responsibility engage with and discover, through active organizational involvement, those networks that are best suited to respond to problems in creative, surprising, and artful ways—those who think "outside the box." Emergence is tied to unleashing constructive energy rather than constraining energy.

Think Systematically. The principles of systems thinking theory have been characterized by Anderson and Johnson (1997) as:

- *Thinking of the "Big Picture"* The nurse who looks past his or her assignment and comprehends the needs of all units of the hospital, who can focus on the needs of all the residents in a long-term care facility, or who can think through the complications of emergency department overcrowding in an urban setting is seeing the big picture.
- *Balancing Short-Term and Long-Term Objectives* The nurse who recognizes the consequences of actions taken today on the long-term effect of the organization or patient care, such as the decision not to perform cancer treatment, can guide thinking about how to balance decision making for quality outcomes.

- *Recognizing the Dynamic, Complex, and Interdependent Nature of Systems* Everything is simply connected to everything. Patients are connected to families and friends. Together, they are connected to communities and cultures. Communities and cultures make up the fabric of society. The cost of health care is linked to local economies, and local businesses are connected to global industries. Identifying and understanding these relationships helps solve problems with full recognition that small decisions can have a large impact.
- *Measurable versus Non-measurable Data* Systems thinking triggers a "tendency to 'see' only what we measure. If we focus our measuring on morale, working relationships, and teamwork, we might miss the important signals that only objective statistics can show us. On the other hand, if we stay riveted on 'the numbers,' on how many 'widgets' go out the door, we could overlook an important, escalating conflict between the purchasing and production departments" (Anderson and Johnson, 1997, p. 19).

EXERCISE 1-3

Identify a clinical scenario in which a complex problem needs to be addressed. Who would you include in a network to engage in creative problem solving? How would you go about linking to other social networks if the problem were "bigger than" your immediate contacts? Identify one member of the network, and map the potential connections of that individual that could influence problem resolution. Concentrate on the power of these influencing individuals. The patient/family is part of the network. What role would they play in co-creating the resolution strategies? How would you encourage non-hierarchical interaction among workers? Cite instances (personally or professionally) in which a small change in a system has had a big effect.

TASKS OF LEADING, MANAGING, AND FOLLOWING

When dealing with theory and concepts, developing professionals can lose sight of the practical behaviors that are needed to put these ideas into practice. Gardner (1990) recognized this and described tasks of leadership in his book *On Leadership*. The purpose of describing tangible behaviors associated with leading, managing, and following is to facilitate an understanding of the distinctions between the tasks and the definitions of leadership, management, and followership presented earlier in the chapter.

Gardner's Tasks of Leadership

Gardner's leadership tasks are presented in Table 1-1 to demonstrate that leading, managing, and following are relevant for nurses who hold clinical positions, formal management positions, and executive positions. Note that each role represents the interests of the organization, although the locus of attention is different.

Envisioning Goals

Leading requires envisioning goals in partnership with others. At the point of care, leading helps patients envision their life journey when health outcomes are unknown. It might help a patient envision walking again, participating in family events, or changing a lifestyle pattern. In the case of leading peers (not dissimilar to working with patients and family members), leader competence, trustworthiness, self-assuredness, decision-making ability, and prioritization skills envision crafting solutions to care delivery problems. Imagine leading a change to an electronic health record from a traditional paper record: the leader uses the aforementioned abilities to engage with, convince, or persuade colleagues about the relevance of this change and proceeds with setting direction. Envisioning goals is contingent upon trustful relationships, shared information, and agreement on mutual expectations.

Establishing a shared **vision** is an important leadership concept. "Visioning" requires the leader to engage with others to assess the current reality, determine and specify a desired end-point state, and then strategize to reduce the difference. When this is done well, the nurse and the patient or nurses within an organization experience creative tension. Creative tension inspires the patient and others to work in concert to achieve a desired goal. Shared visioning gives direction to accelerate change.

Affirming Values

Values are the connecting thoughts and inner driving forces that give purpose, direction, and precedence to

TABLE 1-1	CONTRASTING LEADING/MANAGING BEHAVIORS OF NURSES IN CLINICAL, MANAGEMENT, AND EXECUTIVE POSITIONS		
GARDNER'S TASK	**BEHAVIORS**		
	CLINICAL POSITION	**MANAGEMENT POSITION**	**EXECUTIVE POSITION**
Envisioning goals	Visioning patient outcomes for single patient/families; assisting patients in formulating their vision of future well-being	Visioning patient outcomes for aggregates of patient populations and creating a vision of how systems support patient care objectives; assisting staff in formulating their vision of enhanced clinical and organizational performance	Visioning community health and organizational outcomes for aggregates of patient populations to which the organization can respond
Affirming values	Assisting the patient/family to sort out and articulate personal values in relation to health problems and the effect of these problems on lifestyle adjustments	Assisting the staff in interpreting organizational values and strengthening staff members' personal values to more closely align with those of the organization; interpreting values during organizational change	Assisting other organizational leaders in the expression of community and organizational values; interpreting values to the community and staff
Motivating	Relating to and inspiring patients/families to achieve their vision	Relating to and inspiring staff to achieve the mission of the organization and the vision associated with organizational enhancement	Relating to and inspiring management, staff, and community leaders to achieve desired levels of health and well-being and appropriate use of clinical services
Managing	Assisting the patient/family with planning, priority setting, and decision making; ensuring that organizational systems work in the patient's behalf	Assisting the staff with planning, priority setting, and decision making; ensuring that systems work to enhance the staff's ability to meet patient care needs and the objectives of the organization	Assisting other executives and corporate leaders with planning, priority setting, and decision making; ensuring that human and material resources are available to meet health needs
Achieving workable unity	Assisting patients/families to achieve optimal functioning to benefit the transition to enhanced health functions	Assisting staff to achieve optimal functioning to benefit transition to enhanced organizational functions	Assisting multidisciplinary leaders to achieve optimal functioning to benefit patient care delivery and collaborative care
Developing trust	Keeping promises to patients and families; being honest in role performance	Sharing organizational information openly; being honest in role performance	Representing nursing and executive views openly and honestly; being honest in role performance
Explaining	Teaching and interpreting information to promote patient/family functioning and well-being	Teaching and interpreting information to promote organizational functioning and enhanced services	Teaching and interpreting organizational and community-based health information to promote organizational functioning and service development

Continued

TABLE 1-1	CONTRASTING LEADING/MANAGING BEHAVIORS OF NURSES IN CLINICAL, MANAGEMENT, AND EXECUTIVE POSITIONS—cont'd		
	BEHAVIORS		
GARDNER'S TASK	**CLINICAL POSITION**	**MANAGEMENT POSITION**	**EXECUTIVE POSITION**
Serving as symbol	Representing the nursing profession and the values and beliefs of the organization to patients/families and other community groups	Representing the nursing unit service and the values and beliefs of the organization to staff, other departments, professional disciplines, and the community at large	Representing the values and beliefs of the organization and patient care services to internal and external constituents
Representing the group	Representing nursing and the unit in task forces, total quality initiatives, shared governance councils, and other groups	Representing nursing and the organization on assigned boards, councils, committees, and task forces, both internal and external to the organization	Representing the organization and patient care services on assigned boards, councils, committees, and task forces, both internal and external to the organization
Renewing	Providing self-care to enhance the ability to care for staff, patients, families, and the organization served	Providing self-care to enhance the ability to care for staff, patients, families, and the organization served	Providing self-care to enhance the ability to care for patients, families, staff, and the organization served

life priorities. An organization, through its members, shares collective values that are expressed through its mission, philosophy, and practices. Leaders influence decision making and priority setting as an expression of their values. People (either patients or peers being influenced by the leader) also use their values to achieve their goals, which are then manifested through behavior.

The word *value* connotes something of worth; intentional actions reflect our values. A leader continuously clarifies and acknowledges the values that draw attention to a problem and the resources in human and material terms to solve it. Values are powerful forces that promote acceptance of change and drive achievement toward a goal.

Motivating

When values drive our actions, they become a source of motivation. Motivation energizes what we value, personally and professionally, and stimulates growth and movement toward the vision. Motivators are the reinforcers that keep positive actions alive and sustained, fueling the desire to engage in change.

Theories of motivation identify and describe the forces that motivate people. Examples of motivation theory are presented in the Theory Box on Motivation on pp. 9-11.

Managing

The ability to manage is an important aspect of organizational functioning, because management requires determining routines and practices that offer structure and stability to others. This is especially true in certain positions of influence within a clinical setting, such as a nurse manager, clinical nurse specialist, or clinical nurse leader, all of whom share responsibility for creating effective structures that support clinical and organizational outcomes. Being effective as a manager requires behaviors different from those associated with effective leadership, and vice versa. Ideally, those charged with managing are good leaders and followers, because no organizational position is limited to one exclusive set of behaviors over another. Good leaders need management skills and abilities, and good managers need leading skills and abilities. The tasks of management are discussed on p. 18.

BOX 1-2   PRINCIPLES OF CONFLICT RESOLUTION

1. Put the focus on interests:
   - Examine the real issues of all parties.
   - Be expedient in responding to the issues.
   - Use negotiation procedures and processes such as ethics committees and other neutral sources.
2. Build in "loop-backs" to negotiation:
   - Allow for a "cooling-off" period before reconvening if resolution fails.
   - Review with all parties the likely consequences of not proceeding so that they understand the full consequences of failure to resolve the issue.
3. Build in consultation before and feedback after the negotiations:
   - Build consensus and use political skills to facilitate communication before confrontation, if anticipated, occurs.
   - Work with staff or patients after the conflict to learn from the situation and to prevent a similar conflict in the future.
   - Provide a forum for open discussion.
4. Provide necessary motivation, skills, and resources:
   - Make sure that the parties involved in conflict are motivated to use procedures and resources that have been developed; this requires ease of access and a nonthreatening mechanism.
   - Ensure that those working in the dispute have skills in problem solving and dispute resolution.
   - Provide the necessary resources to those involved to offer support, information, and other technical assistance.

Modified from Ury, W., Brett, J., & Goldberg, S. (1988). *Getting disputes resolved: Designing systems to cut the costs of conflict.* San Francisco: Jossey-Bass.

Achieving Workable Unity

Another leadership challenge is to achieve workable unity between and among the parties being affected by change and to avoid, diminish, or resolve conflict so that vision can be achieved (see Chapters 17 and 23). Conflict-resolution skills are essential for leaders. When a dispute occurs as a result of conflicting values or interests, following a defined set of principles to guide conflict resolution is an excellent aid. In their classic work, Ury, Brett, and Goldberg (1988) describe a highly effective approach for restoring unity and movement toward positive change, as shown in Box 1-2.

Developing Trust

A hallmark task of leadership is to behave with consistency so that others believe in and can count on the leader's intentions and direction. Trust develops when leaders are clear with others about this direction, and the way to achieve high performance is through building on strengths and mitigating poor performance. Inherent in this concept is the behavior of truth telling. Although leaders cannot always share all information, it is unwise to misdirect others in their thinking and actions. Trust, according to Lencioni (2002), is the key component of a team. Without it, the team is dysfunctional. Trustworthiness is reflected in actions and communications.

Explaining

Leading and managing require a willingness to communicate and explain—again and again. The art of communication requires the leader to do the following:

1. Determine what information needs to be shared.
2. Know the parties who will receive the information. Ask, "What will they 'hear' in the process of the communication?" Information that addresses the listener's self-interest must be presented.
3. Provide the opportunity for dialogue and feedback. Face-to-face communication is preferred when the situation requires immediate feedback because it offers the opportunity to clarify information. Written communications through e-mail and text messages increasingly are used as primary communication mechanisms. Although expedient, these mechanisms have their limitations that must be acknowledged.
4. Plan the message. Giving too much information can temporarily paralyze the listener and divert energy away from key responsibilities.
5. Be willing to repeat information in different ways, at different times. The more diverse the group being addressed, the more important it is to avoid complex terms, concepts, or ideas. Information should be kept simple. Remember, a message is heard when a person is ready to hear it, not before.
6. Always explain why something is being asked or is changing. The values behind the change should be reinforced.

7. Acknowledge loss, and provide the opportunity for honest communication about what will be missed, especially if change is involved.

8. Be sensitive to nonverbal communication. It may be necessary in complex situations to have someone reinterpret key points and provide feedback about the clarity of the message after the meeting. Leaders must use every opportunity for explaining as a vehicle to fine-tune communication skills. (See Chapter 18 for additional discussion of communication.)

Serving as Symbol

Every leader has the opportunity to be an ambassador for those he or she represents. Nurses may be symbolically present for patients and families, represent their department at an organizational event, or be involved in community public relations events. Serving as a symbol reflects unity and collective identity.

Representing the Group

More than being present symbolically, many opportunities exist for leaders to represent the group through active participation. Progressive organizations create opportunities for employees to participate in and foster organizational innovation (e.g., organizations seeking Magnet™ recognition). Nurses may participate on human resource committees, patient safety task forces, improvement committees, and departmental initiatives. When nurses offer their "voice" in each of these leadership opportunities, it is imperative to think beyond personal needs and stay clear on group outcomes. When decision making is decentralized and layers of management are compressed, nurses have more leadership accountability. A leader treats these newfound opportunities with respect and represents the group's interests with openness and integrity. Ultimately, leaders must understand the organization's objectives and contribute to its mission and purpose.

Renewing

Leaders can generate energy within and among others. A true leader attends to the group's energy and does not allow it to lose focus. In organizations and nursing practice, there is a constant need to balance problem solving (energy-expending) with vision setting (energy-producing). When changes are made based on a shared vision, they can be made with renewed spirit and purpose. Taking time to celebrate individual accomplishments or creating a "Hall of Honor" to post photos, letters, and other forms of positive feedback renews the spirit of workers.

Furthermore, leaders must be proponents of self-care—eat a balanced diet, get adequate sleep and exercise, and participate in other wellness-oriented activities—to maintain their perspective and the necessary energy level. Likewise, they must ensure that their constituents are given similar opportunities for physical and mental renewal. Gardner (1990) states, "The consideration leaders must never forget is that the key for renewal is the release of human energy and talent" (p. 136). This requires focused energy and personal well-being.

Bleich's Tasks of Management

The ability to manage is very much aligned with how an organization structures its key systems and processes to deliver service.

A care delivery system is composed of multiple processes to achieve all of the requisite components required by patients. Some of the key processes relate to medication procurement, ordering, and administration; patient safety practices; patient education; and discharge planning and care coordination. A process of care specifies the desired sequence of steps to achieve clinical standardization, safety, and outcomes. Effective management depends on knowing, adhering to, and improving processes for efficiency and effectiveness. Each person must respect and act on his or her prescribed role in a process of care. Data-driven outcome measurements add to good management and support feedback, coaching, and mentoring opportunities. Rewards for individual and team effectiveness reinforce desired behaviors.

Box 1-3 lists tasks of management that are essential to effective functioning.

Followers complement leaders and managers with their skills. Followers and leaders fill in the gaps that exist to build on each other's cognitive, technical, interpersonal, and emotional strengths. Followers, showing sensitivity to leaders, offer respite in times of stress. Followers need and respond to feedback from

---

BOX 1-3 BLEICH'S TASKS OF MANAGEMENT

1. Identify systems and processes that require responsibility and accountability, and specify who owns the process.
2. Verify minimum and optimum standards/specifications, and identify roles and individuals responsible to adhere to them.
3. Validate the knowledge, skills, and abilities of available staff engaged in the process; capitalize on strengths; and strengthen areas in need of development.
4. Devise and communicate a comprehensive "big picture" plan for the division of work, honoring the complexity and variety of assignments made at an individual level.
5. Eliminate barriers/obstacles to work effectiveness.
6. Measure the equity of workload, and use data to support judgments about efficiency and effectiveness.
7. Offer rewards and recognition to individuals and teams.
8. Recommend ways to improve systems and processes.
9. Use a social network to engage others in decision making and for feedback, when appropriate or relevant.

BOX 1-4 BLEICH'S TASKS OF FOLLOWERSHIP

1. Demonstrate individual accountability while working within the context of organizational systems and processes; do not alter the process for personal gain or shortcuts.
2. Honor and implement care to the standards and specifications required for safe and acceptable care/service.
3. Offer knowledge, skills, and abilities to accomplish the task at hand.
4. Collaborate with leaders and managers; avoid passive-aggressive or nonassertive responses to work assignment.
5. Include evidence-based feedback as part of daily work activities as a self-guide to efficiency and effectiveness and to contribute to outcome measurement.
6. Demonstrate accountability to the team effort.
7. Take reasonable risks as an antidote for fearing change or unknown circumstances.
8. Evaluate the efficiency and effectiveness of systems and processes that affect outcomes of care/service; advocate for well-designed work.
9. Give and receive feedback to others to promote a nurturing and generative culture.

EXERCISE 1-4

Examine one structured process in the delivery of patient care from start to finish (e.g., food ordering, preparation, and delivery). How is the process organized? How many steps does the process take? Who is responsible for each step in the process? Who has the responsibility and authority for managing the process? What data are available in the organization to measure how well the process is working?

Images associated with followers portray workers who are passive, uninspired, not intellectual, and waiting for direction. In reality, the effective follower is willing to be led, to share time and talents, to create and innovate solutions to problems synergistically, and to take direction from the manager. Simultaneously, followers must perform their assigned structured duties. These duties are not devoid of critical thinking or decision making (see Box 1-4).

---

leaders to stay on course. The follower must acquiesce to the skills and abilities of the leader or manager to promote teamwork. This does not mean that the follower does not have the skills and abilities of the leader or manager, because the follower may be thrust into one of those roles when circumstances demand. Box 1-4 lists the tasks of followership.

The relationship between followers and leaders or managers is complex. "Transformational leaders recognize a clear, consistent focus on the vision by the team and an ability to keep the dream bigger than any fears are a key ingredient to success." (Marshall, 2011, p. ix).

There are also times when the leader is the follower and vice versa. In any given work shift, a charge nurse may hold a leading/managing role. During a shift, the charge nurse assesses resources needed, sees the unit as a complete entity, notes where patients may be admitted or discharged, and delegates according to this "big picture" view. Throughout the shift, critical clinical events arise that are better led by one of the senior staff nurses. Ideally, the charge nurse and senior staff nurse shift their relationship so that the functioning of the unit is balanced. As the system adapts, an examination of complexity, respect, and team achievement factors is at play.

LEADING, MANAGING, AND FOLLOWING IN A DIVERSE ORGANIZATION

The healthcare industry is spiraling through unparalleled change, often away from the traditional industrial models that have reigned throughout the twentieth century. The culture in most healthcare organizations today is more ethnically diverse; has an expansive educational chasm, from non–high school graduates to doctorally prepared clinicians; has multiple generations of workers with varying values and expectations of the workplace; involves the increased use of technology to support all aspects of service functioning; and challenges workers, patients, families, and communities environmentally with medical waste, antibiotic-resistant strains of microorganisms, and other risks.

The complexity of the healthcare system is marred with chronic problems, information imbalance (sometimes too much, sometimes not enough), an abundance of job roles that challenge resource allocation, intense work that makes examining patterns of practice difficult, increased consumer and regulatory demands, and fatigue from too many queues and reminders! Reforms will exacerbate this problem.

These and other variables make leading, managing, and following increasingly challenging. A leader must address the needs of the diverse community of those seeking care. Language and cultural barriers create the opportunity for misunderstanding. Those who manage the systems and processes of care may find a temporary workforce—individuals unfamiliar with organizational standards of care and practice—as their primary resource. Followers may have leaders of other generations with values different from their own, and therefore the opportunity for conflict is omnipresent.

Developing the leading, managing, and following skills and abilities noted throughout this chapter will sustain professional nurses to adapt to and accept differences as a positive rather than a negative force in daily work life. Building on gender strengths; generational values, gifts, and talents; cultural diversity; varying educational and experiential perspectives; and a mobile and flexible workforce is rewarding. It is also rewarding to be led in different ways, to experience the strength of a good manager, and to achieve positive outcomes as a follower knowing that the team approach generated a successful work experience.

THE SOLUTION

The first step in any formal or informal management role is to engage with those who will fulfill followership functions. I tackled this problem by scheduling one-to-one conversations with each staff member, including physicians, during *their* workday, not mine (which included weekends). The conversation was structured by three questions:

1. What is it that keeps you here?
2. Where do you see yourself in 5 years?
3. What would make this unit even better?

These questions helped me understand the culture within the environment. By asking, "What is it that keeps you here?" I identified those whose motivation centered on pay; those with other motivations, such as being close to where they live or being part of this team; and those who had a passion for ED nursing. Those with a strong alignment to the work culture were placed on my mental list as those to tap into when the collective vision was formed around improving patient flow.

The next question, "Where do you see yourself in 5 years?" revealed the morale across the spectrum of seniority. The senior nurses all identified intent to stay until retirement, but those with less than 10 years' experience all suggested they would move on because of the current environment and a feeling of powerlessness in the face of the senior staff. The importance of this information was that, given opportunity and support, the less senior staff could help diffuse cultural power holders.

"What would make this unit even better?" revealed three or four common issues that became my priority for incorporating into a change process.

After the interviews were complete, I met with staff and handed out a "Top 5 Things I Learned About You" list. Although difficult, I led the group through a crucial conversation regarding fear of confronting the more senior nurses because of retaliation. After discerning the differences between a professional or punitive environment, the staff engaged in shaping their vision for what a professional environment would look like, and the "fear of retaliation" was framed as unacceptable. After the meeting, relationships continued to unfold and nonthreatening changes were introduced so that all could see that unit change *was* possible. I was vigilant for signs of retaliation and managed through those events that had that appearance. After 6 months of shaping the culture for change, I was able to appoint both senior and junior staff to review the patient placement policy and revamp it using evidence-based literature. This process was not without challenges, but it did result in standardized patient assignments done in the same manner, each shift, by each charge nurse. The result was not just buy-in but, rather, true collaborative ownership of the problem and the solution.

—*Ruby R. Jason*

Would this be a suitable approach for you? Why or why not?

THE EVIDENCE

- The use of top-down-only organizational structures is no longer sustainable in creating change. It must be complemented with change led from the bottom up and from webs of interested and committed individuals who form teams.
- Collaboration requires a set of special conditions between leaders and followers. Among these conditions is the idea that each voice will be valued in an equitable manner, that power is evenly distributed among all of the stakeholders, and that conditions exist for innovation to occur.
- Organizations often can function with effective leaders and managers who preside over work groups with a common short-term goal, rather than teams, which require development over time and with long-term goals.
- Complexity science does not refer to the complexity of the decision to be made or to the work environment but, rather, to examining how systems adapt and function—where co-creation of ideas and actions unfold in a non-prescriptive manner.
- The goal of leadership and management should be to reduce the complexity of the work itself. Only in simplicity does compliance and useful "fit for practice" occur.
- Social networking is being recognized as a web of relationships that can be tapped and used for communication, problem solving, support, and real-time information, critical to decision making. It is a real tool for individuals to use when leading, managing, or following.

NEED TO KNOW NOW

- Know that new employees are expected to be competent followers and self-managers.
- Develop trust early with your teammates and the clinical manager/director.
- Remember that followership employs the same level of knowledge, skills, and abilities as required of leaders and managers but is the acquiescence of leading and managing for the benefit of organizational and team cohesion.
- Understand the organization and organizational functioning because clinical care is delivered in these settings and with interdisciplinary teams.
- Be willing to make decisions and then take action. Without action, no leadership or management has occurred.
- Social networking creates a web of relationships and resources needed for effective leading and managing.

CHAPTER CHECKLIST

This chapter addresses the attributes and tasks of leading, managing, and following and presents the case that professional nurses require the knowledge, skill, and ability to move in and out of these roles with ease, whether in clinical or management positions.

Emotional intelligence is defined in terms of self-understanding, and the argument is made that emotional intelligence is as critical to professional practice as are cognitive and technical skills. Healthcare organizations are experiencing major changes and increasing diversity in those being served and those serving; diversity presents new challenges and opportunities for leaders, managers, and followers. Multiple theories are used in today's healthcare system to address emerging organizational and care needs.

- The personal attributes needed for effective leading and managing include the following:
  - Focused energy and stamina to accomplish the vision
  - Ability to make decisions in an intelligent manner
  - Willingness to use intuition, backed up with facts
  - Willingness to accept responsibility and to follow up
  - Sincerity in identifying the needs of others
  - Skill in dealing with people; for example, through coaching, communicating, or counseling
  - Comfortable standard setting and boundary setting
  - Flexibility in examining multiple options to accomplish the objective at hand
  - Trustworthiness and a good "steward of information"
  - Assertiveness in motivating others toward the objective at hand
  - Demonstrable competence and quick learning in the arena in which change is desired
- The tasks of leading include the following:
  - Envision goals
  - Affirm values
  - Motivate
  - Manage
    - Planning and priority-setting
    - Organizing and institution-building
    - Keeping the system functioning
    - Setting agendas and making decisions
    - Exercising political judgment
  - Achieve workable unity
  - Develop trust
  - Explain
  - Serve as symbol
  - Represent the group
  - Renew
- The tasks for managing include the following:
  - Identify systems and processes
  - Verify minimum and optimum standards/specifications
  - Validate the knowledge, skills, and abilities of available staff
  - Devise and communicate a comprehensive "big picture" plan
  - Eliminate barriers/obstacles to work effectiveness
  - Measure the equity of workload
  - Offer rewards and recognition to individuals and teams
  - Recommend ways to improve systems and processes
  - Involve others in decision making
- The tasks for following include the following:
  - Recognize how individual responsibilities fit into organizational systems
  - Honor the standards and specifications
  - Offer knowledge, skills, and abilities
  - Collaborate willingly with leaders and managers
  - Include data collection as part of daily work activities
  - Demonstrate accountability for individual actions
  - Take reasonable risks
  - Give feedback on the efficiency and effectiveness of systems
  - Give and receive feedback to and from other team members, leaders, and managers

TIPS FOR LEADING, MANAGING, AND FOLLOWING

- Recall that leading and managing is about decision making and collective action. Does the scenario deal primarily with known or unknown circumstances? If it is known, then the Tasks of Management will be useful; if unknown, reference the Tasks of Leadership.

- Clinical acumen alone is insufficient to address clinical care—leading, managing, and following behaviors must complement clinical acumen.
- Basic knowledge of theory can provide a leading and/or managing framework that leads to effective action, as demonstrated above. Effective clinical

outcomes can be derived only from shared vision, values, actions, and outcomes. This requires knowledge of human motivation, organizational systems, and effective decision making. The theories presented in this chapter all have useful clinical applications.

REFERENCES

Anderson, V., & Johnson, L. (1997). *Systems thinking basics: From concepts to causal loops.* Waltham, MA: Pegasus Communications.

Bass, B. M. (1990). From transactional to transformational leadership: Learning to share the vision. *Organizational Dynamics, 18,* 19-31.

Bennis, W. G., & Nanus, B. (2007). *Leaders: The strategies for taking charge.* (2nd ed.). New York: Harper Business.

Blake, R. R., & Mouton, J. S. (1985). *The managerial grid III.* Houston: Gulf Publishing.

Chaboyer, W., McMurray, A., Johnson, J., Hardy, L., Wallis, M., & Chu, F. (2009). Bedside handover: Quality improvement strategy to "transform care at the bedside." *Journal of Nursing Care Quality, Apr-Jun*; 24(2), 136-142.

Chen, C., Wang, S., Chang, W., & Hu, C. (2008). The effect of leader-member exchange, trust, supervisor support on organizational citizenship behavior in nurses. *Journal of Nursing Research: JNR, 16*(4), 321-327.

Cross, R., & Parker, A. (2004). *The hidden power of social networks: Understanding how work really gets done in organizations.* Boston: Harvard Business School Publishing Corp.

Fiedler, F. A. (1967). *A theory of leadership effectiveness.* New York: McGraw-Hill.

Gardner, J. W. (1990). *On leadership.* New York: Free Press.

Goleman, D. P. (2000). *Working with emotional intelligence.* New York: Bantam Books.

Herzberg, F. (1991). One more time: How do you motivate employees? In M. J. Ward & S. A. Price (Eds.), *Issues in nursing administration: Selected readings.* St. Louis: Mosby.

House, R. J., & Mitchell, T. R. (1974, Autumn). Path-goal theory of leadership. *Journal of Contemporary Business, 3,* 81-97.

Kellerman, B. (Fall, 2012). What every leader needs to know about followers. *Harvard Business Review,* 96-103.

Kerfoot, K. M. (2009). Leadership: Social identity and guiding from within. *Dermatology Nursing, 21*(1), 45-47.

Lencioni, P. M. (2002). *The five dysfunctions of a team: A leadership fable.* San Francisco: Jossey-Bass.

Likert, R. (1987). *New patterns of management.* New York: Garland.

Luthans, F. (2008). *Organizational behavior.* New York: McGraw-Hill.

Marion, R., & Uhl-Bien, M. (2001). Leadership in complex organizations. *The Leadership Quarterly, 12,* 389-418.

Marshall, E. S. (2011). *Transformational leadership in nursing: from expert clinician to influential leader.* New York, NY: Springer.

Maslow, A. (1943). A theory of human motivation. *Psychological Review, 50,* 370-396.

Meleis, A. I. (2011). *Theoretical nursing: development and progress* (5th ed.). Philadelphia, PA: Lippincott.

Melnyk, B. M. & Fineout-Overholt, E. (2011). *Evidence-based practice in nursing and health care: a guide to best practice.* Philadelphia, PA: Lippincott.

Meyer, G., & Lavin, M. A. (2005). Vigilance: The essence of nursing. *Online Journal of Issues in Nursing, 10*(1). Retrieved September 18, 2009, from www.nursingworld.org/MainMenuCategories/ANAMarketplace/ANAPeriodicals/OJIN/TableofContents/Volume102005/No3Sept05/ArticlePreviousTopic/VigilanceTheEssenceofNursing.aspx.

Porter-O'Grady, T., Clark, J. S., & Wiggins, M. S. (2010). The case for clinical nurse leaders: guiding nursing practice into the 21st century. *Nurse Leader, 8*(1), 37-41.

Shartle, C. L. (1956). *Executive performance and leadership.* Englewood Cliffs, NJ: Prentice Hall.

Stogdill, R. M. (1948). Personal factors associated with leadership: A survey of the literature. *Journal of Psychology, 25,* 35-71.

Stogdill, R. M. (1963). *Manual for the leader behavior description questionnaire, form XII.* Columbus: The Ohio State University, Bureau of Business Research.

Tichy, N. M., & Devanna, M. A. (1997). *The transformational leader.* New York: John Wiley & Sons.

Ury, W., Brett, J., & Goldberg, S. (1988). *Getting disputes resolved: Designing systems to cut the costs of conflict.* San Francisco: Jossey-Bass.

Vroom, V. H. (1994). *Work and motivation.* New York: John Wiley & Sons.

Vroom, V. H., & Yetton, P. (1973). *Leadership and decision-making.* Pittsburgh, PA: University of Pittsburgh Press.

SUGGESTED READINGS

Anklam, P. (2007). *Net work: A practical guide to creating and sustaining networks at work and in the world.* Burlington, MA: Butterworth-Neinemann.

Bass, B. M., & Avolio, B. J. (1994). *Improving organizational effectiveness through transformational leadership.* Thousand Oaks, CA: Sage Publications.

Birute, R., & Lewin, R. *Third possibility leaders: The invisible edge women have in complex organizations.* Retrieved September 23, 2009, from http://plexusinstitute.org/services/stories/show.cfm?id=28.

Brafman, O., & Beckstrom, R. (2006). *The starfish and the spider: The unstoppable power of leaderless organizations.* New York: Penguin Group.

Brafman, O., & Brafman, R. (2008). *Sway: The irresistible pull of irrational behavior.* New York: Doubleday.

Bridges, W. (1991). *Managing transitions: Making the most of change.* Reading, MA: Addison-Wesley.

Cohen, A. R., & Bradford, D. L. (1989). *Influence without authority.* New York: John Wiley & Sons.

Covey, S. (1991). *Principle-centered leadership.* New York: Summit.

DeLong, D. (2004). *Lost knowledge: Confronting the threat of an aging workforce.* New York: Oxford University Press.

Gladwell, M. (2000). *The tipping point.* Boston: Little, Brown.

Grossman, R. J. (2000). Emotions at work: Health care organizations are just beginning to recognize the importance of developing a manager's emotional quotient, or interpersonal skills. *Health Forum Journal, 43,* 18-22.

Katzenbach, J. R., & Smith, D. K. (1993). *The wisdom of teams: Creating the high-performance organization.* New York: Harper Business.

Kellerman, B. (1999). *Reinventing leadership: Making the connection between politics and business.* New York: State University of New York Press.

Lentz, S. (1999). The well-rounded leader: Knowing when to use consensus and when to make a decision is crucial in today's competitive health care market. *Health Forum Journal, 42,* 38-40.

Maeda, J. (2006). *The laws of simplicity.* Cambridge, MA: The MIT Press.

McDaniel, R. R. (1997). Strategic leadership: A view from quantum and chaos theories. *Health Care Management Review, 22,* 21-37.

Nelson, E., Batalden, P., & Godfrey, M. (2007). *Quality by design: A clinical microsystems approach.* San Francisco: Jossey-Bass.

Noll, D. C. (1997). Complexity theory 101. *Medical Group Management Journal, 44*(3), 22, 24-26, 76.

Northouse, P. G. (2007). *Leadership theory and practice* (4th ed.). Thousand Oaks, CA: Sage Publications.

Plsek, P. E., & Wilson, T. (2001). Complexity, leadership, and management in healthcare organisations, *BMJ, 323,* 746-749.

Pugh, D. S., & Hickson, D. J. (1997). *Writers on organizations* (5th ed.). Thousand Oaks, CA: Sage Publications.

Rainey, H. G., & Watson, S. A. (1996). Transformational leadership and middle management: Towards a role for mere mortals. *International Journal of Public Administration, 19,* 764-800.

Runde, C., & Flanagan, T. (2007). *Becoming a conflict competent leader: How you and your organization can manage conflict effectively.* San Francisco: Jossey-Bass.

Trott, M. C., & Windsor, K. (1999). Leadership effectiveness: How do you measure up? *Nursing Economic$, 17,* 127-130.

Useem, M. (1998). *The leadership moment.* New York: Three Rivers Press.

Weeks, D. (1994). *The eight essential steps to conflict resolution.* New York: G. Putney Sons.

2

Patient Safety

Patricia S. Yoder-Wise

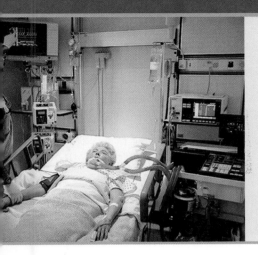

In any discipline, most practitioners think of a leader as someone with positional authority. Terms such as manager, director, chief, *and* leader *convey positional authority. In healthcare organizations, a hierarchy exists of "who is in charge." Realistically, however, every registered nurse is seen by law as a leader—one who has the opportunity and authority to make changes for his or her patients. Even as far back as Florence Nightingale's era, patient safety was important. She focused on changing the way health care was delivered to make a difference in the outcomes of care for those who served in the Crimean War. Yet, in the United States, it was not until the end of the twentieth century that major efforts refocused on the basic safety and quality outcomes of care for patients. This shift to being consumed with a passion for patient safety is a hallmark of today's healthcare delivery and the target for the care of tomorrow. This chapter provides an overview of the key thoughts about patient safety as the basis for all aspects of leading and managing in nursing. Patient safety, and subsequently quality of care, is why the public entrusts us with licensure and why we use our passion for caring.*

OBJECTIVES

- Identify the key organizations leading patient safety movements in the United States.
- Value the need for a focus on patient safety.
- Apply the concepts of today's expectations for how patient safety is implemented.

TERMS TO KNOW

Agency for Healthcare Research and Quality (AHRQ)
DNV (Det Norske Veritas)
Institute for Healthcare Improvement (IHI)

Institute of Medicine (IOM)
Magnet Recognition Program®
National Quality Forum (NQF)
The Joint Commission

Quality and Safety Education for Nurses (QSEN)
TeamSTEPPS (an AHRQ strategy to promote patient safety)

Vickie S. Simpson, BA, BSN, RN, CCRN, CPN
Dell Children's Medical Center of Central Texas, Austin, Texas

Over the years, our hospital has focused on pressure ulcers. In 2002, for example, we reviewed literature on pediatric pressure ulcer risk assessment scales and prevention interventions. A couple of years later, as we were doing our pediatric pressure ulcer risk policy, we realized that pressure ulcers were not tracked. So it was impossible to determine the true incidence. Thus we instituted a tracking system. We also developed a pediatric SKIN bundle. SKIN stands for **S**urface selection, **K**eep turning, **I**ncontinence management, and **N**utrition.

Many of these efforts included broad interdisciplinary teams. For example, after moving to our new facility in 2007, we noticed a trend of pressure ulcer development in nasally intubated patients.

When a root cause analysis was completed with members of the anesthesia and respiratory therapy departments, staff in the critical care unit, and the cardiovascular surgeon, numerous issues were identified. These issues included not purchasing arms for the new ventilators and identification of the need for a different taping process for nasally intubated children, which was developed by our respiratory therapists. Our outcome is that now we have no pressure ulcers on nasally intubated children in our facility.

In 2009, we identified a new trend in our patient population. It was including more overweight teenagers. We had to decide what to do.

What do you think you would do if you were this nurse?

INTRODUCTION

In Chapter 1, the concepts of leading and managing were presented. The question is, however, leading for what? No issue is more prominent in the literature or in healthcare organizations than the concern for patient safety. Although many other aspects of health care are discussed, they all center on patient safety. Many factors and individuals have influenced both the nursing profession's and the public's concerns about patient safety, but the seminal work was *To Err Is Human: Building a Safer Health System* (2000), produced by the Institute of Medicine (IOM). The Web site QSEN.org shows how important patient safety is to the foundation of quality. Even more popularized publications, such as *How Doctors Think* (Groopman, 2007) and *The Best Practice: How the New Quality Movement is Transforming Medicine* (Kenney, 2008), show how important the basic building block of quality—patient safety—is. This focus fits well with the basic patient advocacy role that nurses have supported over decades.

Because the core of concern in any healthcare organization is safety, it also is the core for leaders and managers in nursing. Safety, and subsequently quality, should drive such aspects of leading and managing as staffing and budgeting decisions, personnel policies and change, and information technology and delegation decisions. Most professionals would agree that

three major driving forces are behind the current emphasis on quality: IOM, the Agency for Healthcare Research and Quality (AHRQ), and The National Quality Forum (NQF). Also, other groups such as The Joint Commission, the new accrediting organization (the Det Norske Veritas [DNV]), the QSEN Institute, and the Magnet Recognition Program® have incorporated specific standards and expectations about safety and quality into their respective work. Additionally, specifically focused efforts such as those of the Quality and Safety Education for Nurses (QSEN), which provides expected competencies and resources for both undergraduate and graduate nursing students on the topics of safety and quality, and TeamSTEPPS initiatives have addressed patient safety issues. Also, the **American Board of Quality Assurance and Utilization Review Physicians** provides a certification program for physicians, nurses, and other healthcare professionals. No nurse can function today without a focus on patient safety, nor can any nurse leader or manager.

THE CLASSIC REPORTS AND EMERGING SUPPORTS

Several reports are reflective of the efforts to refocus healthcare to quality. Numerous other reports and supports exist. Table 2-1 highlights the key groups.

TABLE 2-1   MAJOR FORCES INFLUENCING PATIENT SAFETY

ELEMENT	CORE RELEVANCE	IMPLICATIONS FOR LEADERS AND MANAGERS
Institute of Medicine Reports	*To Err Is Human* (2000): Defined the number of deaths attributed to patient safety issues.	Moved safety issues from the incident report level to an integrated patient safety report for the organization.
	Crossing the Quality Chasm (2001): Identified the six major aims in providing health care (See Box 2-1)	Moved care from discipline centric foci to patient centered foci.
		Reinforced the disparities that occur within health care, which, in turn, led to a focus on best practices (and reinforced the need to be patient centered).
		Addressed issues such as healing environments, evidence-based care and transparency, which led to a more holistic environment that was build on evidence and that was transparent.
	Health Professions Education: A Bridge to Quality (2003): Addressed the issue of silo education among the health professions in basic and continuing education (see Box 2-2)	Attempted to shrink the chasm between education and practice so that interprofessional teams would work more effectively together.
		Increased expectation for participation in lifelong learning.
	Keeping Patients Safe: Transforming the Work Environment of Nurses (2004): Identified many past practices that had a negative impact on nurses and thus on patients	Focused on direct care nurses, supporting their involvement in decision making related to their practice.
		Supported the concept of shared governance.
		Provided a framework for considering how nurses could determine staffing requirements.
		Moved the Chief Nursing Officer into the Boardroom as a key spokesperson on safety and quality issues.
	Improving the Quality of Health Care for Mental and Substance-Use Conditions (2005): Addressed issues related to this patient population, including those who can be found among a general care population	Provided a focus on mental health needs of patients who were not admitted for the primary reason of mental health issues.
	Preventing Medication Errors (2006): Addressed many of the issues surrounding the use of medications	Validated the complexity of providing medications to patients.
	Future of Nursing: Leading Change, Advancing Health (2010): Identified 8 recommendations based on evidence that the profession must attend to. (See Box 2-3)	Created state coalitions focused on improving nursing.
		Created nursing/community/business coalitions to accomplish the work.
		Moved the issue of nurses as leaders to a more visible level.
Agency for Healthcare Research and Quality	Federal agency devoted to improving quality, safety, efficiency, and effectiveness (2008) www.ahrq.gov	Outcomes research sections provide resources for nurses.
		Source of Five Steps to Safer Health Care (www.ahrq.gov/consumer/5step.htm) (See Box 2-3)
		Source of Stay Healthy checklists for men and women
		Source of TeamSTEPPS

Continued

TABLE 2-1	MAJOR FORCES INFLUENCING PATIENT SAFETY—cont'd	
ELEMENT	**CORE RELEVANCE**	**IMPLICATIONS FOR LEADERS AND MANAGERS**
National Quality Forum	Membership-based organization related to quality measurement and reporting www.nqf.org	Source for Centers for Medicare and Medicaid's never events Resource for Healthcare Facilities Accreditation Program (a CMS-deemed authority) (uses NQF's Safe Practices) Source of nurse sensitive care standards
The Joint Commission	Not-for-profit organization that accredits healthcare organizations internationally www.jointcommission.org	Focused on outcomes redirected accreditation processes and thus nurses' roles with the process Changed to unannounced visits and thus changed the way organizations prepared for accreditation. Issues annual patient safety goals Issues sentinel event announcements
Det Norske Veritas/ National Integrated Accreditation for Healthcare Organizations	Internationally based organization that accredits many fields, including healthcare. www.dnvaccreditation.com	Based on an internationally understood set of standards known as ISO (International Organization for Standardization) Visits annually and thus changed the way accreditation is viewed.
Quality and Safety Education for Nurses	Comprehensive resource, including references and video modules www.qsen.org	Created knowledge, skills, and attitudes for students and graduates related to safety.
Magnet Recognition Program ™	A designation build on and evolving through research. Emphasizes outcomes nursecredentialing.com/Magnet/ ProgramOverview.aspx	Created unified approaches to seek this designation Redirected focus to outcomes, including data and efforts related to patient safety
Institute for Healthcare Improvement	Independent, not- for- profit Source of TCAB (Transforming Care at the Bedside)	Provides rapid cycle change projects designed to improve care rapidly (See Theory Box)

THE INSTITUTE OF MEDICINE REPORTS ON QUALITY

Although many reports about quality and safety had been issued before 2000, *To Err is Human* is the report credited with causing sufficient alarm about how widespread the issue of patient safety concerns was. When the number of deaths (98,000 annually) attributable to medical error was announced, the interest in safety intensified. Suddenly this issue was not related to just a few isolated instances nor was it likely to diminish without some concerted action. Probably the hallmark of this publication was the acknowledgment that errors commonly occurred because of system errors rather than individual practitioner incompetence. This insight, that it was the system and not the practitioners that needed to be addressed, placed even more emphasis on roles such as chief medical officers and chief nursing officers. Hospital boards that once focused almost exclusively on finances suddenly wanted more of their agendas devoted to discussions about quality and patient safety. The call for a comprehensive approach to the issue of improving patient safety really spurred the release of a second IOM report.

This next report, *Crossing the Quality Chasm*, was released the subsequent year (IOM, 2001). The intent of this second book was to improve the systems within which health care was delivered; after all, the first report identified that systems rather than

BOX 2-1 THE AIMS OF PROVIDING HEALTH CARE

- Safe
- Effective
- Patient-centered
- Timely
- Efficient
- Equitable

From Institute of Medicine (IOM). (2001). *Crossing the quality chasm: A new health system for the 21st century.* Washington, DC: National Academy Press.

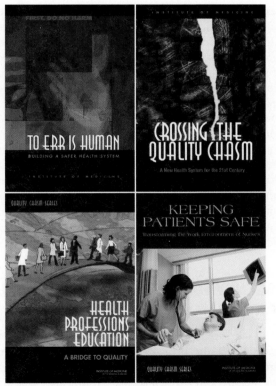

Knowing the relevant literature about safe patient care guides nursing practice.

incompetent people were the major concern. The report spelled out six major aims in providing health care, as shown in Box 2-1.

These aims were designed to enhance the quality of care that was delivered. Most are well documented in the literature, and two of them seem to be receiving much attention. One, patient-centered care, has lessened the past practices of disciplines (e.g., nursing and pharmacy) and services (e.g., orthopedics and urology) vying for control of the patient. Now, because care is to be rendered *with* the patient rather than *to* the patient, the emphasis of care is about what is provided—not who controls the decision about care. The second aim, equitable, has emphasized what the literature refers to as *disparities* and has led to thoughtful consideration of what best practices are and how they can be provided to the masses.

The report went on to acknowledge elements of care that nurses commonly value. For example, the report cited the idea of a healing environment, individualized care, autonomy of the patient in making decisions, evidence-based decision making, and the need for transparency. Although those elements of a healthcare delivery system might not seem so dramatic today, they were fairly revolutionary in 2001. This report also provided substantive support for the use of information technology within health care. In addition, it provided the impetus for payment methods being based on quality outcomes and addressed the issue of preparing the future workforce. This latter recommendation formed the basis for another IOM report, *Health Professions Education: A Bridge to Quality* (IOM, 2003).

Unlike the earlier reports, the *Health Professions Education* report emerged as the work of an invitational summit. In this report, one of the major concerns about safety was exposed publicly, namely that we educate disciplines in silos and then expect them to function as an integrated whole. This is true of both basic and continuing professional education. The report stated, "All health professionals should be educated to deliver patient-centered care as members of an interdisciplinary team, emphasizing evidence-based practice, quality improvement approaches, and informatics" (IOM, 2003, p. 3). Box 2-2 emphasizes those five competencies about health professional education.

The idea of this report was to shrink the chasm between learning and reality so that learning was enhanced and reality was more closely aligned with that learning. A commitment to this redirection of learning is critical for "learning organizations," a term coined by Peter Senge. Thus constant learning is a commitment every healthcare professional must have. Although it is the individual's accountability to maintain competence and participate in learning, the organization can hinder or enhance that individual's need to meet this expectation. Learning organizations exhibit a positive commitment to enhance people's learning and changing.

After looking at safety, the system and core competencies of health professionals, the IOM turned its attention to the workplace itself. As a result, many nurses think of the IOM report *Keeping Patients Safe: Transforming the Work Environment of Nurses* (IOM, 2004) as the major impetus behind many changes that improved the working conditions for nurses. Because nurses are so inextricably linked with patients, it was logical that the importance of the role of nurses in health care emerged as an area of focus. This report identified that nurses had lost trust in the organizations in which they worked and that "flattening" the organization resulted in fewer clinical leaders being available to advocate for staff and patients and to provide resources to those delivering direct care. Further, numerous sources of unsafe equipment, supplies, and practices were discussed. Finally, so many organizations were still engaged in punitive practices related to errors rather than redirecting attention to the broader view of the system.

This report focused on direct-care nurses being able to participate in decisions that affected them and their provision of care, which helped reinforce the ongoing work of shared governance. Addressing staffing issues was accomplished on a broad scale. In other words, the broad processes for determining staffing requirements and how to address those were identified. Average hours per patient day of care, staffing levels, turnover rates, public reporting about those data, support for annual and planned education, and specifics, such as handwashing and medication administration, were addressed. Also, this report

identified the importance of governing boards understanding the issues of safety and propelled the idea of the chief nursing officer participating in board meetings in organizations that had not already embraced this practice. Redesigning both the work of nurses and the workspace was acknowledged as critical to maximizing a positive workforce.

The more recent report, The Future of Nursing: Leading Change, Advancing Health (IOM, 2010), also provides guidance to nursing. Although this report does not focus specifically on quality and safety, the evidence used to build the recommendations includes much that addresses safe, quality practices. For example, the evidence regarding the outcomes of advanced practice registered nurses shows both safety and quality in terms of care. Additionally, the call for more nurses holding bachelors and higher degrees relates to the outcomes evident in the literature about lowered morbidity and mortality with a better prepared workforce.

Each of these reports fits within the IOM's focus on quality and an attempt to make health care a quality endeavor. Together, these reports and others to be developed provide direction for the delivery of care and contain implications, if not outright recommendations, for nursing. These reports form the core of the work around quality in most organizations today. Further, they support many issues nurses have identified as key to quality care.

AGENCY FOR HEALTHCARE RESEARCH AND QUALITY

The Agency for Healthcare Research and Quality (AHRQ) is the primary Federal agency devoted to improving quality, safety, efficiency, and effectiveness of health care (Agency for Healthcare Research and Quality [AHRQ], 2008). As seen in numerous IOM reports, recommendations about what AHRQ could do to enhance safety were prominent. AHRQ's website *(www.ahrq.gov)* is an information-rich source for providers and consumers alike. For example, several healthcare conditions are identified in the outcomes research section. Because AHRQ maintains current information, it is a readily available source, even if the number of conditions is limited. Another example of AHRQ's work is the fairly well-known

BOX 2-3 FIVE STEPS TO SAFER HEALTH CARE

1. Ask questions if you have doubts or concerns.
2. Keep and bring a list of ALL medications you take.
3. Get the results of any test or procedure.
4. Talk to your doctor about which hospital is best for your health needs.
5. Make sure you understand what will happen if you need surgery.

From www.ahrq.gov/consumer/5steps.htm. Retrieved May 10, 2010.

"Five Steps to Safer Health Care," which is available at *www.ahrq.gov/consumer/5step.htm*. Nurses who work in clinics will find these steps especially helpful in working with patients. This list identifies ways in which nurses can support people in assuming a more influential role in their own care. Further, supporting people in assuming a larger role helps them receive care that is patient-centered. Box 2-3 lists the five steps.

If a patient does not volunteer the above information, a nurse could readily seek clarification by asking questions related to each of those items. This is an example of reinforcing work that has been judged to benefit patients.

AHRQ is also the source for the *stay healthy* checklists for men and women. These checklists can be useful in any clinical setting in helping people assume a greater understanding of their own care.

EXERCISE 2-1

Go to *www.ahrq.gov/consumer* and review what sources of information are available to people for whom you may provide care. Click on "Staying Healthy," and then scroll to "Preventing Disease & Improving Your Health" and click on "Men: Stay Healthy at 50+." Review the information there, and then use the back button to return to the prior page and click on "Women: Stay Healthy at 50+." What are the differences in the checklists based on gender?

THE NATIONAL QUALITY FORUM

The National Quality Forum (NQF) is a membership-based organization designed to develop and implement a national strategy for healthcare quality measurement and reporting. As a result, the Centers

for Medicare & Medicaid Services (CMS) formed its no-pay policy based on the growing work of NQF of "never events." In other words, CMS will no longer pay for certain conditions that result from what might be termed *poor practice* or events that should never have occurred while a patient was under the care of a healthcare professional. The NQF brings together providers, insurers, patient groups, federal and state governments, and professional associations and purchasers, to name a few of the groups comprising the membership. This diversity provides a venue for open discussion about healthcare quality that does not normally happen. Having the patients' perspectives at the same time as the perspectives of the insurers and providers allows for a broad view of any issue. The Healthcare Facilities Accreditation Program, a CMS-deemed authority, has adopted the NQF's 34 Safe Practices.

NQF refers to nurses as "the principal caregivers in any healthcare system" (National Quality Forum [NQF], 2008). This acknowledgment, while welcomed, is also a challenge for nurses to perform in the best manner possible to lead organizations in their quests for quality.

Through its consensus process, NQF created a list of endorsed nurse-sensitive care standards. These standards are divided among three key areas: patient-centered outcome measures, nursing-centered intervention measures, and system-centered measures. The first group includes fall and pressure ulcer prevalence; the second, smoking cessation programs with three diagnosis groups; and the third, skill mix, turnover rates, nursing care hours per patient day, and a practice environment scale. Box 2-4 lists the nurse-sensitive care standards from 2008. These standards create a common definition of measures so that any group can collect and report data in a manner comparable to other groups. As a result, those measures form the basis for comparison of quality.

EXERCISE 2-2

Do an online search regarding the concept of "BSN in 10" and read the rationale behind this movement. Assume that you work in a facility that does not provide support (time off, tuition reimbursement, recognition of educational achievement). How could you use this information to change workplace policies and practices?

BOX 2-4   NURSE-SENSITIVE CARE STANDARDS

Patient-Centered Outcome Measures
- Death among surgical inpatients with treatable serious complications (failure to rescue)
- Pressure ulcer prevalence
- Patient falls
- Falls with injury
- Restraint prevalence (vest and limb)
- Urinary catheter–associated infections (CAUTI) rate for intensive care unit (ICU) patients
- Central line catheter–associated bloodstream (CLABSI) infection rate for intensive care unit (ICU) and neonatal intensive care unit (NICU) patients
- Ventilator-associated pneumonia (VAP) rate for intensive care unit (ICU) and neonatal intensive care (NICU) patients

Nursing-Centered Intervention Measures
- Smoking cessation counseling for acute myocardial infarction (AMI)
- Smoking cessation counseling for heart failure (HF)
- Smoking cessation counseling for pneumonia (PN)

System-Centered Measures
- Skill mix
- Nursing care hours per patient day
- Practice environment scale-nursing work index (PES-NWI)
- Voluntary Turnover

Reproduced with permission from the National Quality Forum, copyright © 2004.

ACCREDITING BODIES (TJC AND DNV)

The Joint Commission, formerly known as the *Joint Commission on Accreditation of Healthcare Organizations (JCAHO)*, and the det norske veritas (DNV), are not-for-profit organizations. Both have deemed status from CMS, which means an organization accredited by a deemed body meets the same expectations that CMS sets.

The Joint Commission focuses on outcomes and now uses an unannounced visit approach in an attempt to be certain organizations are meeting expectations at any point in time. This change in emphasis, from one of processes and a regular basis to one of outcomes and unannounced visits has been seem to be of value to hospitals and other organizations as they attempt to meet high standards. TJC issues annual patient safety goals, which can be found on their web site (www.jointcommission.org).

The DNV work is based on a set international standards known as International Organization for Standardization (ISO). The DNV surveys its accredited organizations annually. Because of its extensive work in other fields, the DNV employs similar approaches in health care in meeting the ISO standards.

QSEN INSTITUTE

In addition to defining competencies for prelicensure and graduate students, QSEN, which stands for Quality and Safety Education for Nurses, provides comprehensive resources that are competency based. These resources include bibliographies and videos to enhance our understanding of quality and safety. They have no authority; however, most educational programs subscribe to their efforts to promote both quality and safety as key elements in nursing education.

MAGNET RECOGNITION PROGRAM®

The Magnet Recognition Program® is the only national designation built on and evolving through research. This program is designed to acknowledge nursing excellence. Through the 14 Forces of Magnetism *(www.nursecredentialing.org/Magnet/ProgramOverview/ForcesofMagnetism.aspx)*, organizations must demonstrate how they provide excellence. Although each of the forces contributes to patient safety, two are specifically focused on quality: quality of care and quality improvement. In the model created in 2008, the core of the model is empirical outcomes. Magnet™, like other organizations mentioned here, focuses on quality care *(www.nursecredentialing.org/Magnet/NewMagnetModel.aspx)*.

INSTITUTE FOR HEALTHCARE IMPROVEMENT

The Institute for Healthcare Improvement (IHI) is dedicated to rapidly improving care through a variety of mechanisms including rapid cycle change projects. (See the Theory Box on p. 33.) IHI is an independent, not-for-profit organization. Working with the Robert Wood Johnson Foundation (RWJF), IHI created an

THEORY BOX

Diffusion Theory

THEORY/CONTRIBUTOR	KEY IDEA	APPLICATION TO PRACTICE
Rogers (2003)	• A process of communication about innovation to share information over time and among a group of people. • Allows for non-linear change. • More complex change is less likely to be adopted. • Early adopters serve as role models	• Engage key leaders in a change to infuse the energy from early adopters. • Using Twitter in the hospital culture to engage employees communicates changes quickly.

innovative project called *Transforming Care at the Bedside (TCAB)*. Although TCAB currently is applied only to medical-surgical inpatient units, it addresses safety and reliability, care team vitality, patient-centeredness, and increased value. Spreading innovative approaches to patient safety issues is critical to achieve major patient safety goals.

MEANING FOR LEADING AND MANAGING IN NURSING

Many of the approaches to patient safety and, before that, aviation and nuclear energy safety, consist of strategies to alert us to safety issues. For example, the use of SBAR (See Box 2-5) and checklists are designed to decrease omission of important information and practices. These practices aren't designed to limit a professional's distinctive contributions. Rather they are designed to increase the likelihood of safe practice.

This concern for patient safety is not limited solely to hospitals or to the United States, as the International Council of Nurses points out. In a position statement issued in 2013, safe staffing levels are a concern across the globe. The document, Safe Staffing Levels: Statement of Principles, reflects principles similar to those issued by the American Nurses Asso-

ciation. This global perspective about nurse staffing as an important element in safe, quality care provides a uniform approach to advocating for strategies that increase the potential for quality outcomes.

Although the errors that nurse leaders and managers make do not typically result in a patient's morbidity or mortality, if each decision that is not related to patient care were treated with this type of focus, we would likely make solid decisions more frequently. Often managerial and leadership tasks, like many others we perform, are squeezed into a hectic day. By stopping to concentrate on the work before us, we increase our chances of understanding the complexity of the situation and the ramifications of various decisions. By thinking through various scenarios, we are likely to eliminate strategies and methods that would not meet our needs and be more likely to narrow our choices of best actions to take. Then, if after an action, we took time to review how well some decision was enacted, we would increase our knowledge about particular types of problems and enhance our skill at making decisions.

Similarly, it is possible to look at the five core competencies defined in the 2003 IOM report and create a professional evaluation system and continuing education program. In essence, these five core competencies could drive the personnel performance within an organization. Using some form of a chart, continuing educators could redesign organizational-sponsored learning activities by illustrating how the proposed learning activities contribute to developing, maintaining, or enhancing the five core competencies. This unified focus would help both the individual and the organization. Further, having geographically accessible or virtual demonstration sites would allow physicians, nurses, and others the opportunity to

BOX 2-5 SBAR

S—Situation
B—Background
A—Assessment
R—Recommendation

http://www.ihi.org/knowledge/Pages/Tools/SBARTechniquefor
CommunicationASituationalBriefingModel.aspx

demonstrate through simulation how the five core competencies relate to specific practice areas. These major overhauls of organizational systems require commitment from the organization's largest department—nursing.

One of the challenges for nurses in any position, and especially for leaders and managers, is the task of keeping current with the literature. For example, Hendrick et al. (2012) identify how a strategic, system-wide effort was made to address quality and safety from chief nurses collaborating. Computer technology has allowed us to gather data, analyze it, share it with other colleagues, and read about studies through online availability. Based on the original IOM observation that the numbers of journals, and thus articles, had multiplied dramatically over the past decades, knowing what to read and where to search is critical. Hoss and Hanson (2008) provided a way to consider evidence available through websites. (See the Literature Perspective below.)

The challenge for competent practice today is to stay well-informed about the best evidence or best practices that exist in any practice situation, including that of management and leadership. As the healthcare professions have focused on creating evidence about various practices, the amount of information has become overwhelming. The Research Perspective below illustrates one study focused on a review of the impact of a comprehensive nursing approach to patient safety. The quantity of citations reviewed, alone, illustrates the importance of nurses and patient safety.

 LITERATURE PERSPECTIVE

Resource: Hoss, B., & Hanson, D. (2008). Evaluating the evidence: Web sites. *AORN Journal, 87*(1), 124, 126-128, 130-132, 134-138, 140-141.

The amount of evidence-based practice-related content has grown dramatically. Thus evaluating websites for bias, validity, and patient population descriptors has become increasingly important.

Several national sources provide quality improvement data. Examples of these are the Agency for Healthcare Research and Quality, the Institute for Healthcare Improvement, and The Joint Commission.

The authors proposed three questions to evaluate websites: (1) Is the information from a recognized authority? (2) Does the website comply with voluntary standards? (3) Who is the intended audience? Examples of recognized authorities are most peer-reviewed journals, the Cochrane Database of Systematic Reviews, and The Virginia Henderson International Nursing Library. An example of the second is the standards of Medline Plus, which requires meeting several criteria to have a link from its site. An example of the third is to consider what the *url* extension is. For example, *.com* refers to commercial enterprises; *.edu* to educational institutions; *.org* to organizations (frequently professional and nonprofit societies); and *.gov* to city, county, state, or federal government.

Questions of validity relate to the following: Is the author biased? Is the information complete and accurate? Are the recommendations valid? Will the information help the patient?

Implications for Practice
Knowing what sources provide quality information helps nurses use their time effectively.

 RESEARCH PERSPECTIVE

Resource: Richardson, A. & Storr, J. (2010). Patient safety: a literative review of the impact of nursing empowerment, leadership and collaboration. *International Nursing Review. 57*:12-21. doi: 10.1111/j.1466-7657.2009.00757.x

The purpose of this study was to determine how and in what intensity empowerment, leadership, and collaboration were linked to patient safety. The authors made a comprehensive study of electronic databases from 1998 to 2008. This initial search produced 1,788 articles and abstracts. Sixty five (65) articles had full text available. Specific criteria allowed an item to be included, for example the presence of one of the terms and a measure of impact. As a result, eleven reports were studied in greater detail. All of the papers were from English-speaking countries, with the United States most prevelant as the source (n = 7). Although limited evidence was found, this study was the initiation of a new approach to looking at these various issues and how they interrelated.

Implications for Nursing Practice
Although few reports were available and they varied in quality of contribution to understanding how empowerment, leadership and collaboration work with patient safety, one conclusion was evident. Much work needs to be done before the relationships of these elements to patient safety can be understood. Because nurses have such intimate involvement in care, the need to further studies in this area is great.

THE SOLUTION

A multidisciplinary group was formed to address the problem. Our facility did not have some of the necessary equipment such as lift equipment, adult-size positioning devices, and beds large enough to accommodate larger patients. We purchased the necessary equipment, and we also implemented a safe patient-handling program. The facility "skin champions "also developed an incontinence protocol and a friction/shear protocol.

Participation by our hospital in a multisite research study on pressure ulcer development in critically ill children has shown that our pressure ulcer incidence is significantly lower than that of other participating children's hospitals.

Success of the pediatric pressure ulcer prevention program is the result of extensive multidisciplinary collaboration—support from hospital administration, physicians, and frontline nurses. Utilization of evidence-based practice and research has also driven successful changes in our program. The desire to continually improve pressure ulcer prevention strategies has become the culture within our hospital.
—*Vickie S. Simpson*

Would this be a suitable approach for you? Why?

CONCLUSION

Creating a culture of safety is everybody's business; and nurses, who are so integral to care, are key players in this important work. Every nurse has the accountability to challenge any act that appears unsafe and to stop actions that do not concur with the patient's best interest. Being proactive is insufficient in itself; examining practices and conditions that support errors is critical, as is sharing knowledge that can redirect care. In this challenging context, nurses continue to provide care and provide the organizational "glue" that supports patient care being accomplished in a safe, effective, and efficient manner.

THE EVIDENCE

The Nurse-Sensitive Care Standards, developed by the National Quality Forum (2008), are conditions associated with the quality of nursing care. These form the evidence associated with the care nurses provide.

- Death among surgical inpatients with treatable serious complications (failure to rescue)
- Pressure ulcer prevalence
- Patient falls
- Falls with injury
- Restraint prevalence (vest and limb)
- Urinary catheter–associated infections (CAUTI) rate for intensive care unit (ICU) patients
- Central line catheter–associated bloodstream (CLABSI) infection rate for intensive care unit (ICU) and neonatal intensive care unit (NICU) patients
- Ventilator-associated pneumonia (VAP) rate for intensive care unit (ICU) and neonatal intensive care (NICU) patients
- Smoking cessation counseling for acute myocardial infarction (AMI)
- Smoking cessation counseling for heart failure (HF)
- Smoking cessation counseling for pneumonia (PN)
- Skill mix
- Nursing care hours per patient day
- Practice environment scale-nursing work index (PES-NWI)
- Voluntary turnover

NEED TO KNOW NOW

- Know how to retrieve literature related to best practice and evidence in your area of practice.
- Practice precautionary strategies such as the STAR approach.
- Select workplaces based on the support for the core competencies as defined by IOM.
- Practice what to say to stop an unsafe practice.

CHAPTER CHECKLIST

This chapter focused on the core of leading and managing in nursing, namely an intense passion for patients and their safety. To lead and manage effectively, a nurse must be passionate about quality and patient safety. The nurse leader and manager, as well as followers, must be able to identify potential safety issues, intervene quickly when a safety issue exists, and think skillfully after a safety violation so that all may learn.

- The key organizations dealing with the patient safety movement are the following:
  - The Institute of Medicine
  - The Agency for Healthcare Research and Quality
  - The National Quality Forum
- Accrediting Bodies
  - The Joint Commission
  - The DNV/NIAHO^{SM}
- QSEN Institute
- The Magnet Recognition Program®
- The Institute for Healthcare Improvement
- Considerable potential to capitalize on the information in the IOM reports and in evidence-based research and best practices exists.
- Keeping current with the literature is a challenge we must meet.
- Creating a culture of safety is everyone's job.

TIPS FOR PATIENT SAFETY

- Use the STAR approach: Stop, Think, Act, Review.
- Use the IOM competencies to frame your actions.
- Keep current with the evidence and best practices.
- Use only quality sources, especially websites.
- Read general nursing literature regarding other organizations' work related to safety.

REFERENCES

Agency for Healthcare Research and Quality (AHRQ). *AHRQ mission*. Retrieved December 1, 2008, from www.ahrq.gov/.

Det Norske Veritas (DNV). *Managing risk to improve patient safety*. Retrieved September 23, 2009, from www.dnv.us/consulting/generalindustries/publicsector/Managingrisktoimprovepatientsafety.asp.

Henderson, A. L., Batcheller, J., Ellison, D. A., Janik, A. M., Jeffords, N. B., Miller, L., Perlich, B. L., Stafflileno, G., Storm, M., & Williams, C. (2012). The Ascension Health experience: maximizing the chief nursing officer role in a large, multihospital system to advance patient care quality and safety. *Nursing Administration Quarterly, 36*(4), 277-288.

Hoss, B., & Hanson, D. (2008). Evaluating the evidence: Web sites. *AORN Journal, 87*(1), 124-141.

Institute for Healthcare Improvement. SBAR technique for communication: a situational briefing model. Retrieved July 26, 2013 from http://www.ihi.org/knowledge/Pages/Tools/SBARTechniqueforCommunicationASituationalBriefingModel.aspx

Institute of Medicine (IOM). (2000). *To err is human: Building a safer health system*. Washington, DC: National Academy Press.

Institute of Medicine (IOM). (2001). *Crossing the quality chasm: A new health system for the 21st century*. Washington, DC: National Academy Press.

Institute of Medicine (IOM). (2003). *Health professions education: A bridge to quality*. Washington, DC: National Academy Press.

Institute of Medicine (IOM). (2004). *Keeping patients safe: Transforming the work environment of nurses*. Washington, DC: National Academy Press.

Institute of Medicine (IOM). (2010). *The future of nursing: leading change, advancing health*. Washington, DC: National Academy Press.

International Council of Nurses. (••). *Safe staffing levels: statement of principles*. Geneva, CH: The Council.

Lee, C. (2009). The new hospital accreditation: Case in point. *Nurse Leader, 7*(5), 30-32.

National Quality Forum. (2008). *Nursing care quality at NQF*. Retrieved September 23, 2009, from www.qualityforum.org/nursing.

Richardson, A., & Storr, J. (2010). Patient safety: a literative review on the impact of nursing empowerment, leadership and collaboration. *International Nursing Review, 57*, 12-21.

Rogers, E. M. (2003). *Diffusion of innovations* (5th ed.). New York: The Free Press.

SUGGESTED READINGS

Agency for Healthcare Research and Quality: https://subscriptions.ahrq.gov/service/multi_subscribe.html?code=USAHRQ.

Institute for Healthcare Improvement: www.ihi.org/ihi.

Institute of Medicine: *IOM news*: www.iom.edu/CMS/3238.aspx.

Schnall, R., Stone, P., Currie, L., Desjardins, K., John, R. M., & Bakken, S. (2008). Development of a self-report instrument to measure patient safety attitudes, skills and knowledge. *Journal of Nursing Scholarship, 40*(4), 391-394.

Shaffer, F. A., & Tuttas, C. A. (2009). Nursing leadership's responsibility for patient quality, safety and satisfaction: Current review and analysis. *Nurse Leader, 7*(5), 34-38.

Wagner, L. M., Capezuti, E., & Rice, J. C. (2009). Nurses' perceptions of safety culture in long-term care settings. *Journal of Nursing Scholarship, 41*(2), 184-192.

Walrath, J. M., & Rose, L. E. (2008). The medication administration process: Patients' perspectives. *Journal of Nursing Care Quality, 23,* 345-352.

Wolf, D., Lehman, L., Quinlin, R., Rosenzweig, M., Friede, S., Zullo, T., & Hoffman, L. (2008). Can nurses impact patient outcomes using a patient-centered care model? *Journal of Nursing Administration, 38*(12), 532-540.

Developing the Role of Leader

Michael L. Evans

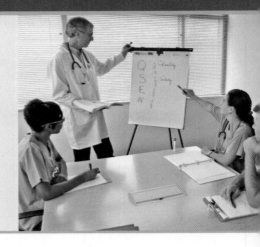

This chapter focuses on leadership and its value in advancing the profession of nursing. Leadership development is explained with examples of how to survive and thrive in a leadership position. The differences between the emerging and entrenched workforce generations are explored, and the desired characteristics of a leader for the emerging workforce are described. Leadership in a variety of situations, such as clinical settings, community venues, organizations, and political situations, is described. This chapter provides an introduction to the opportunities, challenges, and satisfaction of leadership.

OBJECTIVES

- Analyze the role of leadership in creating a satisfying working environment for nurses.
- Evaluate transactional and transformational leadership techniques for effectiveness and potential for positive outcomes.
- Value the leadership challenges in dealing with generational differences.
- Compare and contrast leadership and management roles and responsibilities.
- Describe leadership development strategies and how they can promote leadership skills acquisition.
- Analyze leadership opportunities and responsibilities in a variety of venues.
- Explore strategies for making the leadership opportunity positive for both the leader and the followers.

TERMS TO KNOW

emerging workforce	management	transactional leadership
entrenched workforce	mentor	transformational leadership
leadership		

Rosemary Luquire, PhD, RN, FAAN
Senior Vice President and Chief Nurse Executive, Baylor
Healthcare System, Dallas, Texas
Formerly Senior Vice President, Patient Care & Chief Quality
Officer, St. Luke's Episcopal Health System, Houston, Texas

Houston, known as the *Bayou City,* is accustomed to frequent flooding. Located 60 miles from the Gulf of Mexico, tropical storms and hurricanes are not uncommon for the region. On Tuesday, June 5, 2001, Tropical Storm Allison moved across the city and dropped 2.5 inches of rain, causing some street flooding. St. Luke's Episcopal Hospital, a 948-bed tertiary hospital (26 stories high) in the Texas Medical Center, established an emergency command center in accordance with its emergency preparedness plan. Tropical Storm Allison then moved northward, and the skies cleared. On Friday, June 8, the storm turned and moved back over Houston, creating massive flooding and loss of power throughout the Texas Medical Center. Between 5 PM on June 8 and 5 AM on June 9, 14 inches of rain fell; 36 inches of rain fell within 24 hours in northern Houston. The Bayou City was completely overwhelmed with this "500-year

flood" as families fled to their rooftops to be saved by emergency personnel.

On the evening of Friday, June 8, St. Luke's had approximately 600 patients, 110 of whom were critically ill; many were on life-support devices such as ventilators. I arrived at the hospital before flooding isolated the Texas Medical Center. I was the only senior executive on site. The evening staff was asked to stay and provide patient care, because the storm precluded the arrival of any additional help. In the early morning hours, authorities notified me that the facility would lose all electrical power within an hour. Amid an environment of crisis, isolation, and uncertainty, critical decisions needed to be made quickly. Should patients be evacuated? Who should be evacuated while elevators were still functioning? How could the safety of patients and staff be ensured? When everything is a priority, how do you decide what is truly a priority?

What do you think you would do if you were this nurse?

WHAT IS A LEADER?

A leader is an individual who works with others to develop a clear vision of the preferred future and to make that vision happen. Oakley and Krug (1994) call that type of leadership *enlightened leadership,* or the ability to elicit a vision from people and to inspire and empower those people to do what it takes to bring the vision into reality. Leaders bring out the best in people.

Leadership is a very important concept in life. Great leaders have been responsible for helping society move forward and for articulating and accomplishing one vision after another throughout time. Dr. Martin Luther King, Jr., called his vision a *dream,* and it was developed because of the input and lived experiences of countless others. Mother Teresa called her vision a *calling,* and it was developed because of the suffering of others. Steven Spielberg calls his vision a *finished motion picture,* and it is developed with the collaboration and inspiration of many other people. Florence Nightingale called her vision *nursing,* and it was developed because people were experiencing a void that was a barrier to their ability to regain or establish health.

Atchison (2004) asserts that leaders have followers. An individual can have an impressive title, but that title does not make that person a leader. No matter what the person with that title does, he or she can never be successful without having the ability to inspire others to follow. The leader must be able to inspire the commitment of followers.

Covey (1992) identifies eight characteristics of effective leaders (Box 3-1). Effective leaders are continually engaging themselves in lifelong learning. They are service-oriented and concerned with the common good. They radiate positive energy. For people to be inspired and motivated, they must have a positive leader. Effective leaders believe in other people. They lead balanced lives and see life as an adventure. Effective leaders are synergistic; that is, they see things as greater than the sum of the parts and they engage themselves in self-renewal.

EXERCISE 3-1
List Covey's eight characteristics of effective leaders on the left side of a piece of paper. Next to each characteristic, list any examples of your activities or attributes that reflect the characteristic. Some areas may be blank; others will be full. Think about what this means for you personally.

BOX 3-1	COVEY'S EIGHT CHARACTERISTICS OF EFFECTIVE LEADERS

1. Engage in lifelong learning
2. Are service-oriented
3. Are concerned with the common good
4. Radiate positive energy
5. Believe in other people
6. Lead balanced lives and see life as an adventure
7. Are synergistic; that is, they see things as greater than the sum of the parts
8. Engage themselves in self-renewal

Healthcare organizations are complex. In fact, health care is complex. Continual learning is essential to stay abreast of new knowledge, to keep the organization moving forward, and to continue delivering the best possible care. There is an emphasis on organizations becoming learning organizations, providing opportunities and incentives for individuals and groups of individuals to learn continuously over time. A learning organization is one that is continually expanding its capacity to create its future (Senge, 2006). Leaders are responsible for building organizations in which people continually expand their ability to understand complexity and to clarify and improve a shared vision of the future—"that is, they are responsible for learning" (Senge, 2006, p. 340).

The roles of manager and leader are often considered interchangeable, but they are actually quite different. The manager may also be a leader, but the manager is not required to have leadership skills within the context of moving a group of people toward a vision. The term *manager* is a designated leadership position. *Leadership* is an abilities role, and it is most effective if the manager is also a leader. Management can be taught and learned using traditional teaching techniques. Leadership, however, can also be taught but is usually a reflection of rich personal experiences.

Management and leadership are both important in the healthcare environment. The problem facing healthcare organizations is that they are overmanaged and underled (Atchison, 1990). We can teach new managers, but our leaders are developed over time and through experience. Thus it is important that we value, support, and provide our leaders with the one thing vital for good leadership—good followership. Leadership is a social process involving leaders and followers interacting. Followers need three qualities from their leaders: direction, trust, and hope (Bennis, 2009). The trust is reciprocal. Leaders who trust their followers are, in turn, trusted by them.

The manager is concerned with doing things correctly in the present. The role of manager is very important in work organizations because managers ensure that operations run smoothly and that well-developed formulas are applied to staffing situations, economic decisions, and other daily operations. The manager is not as concerned with developing creative solutions to problems as with using strategies to address today's issues. Covey (1992) believes that a well-managed entity may be proceeding correctly but, without leadership, may be proceeding in the wrong direction.

Leadership as an Important Concept for Nurses

Nurses must have leadership to move forward in harmony with changes in society and in health care. Within work organizations, certain nurses are designated as managers. These individuals are important to ensuring that care is delivered in a safe, efficient manner. Nurse leaders are also vital in the workplace to elicit input from others and to formulate a vision for the preferred future.

Moreover, leadership is key for nursing as a profession. The public depends on nurses to advocate for the public's needs and interests. Nurses must step forward into leadership roles in their workplace, in their professional associations, and in legislative and policy-making arenas. Nurses depend on their leaders to set goals for the future and the pace for achieving them. The public depends on nurse leaders to move the consumer advocacy agenda forward.

Leadership as a Primary Determinant of Workplace Satisfaction

Nurse satisfaction within the workplace is an important construct in nursing administration and healthcare administration. Turnover is extremely costly to any work organization in terms of money, expertise, and knowledge, as well as care quality. Thus being mindful of nurse satisfaction is an economic, as well as professional, concern.

THEORY BOX

A Comparison of Outcomes in Transactional and Transformational Leadership

TRANSACTIONAL LEADERSHIP	TRANSFORMATIONAL LEADERSHIP
Leader Behaviors • Contingent reward *(quid pro quo)* • Punitive • Management by exception (active)—monitors performance and takes action to correct • Management by exception (passive)—intervenes only when problems exist	**Leader Behaviors** • Charismatic • Inspiring and motivating • Intellectual stimulation • Individualized consideration
Effect on Follower • Fulfills the contract or gets punished • Does the work and gets paid • Errors are corrected in a reactive manner	**Effect on Follower** • A shared vision • Increased self-worth • Challenging and meaningful work • Coaching and mentoring happens • Feeling valued
Organizational Outcomes • Work is supervised and completed according to the rules • Deadlines are met • Limited job satisfaction • Low to stable levels of commitment	**Organizational Outcomes** • Increased loyalty • Increased commitment • Increased job satisfaction • Increased morale • Increased performance

Modified from McGuire, E., & Kennerly, S. M. (2006). Nurse managers as transformational and transactional leaders. *Nursing Economic$, 24*(4), 179-185.

An analysis of several dozen interviews of healthcare workers (including physicians), when asked what followers desire from leaders, produced the following responses in rank order (Atchison, 2004):

1. Respect
2. Control of the decisions that most affect me
3. Rewards and recognition
4. Balance of life—colleagues and family, job and home, work and play
5. Professional development

The effective leader in healthcare settings needs to be aware of these important facets of work life that influence followers. The leader should also work with followers to find a way to actualize these important aspects of work life.

The leader, not the manager, inspires others to work at their highest level. The presence of strong leadership sets the tone for achievement in the work environment. Effective leadership is the basis for an effective workplace, and therefore creating leadership succession is an important consideration. This means that, in addition to supporting current leaders in their roles, new leaders must be encouraged and developed.

EXERCISE 3-2
Follower behavior nurtures and supports—or deteriorates—leader behavior. Identify the behavior you exhibited during your most recent clinical experience. What was supportive? What did not support the leader?

THE PRACTICE OF LEADERSHIP

Leadership Approaches

How one approaches leadership depends on experience and expectations. Many leadership theories and styles have been described. Two of the most popular theory-based approaches are transactional leadership and transformational leadership. (See the Theory Box above.)

Transactional Leadership

A transactional leader is the traditional "boss" image. In a transactional leadership environment, employees understand that a superior makes the decisions with little or no input from subordinates. Transactional leadership relies on the power of organizational position and formal authority to reward and punish performance. Followers are fairly secure about what will happen next and how to "play the game" to get where they want to be. A transactional leader uses a *quid pro quo* style to accomplish work (e.g., I'll do *x* in exchange for your doing *y*). Transactional leaders reward employees for high performance and penalize them for poor performance. The leader motivates the self-interest of the employee by offering external rewards that generate conformity with expectations. The status quo is continually reinforced in organizations in which transactional leadership is practiced (Weston, 2008).

Transformational Leadership

Transformational leadership is based on an inspiring vision that changes the framework of the organization for employees. Employees are encouraged to transcend their own self-interest. This style of leadership involves communication that connects with employees' ideals in a way that causes emotional engagement. The transformational leader can motivate employees by articulation of an inspirational vision; by encouragement of novel, innovative thinking; and by individualized consideration of each employee, accounting for individual needs and abilities. The result of such leadership is that both leaders and followers have a higher level of motivation and a greater sense of purpose (Weston, 2008). Covey (1992) states, "The goal of transformational leadership is to transform people and organizations in a literal sense, to change them in mind and heart; enlarge vision, insight, and understanding; clarify purposes; make behavior congruent with beliefs, principles, or values; and bring about changes that are permanent, self-perpetuating, and momentum-building" (p. 287).

Kouzes and Posner (2007) identify five key practices in transformational leadership, as follows:

1. Challenging the process, which involves questioning the way things have been done in the past and thinking creatively about new solutions to old problems
2. Inspiring shared vision or bringing everyone together to move toward a goal that all accept as desirable and achievable
3. Enabling others to act, which includes empowering people to believe that their extra effort will have rewards and will make a difference

4. Modeling the way, meaning that the leader must take an active role in the work of change
5. Encouraging the heart by giving attention to those personal things that are important to people, such as saying "thank you" for a job well done and offering praise after a long day

A transformative leader seems particularly suited to the nursing environment.

There is additional evidence in the literature that transformational leadership produces very positive results in the workplace. Robbins and Davidhizar (2007) link transformational leadership qualities with staff satisfaction, staff retention, and patient satisfaction. Raup (2008) found that nurse managers with effective leadership skills are an essential component to addressing the nursing shortage because lower staff turnover resulted from transformational leadership, although no correlation existed between leadership style and patient satisfaction. Another study found that there was great benefit in spending resources to develop clinical leaders. After transformational leadership development, the nursing team derived benefit because the more effective leadership promoted effective communication, greater responsibility, empowerment, job clarity, continuity of care, and interdisciplinary collaboration (Dierckx de Casterle, Willemse, Verschueren, & Milisen, 2008).

Another study found that a transformational leadership style was closely associated with followers' working conditions, namely involvement, influence, and meaningfulness. This study also found a direct path between leadership behavior and employee well-being (Nielsen, Yarker, Brenner, Randall, & Borg, 2008). Marchionni and Ritchie (2008) found that the presence of a supportive culture in which learning is valued, coupled with transformational leadership, is a key factor in the implementation and sustainability of best practice guidelines.

Positive outcomes are derived from effective leadership in organizations. Transformational leadership is hard work; investment of time and energy is required to bring out the best in people. Transformational leadership is not unique to nursing as the Research Perspective on p. 43 illustrates.

Leadership is the ability to influence people to work toward meeting certain goals. Often this influence requires an ongoing commitment to role-modeling and reinforcing behaviors. The intensity of

RESEARCH PERSPECTIVE

Resource: Snodgrass, J., Douthitt, S., Ellis, R., Wade, S., & Plemons, J. (2008). Occupational therapy practitioners' perceptions of rehabilitation managers' leadership styles and the outcomes of leadership. *Journal of Allied Health, 37*(1), 38-44.

This was a pilot study that investigated the linkage between occupational therapy practitioners' perceptions of rehabilitation managers' leadership styles and the outcomes of leadership. The sample of occupational therapy (OT) practitioners was an *n* of 73. Data for the study were collected using two different survey instruments.

Findings reveal that transformational and transactional leadership styles were associated with leadership outcomes. Transformational leadership had a significant ($p < 0.01$) positive association with leadership outcomes. Transactional leadership had a significant ($p<0.01$) negative association with the leadership outcomes.

Implications for Practice
Nurse executives who function in a transformational leadership style tend to have better leadership outcomes. The existing cadre of transformational leaders need to serve as mentors and role models to other nurse executives, as well as to young nurses, so that the next generation of nurse executives will assume a transformational leadership style. An empowering, receptive environment is essential to the recruitment and retention of young nurses.

repeating such influence multiple times can be wearing. In the chaos of health care, nurse leaders face constant change and many challenges. The leader who lasts through these relationships is influential.

Barriers to Leadership

Leadership demands a commitment of effort and time. Many barriers exist to both leading and following. Good leadership and good followership go hand in hand, and both strengthen the mission of the organization.

False Assumptions

Some people have false assumptions about leaders and leadership. For example, some believe that position and title are equivalent to leadership. Having the title of Chief Executive Officer or Chief Nursing Officer does not guarantee that a person will be a good leader. Inspired and forward-moving organizations often select these executives specifically because of their ability to forge a vision and lead others toward

it. However, a good executive is not necessarily a good leader. Furthermore, assuming a management or administrative role does not automatically confer the title of leader on an individual. Leadership is an earned honor and an action-oriented responsibility.

Others believe that workers who do not hold official management positions cannot be leaders. Some nursing units are managed by the nurse manager but led by the unit clerk. Leaders are those who do the best job of sharing their vision of where the followers want to be and how to get there. Many new nurse managers make the mistake of assuming that along with their new job comes the mantle of leadership. Leadership is an earned right and privilege.

Time Constraints

Leadership requires a time commitment; it does not just happen. The leader must fully comprehend the situation at hand, investigate and research options, assume the responsibility to communicate the vision to others, and continually reevaluate the organization or the team to ensure that the vision remains relevant and attainable. All of these activities take time. The twenty-first century has been described as the period of doing more with less. Everyone is busy. Finding time to lead is, therefore, a barrier for many who have inspirational ideas but lack time to develop the skills needed to lead effectively.

EXERCISE 3-3
Define a clinical or management issue that sparks your passion. Assume you have 6 weeks to make a difference. Create a plan identifying your leadership tasks, the support required from others, and the time frame to move the issue toward resolution. Think about what your message is and how and when you will deliver it. Think about what you would do if no one was responsive to your issue. Think about why the issue may be important for you but not for others.

LEADERSHIP DEVELOPMENT

Leadership effectiveness depends on mastering the art of persuasion and communication. Success depends on persuading followers to accept a vision by using convincing communication techniques and making it possible for the followers to achieve the shared goals. Several important leadership tasks, when used effec-

BOX 3-2   LEADERSHIP DEVELOPMENT TASKS

1. Select a mentor.
2. Lead by example.
3. Accept responsibility.
4. Share the rewards.
5. Have a clear vision.
6. Be willing to grow.

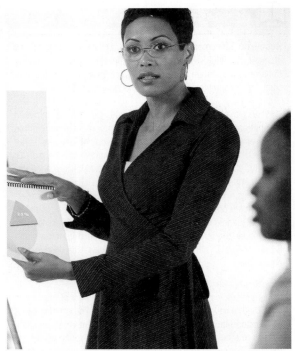

Leading by example helps developing leaders see the mission in action.

tively, will help ensure success (Box 3-2). These are discussed in the following sections.

Select a Mentor

A mentor is someone who models behavior, offers advice and criticism, and coaches the novice to develop a personal leadership style. A mentor is a confidante and coach, as well as a cheerleader and teacher. In other words, a mentor is knowledgeable and skilled. Where do you find a mentor? Usually, a mentor is someone who has experience and some success in the leadership realm of interest, such as in a clinical setting or in an organization. A respected faculty member; a nurse manager, director, or clinician; or an organizational officer or active member may be a mentor. Mentorship is a two-way street. The mentor must agree to work with the novice leader and must have some interest in the novice's future development. A mentor can be close enough geographically to allow both observation and practice of leadership behaviors, as well as timely feedback. A mentor may also be geographically remote and yet well-connected to the mentee. A mentor should provide advice, feedback, and role-modeling. In addition, the mentor has a right to expect assistance with projects, respect, loyalty, and confidentiality. In a mentoring relationship, aspiring leaders soak up knowledge and experience and should expect to return it by serving as a mentor to a young, aspiring leader in the future.

Lead by Example

An effective leader knows that the most effective and visible way to influence people is to lead by example. Desired behavior can be modeled. For example, if an organization has a vision of becoming a political player in the state or community, the leader should be seen engaging in political activities. If the goal is to have improved relationships among followers, the leader must exhibit respect and patience with followers. A key skill to develop is the ability to understand that the leader serves the followers. The effective leader does not send members to do a job but, rather, leads them toward a mutual goal as a team.

Accept Responsibility

Even when the outcome is below expectations, the leader is ultimately responsible for the organization or activity. Effective leaders sometimes react in strange ways when negative outcomes occur. Sometimes these leaders seek to blame others or to make excuses for undesirable or unintended outcomes. Some refuse to accept any responsibility at all. In accepting responsibility, the leader needs to know that there is reward in victory and growth in failure. No one plans to fail, but an effective leader sees failures as opportunities to learn and grow so that previous failures are never repeated. This is called *experience*.

Share the Rewards

An effective leader is as eager to share the glory as to receive it. The more that respect and trust are shared with others, the more they are returned to the leader. Followers who believe their major task is to make the leader look good will soon tire of the task. Empowerment, the act of sharing power with others, is a dynamic process. In essence, sharing power has a synergistic effect that increases power overall. Followers who think the leader is working to make them look good will follow eagerly. Followers form a network and a support base for the leader.

Have a Clear Vision

Leaders see beyond where they are and see where they are going. Strong leaders are proactive and futuristic. The effective leader knows why the journey is necessary and takes the time and energy to inspire others to go along. The ability to communicate and promote the vision is a vital part of achieving it. Effective leaders share their vision and empower followers to come along to achieve it. They also share their leadership skills and successes toward achievement of a goal.

Be Willing to Grow

Thinking that growth for the person or organization is automatic is a misconception. Complacency leads to stagnation. Leaders must continually read about new ideas and approaches, experiment with new concepts, capitalize on a changing world, and seek or create continuing education opportunities to enhance their abilities to lead. Growth takes risk, planning, investment, and work. Setting goals that complement the vision will help the aspiring leader know where to invest time and energy to grow into the desired role.

Leadership development is a lifetime endeavor. Effective leaders are constantly striving to improve their leadership skills. The good news is that leadership skills can be learned and improved. A commitment to improvement strengthens the leader's ability to lead effectively and raises the bar for followers to achieve. As organizations and health care change, the leader is better able to work effectively with an increasingly diverse workforce. The best leaders bring out the best in their followers, as seen in the Literature Perspective on p. 46.

DEVELOPING LEADERS IN THE EMERGING WORKFORCE

Generational differences have always created challenges in the workplace. At the dawn of the twenty-first century, the workplace found an emerging workforce with goals, priorities, and work preferences that were vastly different from those of their Baby Boomer parents. Helping each generation understand and tolerate others is often a delicate orchestration of needs and wants, incentives and motives. Transgenerational leadership must focus on building an understanding and acceptance of each other.

The Emerging Workforce: The 1965 to 1995 Generation

Part of this cohort, born between 1965 and 1976, represents the smallest workforce entry pool since 1930, with just 44 million, compared with the 77 million Baby Boomers preceding them and the 70 million Generation Ys following them. They have a mindset and work ethic that Baby Boomers do not understand. They are hard workers, but unlike the Baby Boomers, they do not have confidence in leaders and institutions. They tend to change jobs more frequently and stay with an employer only as long as there is something that benefits them (Wilcox, 2009).

Their younger siblings, the Generation Ys (also known as *Generation Net, Nexter,* or the *Millennium Generation*), who were born between 1977 and 1995, share many of the same approaches to work but bring their own challenges with no brand loyalty and a blatant disregard for status symbols. Although many of this generation are still children, those in their 20s are already in or entering work settings. This generation represents a large number whose parents are Baby Boomers. They are very technology-savvy, and they tend to be optimistic and interactive (Wilcox, 2009).

In looking at what these emerging workforce members want in their leaders, a study of a national sample of student nurses indicated that they want a leader who is receptive to people, a team player, honest, a good communicator, approachable, knowledgeable, motivating, and competent and has a positive attitude and good people skills (Wieck, Prydun, & Walsh, 2002). Rather than managing details of

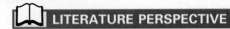

Resource: Gordon, J. (2008). *The no complaining rule: Positive ways to deal with negativity at work.* Hoboken, NJ: John Wiley & Sons.

The role of leader includes creating a workplace that is highly satisfying. There is an abundance of literature on leadership theory and also literature that helps leaders positively impact the workplace through their positive leadership. Jon Gordon is a speaker, consultant, and author of several books inspiring people to create positive energy in the workplace and in life. In his recent book about complaining in the workplace, Gordon describes a fictitious workplace that is steeped in negative energy. The workers in this company complain constantly, and complaining had become a part of the culture of the workplace. The focus on problems was preventing the development of solutions. Gordon suggests that the solution is for leaders to focus on the individual in the workplace instead of the workplace itself and to heighten the self-awareness of employees about the negative power of complaining and the positive power of finding solutions and a positive attitude in the workplace.

Leaders focus on the five things all employees should do instead of complaining, as follows:

1. Be grateful and reflect on things one is grateful about instead of focusing on things that cause stress—the positive energy is reflected in individual behaviors.
2. Focus on praising co-workers instead of only finding things wrong with what they are doing—the result is that those being praised will create more success and will work hard to live up to the praise.
3. Reflect on those things that go right every day instead of on those things that are not ideal—the result is that the individual will focus every day on creating more success tomorrow.
4. Focus on things one has the power to change and let go of those things that are beyond one's control—when one lets go of things they cannot change, stress is naturally reduced.
5. Stepping back and breathing, reflecting, and meditating reduce stress and boost positive energy—stopping to meditate when tempted to complain recharges and redirects energy.

Gordon describes the transformation of the organization when leaders develop concrete ways for employees to think in terms of solutions, not just continually complaining about problems.

Implications for Practice

The nursing workplace environment is full of reasons to be stressed. Students and new graduates entering the nursing workplace notice the culture of individual nursing units. All of them have noticed differences in the attitudes of staff, and they tend to choose workplaces in which there is not the pervasive negativity and constant complaining. To recruit new nurses into nursing and to keep them there, leaders in nursing must redirect negative energy in the workplace into the desire to choose the things one can do something about and work positively toward finding solutions. The culture of the workplace reflects the effectiveness of the leader.

---

work, nurse managers have to be able to lead the group through coaching and mentoring.

Successfully leading the emerging workforce means the leader must shape a vision and win the 20-somethings to it. The vision must be one that excites them, because fun and balance are an important part of their lives. A vision that is powerful enough can transform the workplace.

The successful leader must mobilize the followers to act. The required actions must provide value to the followers (e.g., learning a new skill or attaining certification or recognition). The younger generations are happy to follow as long as they can retain balance in their lives, have information about and input into the decisions that affect them, and see some benefit in the activity. It is the leader's challenge to provide the type of environment in which younger-generation followers want to follow.

The Entrenched Workforce: The 1946 to 1965 Generation

Baby Boomers, born after World War II, see work life very differently compared with the emerging workforce. Boomer workers are much more likely to believe in the power of collective action, based on their successes with social movements in their formative years in the 1960s. They tend to mistrust authority and are very comfortable with the process of getting to a goal. They find the journey of getting to the goal almost as important as reaching the goal. They are tolerant of, even depend on, meetings and ongoing discussions that the younger generation finds tedious and wasteful.

The preferred leader of the entrenched workforce shares some of the characteristics of the younger generation's leader, such as being motivational, honest, approachable, competent, and knowledge-able. However, Baby Boomers also expect their leader to be professional and supportive and have high integrity, a concept not even mentioned by the younger generation (Wieck, Prydun, & Walsh, 2002).

Challenges for the entrenched workforce are sharing leadership with the younger generation, empowering them to lead in their own model rather than trying to make them into second-generation Baby Boomers, and retaining the younger leaders in leadership ranks. Many younger employees are opting out of traditional work roles to become entrepreneurs. They take their leadership potential with them where there are few older role models for them to follow. A risk for aging Boomers is that the best and the brightest potential leaders will lose interest in leading and will opt for personal satisfaction and wealth accumulation rather than leadership and service roles.

The challenges of generational acceptance are some of many facing twenty-first century leaders. Attention to the needs of both the leader and the follower will create an environment in which everyone thrives.

EXERCISE 3-4

List the names of the people with whom you work most frequently. Determine to which workforce (emerging or entrenched) each belongs. Describe known benefits of the workplace that support each generation's view. (One list may be longer than the other.) What elements of benefits are present in the personnel policies and workplace practices that benefit each? What elements are absent?

SURVIVING AND THRIVING AS A LEADER

The keys to leadership are to believe in the vision and to enjoy the journey. The leader has a responsibility to self and followers to stay healthy and enthusiastic for the mission of the group. Surviving and thriving as a leader are based on the rules in Box 3-3. Each element is discussed in the following sections.

The Leader Must Maintain Balance

Time management is essential for an effective leader. Many new leaders, in their zeal to be accessible to

---

BOX 3-3 THE FIVE RULES OF LEADERS

1. Maintain balance.
2. Generate self-motivation.
3. Build self-confidence.
4. Listen to constituents.
5. Maintain a positive attitude.

---

their constituents, lose control of their lives. A good strategy for retaining or regaining control is to get control of communication. Good leaders use the simplest and fastest method of communication that makes them accessible but does not tie them down. The keys to success are setting priorities and keeping in control. Planned telephone time and e-mail are excellent ways to keep control of time. Attending to matters as they arise, handling each question or piece of mail once and only one at a time, and focusing on the task at hand without distractions are just some of the time-management strategies used by effective leaders. Saving time, like wasting time, is a learned habit and can therefore be unlearned or relearned.

The Leader Must Generate Self-Motivation

Leaders who expect their followers to provide them with motivation, to be grateful for the time spent on followers' needs, and to offer frequent and lavish praise are in for a painful awakening. Followers in organizations, work situations, and elected constituencies feel they have earned the right to criticize the leader by being followers. Followers will have an opinion about everything. Sometimes the comments are favorable, and sometimes they are unfavorable. The reason that self-motivation is so essential is because the leader can expect very little external motivation. Most leaders are risk takers and self-starters who are enthused by and believe in the vision they have created. Enthusiasm leads to an energized base, which is a hallmark of a vibrant, healthy organization.

The Leader Must Work to Build Self-Confidence

An effective leader must have self-confidence. This confidence comes from an acceptance of self, despite imperfections. Self-confidence is a self-perpetuating virtue. Effective leaders perform an honest self-appraisal on a regular basis and work to feel good about the job they are doing. A leader who is surrounded by people who enhance the leader's own characteristics makes a formidable leader and strengthens self-confidence in the ability to lead.

The more confident a leader feels, the more likely that success will follow. Success builds self-confidence. Two important factors are related to developing self-confidence. One is avoiding the tendency to become arrogant. The other is maintaining self-confidence despite setbacks.

The Leader Must Listen to His or Her Constituents

Followers always have something to say. Leaders must listen to their constituents and determine whether action is indicated. Active listening, which in the U.S. culture includes looking the person in the eye and offering questioning probes, shows an interest in what a person is saying. However, listening does not obligate the leader to any course of action. Clear boundaries must be communicated. A smart leader listens to all sides and makes decisions based on the vision and direction that is best for the group.

The Leader Must Have a Positive Attitude

Positive attitude is vital to leadership success. No one wants to follow a pessimist anywhere. People expect the leader to have the answers, to know where the organization is going, and to take the initiative to get the group to its goal. A positive attitude can be a great ally in sharing and maintaining the vision. Attitude is a choice, not a foregone conclusion. The effective leader uses positive thinking and positive messages to create an environment in which followers believe in the organization, the leader, and themselves. The problems and challenges in health care demand that nurses seek and fill leadership positions in a positive and future-oriented manner.

EXERCISE 3-5
Using the five rules for leaders, create a personal description of how you maintain balance, generate self-motivation, build self-confidence, listen to constituents, and maintain a positive attitude.

THE NURSE AS LEADER

Leadership Within the Workplace

Staff Nurse as Leader

A common misconception is that leaders within the workplace are the managers. Leaders within the workplace are not necessarily those who are entrusted with the role and title of manager. The role of the workplace manager is one who is a status quo maintainer; that is, the focus is on the day-to-day operations. The manager is concerned about budgets, financial performance, staffing, employee evaluations, and employee education and training. All of these important activities are paramount concerns of the manager of an operational unit in health care. In contrast, the workplace leader is one who has the ability to envision a preferred future for the quality of the working environment. The leader understands that nurse satisfaction is a central construct of many of the most successful nursing-service delivery systems. A manager may also be an effective leader, and thus others, including staff nurses, can emerge in leadership roles.

Workplace leaders create an environment in which nurses can experience satisfaction and have ideas for increasing the level of workplace satisfaction for nurses on the team. Leaders are those who creatively pose solutions to problems and capitalize on opportunities in the workplace. Furthermore, they support staff nurses, who offer numerous ideas about patient safety issues. Nurses who believe that they have good ideas for future improvements should volunteer for opportunities to lead. There might be practice councils, clinical unit standards committees, or legislative committees to pose new solutions. If the hospital or other workplace has no formalized mechanism for nurse input into organizational decision making, staff nurses who are leaders should clarify their vision and work to create such mechanisms.

Developing leadership skills for staff nurses can happen in several ways. Some of these may be employment opportunities (e.g., practice councils), others may be professional opportunities (e.g., the district nurses association), and still others may be clinical opportunities (e.g., the heart association). Leadership can be developed, and staff nurse leaders can help establish workplaces that are satisfying and rewarding. Magnet™ facilities, for example, depend on staff nurse leadership to create the intensity of quality work.

Nurse Manager as Leader

Management and leadership, although different constructs, can be a strong combination for success. The nurse in the role of manager ensures that the day-to-day elements of the workplace are done correctly. Just as the effective manager pays attention to employee selection, hiring, orientation, continuing employee development, and financial accountability, in the role of leader, the manager raises the level of expectations and helps employees reach their highest level of potential excellence. A primary role of the leader is to inspire (Atchison, 1990).

Developing with staff nurses a shared vision of the preferred future is a goal of the nurse manager in the role of leader. Staff members tend to resist change that is thrust upon them. When nurses are active participants in change, from its inception, they are far more likely to be invested in outcomes.

An essential element of success for the nurse manager as a leader is the inclusion of staff nurses in decision making. This contribution can enhance their organizational commitment and create a sense of pride in successful outcomes. The nurse manager inspires staff by involving them in changing the workplace to make it more satisfying. In so doing, the nurse manager also develops personal leadership skills.

Nurse Executive as Leader

A primary goal of the nurse executive is leadership within the workplace. The nurse executive has an outstanding opportunity to shape the future of professional practice within a working environment by creating opportunities for staff nurses and managers to have optimal input into organizational decision making related to the future. The nurse executive thus helps create a shared vision of the preferred future.

The concept of empowerment is important to the role of leadership for the nurse executive in a work organization. Empowerment theory suggests that power must be given away or shared with others in the organization. Staff nurses may be encouraged to have input into decisions, or they may be given considerable information about how decisions are made. The ability to make or influence changes in the orga-

nization is a powerful tool. Nurses must believe that their input and ideas are considered when change occurs. Having input in decisions, having some control over the environment, and receiving feedback about actions taken or not taken all contribute to a feeling of being empowered to have control over one's practice and one's life.

The importance of managers and executives being leaders rather than managers is a recurring theme in nursing literature. The fact is that both management and leadership skills in the nurse executive are essential. The ability to balance the day-to-day operating knowledge with the ability to lead a nursing service organization into the future is a winning combination.

Nursing Student as Leader

Students have many opportunities to learn and practice leadership skills. The goals for leadership at the student level should be kept within a realistic framework. Helping students to practice novice leadership skills within the security of an educational program is a reasonable expectation. Novice leadership skills that contribute to future leadership success involve learning how to work in groups, deal with difficult people, resolve conflict, reach consensus on an action, and evaluate actions and outcomes objectively (Figure 3-1). These opportunities create skills that can lead to some expertise that could transfer to initial practice.

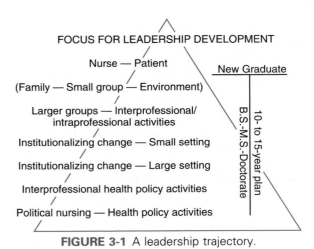

FIGURE 3-1 A leadership trajectory.

Fagin (2000) describes a 10- to 15-year leadership development plan for neophyte nurses that builds on their leadership skills from their beginning nurse-patient experiences. The reality of student development toward true leadership expertise takes place over a long period and should not be expected during the first year or two of nursing school or nursing practice. Nevertheless, every leader started somewhere. Movement toward an increasingly complex leadership experience allows the new nurse to move from leading and planning with an individual to working with groups, such as families or communities. Further leadership development occurs during interactions with larger groups and through instituting changes in research and application of new techniques and moving toward health policy and political activities. With increasing educational achievement and career experience comes increasing complexity of leadership capabilities.

Most countries have some type of national student nurses' association, as well as regional, state, and school-based associations. These types of organizations offer an opportunity for student nurses to become involved in service to their future profession. Programs of study in schools of nursing are appropriately heavy on nursing theory and clinical practice. Through involvement in the student association, the nursing student can understand the bigger picture of nursing as a profession.

The best way to begin involvement is to become active in the local chapter of the student association. If the student is interested in student association activities, opportunities exist to serve on committees or in elected positions on the board of directors at local, regional, state, and national levels. Examples of leadership development at the national level include serving on liaison committees with nurse leaders; attending leadership development educational programs; attending and leading events at local, state, and national meetings and conventions; and interacting with the leaders of complementary professional nursing organizations.

Leadership in Professional Organizations

In the United States, the best and most important step to take in becoming a leader within the nursing profession is to join a professional organization. Many nurses today take part in several organizations.

However, membership in the American Nurses Association (ANA) and the state constituent member associations shapes career growth and mobility. Volunteering for local or committee memberships is a valued and useful way to learn and to grow within the association.

Professional nursing specialty organizations play an important role in disseminating information to members in such areas as clinical practice (e.g., Oncology Nursing Society), role area (e.g., American Organization of Nurse Executives), and interest groups (e.g., Southern Nursing Research Society). Many of the professional specialty organizations maintain a national or regional presence rather than have state or local chapters. Some of them have local chapters (e.g., Association of periOperative Registered Nurses), especially in the larger, more populated areas across the country. The major impact of the professional specialty organization is sharing and dissemination of information, discussion of mutual clinical or role concerns, and education regarding the latest technical innovations in the field. Leadership opportunities are available to present posters or papers at local, regional, or national conferences, as well as to serve on committees and boards.

After becoming established and known in the local association, running for elected office in the local district or chapter association is a way many leaders within professional associations start their leadership careers. It is not unusual to be unsuccessful in the first attempt at running for an elective office in a professional association, but persistence can do two things: (1) it can help with name recognition, and (2) it can let members know that you are serious about being an association leader.

Leaders, often from district or chapter levels, later hold office at the state level. Volunteering for committee assignments and running for elected office in the state association establish leadership interest within the professional association. Leadership efforts at the national association level are usually more successful after establishing a record of successful leadership in the state constituent member association.

This pathway of professional involvement and leadership, from the student association to the district or chapter association to the state association and subsequently to the national association, may seem like a linear progression to more global opportunities for leadership in the profession. However, many successful nursing leaders conceptualize the progression as circular rather than linear. Many well-known leaders who have held high offices at the national or state level take their experience and expertise to return to offices and committee appointments at the local and state levels.

Leadership in the Community

Nurses as Community Opinion Leaders

Nurses are valued and respected members of their communities. As trusted professionals, nurses have an opportunity to serve as catalysts in leadership opportunities in the community. In partnership with others in the community, nurses can help build a more just, more peaceful, and more healthful society.

Many avenues are available for nurses to serve as community opinion leaders. Attendance at civic gatherings, such as city commission and school board meetings, is an excellent way to be aware of what is happening and to offer input from a nursing perspective. For instance, when the school board begins deliberating whether the budget will accommodate a registered nurse for every school or whether to replace a registered nurse with a trained clerk who can record vaccinations, a nursing voice in the audience could clarify the importance of school nurses to a school population. Writing letters to the editor of a newspaper and participating in public forums give the nurse an avenue to share expertise and mold community opinion.

Nurses as Community Volunteers

Many opportunities exist for volunteer participation in the community. Nurses bring a unique leadership skill set to community activities. The ability to understand complex systems, as well as to understand interpersonal dynamics and communication techniques, constitutes knowledge that is valuable in community volunteer opportunities.

Leadership in mobilizing volunteers for health fairs, screening activities, and educational events is a community need that nurses can and do fill. Such activities promote health and advance the health of the community in important ways. Nurses can also lead efforts to engage others in the community in volunteer activities. In addition, nurses can organize individuals in the community to help develop a vision

for the future of the community's health, healthcare opportunities, and healthcare delivery.

From the perspective of the nurse as a community leader, a unique opportunity exists to work with schools, city or county governments, and other community entities to formulate a vision for improving the health of the community through disease prevention and health promotion. The nurse can be a catalyst for a community to recognize present problems and to develop a plan to reach a preferred future.

Leadership Through Appointed and Elected Office

Nurses are valuable leaders in elected and appointed offices at the local, state, and national levels. Because of the trustworthiness of nurses in general, nurses should be able to mobilize resources to raise monies, develop support, and get elected to offices. The numbers of nurses in offices at all three levels of government are continually growing. The ANA Political Action Committee (PAC) and the state constituent member association PACs provide assistance to nurses who want to run for office. Nurses who are elected members of governmental bodies can exert their leadership to shape the vision of the government to help meet the needs of the citizens.

Local Offices

Leadership opportunities in elected or appointed positions in the local government include school boards, city councils, and community boards dealing with various community initiatives. At the local level, nurses who serve on elected or appointed boards and councils bring a unique perspective, even when the major focus of the entity appears to be totally unrelated to health care. Leadership in this case is casting a vision of a healthy, thriving community.

State Offices

Leadership opportunities at the state level in elected or appointed positions include being elected to state legislatures or appointed to state boards, such as the state board of nursing or the state board of health. Each state constituent member association of the ANA often has a role in recommending names of qualified members to be considered for appointment to various boards and committees in the state. Nurses who are members have the highest likelihood of being supported or recommended by the state association or national association.

National Offices

A few nurses have been successful in getting elected to the U.S. Congress as representatives. No nurse has yet been elected U.S. senator, but many opportunities exist for nurses to be appointed to Federal boards and commissions. The ANA and the state constituent member associations often play a role in putting forth nominations of members for appointment to such bodies.

The Challenge of Leading

The nurse is in a trusted role as nurturer and provider of care to the most vulnerable in our society. Nurses who choose leadership roles have many of the needed talents to serve their followers and their profession. Visionary and responsible leadership is vital to the future success of nursing as an art and a science. Professional nursing has been blessed with excellent leaders in the past and will continue to be led by the visionary nurse leaders of tomorrow.

THE SOLUTION

The following priorities were set:
- Patient safety
- Occupant safety
- Return to normal function as quickly as possible

Unit nursing staff were instructed to review their emergency preparedness manuals the evening of June 8 and ensure that they had flashlights and water. They were instructed to divide into teams and watch each other's patients, allowing some of the staff to rest. It was clear that the staff needed to pace themselves because it would be hours before additional personnel would arrive. Staff were reassured by frequent rounds made by the supervisors and calls to the units from the Command Center.

As water rushed into the basement of the facility, the departments of pharmacy and radiology moved their supplies higher and dry cereal, bread, and milk were obtained from the cafeteria to sustain patients over the coming hours. The Network Services Department (hospital telephone and page operators) was relocated to higher ground. At 3 AM, as a power shortage became imminent, the decision to triage stable patients who were on life support devices was made. These patients were located on four different floors and were evacuated, starting at the highest floor and working down before elevators lost power. Patients were transferred to an adjacent medical tower building that had an outpatient ambulatory surgery center linked to the hospital via a skybridge. Anesthesiologists, residents, respiratory therapists, and nurses worked collaboratively to triage patients. Some critical care patients were evacuated down stairwells as elevators failed. All critically ill

patients who were too unstable to evacuate were placed on ventilators with battery backup. It became apparent that power was needed quickly to maintain ventilator support because batteries would be drained. As soon as roads were passable, external diesel generators were obtained and connected to provide power to ventilators, which then created the need to test for carbon dioxide levels. A human chain was created to deliver medical supplies, water, food, and lights to staff.

Staff were educated to deliver IVs without pumps and to take blood pressures the old-fashioned way, with a manometer and a flashlight. Food was provided to patients and staff from volunteer agencies such as the Salvation Army. Patient and staff comfort was difficult to maintain in an un–air-conditioned, 26-story tower in the summertime. Patients were triaged for discharge; all admissions were carefully screened by a medical director and nurses because the city of Houston was short 3000 hospital beds for an extended period. Nine days after the flood, all beds and essential services were functioning and the hospital was open for all admissions.

Nurses often have not learned the necessary skills for triage and disaster response. An understanding of emergency plans and quick critical-thinking skills are imperative to surviving a natural disaster.

—*Rosemary Luquire*

Would this be a suitable approach for you? Why?

THE EVIDENCE

- More effective leadership promotes effective communication, greater responsibility, empowerment, job clarity, continuity of care, and interdisciplinary collaboration.
- A transformational leadership style is closely associated with followers' working conditions—

namely involvement, influence, and meaningfulness.
- Nurse managers with effective leadership skills are an essential component to addressing the nursing shortage, because lower staff turnover results from transformational leadership.

- The presence of a supportive culture in which learning is valued and the presence of transformational leadership are key factors in the implementation and sustainability of best practice guidelines.

- Emerging workforce members want a leader who is receptive to people, a team player, honest, a good communicator, approachable, knowledgeable, motivating, and competent and has a positive attitude and good people skills.

NEED TO KNOW NOW

- Work with others to create a positive environment so students and others will want to work there.
- Look for leaders, not titles. Communicate with all people you deal with, including patients and their families, by taking generational differences into consideration.

- Leading in the community has great potential to strengthen your skills quickly.
- Leading in professional organizations improves the profession and provides personal connections.

CHAPTER CHECKLIST

The role of the nurse leader is to share a vision and provide the means for followers to reach it. When the group succeeds, the leader succeeds. Members of different generations have expectations and needs that are different from those of a leader. Various leadership opportunities are available; it is up to the nurse to take advantage and contribute to the progress of the nursing profession.

- Excellent leadership in any working environment can improve recruitment and retention efforts and result in satisfied employees.
- Two leadership approaches contrast the leader role, as follows:
  - Transactional leaders rely on the power of the organizational position to reward or punish performance to control employees.
  - Transformational leaders ascribe power to interpersonal skills and personal contact in transforming people to make them want to progress.
- Key elements to becoming an effective leader can be learned and practiced, as follows:

- Select an effective and willing mentor.
- Lead by example through role-modeling.
- Share the rewards with followers.
- Have a clear vision that followers can support.
- Be willing to grow and change to meet current needs.
- The emerging workforce (born 1965 to 1995) wants a leader who has good people skills and a nurturing attitude. The entrenched workforce (born 1946 to 1965) wants a leader who is tolerant of the process of change and who exhibits high integrity and professionalism.
- Many opportunities exist to lead in nursing. To thrive in a leadership position, the nurse must do the following:
  - Maintain balance.
  - Generate self-motivation.
  - Build self-confidence.
  - Listen to constituents.
  - Maintain a positive attitude.

TIPS FOR BECOMING A LEADER

- Take advantage of leadership opportunities, and practice your leadership skills.

- Expect to stumble occasionally, but learn from your mistakes and continue. Every leader has made mistakes. The truly inspired leaders have learned from them and moved forward.

- Get some help—having a caring mentor is the best way to develop leadership ability. The mentor can give you the benefit of experience and will serve as a resource to get feedback on actions and to explore options.

- Take risks. A person does not become a leader by maintaining the status quo. Leaders forge a vision and bring followers forward. However, change involves risks. Do not be foolhardy, but do not be complacent either.

REFERENCES

Atchison, T. A. (1990). *Turning health care leadership around.* San Francisco: Jossey-Bass.

Atchison, T. A. (2004). *Followership: A practical guide to aligning leaders and followers.* Chicago: Health Administration Press.

Bennis, W. (2009). *On becoming a leader.* New York: Basic Books.

Covey, S. R. (1992). *Principle-centered leadership.* New York: Simon & Schuster.

Dierckx de Casterle, B., Willemse, A., Verschueren, M., & Milisen, K. (2008). Impact of clinical leadership development on the clinical leader, nursing team and care-giving process: A case study. *Journal of Nursing Management, 16*(6), 753-763.

Fagin, C. (2000*). Essays on nursing leadership.* New York: Springer Publishing.

Gordon, J. (2008). *The no complaining rule: Positive ways to deal with negativity at work.* Hoboken, NJ: John Wiley & Sons.

Kouzes, J., & Posner, B. (2007). *The leadership challenge.* San Francisco: Jossey-Bass.

Marchionni, C., & Ritchie, J. (2008). Organizational factors that support the implementation of a nursing best practice guideline. *Journal of Nursing Management, 16*(3), 266-274.

Nielsen, K., Yarker, J., Brenner, S., Randall, R., & Borg, V. (2008). The importance of transformational leadership style for the well-being of employees working with older people. *Journal of Advanced Nursing, 63*(5), 465-475.

Oakley, E., & Krug, D. (1994). *Enlightened leadership.* New York: Simon & Schuster.

Raup, G. H. (2008). The impact of ED nurse manager leadership style on staff nurse turnover and patient satisfaction in academic health center hospitals. *Journal of Emergency Nursing, 34*(5), 403-409.

Robbins, B., & Davidhizar, R. (2007). Transformational leadership in health care today. *Health Care Manager, 26*(3), 234-239.

Senge, P. M. (2006). *The fifth discipline: The art and practice of the learning organization.* New York: Doubleday.

Snodgrass, J., Douthitt, S., Ellis, R., Wade, S., & Plemons, J. (2008). Occupational therapy practitioners' perceptions of rehabilitation managers' leadership styles and the outcomes of leadership. *Journal of Allied Health, 37*(1), 38-44.

Weston, M. J. (2008). Transformational leadership at a national perspective. *Nurse Leader, 6*(4), 41-45.

Wieck, K. L., Prydun, M., & Walsh, T. (2002). What emerging workforce nurses want in their leaders. *Journal of Nursing Scholarship, 34*(3), 283.

Wilcox, J. (2009). Challenges of nursing management. In J. Zerwekh & J. C. Claborn (Eds.), *Nursing today* (6th ed.). St. Louis: Saunders.

SUGGESTED READINGS

Barger, S. E. (2000). Professional practice: The practice of leadership. *Journal of Professional Nursing, 16*(2), 72.

Bower, F. L. (2000). *Nurses taking the lead: Personal qualities of effective leadership.* St. Louis: Mosby.

Labarre, P. (2000, March). Do you have the will to lead? *FastCompany,* 222-230.

Northouse, P. G. (2009). *Leadership: Theory and practice* (3rd ed.). Thousand Oaks, CA: Sage Publishers.

Shtogren, J. A. (Ed.), (1999). *Skyhooks for leadership.* New York: American Management Association.

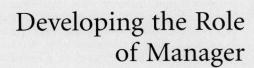

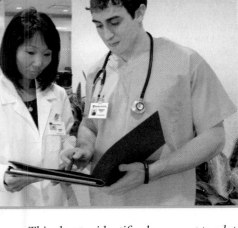

Developing the Role of Manager

Angela L. Stalbaum and Ana M. Valadez

This chapter identifies key concepts related to the roles of the nurse manager. It describes basic manager functions, illustrates management principles that are inherent in the role of professional practice, and identifies descriptive competencies for the nurse manager. Role development is crucial to forming the right questions to ask in a management or clinical situation that will help the practitioner identify problems and anticipate needs. This chapter provides an overview for the further development of practical skills.

OBJECTIVES

- Analyze roles and functions of a nurse manager.
- Analyze the relationship of the nurse manager with others.
- Analyze management of healthcare settings.
- Evaluate management resource allocation/distribution.
- Evaluate behaviors of professionalism of the nurse manager.

TERMS TO KNOW

case management	manager	role
follower	organizational culture	role theory
leader	quality indicators	
managed care	quantum theory	

THE CHALLENGE

Donna McKinster, RN, BSN
Tiffany Thornton, RN, BSN
Co-Clinical Managers, Seton Medical Center—Austin,
Austin, Texas

In today's changing healthcare world, opportunities continually come about in response to a particular "crisis" situation. On our 64-bed medical/surgical unit, the average census is at budget, but the day-to-day volume of patients varies widely. Both flexibility and creativity are needed for processes related to optimal staffing for patient safety while meeting budget expectations. A 40% patient occupancy turnover can occur daily in this very busy medical/surgical unit (e.g., if the unit is full with 64 patients, 25 patients may be discharged and 25 admitted in a 24-hour period). Over the past several months, such has been the case. In addition, with increased budgetary constraints, partly because of the overall economic downturn across the country, it became important to see how to make particular changes in staffing that could influence our budget in a positive way and at the same time maintain and even improve staff satisfaction. Our goal was to not cut any positions at the bedside and to not increase the number of patients to whom a nurse would be assigned. As managers of this unit, we were forced to look at our current processes and develop a plan unique to our unit.

What do you think you would do if you were one of these nurses?

INTRODUCTION

Chapter 1 provided a general overview of leading and managing. This chapter looks at management from different perspectives. The core of role theory began with management theory—a science that has undergone numerous changes in the past century. In the early 1900s, the theory of scientific management was embraced—a theory based on the idea that there is one best way to accomplish a task. Practice in the 1930s through the 1970s was dominated by participative, humanistic leadership theories. Although changes in healthcare delivery no doubt are affecting the roles of nurse managers, the relevance of role theory remains a constant. Conway's (1978) historic definition, "**role theory** represents a collection of concepts and a variety of hypothetical formulations that predict how actors will perform in a given role, or under what circumstances certain types of behaviors can be expected" (p. 17), is still appropriate.

The evolutionary process of management theories has affected how managers address workers' concerns and needs. The beginning management theories discounted concern for workers' psychological needs and focused on productivity and efficiency. When theories relating to human relations came about, workers' needs and motivations became focal points for the nurse manager. Conversely, situational theories, such as the Path-Goal theory, focused on the environment, clarifying the relationship between the pathway employees take and the outcome or goal they wish to obtain.

What is involved in management? A self-appraisal might lead a potential nurse manager to ask himself or herself the following questions: Do I have career goals that include gaining experience and education to become a nurse manager? What specific knowledge, skills, and personal qualities do I need to develop to be most effective in practice? Do I have a mentor who can guide me in this direction? Does the organization I currently work for have succession planning? If changes need to be made, they must be matched with changes in healthcare agencies and within the larger social system. A nurse manager must recognize the need for growth within, which then translates into improvement of one's practice. A prerequisite for self-actualization is a bond between the nurse and the community, because a nurse manager's patients and staff make up the community. Consider also, what is the role of the nurse manager? Practicing nurse managers illustrate role perceptions. Some nurse managers would cite decision making and problem solving as major roles, for which maintaining objectivity is sometimes a special challenge. Others would identify collaboration, especially with other departments, to enhance quality patient outcomes. Truly effective care is the result of efforts by the total healthcare team. Effective collaboration includes honesty, directness, and listening to others' points of view. However, management is more complex than this.

THE MANAGEMENT ROLE

Management is a generic function that includes similar basic tasks in every discipline and in every society. However, before the nurse manager can be effective, he or she must be well-grounded in nursing practice. Drucker (1974), in his classic writings, identified the following five basic functions of a manager, which are still true today:

- Establishes objectives and goals for each area and communicates them to the persons who are responsible for attaining them
- Organizes and analyzes the activities, decisions, and relations needed and divides them into manageable tasks
- Motivates and communicates with the people responsible for various jobs through teamwork
- Analyzes, appraises, and interprets performance and communicates the meaning of measurement tools and their results to staff and superiors
- Develops people, including self

Table 4-1 shows how these basic management functions apply to the nurse manager.

Managers develop efforts that focus on the individual. Their aim is to enable the person to develop his or her abilities and strengths to the fullest and to achieve excellence. Thus a manager has a role in helping people develop realistic goals. Goals should be set high enough yet be attainable. Active participation, encouragement, and guidance from the manager and from the organization are needed for the individual's developmental efforts to be fully productive. Nurse managers who are successful in motivating staff are often providing an environment that facilitates accomplishment of goals, resulting in personal satisfactions.

The nurse manager must possess qualities similar to those of a good leader: knowledge, integrity, ambition, judgment, courage, stamina, enthusiasm, communication skills, planning skills, and administrative abilities. The arena of management versus leadership has been addressed by numerous authors, and although points of view differ, some similarities exist between managers and leaders.

Managers address complex issues by planning, budgeting, and setting target goals. They meet their goals by organizing, staffing, controlling, and solving problems. By contrast, leaders set a direction, develop a vision, and communicate the new direction to the staff. Managers address complexity, whereas leaders address change. Another way of looking at management in contrast to leadership and followership is to look at the common traits of each. In Table 4-2, the characteristics of a leader are compared with those of a manager and a follower.

TABLE 4-1	BASIC MANAGER FUNCTIONS AND NURSE MANAGER FUNCTIONS
BASIC MANAGER FUNCTIONS	**NURSE MANAGER FUNCTIONS**
Establishes and communicates goals and objectives	Delineates objectives and goals for assigned area Communicates objectives and goals effectively to staff members who will help attain goals
Organizes, analyzes, and divides work into tasks	Assesses and evaluates activities on assigned area Makes sound decisions about dividing up daily work activities for staff
Motivates and communicates	Stresses the importance of being a good team player Provides positive reinforcement
Analyzes, appraises, and interprets performance and measurements	Completes performance appraisals of individual staff members Communicates results to staff and management
Develops people, including self	Addresses staff development continuously through mentoring and preceptorships Furthers self-development by attending educational programs and seeking specialty certification credentialing

TABLE 4-2   LEADER, MANAGER, AND FOLLOWER TRAITS

LEADER TRAITS	MANAGER TRAITS	FOLLOWER TRAITS
Values commitments, relationships with others, and esprit de corps in the organization	Emphasizes organizing, coordinating, and controlling resources (e.g., space, supplies, equipment, people)	Perceives the needs of both the leader and other staff
Provides a vision that can be communicated and has a long-term effect on the organization that moves it in new directions	Attends to short-term objectives/goals	Demonstrates cooperative and collaborative behaviors
Communicates the rationale for changing paths; charts new paths that lead to progress	Maximizes results from existing resources	Exerts the power to communicate through various channels
Endorses and thrives on taking risks that bring about change	Interprets established policy, procedures, and mandates	Remains fully accountable for actions while relinquishing some autonomy and conceding certain authority to the leader
Demonstrates a positive feeling in the workplace and relates the importance of workers	Moves cautiously; dislikes uncertainty	Exhibits willingness to both lead and follow peers, as the situation warrants, allowing for competency-based leadership
	Enforces policy mandates, contracts, etc. (acts as a gatekeeper)	Assumes responsibility to understand what risks are acceptable for the organization and what risks are unacceptable

The literature abounds with complexities that nurse managers face in the everyday roles they encounter when leading their staff. One of those roles is creating a positive workplace environment that now includes four generations of nurses (Veterans, Baby Boomers, Generation X-ers, and Millennials [Generation Y-ers]). Carver and Candela (2008) discuss the importance of nurse managers having a strategy to increase job satisfaction, decrease nurse turnover, and increase organizational commitment by considering the generational differences. Managers who know how to relate to the different generations can improve work environments for nursing. The concept was validated in a study conducted by Widger, Pye, Wilson, Squires, Tourangeau, and Cranley (2007). Data were collected from 6541 registered nurses comprising the Baby Boomers, Generations X-ers, and Generation Y-ers). Although the Baby Boomers showed a high degree of job satisfaction, such was not the case for the Generation X-ers and Millennials. If managers want to be successful in establishing job satisfaction for the younger generations, the study concluded, the following must be considered: (1) creating a shared governance structure in which nurses are encouraged to make decisions; (2) providing opportunities for self-scheduling; and (3) providing opportunities for career development and supporting education.

The nurse manager is the environmentalist of the unit. In other words, the manager is always assessing the context in which a practice and work environment that is positive and healthy can affect people's performance. Thus the nurse manager's role is to ensure that the nine principles and elements of such an environment are present as defined by the American Organization of Nurse Executives (2004):

1. A culture that promotes collaboration through trust, diversity, and team orientation

2. A culture with clear, respectful, open, and trusting communication

3. A culture in which everyone is accountable and knows what is expected

4. Adequate numbers of qualified staff to meet patient expectations and provide balance to the work and home life of staff

5. Presence of leadership who serves as an advocate for nursing, supports empowerment of nurses, and ensures availability of resources

6. A structure for participation in shared decision making

7. Ongoing education and professional development

8. Recognition of contributions of nursing staff

9. Recognition by nurses of the contributions they provide to practice

Quantum theory speaks to the uncertainty and the vast number of possibilities that can be used in different situations. Valentine (2002) included Quantum theory when addressing nursing leadership theories. She referred to the work of Porter-O'Grady and his observations that leaders display various roles according to the needs of the system and can be seen in a number of places in the system. Thus his work has opened up new horizons when thinking about leadership and how the ever-changing healthcare environment is requiring new leadership characteristics. Valentine refers to what Porter-O'Grady has written regarding technology and how it has changed the way leadership is viewed. Historically, knowledge increased as the position of the person increased and nurse growth was vertical up the chain of command. Now, when new nurses enter the workforce with enormous technologic knowledge and skills, their professional growth is on a horizontal plane. Thus Quantum theory may be the most significant theory for the nurse manager of the twenty-first century.

To be successful in day-to-day operations, a manager must be concerned with relationships. Chaleff (2009) developed one of the early models of followership to reorient individuals: "Courageous followership is built on the platform of courageous relationship. The courage to be right, the courage to be wrong, the courage to be different from each other. Each of us sees the world through our own eyes and experiences" (p. 4). Chaleff describes five dimensions of the relationship: the courage to assume responsi-

TABLE 4-3	THE MANAGER'S COROLLARY TO THE COURAGE OF FOLLOWERS
DIMENSION OF THE RELATIONSHIP	
FOLLOWER	**MANAGER**
Courage to assume responsibility	Demonstrates trust in individual autonomy
Courage to serve	Advocates for service role
Courage to challenge	Poses dilemmas to encourage behavior
Courage to participate in transformation	Designs opportunities to develop transformational abilities
Courage to leave by separating from a leader or group	Risks separation

Reprinted with permission of the publisher. From Chaleff, I. (1995). *The courageous follower: Standing up to and for our leaders.* San Francisco: Berrett-Koehler Publishers. All rights reserved. Website: www.bkconnection.com.

bility, the courage to serve, the courage to challenge, the courage to participate in transformation, and the courage to leave by separating from a leader or group. Table 4-3 poses the possible corollary role of the manager for supporting this courage development in followers.

CONSUMING RESEARCH

The nurse manager's role calls for a twofold responsibility: that of being a participant in research and that of being an interpreter of research. Nursing literature, especially in nursing administration journals, reflects that nurse managers are contributing to research either by doing unit research or contributing to large-scale agency research projects. (See the Research Perspective on p. 60.) Likewise, the nurse manager also interprets published research findings that have implications for the staff or the patients and makes every effort to incorporate the findings into unit activities so that both staff and patients can benefit from evidence-based care. Nurse managers, as first-line managers, are also in the position of identifying best nursing practices that can be researched through collaborative efforts of service and educational insti-

RESEARCH PERSPECTIVE

Resource: Mackoff, B. L., & Triolo, P. K. (2008). Why do managers stay? Building a model of engagement. Part 1. Dimensions of engagement; Part 2. Cultures of engagement. *Journal of Nursing Administration, 38*(3/4), 118-124; 166-171.

This descriptive study addresses high-performing nurse managers in six hospital settings. The researchers chose study participants who met two criteria: (1) the nurse manager had been in the position at least 5 years and (2) had been rated as outstanding in the nurse manager role. A convenience sample of 30 nurse managers participated in 90-minute interviews.

The data collected were analyzed from the perspective of individual and organizational signature elements (factors). Ten individual nurse factors were linked to the nurse managers' engagement, longevity, and vitality. The factors included the following:

1. Mission driven—The mission was meaningful to the manager.
2. Generativity—The manager was delighted to help and contribute to the next nurse generation.
3. Ardor—The manager exhibited enthusiasm and excitement toward his or her colleagues and was dedicated to patient care and the organization.
4. Identification—The nurse manager identified and appreciated how the work of others, such as patient care, affected his or her functioning in a positive manner.
5. Boundary clarity—The nurse manager had strong connections with others without losing a sense of self.
6. Reflection—The nurse manager stood back and learned from both positive and negative experiences.

7. Self-regulation—The nurse manager controlled his or her emotions and chose battles wisely.
8. Atonement—The nurse manager had the insight to appreciate the other person's perspective and learn to walk a mile in the other person's shoes before passing judgment.
9. Change agility—The nurse manager addressed change in more than one way, through new knowledge and by challenging the process.
10. Affirmative framework—The nurse manager met the challenges without burnout and remained optimistic and upbeat.

The data collected also yielded the following five organizational elements or signature factors that contribute to nurse manager longevity: culture of learning, culture of regard, culture of meaning, culture of generativity, and culture of excellence.

The results of the study indicate that the individual and organizational elements are viewed by the nurse managers in the study as the "glue" that contributes to their long-term engagement and success.

Implications for Practice

It is imperative that, with the nursing shortage and the leadership voids that are seen throughout nursing, the executive leadership of the organization address the study findings. As the researchers have pointed out: by addressing nurse manager engagement versus retention, the nurse leader who produces a healthy worksite can continue to contribute in numerous ways including development of the next generation of nursing leaders. The nurse manager position is a crucial one that can either greatly enhance or hinder the development of the organization

---

tutions. Nurse managers should also provide and support staff nurses to conduct nursing research studies, as well as present their own findings of current evidence-based practice in the literature.

MENTORING

A manager also should be concerned about preparing successors. Cherry and Jacob (2008) include the role of mentoring as another role that nurses in leadership/management positions must embrace. They view mentoring as an interactive, multifaceted role that assists the staff with setting realistic, attainable goals. Through mentoring their staff, nurse managers can help boost staff self-confidence, thereby helping them gain professional satisfaction as they reach their goals. Nurse managers give clinical guidance to their staff,

and they can be instrumental in assisting them with their present work and their career development.

ORGANIZATIONAL CULTURE

In the ever-changing environment of health care, nurse managers need to know the organizational culture of their hospitals and how it supports their unit's mission and goals. Laschinger (2004) reports on a study conducted on a random sample of 500 staff nurses working in the Ontario teaching hospitals. The study looked at the nurses' perception of respect and organizational justice. The instrument used addressed interactional justice (the perceptions of the quality of interactions among persons who are affected by decisions and subsequent outcomes), structural empowerment, respect, work pressures, emotional exhaustion, and work effectiveness. Two hundred and eighty questionnaires were returned, yielding a 52% response rate. The results revealed that the nurses did not perceive their managers as sharing information about eminent changes in their work environment or showing any compassion for the nurses' response to the changes. The nurses also felt that the managers rarely provided them with rationale for changes in their work environment, showed little concern, and did not deal with them in a truthful way. The study highlighted the importance of a positive organizational environment for nurses to feel respected in their work environment. A consistent factor in the results was the importance of good interpersonal relationships with both managers and colleagues in the organization.

DAY-TO-DAY MANAGEMENT CHALLENGES

The nurse manager who meets the day-to-day management challenges must be able to balance three sources of demand: upper management requests, consumer demands, and staff needs. The manager (1) has to ensure that the staff members have opportunities for providing upper management with input regarding changes that affect them and (2) has to make unit and staff needs known to upper management. The consumers of health services today are much better educated and accustomed to providing input into decisions that affect them. The nurse manager needs to respect their requests yet maintain care in the broad context of safety and efficiency. The staff members need recognition and independence when carrying out their roles and responsibilities. The nurse manager needs to have a sense of when to relinquish control, thus allowing decision making at the point of service. Furthermore, the nurse manager influences staff nurses' satisfaction/dissatisfaction with the work environment.

Nurse managers also must be credible clinicians in the areas they manage. A critical factor in being an excellent nurse manager is to understand how to ensure optimal patient outcomes, involve families or significant others in the plan of care, and allocate resources and technology in a fair and ethical manner. The nurse manager-clinician is confronted with complex and ambiguous patient-care situations. Sometimes, decisions are made to meet one important patient care need at the expense of another. That is an important message to convey to staff.

> **EXERCISE 4-2**
> Select a nurse manager and a staff nurse follower in one of your clinical facilities. Observe them over a certain time (e.g., 2 to 4 hours). Compare the styles they exhibit. Is power shared or centralized? Are interactions positive or negative? What is the nature of their conversations? How does your summation of this observation relate to managerial, leadership, and followership characteristics?

Workplace Violence

Nurse managers continue to be responsible for ensuring the safety of their staff and patients. Workers in high-risk areas, such as the emergency department, require special attention. For the nurse manager, "special attention" translates to his or her staff receiving adequate on-the-job training. Such training may include effective techniques relating to crisis intervention and handling highly agitated people who may be armed. From the point of hiring through the potential disciplinary process, nurse managers who assess both employees and the workplace can help avert violence and the conditions that lead to it. Top-level administrators are ultimately responsible for employee violence in their own setting; however, managers who lack training in policy practices have an increased risk for nonadherence to state/federal employee selection requirements. Refer to Chapter 25 (Workplace Violence) for additional information on this topic.

MANAGING HEALTHCARE SETTINGS

Managing healthcare settings is always challenging for the nurse manager, and the current nursing shortage has made the challenge paramount. The nurse manager is a key person in creating and maintaining a healthy work setting that keeps stress to a minimum so that the staff can achieve optimal work satisfaction. However, before the manager can help the staff, he or she must be able to work in a relatively stress-free environment. (See the Research Perspective on p. 62.)

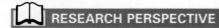

Resource: Shirey, M. R., Ebright, P. R., & McDaniel, A. M. (2008). Sleepless in America: Nurse managers cope with stress and complexity. *Journal of Nursing Administration, 38*(3), 125-131.

Shirey, Ebright, and McDaniel (2008) through a qualitative, descriptive study looked at what factors contribute to stress in nurse managers. The investigators interviewed five nurse managers ranging in age from 39 to 51 years; their tenure as nurse managers ranged from 5 to 17 years. Interviews with the nurse managers lasted up to 2 hours and produced data that emerged into the following eight common themes:

1. Nurse manager work—All the participants saw themselves as "clearing houses" for information affecting the staff. They felt that expectations of them were unrealistic, including "putting out fires" and simultaneously being asked to allow time for strategic planning and innovation.
2. Sources of stress—These included such things as demands of the role with not enough resources, leading to unclear role expectations; confusing reporting organizational lines; and workload that allowed no down time.
3. Emotions—Nurse managers felt that their own emotions took a back seat to the emotions of the staff, and therefore stress was produced when turning "on and off" their own emotional needs.
4. Value conflicts—The managers felt that a great source of stress for them was being pushed almost over the line, especially in relation to budgets and what might be best for patients.
5. Coping strategies—The managers used two types of coping strategies: emotion-focused, such as anger used with negative situations; and problem-focused for solving specific stress-related problems, such as returning to school.
6. Social support—Most of the managers believed that their support came mostly from individuals not connected with their job, such as family, and all of them cited giving more support to staff than they themselves received.
7. Relationships and communication—The managers rated building relationships with their staff as a top priority; however, they believed that this category of work was "invisible work" and often sacrificed because of other commitments away from their unit.
8. Health outcomes—This theme brought to light how stress affected outcomes such as not being able to sleep, feeling stressed out, being emotionally exhausted, and experiencing physical symptoms of stress such as shortness of breath, palpitations, and tensed muscles.

Although all of the managers loved their jobs, they did feel a work-life imbalance, and although more studies are needed pertaining to stress in nurse managers, this study supports the need that other studies have found—that is, to reexamine and redesign the nurse manager position, which is crucial to their contributions to the overall organization.

Implications for Practice

The findings of the study clearly demonstrate that the stress that nurse managers feel affects not only their physical well-being but also their family life. Several other studies have consistently shown similar results, and the nursing profession needs to address the study findings and develop concrete plans that reduce nurse manager stress. Nurse managers are not expendable, and nursing needs to reexamine and develop mechanisms that reduce the stress in these essential management leaders.

The Institute of Medicine (IOM) report *Keeping Patients Safe* (2004) spoke to the creation of work environments that are more conducive to nurses providing safer patient care. For this to happen, many changes are required of those in leadership roles, beginning with top-level administration and filtering through the hierarchy to unit managers. Managers need to address the five management practices that have been found to be effective when instituting change and achieving patient safety in high-risk organizations. These practices are as follows:

1. Managing the change process actively
2. Balancing the tension between efficiency and reliability
3. Creating a learning environment
4. Creating and sustaining trust

5. Involving the workers in the work-redesign and the workflow decision making

Keeping Patients Safe also addressed and supported the use of evidence-based management. Evidence-based practice is supported from systematic research findings, and the same should apply to management practices. Evidence-based management should reflect application of empirical research into everyday managing practices. Another IOM report that remains significant for nurse managers is *Crossing the Quality Chasm: A New Health System for the 21st Century* (2001). This report proposes six "improvement" aims for today's lower-performing healthcare system. Those aims are identified in Chapter 2.

High technology will continue to modify nurse managers' roles. For example, because of the ability to perform more complex surgery through surgicenters, nurse managers will find themselves practicing with short-term or ambulatory-care admissions. A key to successful management is interdependence. A critical component of interdependence is collaboration, which uses the different strengths of each person. Collaboration requires one to be flexible and broadminded and to have a strong self-concept. Sullivan and Decker (2005) addressed the concept of collaboration from the perspective of conflict management. When collaboration is used to solve a conflict, the energies of all parties are focused on solving the problem versus defeating the opposing party.

The staff members often look to the nurse manager to lead them in addressing workplace issues with higher levels of administration. To do this, the nurse manager must possess two sets of skills: (1) the ability to address power sources in one's work environment and define power-based strategies, such as in organizing a following of other nurse managers with similar concerns; and (2) the ability to effectively place pressure on the power holders so that needed changes can occur. Employees' "buy in" to a change sometimes needs to be thought out carefully.

The staff members also look to the nurse manager to lead them in ethical, value-based management. The manager's commitment to the mission, vision, and purpose must be demonstrated in everyday behavior, not merely recited on special occasions. This ongoing commitment lends stability in a time of constant change. In other words, although the approach to an issue may change, the core values remain, and the nurse manager is the one who must lead the group in the changed behavior to reflect the mission, vision, and purpose. Without this evidence that is almost palpable, staff nurses may be skeptical about the manager's commitment to the organization and to them. This contemporary commitment reflects an understanding of the core values and a relationship with the world as it is today. The nurse manager then must translate this commitment to the staff members so that they know they are valued in accomplishing the work of the unit that furthers the mission of the organization. One way of demonstrating that employees are valued is by recognizing staff through various means. Employees who have gone beyond the scope of their job to meet the needs of the patient, department, or institution deserve recognition. An award may reflect the institution's philosophy, beliefs, and mission, as exemplified in one institution's "Quality Credo"—communication, competent performance, personal leadership, respect, and teamwork.

EXERCISE 4-3

The Vice-President for Patient Care Services for the local health department has just undergone a tremendous challenge because of a natural disaster of a hurricane in the vicinity. Many staff members, despite their own family needs, assisted victims with their needs, which ranged from crisis care to adequate follow-up of chronic disorders. The Vice-President for Patient Care Services wants to establish a recognition program for the staff members who gave endless hours to their community. How would you approach establishing this recognition program? What resources would you need, and where would you go to seek the needed resources? How do you want to be recognized?

MANAGING RESOURCES

Each of these concepts inherent in managing resources is addressed in depth elsewhere in this book, but the key point is that the manager must manage each and integrate each with the others. The practice settings of tomorrow will no doubt continue to include in-hospital care; however, numerous innovative practice models operating from a community-based framework also may be found. Predictors of effective outcomes to ensure quality patient care include (1) rationed and multitiered distribution of healthcare services, such as health maintenance organizations (HMOs), preferred provider organizations (PPOs), and independent private payment plans; (2) precise outcome-oriented quality-assurance measures, such as critical pathways; and (3) concerted efforts to control spiraling health costs by increasing productivity and efficiency of healthcare providers. Other practice models, differentiated practice, shared governance, and restructured work environments make use of all levels of healthcare personnel.

The manager is responsible for managing all resources designated to the unit of care. This includes all personnel, professionals and others, under the manager's span of control. The wise manager quickly determines that a unit must function economically and, in so doing, realizes that many opportunities exist to reshape how nursing is delivered. Sare and Ogilvie (2010) discussed theories from the perspective of what nursing needs in the twenty-first century as new models of care that empower the profession. They suggested combining existing nursing theories with business theories to depict the nurse as a change agent in universal health care. To accomplish this, nursing needs to operate from a sufficient information baseline that is captured through the use of business theorists working with nursing theorists. Why are business theories important when discussing the role of the manager? The answer is simple yet very germane, because many of the tenets of business theories such as management, leadership, personnel, and systems are inherent in the role of the nurse manager.

Budget and personnel have always been considered critical resources. However, as technology improves, informatics must be integrated with budget and personnel as a critical resource element. Basing practice on research findings (evidence-based care), networking through the Internet with other nurse managers, sharing concerns and difficulties, and being willing to step outside of tradition can assist future managers in decisions about resource utilization.

MANAGED CARE

Managed care was introduced in the 1980s. The goal of managed care is to provide needed services efficiently and at an appropriate cost. In essence, this goal requires nurse managers to know and incorporate business principles into patient-care practices. Nurse managers who know business principles become conduits for ensuring safe, effective, affordable care. The same can be said for the Never Events identified by the Centers for Medicare & Medicaid Services (CMS) (2008). The term *Never Events* refers to conditions for which healthcare organizations will not be paid. They are conditions that are acquired while the patient is institutionalized. Examples of some of the Never Events include a stage 3 or 4 pressure ulcer acquired during a hospital stay, a fall occurring during a hospital stay that results in an injury requiring a longer length of stay, or surgery on the wrong body part or side of the body requiring a return trip to surgery.

CASE MANAGEMENT

Case management, a method used to provide care for many years in outpatient service areas, is now, because of managed care, an option of care in acute care settings (Sullivan & Decker, 2005). The key to effective case management is coordination of care, with identified time frames for accomplishing appropriate care outcomes. The nurse manager is often the overseer of the case managers, and in some settings, the nurse manager is the immediate supervisor of the case managers. Case management involves components of case selection, multidisciplinary assessment, collective planning, coordination of events, negotiation, and evaluation and documentation of the outcomes of patient status in measures of cost and quality. Case managers are employed in acute care settings, rehabilitation facilities, subacute facilities, community-based programs, home care, and insurance companies. These managers must possess a broad range of personal, interpersonal, and management skills.

INFORMATICS

Informatics in health care is in a stage of constant change and growth. Much technology and many systems are available to organizations to assist in improvements. The electronic medical record gives quick and ready access to current and retrospective clinical patient data. The use of electronic patient classification systems allows managers to better measure the acuity of nursing areas, as well as assist in budget planning and need for resources. Smart Beds are actual patient beds being used in the hospital settings that replace the manual process of documentation of patients' vital statistics, creating real time for nurses to think critically about what to do regarding the data. The Smart Bed has the capacity to collect the information for the nurse. The accessibility and use of the Internet facilitates the education of staff, patients, and their families. Nurse managers must stay abreast of and in touch with the changing technology and informatics available in health care and be ready to defend the need for it to make improvements. In addition, managers must be early adapters of the technology to demonstrate its value in performance to staff and to help with generational differences. Older generations of nurses (Veterans and many Baby Boomers) were not exposed to informatics systems for most of their careers and may have a difficult time adapting to new technology, whereas the Generation

X-ers and Millennials do not know how to exist without it.

BUDGETS

Budgetary allocations, whether they are related to the number of dollars available to manage a unit or related to full-time equivalent employee formulas, may be the direct responsibility of nurse managers. For highly centralized organizations, only the administrative group at the executive level decides on the budgetary allocations. As healthcare organizations adopt "flat" organizational structures and decentralize responsibilities to the patient care areas, nurse managers allocate fiscal resources for their designated unit. In the decentralized organizational model, nurse managers must have the business and financial skills to be able to prepare and justify a detailed budget that reflects the short-term and long-term needs of the unit.

Perhaps the most important aspect of a budget is the provision for a mechanism that allows some self-control, such as decision making at the point of service (POS), which does not require previous hierarchical approval and a rationale for budgetary spending.

EXERCISE 4-4

Visit a city health department or an adult daycare facility. What type of information system is used? Are both paper (hard copy) and computer sources used? What can you assume about the budget, based on the physical appearance of the setting? Does any equipment appear dated? How do the employees (and perhaps volunteers) function? Do they seem motivated? Ask two or three to tell you, in a sentence or two, the purpose (vision and mission) of the organization. Can you readily identify the nurse manager? What does the manager do to manage the three critical resources of personnel, finances, and technologic access?

QUALITY INDICATORS

The nurse manager is consistently concerned with the quality of care that is being delivered on his or her unit. The quality indicators developed by the American Nurses Association (ANA), such as the National Database of Nursing Quality Indicators (NDNQI) (www.nursingquality.org), are good resources for the nurse manager. The NDNQI measures are specifically

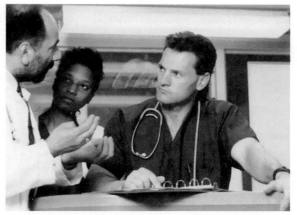

Nurse managers are constantly concerned with the quality of care that is being delivered on their unit.

concerned with patient safety and aspects of quality of care that may be affected by changes in the delivery of care. The quality indicators address staff mix and nursing hours for acute-care settings, as well as other care components. The NDNQI project is designed to assist healthcare organizations in identifying links between nursing care and patient outcomes. The Joint Commission (2008) requires organizations, as part of meeting accreditation, to participate in the collection and adherence to certain core measures. Hospitals are compared with other hospitals across the nation in these measurements. Examples of the core measures required by The Joint Commission are practices associated with acute myocardial infarctions, care for the patient with congestive heart failure, and care associated with the treatment of pneumonia. As with the NDNQI measures, the core measures are concerned with level of quality of care and outcomes of care.

PROFESSIONALISM

Nurse managers must set examples of professionalism, which include academic preparation, roles and function, and increasing autonomy. The ANA's classic "Nursing's Social Policy Statement" (American Nurses Association [ANA], 2003) provides significant ideals for all nurses, specifically autonomy, self-regulation, and accountability. Nurses are guided by a humanistic philosophy that includes the highest

THEORY BOX

Theory X/Theory Y

THEORY/CONTRIBUTOR	KEY IDEA	APPLICATION TO PRACTICE
McGregor (1960)	**Theory X:** Authoritarian • People do not like to work. • People need to have the threat of punishment. • People want to be told what to do.	This style might be useful when quick action or critical decisions must be made in which everyone must perform in the same way. In general, it is ineffective with professionals and creates workplace issues. However, in situations such as violence, this strategy may be necessary.
	Theory Y: Participative • Work is natural, and people like to work. • People use self-control. • People accept responsibility. • People like to solve problems.	This style might be useful when sufficient time is available or when the group must agree to a plan. In general, this approach is effective in health care and helps reinforce the concept of team. It is especially effective when a group is dealing with a quality initiative.

Data from McGregor, D. (1960). *The human side of enterprise.* New York: McGraw-Hill.

regard for self-determination, independence, and choice in decision making, whether for staff or for patients. The policy statement can be used by the nurse manager as a framework for a broader understanding of nursing's connection with society and nursing's accountability to those who receive nursing

---

EXERCISE 4-5

Mr. Jones, a patient who had foot surgery 3 days ago, has asked Donna D., a young nurse on a surgical orthopedic unit, several times during her 12-hour day shift for some medication for pain. Donna D.'s assessment of Mr. Jones leads her to believe that he is not having that much pain. Although the patient does have an oral medication order for pain, Donna D. independently decides to administer a placebo by subcutaneous injection and documents her medication intervention. Mr. Jones does not receive any relief from this subcutaneous medication. When the 12-hour night nurse relieves Donna D., Donna D. gives the nurse a report of her intervention concerning Mr. Jones' pain. The following morning, the night nurse reports Donna D.'s medication intervention to you, the nurse manager. You will have to address Donna D.'s behavior. What will you do? What resources will you use to handle Donna D.'s behavior? How will you demonstrate professionalism?

---

care that facilitates "health and healing" in a caring relationship. For example, a nurse manager's professional philosophy should include the patient's rights. These rights have traditionally identified such basic elements as human dignity, integrity, honesty, confidentiality, privacy, and informed consent.

Professionalism is all-encompassing; the way a manager interacts with personnel, other disciplines, patients, and families reflects a professional philosophy. Professional nurses are ethically and legally accountable for the standards of practice and nursing actions delegated to others. Conveying high standards, holding others accountable, and shaping the future of nursing for a group of healthcare providers are inherent behaviors in the role of a manager.

The nurse manager is the closest link to the direct care staff. That individual sets the tone, creates the environment, and manages within the context while providing professional role modeling to develop future managers and leaders (see the Theory Box above). That person influences staff members in their decisions to stay or leave. The nurse manager is critical to the success of any healthcare endeavor.

THE SOLUTION

Working with our charge nurses, we established flexible staffing guidelines. This process enabled the charge nurses to place a nurse on call for the security of staffing and to flex up for additional patient admissions while helping to keep the unit budget intact. This was the first step of the solution. We then began looking at the hours that our nurses were working to see if there were opportunities for reduction in this area. We noticed that our charge nurses were working up to 9½ hours per shift. When delving further, the reason was that each charge nurse was coming in sometimes as much as an hour earlier than the start of the shift to make assignments. For example, the day-shift charge nurse would come in at 6 AM and make the assignments for that shift to have the assignments ready by 6:45 AM. The process repeated for the other shifts. The charge nurse was also working past the end of the shift to finish duties and give report. This became an obvious area with potential to increase staff satisfaction, as well as help stay on budget. A charge-nurse meeting was held and potential solutions discussed. The team came up with a viable solution. The charge nurses for the previous shift would make the staff assignments for the oncoming shift, and the charge nurses would not need to come in until 15 minutes before the start of their shift. For example, the night shift charge nurse would make the assignment for day shift and the day shift charge nurse would not come in until 6:30 AM, at which time he or she would review the assignment and make any final adjustments. The change was well-received. The charge nurse's work life was positively impacted, since he or she no longer had to start the day as early. There was a definite learning curve for the charge nurses to make assignments for a shift of staff with whom they were not as familiar. For the process to be successful, much work and support were needed from the staff, the charge nurses, and the managers. As managers, we came in early each morning for a couple of weeks to assist the night-shift charge nurses with making day-shift assignments. Each charge nurse knew his or her own staff for that shift but may not have known the particular needs for the shift for which he or she was now making the assignment. Education, understanding, trust, and patience with the change were of utmost importance. The other aspect of this was to ensure that the charge nurse was ready to leave the shift at the appropriate time. This required being present with the charge nurses at shift change and giving them feedback on their process of changing shifts. We worked together to revise shift report and the expectations for handing off tasks that still needed to be completed. By the end of this transformation, we had shaved approximately 3 hours a day off of our daily hours. The charge nurses have reported satisfaction with the new process and being able to leave work on time. The changes (1) did not negatively affect patient safety, (2) increased staff satisfaction, and (3) helped the unit achieve the budget.

—*Donna McKinster*
—*Tiffany Thornton*

Would this be a suitable approach for you? Why?

THE EVIDENCE

Hall, Doran, and Pink (2008) conducted a study in Ontario, Canada, to measure how interventions that are designed to improve the environment of nursing units impacted patient and nurse outcomes. The study involved 16 nursing managers, 1137 patients, and 296 observations by registered nurses using a quasi-experimental design. Baseline data were collected from the participating units, and the interventions of change were completed; follow-up data were collected immediately after introducing the change interventions, at 3 months after the interventions, and then again at 6 months after the interventions. Interventions included improving linen supply, enhancing documentation, providing better availability of patient stock medications, improving communication relating to transfers of patients, and making known basic equipment needs for staff to care for patients. The experience of the nursing staff and managers involved ranged from less than 5 years to more than 25 years. The most significant effect found was an increase of how the nursing staff felt about the quality of their work life after the change interventions were instituted. Patients' perceptions of the quality of care in the participating units significantly increased as a result of the change interventions. The results of the study made it apparent that nursing managers can positively influence the perceptions of nursing staff by introducing change interventions about which staff had a voice. In addition, by positively impacting the nursing staff, patients' perceptions of the quality of care increase as well. Nurse managers greatly influence perceptions of staff, thereby impacting staff retention.

NEED TO KNOW NOW

- Understand and respect the individual needs of the four generations of nurses currently working together at the bedside.
- Engage in a unit-based, shared-governance council inclusive of staff, allowing for empowerment.

- Use professional development opportunities and support for furthering of education.
- Encourage, support, and model the use of evidence-based practice.
- Participate in the reward for and recognition of nursing staff.

CHAPTER CHECKLIST

The role of the nurse manager is multifaceted and complex. Integrating clinical concerns with management functions, synthesizing leadership abilities with management requirements, and addressing human concerns while maintaining efficiency are the challenges facing a manager. Thus the nurse manager's role is to ensure effective operation of a defined unit of service and to contribute to the overall mission of the organization and quality of care by working through others.

- The following are the five basic functions of a manager:
  - Establishing and communicating goals and objectives

- Organizing and analyzing activities and decisions and dividing them into tasks
- Motivating and communicating with others
- Analyzing, appraising, and interpreting performance
- Developing people
- A nurse manager is responsible for the following:
  - Relationships with those above themselves, peers, and staff for whom they are accountable
  - Professionalism
  - Management of resources

TIPS FOR IMPLEMENTING THE ROLE OF NURSE MANAGER

Aspects of the role of the nurse manager include being a leader, as well as a follower. To implement the role, the nurse manager must profess to the following:

- Management philosophy that values people

- Commitment to patient-focused quality-care outcomes that address customer satisfaction
- Desire to learn healthcare changes and their effect on his or her role and functions

REFERENCES

American Nurses Association (ANA). (2003). *Nursing's social policy statement (NP-107)*. Washington, DC: American Nurses Publishing.

American Organization of Nurse Executives (AONE). (2004). *Principles & elements of a healthful practice/work environment*. Retrieved September 23, 2009, from www.aone.org/aone/pdf/PrinciplesandElementsHealthfulWorkPractice.pdf.

Carver, L., & Candela, L. (2008). Attaining organizational commitment across different generations of nurses. *Journal of Nursing Management, 16*(8), 984-991.

Centers for Medicare & Medicaid Services (CMS). (2008). *CMS improves patient safety for Medicare and Medicaid by addressing Never Events*. Retrieved September 23, 2009, from www.cms.hhs.gov/apps/media/press/factsheet.asp?Counter=3224&intNumPerPage.

Chaleff, I. (2009). *The courageous follower: Standing up to and for our leaders* (3rd ed.). San Francisco: Berrett-Koehler.

Cherry, B., & Jacob, S. R. (2008). *Contemporary nursing, issues, trends and management*. St. Louis: Mosby.

Conway, M. E. (1978). Theoretical approaches to the study of roles. In M. E. Hardy & M. E. Conway (Eds.), *Role theory:*

Perspectives for health professionals. New York: Appleton-Century-Crofts.

Drucker, P. F. (1974). *Management tasks, responsibilities and practices.* New York: Harper & Row.

Hall, L. M., Doran, D., & Pink, L. (2008). Outcomes of interventions to improve hospital nursing work environments. *Journal of Nursing Administration, 38*(1), 40-46.

Institute of Medicine (IOM). (2001). *Crossing the quality chasm: A new health system for the 21st century.* Washington, DC: The National Academy Press.

Institute of Medicine (IOM). (2004). *Keeping patients safe: Transforming the work environment of nurses.* Washington, DC: The National Academy Press.

Laschinger, H. K. P. (2004). Hospital nurses' perception of respect and organizational justice. *Journal of Nursing Administration, 34*(7/8), 354-363.

Mackoff, B. L., & Triolo, P. K. (2008). Why do managers stay? Building a model of engagement. Part 1. Dimensions of engagement; Part 2. Cultures of engagement. *Journal of Nursing Administration, 38*(3/4), 118-124; 166-171.

McGregor, D. (1960). *The human side of enterprise.* New York: McGraw-Hill.

Sare, M. V., & Ogilvie, L. A. (2010). *Strategic planning for nurses: Change management in health care* (1st ed.). Boston: Jones and Bartlett Publishers.

Shirey, M. R., Ebright, P. R., & McDaniel, A. M. (2008). Sleepless in America: Nurse managers cope with stress and complexity. *Journal of Nursing Administration, 38*(3), 125-131.

Sullivan, E. J., & Decker, P. J. (2005). *Effective leadership and management in nursing* (5th ed.). Upper Saddle River, NJ: Prentice Hall.

The Joint Commission (TJC). (2008). *A comprehensive review of development and testing for national implementation of hospital core measures.* Retrieved September 23, 2009, from www.jointcommission.org.

Valentine, S. O. (2002). Nursing leadership and the new nurse. Retrieved January 26, 2009, from www.juns.nursing.arizona.edu/articles/Fall%202002/Valentine.htm

Widger, K., Pye, C., Wilson, B., Squires, M., Tourangeau, A., & Cranley, L. (2007). Generational differences in acute care nurses. *Nursing Leadership, 20*(1), 49-61.

SUGGESTED READINGS

Cameron, K. S., & Quinn, R. E. (1994). *PRISM5: Changing organizational culture—A competing values workbook.* Ann Arbor, MI: University of Michigan. In K.R. Jones & R.W. Redman (December 2000). Organizational culture and work redesign: Experiences in three organizations. *Journal of Nursing Administration, 30*(12), 604-610.

Cathcart, D., Jeska, S., & Karmas, J. (2004). Span of control matters. *Journal of Nursing Administration, 34*(9), 395-399.

Duchscher, J. E., & Cowin, L. (2004). Multigenerational nurses in the workplace. *Journal of Nursing Administration, 34*(11), 493-501.

Ferguson, L. M., & Day, R. A. (2004). Supporting new nurses in evidence-based practice. *Journal of Nursing Administration, 34*(11), 490-492.

Greenberg, J., & Baron, R. A. (2008). *Behavior in organizations* (7th ed.). Upper Saddle River, NJ: Prentice Hall.

Lang, T. A., Hodge, M., & Olson, V. (2004). Nurse-patient ratios: A systematic review on the effects of nurse staffing on patient, nurse employee, and hospital outcomes. *Journal of Nursing Administration, 34*(7/8), 326-337.

Lavoit-Tremblay, M. (2004). Creating a healthy workplace: A participatory organizational intervention. *Journal of Nursing Administration, 34*(10), 469-474.

Lunney, M., Delaney, C., & Duffy, M. (2005). Advocating for standardized nursing languages in electronic health records. *Journal of Nursing Administration, 35*(1), 1-3.

Sams, L., Penn, B. K., & Facteau, L. (2004). The challenge of using evidence-based practice. *Journal of Nursing Administration, 34*(9), 407-414.

Tiedeman, M. E., & Lookinland, S. (2004). Traditional models of care delivery: What have we learned? *Journal of Nursing Administration, 34*(6), 291-297.

Vestal, K. (December 2004). Making time for leadership. *Nurse Leader, 2*(6), 8-9.

Wagner, R., & Harter, J. K. (2006). *12: The elements of great managing.* New York: Gallup Press.

Wolf, G., Bradle, J., & Nelson, G. (2005). Bridging the strategic leadership gap: A model program for transformational change. *Journal of Nursing Administration, 35*(2), 54-60.

5

Legal and Ethical Issues

Ginny Wacker Guido

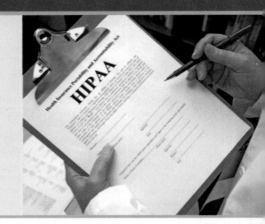

This chapter highlights and explains key legal and ethical issues as they pertain to managing and leading. Nurse practice acts, negligence and malpractice, informed consent, types of liability, selected federal and state employment laws, ethical principles, and related concepts are discussed. This chapter provides specific guidelines for preventing legal liability and guides the reader in applying ethical decision-making models in everyday clinical practice settings.

OBJECTIVES

- Examine nurse practice acts, including the legal difference between licensed registered nurses and licensed practical (vocational) nurses that a nurse manager must know.
- Apply various legal principles, including negligence and malpractice, privacy, confidentiality, reporting statutes, and doctrines that minimize one's liability, in leading and managing roles in professional nursing.
- Analyze the causes of malpractice for nurse managers.
- Examine legal implications of resource availability versus service demand from a manager's perspective.
- Evaluate informed-consent issues, including patients' rights in research and health literacy, from a nurse manager's perspective.
- Analyze key aspects of employment law, and give examples of how these laws benefit professional nursing practice.
- Analyze ethical principles, including autonomy, beneficence, nonmaleficence, veracity, justice, paternalism, fidelity, and respect for others.
- Apply the *Code of Ethics for Nurses* from the manager's perspective.
- Apply the MORAL model in ethical decision making.
- Discuss moral distress and its implications for nurse managers.
- Analyze the role of institutional ethics committees.
- Analyze decision making when legal and ethical situations overlap, using the Theresa M. Schiavo case as the framework for this analysis.

TERMS TO KNOW

apparent agency	health literacy	nonmaleficence
autonomy	indemnification	nurse practice act
beneficence	independent contractor	paternalism
collective bargaining	informed consent	personal liability
confidentiality	justice	privacy
corporate liability	law	respect for others
emancipated minor	liability	respondeat superior
ethics	liable	standard of care
ethics committee	licensure	statute
failure to warn	malpractice	veracity
fidelity	moral distress	vicarious liability
foreseeability	negligence	

THE CHALLENGE

Cynthia Fahy, MN, RN
Assistant Clinical Manager, 6D, Portland Veterans
Administration Medical Center, Portland, Oregon

I am the new acting clinical nurse manager on a busy 28-bed acute-care medicine unit in a major metropolitan hospital acknowledges that retaining competent, qualified, and satisfied nursing staff members presents a continual challenge. Recently, the unit shift leader (USL) in charge of the day shift approached me with concerns about a team member's clinical practice, commenting on the nurse's inability to complete assignments within the time frame of the shift, constantly relying on help from the nursing assistants and other professional nurses, and refusing new patient admissions. The USL was concerned because this nurse has been on the unit for nearly 2 years, seemingly a sufficient time to develop appropriate organizational and physical assessment skills, and asked whether the nurse could need additional education, further orientation, or perhaps a transfer to a less-demanding unit. In addition, the USL questioned the nurse's clinical judgment, noting that the nurse, when caring for a high-risk fall patient, positioned herself at the opposite side of the room and thus was unable to assist the patient as she fell from the bed.

I listened to all of the USL's concerns and then commented that the same nurse had approached me several days earlier about taking on added responsibilities as a charge nurse. The USL expressed concern and asked the question, "How do you orient someone to a leadership role in which the person will serve as a resource to staff members when he or she is not competently functioning as a direct care staff nurse?" I acknowledged this concern and inquired about the current process for orienting charge nurses. The USL stated there was no formal orientation process for a charge nurse within the hospital, noting that occasionally this responsibility was fulfilled by the nurse with the most seniority or the one who volunteers first. Although this practice sounded all too familiar, I quickly recognized the ethical and legal implications inherent in such a clinical practice. We were torn between promoting an individual's interests and goals versus maintaining the standard of competent nursing care.

What do you think you would do if you were this nurse?

INTRODUCTION

The role of professional nursing continues to expand and incorporate increasingly higher levels of expertise, specialization, autonomy, and accountability from both a legal and ethical perspective. This expansion has forced new concerns for nurse managers and nurse leaders and a heightened awareness of the interaction of legal and ethical principles. Areas of concern include professional nursing practice, legal issues, ethical principles, labor-management interactions, and employment. Each of these areas is individually addressed in this chapter.

PROFESSIONAL NURSING PRACTICE

Nurse Practice Acts

The scope of nursing practice, those actions and duties that are allowable by a profession, is defined and guided individually by each state in the nurse practice act. The state nurse practice act is the single most important piece of legislation for nursing because it affects all facets of nursing practice. Furthermore, the act is the law within the state or the United States territory, and state boards of nursing cannot grant exceptions, waive the act's provisions, or expand practice outside the act's specific provisions.

Nurse practice acts define three categories of nurses: licensed practical or vocational nurses (LPNs and LVNs, respectively); licensed registered nurses (RNs); and advanced practice nurses. The nurse practice acts set educational and examination requirements, provide for licensing by individuals who have met these requirements, and define the functions of each category of nurse, both in general and in specific terminology. The nurse practice act must be read to ascertain what actions are allowable for the three categories of nurses. Four states (California, Georgia, Louisiana, and West Virginia) have separate acts for licensed RNs and LPNs/LVNs. In these states, the acts must be reviewed at the same time to ensure that all allowable actions are included in one of the two acts and that no overlap exists between the acts. In addition, nurse managers should understand that individual state nurse practice acts are not consistent in defining or delineating advanced nursing roles.

Each practice act also establishes a state board of nursing. The main purposes of state boards of nursing are, first, to ensure enforcement of the act, serving to regulate those who come under its provisions and prevent those not addressed within the act from practicing nursing and, second, to protect the public, ensuring that those who present themselves as nurses are licensed to practice within the state. The National Council of State Boards of Nursing (NCSBN) serves as a central clearinghouse, further ensuring that individual state actions against a nurse's license are recorded and enforced in all states in which the individual nurse holds licensure.

These various boards of nursing develop and implement rules and regulations regarding the discipline of nursing and must be read in conjunction with the nurse practice act. Often any changes within the state's definition of nursing practice occur through modifications in the rules and regulations rather than in the act itself. This mandates that nurses and their nurse managers periodically review both the state act and the board of nursing rules and regulations.

Because each state has its own nurse practice act and state courts have jurisdiction for the state, nurses are well advised to know and understand the provisions of the state's nurse practice act. This is especially true in the areas of diagnosis and treatment; states vary greatly on whether nurses can diagnose and treat or merely assess and evaluate. An acceptable action in one state may be the practice of medicine in a bordering state.

With the advent of multistate licensure, the need to know and understand provisions of state nurse practice acts has become even more critical. Multistate licensure permits an RN to be licensed in one state and to legally practice in states belonging to the compact without obtaining additional state licenses. For the purposes of the law, the state nurse practice act that regulates the practice of the RN is the state in which the patient or client resides, not the state in which the nurse holds his or her license. Many of the nurses practicing under multistate licensure are working with patients in a variety of states through telenursing, which involves the use of telecommunications technology, such as telephone triage and advice. Others work for agencies or clinics that serve patients across state borders.

All nurses must know applicable state law and use the nurse practice act for guidance and appropriate action. Nurse managers have this same basic responsibility to apply legal principles in their practice. However, they are also responsible for monitoring the practice of employees under their supervision and for ensuring that personnel maintain current and valid licensure. Unless nurse managers remain current with the nurse practice act in their state or with nurse practice acts in all states in which they supervise employees, there is the constant potential for liability.

TABLE 5-1	ELEMENTS OF MALPRACTICE	
ELEMENTS	**EXAMPLES**
Duty owed the patient	Failure to monitor a patient's response to treatment
Breach of the duty owed	Failure to communicate change in patient status to the primary healthcare provider
Foreseeability	Failure to ensure minimum standards are met
Causation	Failure to provide adequate patient education
Injury	Fractured hip and head concussion after a patient fall
Damages	Additional hospitalization time; future medical and nursing care needs and costs

Negligence and Malpractice

Nurse managers frequently serve as mentors and consultants for the nurses whom they supervise. It is imperative that nurse managers have a full appreciation for this area of the law as negligence and malpractice continue to be the major causes of action brought against nursing staff members. Managers cannot guide and counsel their employees unless the managers are fully knowledgeable about this area of the law.

Negligence denotes conduct that is lacking in care and typically concerns nonprofessionals. Many experts equate negligence with carelessness, a deviation from the standard of care that a reasonable person would deliver. Malpractice, sometimes referred to as *professional negligence,* concerns professional actions and is the failure of a person with professional education and skills to act in a reasonable and prudent manner. Issues of malpractice have become increasingly important to the nurse as the authority, accountability, and autonomy of nurses have increased. The same types of actions may be the basis for either negligence or malpractice; *Pender v. Natchitoches Parish Hospital* (2003) specifically noted that for malpractice there must be a dereliction of a professional skill. Usually, six elements must be presented in a successful malpractice suit. All of these factors must be shown before the court will find liability against the nurse or institution. These six elements are shown in Table 5-1.

Negligence and malpractice have two commonalities. Both concern actions that are a result of omission (the failure to do something that the reasonable, prudent person or nurse would have done) and commission (acting in a way that causes injury to the patient). Both also concern nonintentional actions—injury results, but the individual who caused the harm never intended to hurt the patient. Remember: the most important point in determining whether an action was truly malpractice/negligence is the nonintent to do any harm to another.

Elements of Malpractice
Duty Owed the Patient

The first element is duty owed the patient, which involves both the existence of the duty and the nature of the duty. That a nurse owes a duty of care to a patient is seldom hard to establish. Often, this is established merely by showing the valid employment of the nurse within the institution. The more difficult part is the nature of the duty, which involves standards of care that represent the minimum requirements for acceptable practice. Standards of care are established by reviewing the institution's policy and procedure manual, the individual's job description, and the practitioner's education and skills, as well as pertinent standards established by professional organizations, journal articles, and standing orders and protocols. Several sources may be used to determine the applicable standard of care. The American Nurses Association (ANA), as well as a cadre of specialty organizations, publishes standards for nursing practice.

The overall framework of these standards is the nursing process. In 1988, the ANA first published *Standards for Nurse Administrators* (American Nurses Association [ANA], 1988), a series of nine standards incorporating responsibilities of nurse administrators across all practice settings. Accreditation standards, especially those published yearly by The Joint Commission (TJC), also assist in establishing the acceptable standard of care for healthcare facilities. In addition, many states have healthcare standards that affect individual institutions and their employees.

Nurse managers are directly responsible for ensuring that standards of care, as written in the hospital policy and procedure manuals, are current and that all nursing staff follow these standards of care. Should a standard of care be revised or changed, nurse managers must ensure that all staff members who are expected to implement this altered standard are apprised of the revised standard. If the new standard entails new skills, staff members must be educated about this revision before they implement the new standard. For example, if the institution alters a policy regarding nurses removing invasive lines, the nurse manager must first ensure that all nurses who will be performing this skill understand how to perform the skill safely, possible complications that could occur, and the most appropriate interventions to take should those complications occur.

Breach of the Duty of Care Owed the Patient

The second element required in a malpractice case is breach of the duty of care owed the patient. Once the standard of care is established, the breach or falling below the standard of care is relatively easy to show. However, the standard of care may differ depending on whether the injured party is trying to establish the standard of care or whether the hospital's attorney is establishing an acceptable standard of care for the given circumstances. The injured party will attempt to show that the acceptable standard of care is at a much higher level than that shown by the defendant hospital and staff. Expert witnesses give testimony in court to determine the applicable and acceptable standard of care on a case-by-case basis, assisting the judge and jury in understanding nursing standards of care.

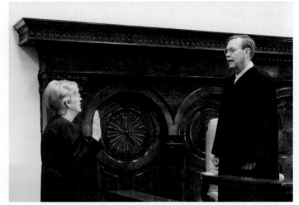

Nurses sometimes serve as expert witnesses whose testimony helps the judge and jury understand the applicable standards of nursing care.

A case example, *Sabol v. Richmond Heights General Hospital* (1996), shows this distinction. A patient was admitted to a general acute care hospital for treatment after attempting to commit suicide by drug overdose. While in the acute care facility, the patient became increasingly paranoid and delusional. A nurse sat with the patient and tried to calm him. Restraints were not applied because the staff feared this would compound the situation by raising the patient's level of paranoia and agitation. The patient jumped out of bed, knocked down the nurse who was in his room, fought his way past two nurses in the hallway, ran off the unit, and jumped from a third-story window, fracturing his arm and sustaining other relatively minor injuries.

Expert witnesses for the patient introduced standards of care pertinent to psychiatric patients, specifically those hospitalized in psychiatric facilities or in acute care hospitals with separate psychiatric units. The court ruled that the nurses in this general acute care situation were not professionally negligent in this patient's care. The court stated that the nurses' actions were consistent with basic professional standards of practice for medical-surgical nurses in an acute care hospital. They did not have nor were they expected to have specialized psychiatric nursing training and would not be judged as though they did.

Foreseeability

The third element needed for a successful malpractice case, foreseeability, involves the concept that certain events may reasonably be expected to cause specific results. The nurse must have prior knowledge or information that failure to meet a standard of care may result in harm. The challenge is to show what was foreseeable given the facts of the case at the time of the occurrence, not when the case finally comes to court. Some of the more common areas concerning foreseeability concern medication errors, patient falls, and failure to adhere to physician orders. For example, in *Christus Spohn v. De La Fuente* (2007), a patient in labor ruptured her uterus when nursing staff failed to appreciate the fact that Pitocin can cause uterine hyperstimulation and the nurses failed to monitor the patient, induced for a vaginal delivery after a prior cesarean section, for such hyperstimulation.

Causation

The fourth element of a malpractice suit is causation, which means that the nurse's actions or lack of actions directly caused the patient's harm; the patient did not merely experience some type of harm. There must be a direct relationship between the failure to meet the standard of care and the patient's injury. Note that it is not sufficient that the standard of care has been breached but, rather, that the breach of the standard of care must be the direct cause-and-effect factor for the injury. For example, *O'Shea v. State of New York* (2007) concerned a patient who sustained an accident in which two fingers were severed while using a power saw. The patient permanently lost the two fingers when the nursing staff failed to follow the order for an immediate orthopedist consultation.

Injury

The resultant injury, the fifth malpractice element, must be physical, not merely psychological or transient. In other words, some physical harm must be incurred by the patient before malpractice will be found against the healthcare provider. Although there are some specific exceptions to the requirement that a physical injury must result, they are extremely limited and usually involve specific relationships, such as the parent-child relationship. Pain and suffering are allowed when they accompany actual physical injuries.

Damages

The injured party must be able to prove damages, the sixth element of malpractice. Damages are vital because malpractice is nonintentional. Thus the patient must show financial harm before the courts will allow a finding of liability against the defendant nurse and/or hospital.

A nurse manager must know the applicable standards of care and ensure that all employees of the institution meet or exceed them. The standards must be reviewed periodically to ensure that the staff members remain current and attuned to advances in technology and newer ways of performing skills. If standards of care appear outdated or absent, the appropriate committee within the institution should be notified so that timely revisions can be made. Finally, the nurse manager must ensure that all employees meet the standards of care. This may be done by (1) performing or reviewing all performance evaluations for evidence that standards of care are met, (2) reviewing randomly selected patient charts for standards of care documentation, and (3) inquiring of employees what constitutes standards of care and appropriate references for standards of care within the institution.

EXERCISE 5-2

Read a policy and procedure manual at a community nursing setting with which you are familiar. Are any policies outdated? Find out who is in charge of revising and writing policies and procedures for the agency. Take an outdated policy and revise it, or think of an issue that you determine should be included in the policy and procedure manual and write such a policy. Does your rewritten or new policy define standards of care? Where would you find criteria for ensuring that your policies and procedures fit a national standard? As the nurse manager within the healthcare setting, how would you go about ensuring that staff members whom you supervise follow the standards of care as outlined in the policy and procedure manual? How would you inform/teach the staff about the new policy?

LIABILITY: PERSONAL, VICARIOUS, AND CORPORATE

Personal liability defines each person's responsibility and accountability for individual actions or omissions. Even if others can be shown to be liable for a patient injury, each individual retains personal accountability for his or her actions. The law, though, sometimes allows other parties to be liable for certain causes of negligence. Known as **vicarious liability**, or *substituted liability*, the doctrine of **respondeat superior** (let the master answer) makes employers accountable for the negligence of their employees. The rationale underlying the doctrine is that the employee would not have been in a position to have caused the wrongdoing unless hired by the employer, and the injured party would be allowed to suffer a double wrong if the employee was unable to pay damages for the wrongdoings. Nurse managers can best avoid these issues by ensuring that the staff they supervise know and follow hospital policies and procedures and continually deliver safe, competent nursing care or raise issues about policies and procedures through formal channels.

Nurses often believe that the doctrine of vicarious liability shields them from personal liability—the institution may be sued but not the individual nurse or nurses. However, patients injured because of substandard care have the right to sue both the institution and the nurse. This includes potentially suing the nurse's nurse manager if he or she knowingly allowed substandard and unsafe care to be given to a patient. In addition, the institution has the right under **indemnification** to countersue the nurse for damages paid to an injured patient. The principle of indemnification is applicable when the employer is held liable based solely on the actions of the staff member's negligence and the employer pays monetary damages because of the employee's negligent actions.

Corporate liability is a newer trend in the law and essentially holds that the institution has the responsibility and accountability for maintaining an environment that ensures quality healthcare delivery for consumers. Corporate liability issues include negligent hiring and firing issues, failure to maintain safety in the physical environment, and lack of a qualified, competent, and adequate staff. In *Wellstar Health System, Inc. v. Green* (2002), a hospital was held liable to an injured patient for the negligent credentialing of a nurse practitioner.

Nurse managers play a key role in assisting the institution to avoid corporate liability. For example, the nurse manager is normally delegated the duty to ensure that staff members remain competent and qualified, that personnel within their supervision

LITERATURE PERSPECTIVE

Resource: Hill, K. (2006). Collaboration is a competency! *Journal of Nursing Administration, 36*(9), 390-392.

Collaboration among disciplines, as the author notes, is a competency and a key to optimal patient care management, regardless of the healthcare setting. This evidence-based article explored ways to ensure that all disciplines were knowledgeable about the role of collaboration and how such collaboration could be successfully incorporated into a comprehensive cancer center. To implement the collaboration project at a leadership level, a redesign of the governance model was undertaken, positioning a physician and a nurse leader at the clinical program and executive levels of each area of the institution. Such collaboration ensured that all decision points, including strategic planning, resource allocation, capital prioritization, and new program development were addressed by the key members of the collaboration team. As new clinical initiatives were started, physicians and nurses shared the leadership roles, enforcing the commitment that the institution had to patient and family-centered care and the importance of clinical co-leadership. This model has led to improved patient care that reinforces accountability and responsibility among all interdisciplinary healthcare members.

Implications for Practice
Being able to work across professions for the benefit of patients and the care delivered is an important skill to develop. Having shared leadership roles (medicine and nursing) reinforces the idea of true collaboration.

have current licensure, and that incompetent, illegal, or unethical practices are reported to the proper persons or agencies. Nurse managers also play a pivotal role in whether a nurse remains employed on the unit or is discharged or reassigned.

Perhaps the key to avoiding corporate liability is ensuring that all members of the healthcare team fully collaborate and work with other disciplines to ensure quality, competent health care, regardless of the care setting. Such collaboration, as the Literature Perspective above notes, is a competency that must be mastered across disciplines.

CAUSES OF MALPRACTICE FOR NURSE MANAGERS

Nurse managers are charged with maintaining a standard of safe and competent nursing care within the institution. Several potential sources of liability for malpractice among nurse managers may be identified; thus guidelines to prevent or avoid these pitfalls should be developed.

Assignment, Delegation, and Supervision

The field of nursing management involves supervision of various personnel who directly provide nursing care to patients. *Supervision* is defined as the active process of directing, guiding, and influencing the outcome of an individual's performance of an activity. The nurse manager retains personal liability for the reasonable exercise of assignment, delegation, and supervision activities. The failure to assign, delegate, and supervise within acceptable standards of professional nursing practice may constitute malpractice. In addition, in a newer trend in the law, failure to delegate and supervise within acceptable standards may extend to direct corporate liability for the institution.

Delegation, used throughout all of nursing history, has evolved into a complex, work-enhancing strategy that has the potential for varying levels of legal liability. Before the early 1970s, nurses used delegation to direct the multiple tasks performed by the various levels of staff members in a team-nursing model. Subsequently, the concept of primary nursing and assignment became the desirable nursing model in acute care settings, with the focus on an all-professional staff, requiring little delegation but considerable assignment of duties. By the mid-1990s, a nursing shortage had again shifted the nursing model to a multilevel staff, with the return of the need for delegation.

It is necessary for the nurse manager to know certain definitions regarding this area of the law. *Delegation* involves at least two people, a delegator and a delegatee, with the transfer of authority to perform some type of task or work. A working definition could be that delegation is the transfer of responsibility for the performance of an activity from one individual to another, with the delegator retaining accountability for the outcome. In other words, delegation involves the transfer of responsibility for the performance of tasks and skills without the transfer of accountability for the ultimate outcome. Examples include an RN who delegates patients' personal care tasks to certified nursing aides who work in a long-term care setting. In delegating these tasks, the RN retains the ultimate accountability and responsibility for ensuring that the delegated tasks are completed in a safe and competent manner.

Typically, delegation involves the tasks and procedures that are given to unlicensed assistive personnel, such as certified nursing aides, orderlies, assistants, attendants, and technicians. However, delegation can also occur with licensed to licensed staff members. For example, if one RN has the accountability for an outcome and asks another RN to perform a specific component of the overall function, that is delegation. This is typically the type of delegation that occurs between professional staff members when one member leaves the unit/work area for a meal break.

Delegation is complex, because it involves relationships and the ability to communicate with all levels of staff personnel (Potter & Grant, 2004). Multiple players, usually with varying degrees of education and experience and different scopes of practice, are involved in the process. Understanding these variances and communicating effectively to the delegatee involve an understanding of competencies and the ability to communicate with all levels of staff personnel.

Assignment is the transfer of both the accountability and the responsibility from one person to another. This is typically what happens between professional staff members. The nurse manager assigns patient care responsibilities to other professional nurses working in the same unit of the institution or community healthcare setting. The level of accountability for the nurse manager who assigns as opposed to delegates is fairly obvious, although there can be some accountability in both instances. The degree of knowledge concerning the skills and competencies of those one supervises is of paramount importance. The doctrine of respondeat superior has been extended to include "knew or should have known" as a legal standard in both assigning and delegating tasks to individuals whom one supervises. If it can be shown that the nurse manager assigned/delegated tasks appropriately and had no reason to believe that the nurse to whom tasks were assigned/delegated was not competent to perform the task, the nurse manager potentially has either no or minimal personal liability. The converse is also true; if it can be shown that the nurse manager was aware of incompetence in a given employee or that the assigned/delegated task was outside the employee's capabilities, the nurse manager becomes substantially liable for the subsequent injury to a patient.

Nurse managers have a duty to ensure that the staff members under their supervision are practicing in a safe and competent manner. The nurse manager must be aware of the staff members' knowledge, skills, and competencies and should know whether they are maintaining their competencies. Knowingly allowing a staff member to function below the acceptable standard of care subjects both the nurse manager and the institution to potential liability. For example, in *Fairfax Nursing Home, Inc. v. Department of Health and Human Services* (2003), a nursing home was held liable for inadequate practices and procedures in monitoring ventilator-dependent patients. In that case, a professional staff member delegated the task of suctioning a ventilator-dependent patient to a nurse's aide. After suctioning the patient, the aide failed to ensure that the ventilator was reconnected to the patient's tracheostomy and the patient subsequently died. The professional nurse was also found to be liable for her failure to ensure that the task had been correctly performed.

Some nurse practice acts also legislate fines and discipline for the nurse manager who assigns/delegates tasks or patient care loads that make a nursing assignment unsafe. Means of ensuring continuing competency are expected and may include continuing education programs and assignment of a staff member to work with a second staff member to improve technical skills.

Duty to Orient, Educate, and Evaluate

Most healthcare institutions have continuing education departments to orient nurses who are new to the institution and to supply in-service education addressing new equipment, procedures, and interventions to existing employees. Nurse managers also have a duty to orient, educate, and evaluate. Nurse managers and their representatives are responsible for the daily evaluation of whether nurses are performing safe and competent care. The key to meeting this requirement is reasonableness and is determined by courts on a case-to-case basis. Nurse managers should ensure that they promptly respond to all allegations, whether by patients or staff, of incompetent or questionable nursing care. Nurse managers should thoroughly investigate allegations, recommend options for correcting the situation, and follow up on recommended options and suggestions.

In *Bunn-Penn v. Southern Regional Medical Corporation* (1997), a male emergency center technician was accused of sexually assaulting a female patient. Before this incident, nurses had complained to the nurse manager that the male technician seemed too eager to assist female patients and that he stayed too long with female patients while they were undressing. The nurse manager spoke to the technician about these concerns. The nurse manager gave him detailed instructions regarding how he was to conduct himself in the future. She then monitored his activities carefully and noted no further evidence of inappropriate behavior. In finding that there was no liability on the part of the hospital, the court was positive in its praise of the nurse manager, noting that she had fulfilled her duty by counseling and monitoring the employee and by acting promptly when the issues were first presented to her. The court also noted that the nurse manager had monitored this employee for an 18-month period and had filed favorable periodic reviews in his personnel folder.

Failure to Warn

A newer area of potential liability for nurse managers is **failure to warn** potential employers of staff incompetencies or impairment. Information about suspected addictions, violent behavior, and incompetency is of vital importance to subsequent employers. If the institution has sufficient information and suspicion to warrant the discharge of an employee or force a resignation, subsequent employers should be advised of those issues. In addition, the state board of nursing or agency that oversees disciplinary actions of professional and nonprofessional nursing staff should also be notified whenever there is cause to dismiss an employee for incompetency or impairment unless the employee voluntarily enters a peer-assistance program.

One means of supplying this information is through the use of *qualified privilege* to certain communications. In general, qualified privilege concerns communications made in good faith between persons or entities with a need to know. Most states now recognize this privilege and allow previous employers to give factual, objective information to subsequent employers. Note, however, that the previous employee must have listed the nurse manager or institution as a reference before this privilege arises.

Staffing Issues

Three issues arise under the general term *staffing*. These include (1) maintaining adequate numbers of staff members in a time of advancing patient acuity and limited resources; (2) floating staff from one unit to another; and (3) using temporary or "agency" staff to augment the healthcare facility's current staffing. Though each area is addressed separately, common to all three of these staffing issues is the requisite of collaboration among nurse managers in addressing the needs for the entire institution or healthcare agency.

Accreditation standards, specifically those of TJC and the Community Health Accreditation Program (CHAP), as well as other state and federal standards, mandate that healthcare institutions provide adequate staffing with qualified personnel. This applies not only to the number of staff but also to the legal status of the staff. For instance, some areas of an institution, such as critical care areas, postanesthesia care areas, and emergency care centers, must have greater percentages of RNs than LPNs/LVNs. Other areas, such as the general nursing areas and some long-term-care areas, may have equal or lower percentages of RNs to LPNs/LVNs or nursing assistants. Whether understaffing exists in a given situation depends on the number of patients, care acuity scores, and number and classification of staff. Courts determine whether understaffing existed on an individual case basis.

California was the first state to adopt legislation that mandated fixed nurse-to-patient ratios, passing this historic legislation in 1999. Although an additional 15 states have introduced similar legislation since that time, California remains the only state that has set requirements for every patient care unit in every hospital in the state (ANA, 2009). These types of ratios require set nurse-to-patient ratios based solely on numbers of patients within given nursing care areas and do not consider issues such as patient acuity, level of staff preparation, or environmental factors. Though a first step toward beginning to ensure adequate numbers of nurses, many states are now moving toward the concept of safe staffing rather than specific nurse-to-patient ratios.

A minority of states have passed safe staffing measures rather than mandating ratios. Generally, these safe staffing measures call for a committee to develop, oversee, and evaluate a plan for each specific nursing unit and shift based on patient care needs, appropriate skill mix of RNs and other nursing personnel, the physical layout of the unit, and national standards or recommendations regarding nursing staffing. Washington State's plan, for example, also includes a provision that the staffing information is posted in a public area of the nursing unit and updated at least once per shift and that the information is available to patients and visitors upon request (Safe Nurse Staffing Legislation, 2008).

Although the institution is ultimately responsible for staffing issues, nurse managers may also incur liability because they directly oversee numbers of personnel assigned to a given unit. Courts have looked to the constant exercise of professional judgment, rather than reliance on concrete nurse-patient ratios, in cases involving staffing issues. Thus nurse managers should exercise sound judgment to ensure patient safety and quality care rather than rely on exact nurse-to-patient ratios. For liability to incur against the nurse manager, it must be shown that a resultant patient injury was directly caused by staffing issues and not by the incompetent or inappropriate actions of an individual staff member. To prevent nurse manager liability, he or she must show that sufficient numbers of competent staff were available to meet nursing needs.

Guidelines for nurse managers in inadequate-staffing issues include alerting hospital administrators and upper-level managers of concerns. First, however, the nurse manager must do whatever is under his or her control to alleviate the circumstances, such as approving overtime for adequate coverage, reassigning personnel among those areas he or she supervises, and restricting new admissions to the area. Second, nurse managers have a legal duty to notify the chief operating officer, either directly or indirectly, when understaffing endangers patient welfare. One way of notifying the chief operating officer is through formal nursing channels, for example, by notifying the nurse manager's direct supervisor. Upper management must then decide how to alleviate the staffing issue, either on a short-term or a long-term basis. Appropriate measures could be closing a unit or units, restricting elective surgeries, hiring new staff members, or temporarily reassigning personnel from other departments. Once the nurse manager can show that he or she acted appropriately, used sound judgment given the circumstances, and alerted his or her supervisors of the serious nature of the situation, the institution and not the nurse manager becomes potentially liable for staffing issues.

Many states now prohibit the use of mandatory overtime by nurses. Generally these laws state that the healthcare facility may not require an employee to work in excess of agreed to, predetermined, and regularly scheduled daily work shifts unless there is an unforeseeable declared national, state, or municipal emergency or catastrophic event that is unpredicted or unavoidable and that substantially affects or increases the need for healthcare services. In addition, many of these laws define "normal work schedule" as 12 or fewer hours; employees are protected from disciplinary action or retribution for refusing to work overtime; and monetary penalties can result from the employer's failure to adhere to the law. Some states also mandate that healthcare facilities are required to have a process for complaints related to patient safety. Note that nothing in these laws negates voluntary overtime.

Floating staff from unit to unit is the second issue that concerns overall staffing. Institutions have a duty to ensure that all areas of the institution are staffed adequately. Units temporarily overstaffed because of low patient census or a lower patient acuity ratio usually float staff to units that are understaffed. Although floating nurses to areas with which they have less familiarity and expertise can increase potential liability for the nurse manager, leaving another area dangerously understaffed can also increase potential liability.

Before floating staff from one area to another, the nurse manager should consider staff expertise, patient-care delivery systems, and patient-care requirements. Nurses should be floated to units as comparable to their own unit as possible. This requires the nurse manager to match the nurse's home unit and float unit as much as is possible or to consider negotiating with another nurse manager to cross-float a nurse. For example, a manager might float a critical care nurse to an intermediate care unit and float an intermediate care unit nurse to a general unit. Or the nurse manager might consider floating the general unit nurse to the postpartum unit and floating a postpartum nurse to labor and delivery. Open communications regarding staff limitations and concerns, as well as creative solutions for staffing, can alleviate some of the potential liability involved and create better morale among the floating nurses. A positive option is to cross-train nurses within the institution so that nurses are familiar with two or three areas and can competently float to areas in which they have been cross-trained.

The use of temporary or "agency" personnel has created increased liability concerns among nurse managers. Until recently, most jurisdictions held that such personnel were considered independent contractors and thus the institution was not liable for their actions, although their primary employment agency did retain potential liability. Today, courts have begun to hold the institution liable under the principle of apparent agency. *Apparent authority* or *apparent agency* refers to the doctrine whereby a principal becomes accountable for the actions of his or her agent. Apparent agency is created when a person (agent) holds himself or herself out as acting in behalf of the principal; in the instance of the agency nurse, the patient cannot ascertain whether the nurse works directly for the hospital (has a valid employment contract) or is working for a different employer. At law, lack of actual authority is no defense. This principle applies when it can be shown that a reasonable patient believed that the healthcare worker was an employee of the institution. If it appears to the reasonable patient that this worker is an employee of the institution, the law will consider the worker an employee for the purposes of corporate and vicarious liability.

These trends in the law make it imperative that the nurse manager considers the temporary worker's skills, competencies, and knowledge when delegating tasks and supervising the worker's actions. If there is reason to suspect that the temporary worker is incompetent, the nurse manager must convey this fact to the agency. The nurse manager must also either send the temporary worker home or reassign the worker to other duties and areas. The same screening procedures should be performed with temporary workers as are used with new institution employees.

Additional areas that nurse managers should stress when using agency or temporary personnel include ensuring that the temporary staff member is given a brief but thorough orientation to institution policies and procedures, is made aware of resource materials within the institution, and is made aware of documentation procedures. It is also advisable for nurse managers to assign a resource person to the temporary staff member. This resource person serves in the role of mentor for the agency nurse and serves to prevent potential problems that could arise merely because the agency staff member does not know the institution routine or is unaware of where to turn for assistance. This resource person also serves as a mentor for critical decision making for the agency nurse.

PROTECTIVE AND REPORTING LAWS

Protective and reporting laws ensure the safety or rights of specific classes of individuals. Most states have reporting laws for suspected child and older adult abuse and laws for reporting certain categories of diseases and injuries. Examples of reporting laws include reporting cases of sexually transmitted diseases, abuse of residents in nursing and convalescent homes, and suspected child abuse. Nurse managers are often the individuals who are responsible for ensuring that the correct information is reported to the correct agencies, thus avoiding potential liability against the institution.

Many states now also have mandatory reporting of incompetent practice, especially through nurse practice acts, medical practice acts, and the National Practitioner Data Bank. In addition, the NCSBN has developed an electronic license verification system called *Nursys* that monitors nurses' licensure status in all states and U.S. territories for discipline issues, competency ratings, and renewals. Reporting incompetent practice often is restricted to issues of chemical abuse, and special provisions prevail if the affected nurse voluntarily undergoes drug diversion or chemical-dependency rehabilitation.

Mandatory reporting of incompetent practitioners is a complex process, involving both legal and ethical concerns. Nurse managers must know what the law requires, when reporting is mandated, to whom the report must be sent, and what the individual institution expects of its nurse managers. When in doubt,

seek clarification from the state board of nursing, hospital administration, or professional association.

INFORMED CONSENT

Informed consent becomes an important concept for nurse managers in three very different instances. First, staff nurses may approach the nurse manager with questions about informed consent; thus the nurse manager becomes a consultant for the staff nurse. Second, and more often, the nurse manager is queried about patients' rights in research studies that are being conducted in the institution. Third, the issue of medical literacy has implications for the provision of valid informed consent by an ever-growing number of patients.

Remember: informed consent is the authorization by the patient or the patient's legal representative to do something to the patient; it is based on legal capacity, voluntary action, and comprehension. Legal capacity is usually the first requirement and is determined by age and competency. All states have a legal age for adult status defined by statute; generally, this age is 18. Competency involves the ability to understand the consequences of actions or the ability to handle personal affairs. State statutes mandate who can serve as the representative for a minor or incompetent adult. The following types of minors may be able to give valid informed consent: emancipated minors, minors seeking treatment for substance abuse or communicable diseases, and pregnant minors.

Voluntary action, the second requirement, means that the patient was not coerced by fraud, duress, or deceit into allowing the procedure or treatment. Comprehension is the third requirement and the most difficult to ascertain. The law states that the patient must be given sufficient information, in terms he or she can reasonably be expected to comprehend, to make an informed choice. Inherent in the doctrine of informed consent is the right of the patient to informed refusal. Patients must clearly understand the possible consequences of their refusal. In recent years, most states have enacted statutes to ensure that the competent adult has the right to refuse care and that the healthcare provider is protected should the adult validly refuse care. This refusal of care is most

BOX 5-1 INFORMATION REQUIRED FOR INFORMED CONSENT

- An explanation of the treatment/procedure to be performed and the expected results of the treatment/procedure
- Description of the risks involved
- Benefits that are likely to result because of the treatment/ procedure
- Options to this course of action, including absence of treatment
- Name of the person(s) performing the treatment/procedure
- Statement that the patient may withdraw his or her consent at any time

BOX 5-2 ELEMENTS OF INFORMED CONSENT IN RESEARCH STUDIES

- A statement that the study involves research, an explanation of the purposes of the research and the expected duration of the subject's participation, a description of the procedures to be followed, and identification of any procedures that are experimental
- A description of any reasonably foreseeable risks or discomforts to the subject
- A description of any benefits to the subjects or others that may reasonably be expected from the research
- A disclosure of appropriate alternative procedures or courses of treatment, if any, that may be advantageous to the subject
- A statement describing the extent, if any, to which confidentiality of records identifying the subject will be maintained
- For research involving more than minimal research, an explanation as to any compensation and an explanation as to whether any medical treatments are available if injury occurs and, if so, what they consist of or where further information may be obtained
- An explanation of whom to contact for answers to pertinent questions about the research and research subjects' rights and whom to contact in the event of a research-related injury to the subject
- A statement that participation is voluntary, refusal to participate will involve no benefits to which the subject is otherwise entitled, and the subject may discontinue participation at any time without penalty or loss of benefits to which the subject is otherwise entitled

From *45 Code of Federal Regulations (CFR)*, Sec. 46.116 (1991).

frequently seen in end-of-life decisions. Box 5-1 lists the information needed for obtaining informed consent.

Nurses often ask about issues concerning informed consent that concern the actual signing of the informed consent document, not the teaching and information that make up informed consent. Many nurses serve as witnesses to the signing of the informed consent document; in this capacity, they are attesting only to the voluntary nature of the patient's signature. There is no duty on the part of the nurse to insist that the patient repeat what has been said or what he or she remembers. If the patient asks questions that alert the nurse to the inadequacy of true comprehension on the patient's part or expresses uncertainty while signing the document, the nurse has an obligation to inform the primary healthcare provider and appropriate persons that informed consent has not been obtained.

Another issue about informed consent concerns the patient who is part of a research study. Federal laws regulate this area because patients are generally considered to come under the heading of *vulnerable populations*. Whenever research is involved, such as a drug study or a new procedure, the investigators must disclose the research to the subject or the subject's representative and obtain informed consent. Federal guidelines have been developed that specify the procedures used to review research and the disclosures that must be made to ensure that valid informed consent is obtained.

The federal government mandates the basic elements of information that must be included to meet the standards of informed consent. Elements of informed consent are enumerated in Box 5-2.

The information given must be in a language that is understandable by the subject or the subject's legal representative. No exculpatory wording may be included, such as a statement that the researcher incurs no liability for the outcomes of the study or any injury to an individual subject. Subjects should be advised of the elements listed in Box 5-3.

Excluded from these strict requirements were studies that use existing data, documents, records, or pathologic and diagnostic specimens, if these sources are publicly available or the information is recorded so that the subjects cannot be identified. Other studies that involve only minimal risks to subjects, such as moderate exercise by healthy adults, may be expedited through the review process (45 CFR, Section

BOX 5-3   ELEMENTS OF CONCERN IN RESEARCH STUDIES

- Any additional costs that they might incur because of the research
- Potential for any foreseeable risks
- Rights to withdraw at will, with no questions asked or additional incentives given
- Consequences, if any, of withdrawal before the study is completed
- A statement that any significant new findings will be disclosed
- The number of proposed subjects for the study

From *45 Code of Federal Regulations (CFR),* Sec. 46.101(b) (1991).

46.110, 1991). Nurse managers must verify that staff members understand any research protocol with which their patients are involved.

The advent of the Health Insurance Portability and Accountability Act (HIPAA) of 1996 (Public Law [P.L.] 104-191) has affected how medical record information can now be used in research studies. No separate permission need be secured from the patient to use medical-record information if de-identified information is used. De-identified information is health information that cannot be linked to an individual; most of the 18 demographic items constituting the protected health information (PHI) must be removed before researchers are permitted to use patient records without obtaining the individual patient's permission to use/disclose PHI. The de-identified data set that is permissible for usage may contain the following demographic factors: gender and age of individuals and a three-digit ZIP code. Note that all individuals 90 years of age or older are listed as 90 years of age.

To prevent the onerous task of requiring patients who have been discharged from healthcare settings to sign such permission forms, researchers are allowed to submit a request for a waiver. The waiver is a request to forego the authorization requirements based on two conditions: (1) the use and/or disclosure of PHI involves minimal risk to the subject's privacy, and (2) the research cannot be done practically without this waiver. Additional information about HIPAA and confidentiality are covered later in this chapter.

Concerns over the past abuses that have occurred in the area of research with children have led to the adoption of federal guidelines specifically designed to protect children when they are enrolled as research subjects. Before proceeding under these specific guidelines, state and local laws must be reviewed for laws regulating research on human subjects. In 1998, Subpart D: Additional Protections for Children Involved as Subjects in Research was added to the code (45 Code of Federal Regulation [CFR] 46.401 et seq., 1998). These sections were added to give further protection to children when they are subjects of research studies and to encourage researchers to involve children, where appropriate, in research.

A final issue with informed consent about which nurse managers should be cognizant concerns health literacy or the degree to which individuals have the capacity to obtain, process, and understand basic health information, including services needed to make appropriate health decisions. Functional health literacy concerns the "ability to read, understand and act on health information" (Andrus & Roth, 2002, p. 282). Comprehending medical jargon is difficult for well-educated Americans; it is virtually impossible for approximately 90 million Americans who have limited health literacy (Maniaci, Heckman, & Dawson, 2008). Comprehending medical instructions and terms may be impossible for individuals whose first language is not English, who cannot read at greater than a second-grade level, or who have vision or cognitive problems caused by aging. These individuals have difficulty following instructions that are printed on medication labels (both prescription and over-the-counter), interpreting hospital consent forms, and even understanding diagnoses, treatment options, and discharge instructions.

Nurse managers play a significant role in addressing this growing problem. The first issue to address is awareness of the problem, because many patients and their family members hide the fact that they cannot read or do not understand what healthcare providers are attempting to convey. A second issue involves ensuring that the information and words nurses use to communicate with patients are at a level that the person can comprehend. One means of assisting staff nurses to ensure that patients do understand patient discharge information and medication instructions is to give the patient the bottle of prescription medication and ask him or her to tell you how he or she would take the medication at home.

PRIVACY AND CONFIDENTIALITY

Privacy is the patient's right to protection against unreasonable and unwarranted interference with his or her solitude. This right extends to protection of the person's reputation as well as protection of one's right to be left alone. Within a medical context, the law recognizes the patient's right to protection against (1) appropriation of the patient's name or picture for the institution's sole advantage, (2) intrusion by the institution on the patient's seclusion or affairs, (3) publication of facts that place the patient in a false light, and (4) public disclosure of private facts about the patient by the hospital or staff. Confidentiality is the right to privacy of the medical record.

Institutions can reduce potential liability in this area by allowing access to patient data, either written or oral, only to those with a "need to know." Persons with a need to know include physicians and nurses caring for the patient, technicians, unit clerks, therapists, social service workers, and patient advocates. Usually, this need to know extends to the house staff and consultants. Others wishing to access patient data must first ask the patient for permission to review a record. Administrative staff of the institution can access the patient record for statistical analysis, staffing, and quality-of-care review.

The nurse manager is cautioned to ensure that staff members both understand and abide by rules regarding patient privacy and confidentiality. "Interesting" patients should not be discussed with others, and all information concerning patients should be given only in private and secluded areas. All nurses may need to review the current means of giving reports to oncoming shifts and policies about telephone information. Many institutions have now added to the nursing care plan a place to list persons to whom the patient has allowed information to be given. If the caller identifies himself or herself as one of those listed persons, the nurse can give patient information without violating the patient's privacy rights. Patients are becoming more knowledgeable about their rights in these areas, and some have been willing to take offending staff members to court over such issues.

The patient's right of access to his or her medical record is another confidentiality issue. Although the patient has a right of access, individual states mandate when this right applies. Most states give the right of access only after the medical record is completed; thus the patient has the right to review the record after discharge. Some states do give the right of access while the patient is hospitalized, and therefore individual state law governs individual nurses' actions. When supervising a patient's review of his or her record, the nurse manager or representative should explain only the entries that the patient questions or about which the patient requests further clarification. The nurse makes a note in the record after the session, indicating that the patient has viewed the record and what questions were answered.

Patients also have a right to copies of the record, at their expense. The medical record belongs to the institution as a business record, and patients never have the right to retain the original record. This is also true in instances in which a subpoena is obtained to secure an individual's medical record for court purposes. A hospital representative will verify that the copy is a "true and valid" copy of the original record.

An issue that is closely related to the medical record is that of incident reports or unusual occurrence reports. These reports are mandated by TJC and serve to alert the institution to risk management and quality assurance issues within the setting. As such, incident reports are considered internal documents and thus not discoverable (open for review) by the injured party or attorneys representing the injured party. In most jurisdictions where this question has arisen, however, the courts have held that the incident report was discoverable and thus open to review by both sides of the suit.

It is therefore prudent for nurse managers to complete and to have staff members complete incident reports as though they will be open records. It is advisable to omit any language of guilt, such as, "The patient would not have fallen if Jane Jones, RN, had ensured the side rails were in their up and locked position." This document should contain only pertinent observations and all care given the patient, such as x-rays that were obtained for a potential broken bone, medication that was given, and consultants who were called to examine the patient. It is also inadvisable to make any notation of the incident report in the official patient record because such a notation incorporates the incident report "by reference," and there is no way to keep the report from being seen by the injured party or attorneys for the injured party.

Protected health information, which includes some 18 individual identifiers, is at the crux of the confidentiality aspect of the law. The privacy standards limit how PHI may be used or shared, mandate safeguards for protecting the health information, and shift the control of health information from providers to the patient by giving patients significant rights. Healthcare facilities must provide patients with a documented Notice of Privacy Rights, explaining how their PHI will be used or shared with other entities. This document also alerts patients to the process for complaints if they determine that their information rights have been violated. Nurse managers have the responsibility to ensure that those they supervise uphold these patient rights as dictated by HIPAA and to take corrective actions should these rights not be upheld.

POLICIES AND PROCEDURES

Risk management is a process that identifies, analyzes, and treats potential hazards within a given setting. The object of risk management is to identify potential hazards and eliminate them before anyone is harmed or disabled. Risk management activities include writing policies and procedures. Written policies and procedures are a requirement of TJC. These documents set standards of care for the institution and direct practice. They must be clearly stated, well

---

EXERCISE 5-3

You are assigned some risk management activities in the nursing facility where you work. In investigating incident reports that were filed by your staff, you discover that this is the third patient this week who has fallen while attempting to get out of bed and sit in a chair. How would you begin to address this issue? Decide how you would start a more complete investigation of this issue. For example, is it a facility-wide issue or one that is confined to one unit? Does it affect all shifts or only one? What safety issues are you going to discuss with your staff, and how are you going to discuss these issues? Do these falls involve the same staff member? Design a unit in-service class for the staff concerning incident reports and patient safety.

---

delineated, and based on current practice. Nurse managers should review the policies and procedures frequently for compliance and timeliness. If policies are absent or outdated, the nurse manager must request the appropriate person or committee to either initiate or update the policy.

EMPLOYMENT LAWS

The federal and individual state governments have enacted laws regulating employment. To be effective and legally correct, nurse managers must be familiar with these laws and how the individual laws affect the institution and labor relations. Many nurse managers have come to fear the legal system because of personal experience or the experiences of colleagues, but much of this concern may be directly attributable to uncertainty with the law or partial knowledge of the law. By understanding and correctly following federal employment laws, nurse managers may actually decrease their potential liability by complying with both federal and state laws. Table 5-2 gives an overview of key federal employment laws.

Equal Employment Opportunity Laws

Several federal laws have been enacted to expand equal employment opportunities by prohibiting discrimination based on gender, age, race, religion, handicap, pregnancy, and national origin. The Equal Employment Opportunity Commission (EEOC) enforces these laws. All states have also enacted statutes that address employment opportunities, and the nurse manager should consider both when hiring and assigning nursing employees.

The most significant legislation affecting equal employment opportunities today is the amended Civil Rights Act of 1964 (1978). Section 703(a) of Title VII makes it illegal for an employer "to refuse to hire, discharge an individual, or otherwise to discriminate against an individual, with respect to his compensation, terms, conditions, or privileges of employment because of the individual's race, color, religion, sex, or national origin." The Equal Opportunities Act of 1972 also amended Title VII so that it applies to private institutions with 15 or more employees, state and local governments, labor unions, and employment agencies.

TABLE 5-2   SELECTED FEDERAL LABOR LEGISLATION

YEAR	LEGISLATION	PRIMARY PURPOSE OF THE LEGISLATION
1935	Wagner Act; National Labor Act	Unions, National Labor Relations Board established
1947	Taft-Hartley Act	Equal balance of power between unions and management
1948	1962 Executive Order 10988	Public employees could join unions
1963	Equal Pay Act	Became illegal to pay lower wages based on gender
1964	Civil Rights Act	Protected against discrimination based on race, color, creed, national origin, etc.
1967	Age Discrimination in Employment Act	Act protected against discrimination based on age
1970	Occupational Safety and Health Act	Ensured healthy and safe working conditions
1974	Wagner Amendments	Allowed nonprofit organizations to unionize
1990	Americans with Disabilities Act	Barred discrimination against workers with disabilities
1991	Civil Rights Act	Addressed sexual harassment in the workplace
1993	Family and Medical Leave Act	Allowed work leaves based on family and medical needs

The Civil Rights Act of 1991 further broadened the issue of sexual harassment in the workplace and supersedes many of the sections of Title VII. Sections of the new legislation define sexual harassment, its elements, and the employer's responsibilities regarding harassment in the workplace, especially prevention and corrective action. The Civil Rights Act of 1991 is enforced by the EEOC; its powers were broadened in the 1972 Equal Employment Opportunity Act. The primary activity of the EEOC is processing complaints of employment discrimination. There are three phases: investigation, conciliation, and litigation. Investigation focuses on determining whether the employer has violated provisions of Title VII. If the EEOC finds "probable cause," an attempt is made to reach an agreement or conciliation between the EEOC, the complainant, and the employer. If conciliation fails, the EEOC may file suit against the employer in federal court or issue to the complainant the right to sue for discrimination under its auspices, including those relating to staffing practices and sexual harassment in the workplace.

The EEOC defines sexual harassment broadly, and this has generally been upheld in the courts. Nurse managers must realize that it is the duty of employers (management) to prevent employees from sexually harassing other employees. The EEOC issues policies and practices for employers to implement, both to sensitize employees to this problem and to prevent its occurrence. Nurse managers should be aware of these policies and practices and seek guidance in implementing them if sexual harassment occurs in their units.

Employers may seek exceptions to Title VII on a number of premises. For example, employment decisions made on the basis of national origin, religion, and gender (never race or color) are lawful if such decisions are necessary for the normal operation of the business, although the courts have viewed this exception very narrowly. Promotions and layoffs based on bona fide seniority or merit systems are permissible, as are exceptions based on business necessity.

Age Discrimination in Employment Act of 1967

The Age Discrimination in Employment Act of 1967 made discrimination against older men and women by employers, unions, and employment agencies illegal. A 1986 amendment to the law prohibits discrimination against persons older than 40 years. The practical outcome of this act has been that mandatory retirement is no longer allowed in the American workplace.

As with Title VII, there are some exceptions to this act. Reasonable factors other than age may be used when terminations become necessary. Reasonable factors may include a performance evaluation system or certain limited occupational qualifications, such as the tedious physical demands of a specific job.

TABLE 5-3	AMERICANS WITH DISABILITIES ACT OF 1990
TITLE	PROVISIONS
I	Employment: defines the purpose of the act and who is qualified under the act as having a disability
II	Public services: concerns services, programs, and activities of public entities as well as public transportation
III	Public accommodations and services operated by private entities: prohibits discrimination against persons with disabilities in areas of public accommodations, commercial facilities, and public transportation services
IV	Telecommunications: intended to make telephone services accessible to individuals with hearing or speech impairments
V	Miscellaneous provisions: certain insurance matters; incorporation of this act with other federal and state laws

From Americans with Disabilities Act of 1990, 42 U.S.C. § 12101 *et seq.* (1990).

Americans with Disabilities Act of 1990

The Americans with Disabilities Act (ADA) of 1990 provides protection to persons with disabilities and is the most significant civil rights legislation since the Civil Rights Act of 1964. The purpose of the ADA is to provide a clear and comprehensive national mandate for the elimination of discrimination against individuals with disabilities and to provide clear, strong, consistent, enforceable standards addressing discrimination in the workplace. The ADA is closely related to the Civil Rights Act of 1991 and incorporates the antidiscrimination principles established in Section 504 of the Rehabilitation Act of 1973.

The act has five titles; Table 5-3 depicts the pertinent issues of each title. The ADA has jurisdiction over employers, private and public; employment agencies; labor organizations; and joint labor-management committees. Disability is defined broadly. With respect to an individual, a disability is (1) a physical or mental impairment that substantially limits one or more of the major life activities of such individual, (2) a record of such impairment, or (3) regarded as having such an impairment (ADA, 1990). The overall effect of the legislation is that persons with disabilities will not be excluded from job opportunities or adversely affected in any aspect of employment unless they are not qualified or are otherwise unable to perform the job. The ADA thus protects qualified individuals with disabilities in regard to job application procedures, hiring, compensation, advancement, and all other employment matters.

The number of lawsuits filed under the ADA since its enactment continues to be extensive. Recent cases have assisted in defining disability eligibility. The following findings have been decided in court regarding disabilities:

1. A nurse with a lifting disability is not qualified for protection under the ADA (*Squibb v. Memorial Medical Center*, 2007; *Storkamp v. Geren*, 2008)
2. Chemical dependency does not require accommodation (*Dovenmuehler v. St. Cloud Hospital*, 2007; *Nicholson v. West Penn Allegheny Health System*, 2007)
3. Depression and anxiety are not disabling conditions (*Cody v. Cigna Healthcare of St. Louis, Inc.*, 1998)
4. Short-term impairment, even if quite severe, with no expected long-term side effects is not a disability (*Garrett v. University of Alabama*, 2007; *Vierra v. Wayne Memorial Hospital*, 2006)
5. Migraine headaches and latex allergies are not disabilities (*Howard v. North Mississippi Medical Center*, 1996)
6. Pregnancy is not a disability (*Equal Employment Opportunity Commission v. Catholic Healthcare West*, 2008)

The ADA requires an employer or potential employer to make reasonable accommodations to employ persons with a disability. The law does not mandate that individuals with a disability be hired before fully qualified persons who do not have a disability; it does mandate that those with disabilities not be disqualified merely because of an easily accommodated disability.

This last point was well illustrated by the court in *Zamudio v. Patia* (1997). The court stated that the employer would be required to inform Ms. Zamudio when a position became available for which the reasonable accommodation she required could be met. She would be allowed to apply, but "as a disabled employee seeking reasonable accommodation she did not have to be given preference over other employees without disabilities who might have better qualifications or more seniority" (*Zamudio v. Patia,* 1997, at 808).

Moreover, the court will not impose job restructuring on an employer if the person needing accommodation qualifies for other jobs not requiring such accommodation. In *Mauro v. Borgess Medical Center* (1995), the court refused to impose accommodation on the employer hospital merely because the affected employee desired to stay within a certain unit of the institution. In this case, an operating surgical technician who tested positive for HIV was offered an equivalent position by the hospital in an area where there would be no patient contact. He refused the transfer, desiring accommodation within the operating arena, and was denied such accommodation by the Michigan court.

The act also provides for essential job functions. These are defined by the ADA as those functions that the person must be able to perform to be qualified for employment positions. Courts have assisted in determining these essential job functions. For example, in *Jones v. Kerrville State Hospital* (1998), the court found that an essential job function for a psychiatric nurse is the ability to restrain patients. In *Laurin v. Providence Hospital and Massachusetts Nurses Association* (1998), the ability to work rotating shifts was held to be an essential job function.

The act also specifically excludes the following from the definition of disability: homosexuality and bisexuality, sexual behavioral disorders, gambling addiction, kleptomania, pyromania, and current use of illegal drugs (ADA, 1990). Moreover, employers may hold alcoholic persons to the same job qualifications and job performance standards as other employees, even if the unsatisfactory behavior or performance is related to the alcoholism (ADA, 1990). As with other federal employment laws, the nurse manager should have a thorough understanding of the law as it applies to the institution and his or her specific job description and should know whom to contact within the institution structure for clarification as needed.

Affirmative Action

The policy of affirmative action (AA) differs from the policy of equal employment opportunity (EEO). AA policy enhances employment opportunities of protected groups of people; EEO policy is concerned with implementing employment practices that do not dis-

criminate against or impair the employment opportunities of protected groups. Thus AA can be seen in conjunction with several federal employment laws. For example, in conjunction with the Vietnam Era Veterans' Re-adjustment Act of 1974, AA requires that employers with government contracts take steps to enhance the employment opportunities of veterans with disabilities and other veterans of the Vietnam Era.

Equal Pay Act of 1963

The Equal Pay Act of 1963 makes it illegal to pay lower wages to employees of one gender when the jobs (1) require equal skill in experience, training, education, and ability; (2) require equal effort in mental or physical exertion; (3) are of equal responsibility and accountability; and (4) are performed under similar working conditions. Courts have held that unequal pay may be legal if it is based on seniority, merit, incentive systems, or a factor other than gender. The main cases filed under this law in the area of nursing have been by nonprofessionals.

Occupational Safety and Health Act

The Occupational Safety and Health Administration (OSHA) Act of 1970 was enacted to ensure that healthful and safe working conditions would exist in the workplace. Among other provisions, the law requires isolation procedures, placarding areas containing ionizing radiation, proper grounding of electrical equipment, protective storage of flammable and combustible liquids, and the gloving of all personnel when handling bodily fluids. The statute provides that if no federal standard has been established, state statutes prevail. Nurse managers should know the relevant OSHA laws for the institution and their specific area. Newer updates are occurring in the areas of methicillin-resistant *Staphylococcus aureus* (MRSA), personal protective equipment, latex allergy, sonography, combustible dust, and occupational exposure to chlorinated solvents. Sonography identifies ergonomic factors, offering a variety of possible solutions for the safer movement and positioning of patients.

Violence in the workplace is an issue that OSHA continues to address in its rules. Violence is perhaps the greatest hidden health and safety threat in the workplace today, and nurses, as the largest group of healthcare professionals, are most at risk of assault at work. In 1996, OSHA developed voluntary guidelines to protect healthcare workers and consumers; these voluntary guidelines are still in effect. Many states, Puerto Rico, and the Virgin Islands have now adopted their own standards and enforcement policies, with the majority of these standards and policies identical to the federal guidelines.

An issue that OSHA has not yet addressed but that nursing is now addressing in-depth is safe patient handling—preventing injury to healthcare workers while ensuring that patients are protected as they are transferred/moved in healthcare settings. The ANA's data show that more than 52% of nurses complain of chronic back pain, 12% leave the profession citing chronic back pain as the determining factor for their leaving, and 20% transfer to a different unit out of direct patient care or other employment settings because of back pain and neck and shoulder injuries (Timmons, 2009). Given these data and recognizing that manual patient lifting simply is not safe, the ANA promotes legislation that would require hospitals and other healthcare institutions to develop programs to prevent work-related musculoskeletal disorders and eliminate manual patient lifting. Toward this end, states are now introducing and passing legislation that mandates healthcare facilities provide the needed equipment and education for a total no-lift policy. The momentum now in place can lead to federal laws that would require mechanical lifting equipment and friction-reducing devices for all healthcare workers, patients, and residents across all healthcare settings.

Family and Medical Leave Act of 1993

The Family and Medical Leave Act of 1993 was passed because of the large numbers of single-parent and two-parent households in which the single parent or both parents are employed full-time, placing job security and parenting at odds. The law also supports the growing demands that aging parents are placing on their working children. The act was written in an attempt to balance the demands of the workplace with the demands of the family, allowing employed individuals to take leaves for medical reasons, including the birth or adoption of children and the care of a spouse, child, or parent who has serious health problems.

Essentially, the act provides job security for unpaid leave while the employee is caring for a new infant or other family healthcare needs. The act is gender-neutral and allows both men and women the same leave provisions.

To be eligible under the act, the employee must have worked for at least 12 months and worked at least 1250 hours during the preceding 12-month period. The employee may take up to 12 weeks of unpaid leave. The act allows the employer to require the employee to use all or part of any paid vacation, personal leave, or sick leave as part of the 12-week family leave. Employees must give the employer 30-days notice, or such notice as is practical in emergency cases, before using the medical leave.

On January 28, 2008, then President George W. Bush signed the Family and Medical Leave Amended Act of 2008, which became effective January 16, 2009. The amendments permit a spouse, son, daughter, parent, or next of kin to take up to 26 work weeks of leave to care for a member of the Armed Forces, including a member of the National Guard or Reserves, who is undergoing medical treatment, recuperation, or therapy, is otherwise in outpatient status, or is otherwise on the temporary disability retired list, for a serious injury or illness. In addition, the act permits an employee to take leave for any qualifying exigency arising out of the fact that the spouse or a son, daughter, or parent of the employee is on active duty (or has been notified of an impending call or order to active duty) in the Armed Forces in support of a contingency operation.

Employment-at-Will and Wrongful Discharge

Historically, the employment relationship has been considered a "free will" relationship. Employees were free to take or not take a job at will, and employers were free to hire, retain, or discharge employees for any reason. Many laws, some federal but predominantly state, have been slowly eroding this at-will employment relationship. Evolving case law provides at least three exceptions to the broad doctrine of employment-at-will.

The first exception is a public policy exception. This exception involves cases in which an employee is discharged in direct conflict with established public policy. Some examples include discharging an employee for serving on a jury, reporting employers' illegal actions (better known as "whistleblowing"), and filing a workers' compensation claim.

Several recent court cases attest to the number of terminations in healthcare settings that serve as retaliation for the employer. More commonly known as "whistleblowing" cases, the healthcare provider in these cases is terminated for one of three distinct reasons: (1) speaking out against unsafe practices, (2) reporting violations of federal laws, or (3) filing lawsuits against employers. Essentially, whistleblower laws state that no employer can discharge, threaten, or discriminate against an employee regarding compensation, terms, conditions, location, or privileges of employment because the employee in good faith reported or caused to be reported, verbally or in writing, what the employee had a reasonable cause to believe was a violation of a state or federal law, rule, or regulation. For example, in *Wendeln v. Beatrice Manor, Inc.* (2006), the issue concerned the improper handling of vulnerable adults by paid caregivers. An aide had previously informed the nursing director and the administrator of a nursing home that another aide was not following the agency's rules regarding the safe transfer of elderly patients. She again reported this information to the staffing coordinator who investigated the matter and reported the aide in question to the state department of health and human services.

Within the week after reporting the aide in question, the staff coordinator came in to find that the locks had been changed on her office and that she was to resign. The Supreme Court in Nebraska upheld her right to sue and endorsed a $79,000 verdict in her favor, holding that improper handling of vulnerable adults constitutes abuse and nurses, physicians, and other healthcare workers have a duty to report such abuse. In reporting such abuse, they are protected by law from employer retaliation for performing their legal duty. Similarly, in 2010 two nurses were fired by the Winkler County Hospital for reporting a physician to the medical board. This complex case resulted in arrests (*www.texasnurses.org/displaycommon.cfm?an=1&subarticlenbr=509*) and a subsequent trial for one of the nurses.

The second exception to wrongful discharge involves situations in which there is an implied contract. The courts have generally treated employee handbooks, company policies, and oral statements made at the time of employment as "framing the employment relationship" (*Watkins v. Unemployment Compensation Board of Review*, 1997). For example, in *Trombley v. Southwestern Vermont Medical Center* (1999), the court found that the employee handbook outlined the procedure for progressive discipline, mandating that such procedure be followed before a nurse could be terminated for incompetent nursing care.

The third exception to wrongful discharge is a "good faith and fair dealing" exception. The purpose of this exception is to prevent unfair or malicious terminations, and the courts use the exception sparingly. Although this exception is rarely seen in nursing, it remains a valid exception to wrongful discharge of an employee.

Nurse managers are urged to know their respective state laws concerning this growing area of the law, particularly in conjunction with whistleblower laws. Managers should review institution documents, especially employee handbooks and recruiting brochures, for unwanted statements implying job security or other unintentional promises. Managers are also cautioned not to say anything during the preemployment negotiations and interviews that might be construed as implying job security or other unintentional promises to the potential employee. To prevent successful suits for retaliation by whistleblowers, nurse managers should carefully monitor the treatment of an employee after a complaint is filed and ensure that performance evaluations are performed and placed in the appropriate files. The nurse manager should also take steps to correct the whistleblower's complaint or refer the complaint to upper management so that it can effectively be addressed.

Collective Bargaining

Collective bargaining, also called *labor relations*, is the joining together of employees for the purpose of increasing their ability to influence the employer and improve working conditions. Usually, the employer is referred to as *management*, and the employees, even professionals, are *labor*. Those persons involved in the hiring, firing, scheduling, disciplining, or evaluating of employees are considered management and may not be included in a collective bargaining unit. Those in management could form their own group but are not protected under these laws. Nurse managers may or may not be part of management; if they have hiring and firing authority, they are part of management.

Collective bargaining is defined and protected by the National Labor Relations Act and its amendments; the National Labor Relations Board (NLRB) oversees the act and those who come under its auspices. The NLRB ensures that employees can choose freely whether they want to be represented by a particular bargaining unit, and it serves to prevent or remedy any violation of the labor laws. Chapter 19 provides further detail regarding collective bargaining and collective action.

Healthcare Reform

Two components of healthcare reform need to be addressed: (1) insurance (or payment) and (2) care (actual services). Most of the initial efforts focused on the insurance component rather than the care. Over the next decade, changes will occur regarding insurance and what in health care will be reimbursed. These changes have the potential to affect the way patients seek care, the way in which care is delivered, the role of the nurse, and the way in which quality will play an increasing role in determining the next steps in health care.

PROFESSIONAL NURSING PRACTICE: ETHICS

Ethics is an area of professional practice in which nurse managers should have a solid foundation, because it is becoming increasingly more prominent in clinical practice settings. However, it remains an area in which many nurses feel the most inadequate. This is partially because ethics is much more nebulous than are laws and regulations. In ethics, there are no right and wrong answers, just better or worse answers, and nurses seek mentorship and counseling from nurse managers when they encounter difficult situations. Thus nurse managers must have a deep understanding of ethical principles and their application.

Ethics may be distinguished from the law because ethics is internal to an individual, looks to the ultimate "good" of an individual rather than society as a whole, and concerns the "why" of one's actions. The law, comprising rules and regulations pertinent to society as a whole, is external to oneself and concerns one's actions and conduct. Ethics concerns the individual within society, whereas law concerns society as a whole. Law can be enforced through the courts, statutes, and boards of nursing, whereas ethics is enforced via ethics committees and professional codes.

Today, ethics and legal issues often become entwined, and it may be difficult to separate ethics from legal concerns. Legal principles and doctrines assist the nurse manager in decision making; ethical theories and principles are often involved in those decisions. Thus the nurse manager must be cognizant of both laws and ethics in everyday management concerns, remembering that ethical principles form the essential base of knowledge from which to proceed, rather than giving easy, straightforward answers.

Ethical Principles

Ethical principles, those incorporated daily in patient care situations, are equally paramount in the effective nurse manager's work. Ethical principles that the nurse manager should consider when making decisions include the eight items listed in Box 5-4. Each of the principles is applied in everyday clinical practice, some to a greater degree than others.

The principle of autonomy addresses personal freedom and the right to choose what will happen to one's own person. The legal doctrine of informed consent is a direct reflection of this principle. Autonomy underlies the concept of progressive discipline because the employee has the option to meet delineated expectations or take full accountability for his or her actions. This principle also underlies the nurse manager's clinical practice because autonomy is reflected in individual decision making about patient care issues and in group decision making about unit operations decisions.

The principle of beneficence states that the actions one takes should promote good. Nurse managers

BOX 5-4	ETHICAL PRINCIPLES
• Autonomy	• Justice
• Beneficence	• Paternalism
• Nonmaleficence	• Fidelity
• Veracity	• Respect for others

employ this principle when encouraging employees to seek more challenging clinical experiences or to take on additional responsibilities as a charge nurse. Progressive discipline focuses on this principle when one incorporates the employee's positive attributes and qualities in developing goals and expected outcomes.

The corollary of beneficence, the principle of non-maleficence, states that one should do no harm. For a nurse manager following this principle, performance evaluation should emphasize the employee's good qualities and give positive direction for growth. Destroying the employee's self-esteem and self-worth would be considered doing harm under this principle.

Veracity concerns telling the truth and incorporates the concept that individuals should always tell the truth. The principle also compels that the truth be told completely. Nurse managers employ this principle when they give all the facts of a situation truthfully and then assist employees to make decisions. For example, with low patient censuses, employees must be informed about potential options and then be allowed to make their own decisions about floating to other units, taking vacation time, or taking a day without pay if the institution has such a policy.

Justice is the principle of treating all persons equally and fairly. This principle usually arises in times of short supplies or when there is competition for resources or benefits. This principle is used by nurse managers when they decide which staff members will have holiday and vacation time or paid attendance at national or local conferences. The staff member's overall performance should be considered rather than who is next on the list to attend a conference or allowed to take a vacation. Justice is also encountered when deciding who should be floated to another unit/service within the institution or which staff member should be moved to a straight day position rather than remaining on a rotating schedule.

The principle of paternalism allows one person to make partial decisions for another and often is seen as a negative or undesirable principle. Paternalism, however, may be used to assist persons to make decisions when they do not have sufficient data or expertise. Paternalism becomes undesirable when the entire decision is taken from the employee. Nurse managers employ this principle in a positive manner by assisting employees in deciding major career moves and plans, helping the staff member more fully understand all aspects of a possible career change, or conversely, assisting staff members comprehend why such a potential change could impact their future growth opportunities within the organization.

Fidelity means keeping one's promises or commitments. Nurse managers abide by this principle when they follow through on any promises they have previously made to employees, such as a promised leave, a certain shift to be worked, or a promotion to a preceptor position within the unit.

Many consider the principle of respect for others as the highest principle. Respect for others acknowledges the right of individuals to make decisions and to live by these decisions. Respect for others also transcends cultural differences, gender issues, and racial

---

📖 LITERATURE PERSPECTIVE

Resource: Failla, K. R., & Stichler, J. F. (2008). Manager and staff perceptions of the manager's leadership style. *Journal of Nursing Administration, 38*(11), 480-487.

Transformational and transactional leadership theories indicate that a relationship exists between the manager's leadership style and the staff members' job satisfaction and motivation. Transformational leaders influence staff members' perceptions using the following five critical strategies:

1. Instilling the staff members' pride in the leader's vision and mission
2. Using leader behaviors to demonstrate his or her values and ethics to staff members
3. Increasing the staff members' awareness and acceptance of desired outcomes
4. Influencing staff members to think in new and more creative ways
5. Mentoring staff members and expressing appreciation when the outcomes are achieved

Conversely, transactional leaders reward staff members by giving constructive recognition for staff members' accomplishment of outcomes and by giving corrective feedback to staff members so that specific tasks are accomplished in such a way as to achieve desired outcomes. Blending these two theories of leadership leads to greater satisfaction among staff members and motivates them to achieve outcomes "beyond what they would ordinarily accomplish in any other style" (p. 481).

Implications for Practice

Nurse managers and staff need to value the benefits of both transformational and transactional leadership. Being able to move between these two approaches produces positive outcomes.

concerns and is the first principle enumerated in the American Nurses Association's *Code of Ethics for Nurses* (2001). Nurse managers positively reinforce this principle daily in their actions with employees, patients, and peers because they serve as leaders and models for staff members and others in the institution. This concept is further developed in the Literature Perspective on p. 92.

Codes of Ethics

Professional codes of ethics are formal statements that articulate values and beliefs of a given professional, serving as a standard of professional actions and reflecting the ethical principles shared by its members. Professional codes of ethics generally serve the following purposes:

- Inform the public of the minimum standards acceptable for conduct by members of the discipline and assist the public in understanding a discipline's professional responsibilities
- Outline the major ethical considerations of the profession
- Provide to its members guidelines for professional practice
- Serve as a guide for the discipline's self-regulation

The *Code of Ethics for Nurses* (ANA, 2001) should be the starting point for any nurse faced with an ethical issue. The first American nursing code was adopted in 1950, and it focused on the character of the nurse and the virtues that were essential to the profession. In 1968, the focus shifted to a duty-based ethical focus, and the current *Code of Ethics for Nurses* (ANA, 2001) has blended these duty-based ethics with a historical focus on character and virtue. The *Code of Ethics for Nurses* (ANA, 2001) has been simplified and updated so that nurses can readily understand and apply its provisions. This nine-point code guides nurses in understanding the extent of their commitment to the patient, themselves, other nurses, and the nursing profession. The code begins with addressing respect for others, as the first provision of the code refers to the "inherent dignity, worth, and uniqueness of every individual" (ANA, 2001, provision 1). Further provisions in the code assist nurses in understanding that patients, whether as individuals or as members of families, groups, or communities, are their first obligation and that nurses must not only ensure quality care but also protect the safety of these patients. Nurses and their nurse managers should ensure that the provisions of the code are incorporated into nursing care delivery in all clinical settings. Along with establishing the ethical standard for the disciplines, the nursing codes of ethics provide a basis for ethical analysis and decision making in clinical situations.

Ethical Decision-Making Framework

Ethical decision making involves reflection on the following:

- Who should make the choice
- Possible options or courses of action
- Available options
- Consequences, both good and bad, of all possible options
- Rules, obligations, and values that should direct choices
- Desired goals or outcomes

When making decisions, nurses need to combine all of these elements using an orderly, systematic, and objective method; ethical decision-making models assist in accomplishing this goal.

For most nurses, formal ethical decision-making models are considered only when complex ethical dilemmas present in clinical settings. In truth, however, nurses use ethical decision-making models each time an ethical situation arises although the decision-making model may not be acknowledged or fully appreciated. Ethical dilemmas involve situations in which a choice must be made between alternatives that an individual perceives he or she can accept and reasonably justify on a moral plane or in which there is not a more favorable or appropriate choice that dominates the situation.

Ethical decision making is always a process. To facilitate this process, the nurse manager must use all available resources, including the institutional ethics committee, and communicate with and support all those involved in the process. Some decisions are easier to reach and support. It is important to allow sufficient time for the process so that a supportable option can be reached.

Moral Distress

Nurses experience stress in clinical practice settings as they are confronted with situations involving ethical dilemmas. Moral distress most often occurs when faced with situations in which two ethical principles compete, such as when the nurse is balancing the patient's autonomy issues with attempting to do what the nurse knows is in the patient's best interest. Moral distress may occur also when the nurse manager is balancing a staff nurse's autonomy with what the nurse manager perceives to be a better solution to an ethical dilemma. Though the dilemmas are stressful, nurses must make decisions and implement those decisions.

Seen as a major issue in nursing today, moral distress is experienced when nurses cannot provide what they perceive to be best for a given patient. Examples of moral distress include constraints caused by financial pressures, limited patient care resources, disagreements among family members regarding patient interventions, and/or limitations imposed by primary healthcare providers. Moral distress may also be experienced when actions nurses perform violate their personal beliefs. The impact of moral distress can be quite serious. The American Nurses Association (2008):

> ... attributes moral distress as a significant cause of emotional suffering, possibly causing nurses to give poor nursing care, change positions frequently or leave the professional entirely ... It may be a significant contributing factor to nurses' feelings of loss of integrity and dissatisfaction with their work. It may also contribute to problems with nurses' relationships with patient and others and may affect the quality, quantity, and cost of nursing care. (paragraph 9)

Nurse managers can best assist nurses experiencing moral distress by remembering that such distress may be lessened through adequate levels of knowledge regarding nursing ethics and its application, acknowledging that such distress does occur, and serving as an advocate for nurses. In this latter role, the nurse manager advocates for improvement in conditions that may directly influence moral distress, such as additional staff during periods of high patient acuity, additional counselors to work with patients' family issues and disputes, and the implementation of ethical in-service education and/or education concerning better communication among all levels of healthcare practitioners. These positive aspects of leadership may significantly reduce the level of moral distress encountered by staff nurses and greatly increase

RESEARCH PERSPECTIVE

Resource: Cummings, G. G., Olson, K., Hayduk, L., Bakker, D., Fitch, M., Green, E., Butler, L., & Conlon, M. (2008). The relationship between nursing leadership and nurses' job satisfaction in Canadian oncology work environments. *Journal of Nursing Management, 16*, 508-518.

Nurses working in these oncology clinical practice settings are challenged by the same factors that challenge nurses in other nursing specialties, including stress, demand for physical work, lack of adequate resources, and strained relationships with other members of the healthcare team. In addition, these authors noted that more than 8% of the nursing workforce is absent each week because of illness. The study's purpose was to develop and estimate a theoretical model of work environment factors that affect these nurses' job satisfaction. Participating in the study were 515 full-time registered nurses, answering a Likert scale questionnaire that addressed features of the professional nurses' practice environment such as perception of nursing practice, quality of care, job satisfaction, and intention to leave the current job.

Demographic findings from the study showed that the majority of the sample (54.4%) were older than 45 years, 97.1% were female, 41.2% had more than 26 years of nursing experience, and 45.2% were certified in oncology nursing. Factors that most influenced a positive job satisfaction were relational leadership, positive physician/nurse relationships, nursing autonomy to make important patient care decisions, and supervisor support in managing conflict. Relational leadership, the ability of the leader to create positive relationships within the organization, had the most significant effect on all variables displaying direct effects on job satisfaction. Relational leadership predicted greater opportunities for staff development, greater perceptions of sufficient numbers of nurses to provide quality care, greater opportunities to participate in policy decisions, and greater nursing autonomy for staff nurses. Visible nursing leadership also led to a greater perception of perceived support for innovation and creativity.

Implications for Practice

Nurse managers have many avenues for creative solutions to job satisfaction. This study would suggest that if managers attended to the ability to create positive relationships, many organizational factors would be affected in a positive manner.

their job satisfaction. (See the Research Perspective above.)

Ethics Committees

With the increasing numbers of ethical dilemmas in patient situations and administrative decisions, healthcare providers are increasingly turning to hospital ethics committees for guidance. Such committees can provide both long-term and short-term assistance. Ethics committees can provide structure and guidelines for potential problems, serve as open forums for discussion, and function as true patient advocates by placing the patient at the core of the committee discussions.

To form such a committee, the involved individuals should begin as a bioethical study group so that all potential members can explore ethical principles and theories. The composition of the committee should include nurses, physicians, clergy, clinical social workers, nutritional experts, pharmacists, administrative personnel, and legal experts. Once the committee has become active, individual patients or patients' families and additional representatives of members of the healthcare delivery team may be invited to committee deliberations.

Ethics committees traditionally follow one of three distinct structures, although some institutional committees blend the three structures. The *autonomy model* facilitates decision making for competent patients. The *patient-benefit model* uses substituted judgment (what the patient would want for himself or herself if capable of making these issues known) and facilitates decision making for the incompetent patient. The *social justice model* considers broad social issues and is accountable to the overall institution.

In most settings, the ethics committee already exists because there are complex issues dividing healthcare workers. In many centers, ethical rounds, conducted weekly or monthly, allow staff members who may later become involved in ethical decision making to begin reviewing all the issues and to become more comfortable with ethical issues and their resolution.

Blending Ethical and Legal Issues

Blending legal demands with ethics is a challenge for nursing, and no case better portrays this type of difficult decision making than does the case of Theresa (Terri) M. Schiavo. Ms. Schiavo suffered a cardiac arrest in February 1990, sustaining a period of approximately 11 minutes when she was anoxic. She was resuscitated and, at the insistence of her husband, was intubated, placed on a ventilator, and eventually received a tracheotomy. The cause of her cardiac arrest was determined to be a severe electrolyte imbalance that was directly caused by an eating disorder. In the 6 years preceding the cardiac event, Ms. Schiavo

had lost approximately 140 pounds, going from 250 to 110 pounds.

During the first 2 months after her cardiac arrest, Ms. Schiavo was in a coma. She then regained some wakefulness and was eventually diagnosed as being in persistent vegetative state (PVS). She was successfully weaned from the ventilator and was able to swallow her saliva, both reflexive behaviors. However, she was not able to eat food or drink liquids, which is characteristic of PVS. A permanent feeding tube was placed so that she could receive nutrition and hydration.

Throughout the early years of her PVS, there was no challenge to the diagnosis or to the appointment of her husband as her legal guardian. Four years after her cardiac arrest, a successful lawsuit was filed against a fertility physician who failed to detect her electrolyte imbalance. A judgment of $300,000 went to her husband for loss of companionship and $700,000 was placed in a court-managed trust fund to maintain and provide care for Ms. Schiavo.

Sometime after this successful lawsuit, the close family relationship that Ms. Schiavo's husband and her parents had began to erode, and the public first became aware of Ms. Schiavo's plight. As her court-appointed guardian noted (Wolfson, 2005):

> Thereafter, what is for millions of Americans a profoundly private matter catapulted a close, loving family into an internationally watched blood feud. The end product was a most public death for a very private individual … Theresa was by all accounts a very shy, fun loving, and sweet woman who loved her husband and her parents very much. The family breach and public circus would have been anathema to her. (p. 17)

The court battles regarding the removal or retention of her feeding tube were numerous. There was adequate medical and legal evidence to show that Ms. Schiavo had been correctly diagnosed and that she would not have wanted to be kept alive by artificial means. Laws in the state of Florida, where Ms. Schiavo was a patient, allowed the removal of tubal nutrition and hydration in patients with PVS. The feeding tube was removed and later reinstated following a court order.

In October 2003, there was a second removal of the feeding tube after a higher court overturned the lower court decision that had caused the feeding tube to be reinserted. With this second removal, the Florida legislature passed what has become to be known as *Terri's Law.* This law gave the Florida governor the right to demand the feeding tube be reinserted and also appoint a special guardian to review the entire case. The special guardian ad litem was appointed in October 2003. Terri's Law was later declared unconstitutional by the Florida Supreme Court, and the U.S. Supreme Court refused to overrule their decision.

In early 2005, during the last weeks of Ms. Schiavo's life, the U.S. Congress attempted to move the issue to the federal rather than Florida state court system. This fiasco ended with the Federal District Court in Florida and the 11th Circuit Court of Appeals ruling that there was insufficient evidence to create a new trial, and the U.S. Supreme Court refused to review the findings of these two lower courts (Wolfson, 2005). Ms. Schiavo died on March 31, 2005; she was 41 years old.

Whichever side of the case one supported, the plight of Terri Schiavo created numerous ethical concerns for the nurses caring for her and for the nurse managers in the clinical setting. Issues that created these conflicts ranged from working with feuding family members, to multiple media personnel attempting to cover the story, to constant editorial and news stories invading the privacy of this individual, to masses of people lined at the borders of the hospice center insisting that she be fed, to individual emotions about the correctness of either keeping or removing the feeding tube. One issue remains clear. The nurse managers and nurses caring for this particular patient had a legal obligation to either remove or reinsert the feeding tube based on the prevailing court decision or legislative act. Their individual reflections about the correctness or justice of such court decrees were secondary to the prevailing court orders.

Nurse managers should ensure that nurses whose ethical values differ from court orders are given opportunities to voice their concerns and feelings, mechanisms for requesting reassignment, and time for quiet reflection. Although there can be no deviance from one's legal obligation, the nurse manager must ensure that the emotional and psychological well-being of those he or she supervises are also recognized. Merely acknowledging that such discord can occur and allowing positive means to express this concern may be the best solution in handling these difficult legal and ethical patient situations.

Future Ethical Concerns for Nurses

Issues of concern in the near future involve autonomy and independent practice among nurses, quality of care in home and community settings, and development of nurses as leaders in the healthcare delivery field. Issues that continue to permeate ethical concerns for nurses include the patient's right to refuse health care; issues surrounding death and dying including the issues of hydration and nutrition for patients in persistent vegetative states; nurses' ability to be patient advocates in today's healthcare structure; and the ability to perform competent, quality nursing care in a system that continuously rewards cost-saving measures rather than quality healthcare delivery and that employs increasingly fewer professional nurses. Nursing must begin to address potential issues in a timely manner, particularly as the nursing shortage continues to escalate, because these issues will become more prominent in the future. As with ethical dilemmas in patient care, the more expertise and time one has to resolve issues, usually, the better the outcome. The Evidence section on p. 97 reinforces this need for nurse leaders to be proficient in ethical decision making.

THE SOLUTION

Realizing there are many components to address in this situation, I began by assessing current practices related to charge nurses' orientation and initiated a staff satisfaction survey addressing this topic. Ideas related to succession planning, a formal orientation process, and shared decision making were discussed at staff meetings. Resoundingly, the message from staff was the need to develop a more formal charge nurse orientation. I then sat down with the nurse and had a crucial conversation, first assessing how the nurse

THE SOLUTION—cont'd

viewed her own practice and then providing feedback based on the manager's and fellow co-worker's observations. I discussed what qualities were necessary for the charge nurse role, including expertise in safe patient care, the ability to prioritize, communication with staff at all levels, and the ability to view the big picture. Throughout this conversation, I focused on techniques that did not demean the nurse, but acknowledged her unique skill set and how these attributes would be incorporated into a performance improvement plan. It became apparent through my observation and the nurse's comments that this nurse had an innate quality for teaching and desire to give back to the nursing community. Together we developed a specific plan that included taking classes that focused on clinical practice updates, developing organizational skills, enhancing communication, and shadowing a current clinical instructor. This conversation gave the nurse a sense of empowerment and autonomy as well as a specific plan that would likely better her current nursing practice. I realized I used the ethical principles of paternalism, beneficence, justice, and respect for others in a most positive manner.

—*Cynthia Fahy*

Would this be a suitable approach for you? Why?

THE EVIDENCE

Many of the issues challenging nurse mangers and leaders in today's environment involve conflict resolution, most often involving ethical conflicts and dilemmas. "The evidence of a leader is the ability to make ethical decisions and to lead the organization along a path of moral integrity" (Piper, 2007, p. 249). This demands that nurse managers and leaders have knowledge of the history of ethics so that they can have a better understanding of ethics within society and healthcare organizations and can better assist members of the healthcare team in making ethical decisions. Preventing ethical conflicts in the future will depend on the manager's knowledge and application of ethical principles, the ability to assert leadership and role modeling, periodic ethics assessment within the institution, support for ethical decision making by higher administration and the governing board of the institution, and the development of ethical policies within the institution.

Nurses need to begin now to look at the issues, professional values, and expectations they face and decide the issues for which they will fight and those that are acceptable as they are. Once these issues are identified, strategies for promoting quality nursing care can be delineated.

NEED TO KNOW NOW

- Understand the legal ramifications of the nurse manager role, especially in terms of federal and state laws. Query the hospital legal staff, administration, and/or the state board of nursing as needed.
- Remember that there are no right and wrong answers in ethical situations, merely better or worse solutions. Consider all aspects and consult with others before proceeding if there are unanswered questions.
- If legal and ethical issues are contradictory, legal aspects are enacted first.

CHAPTER CHECKLIST

This chapter explores multiple legal and ethical issues as they pertain to managing and leading in nursing. Legal areas that nurse managers must understand include the importance of nurse practice acts, elements of negligence and malpractice with particular emphasis on areas of potential liability for nurse managers, informed consent, and selected federal and state employment laws. Ethical areas of concern include ethical theories and principles, codes of ethics, and ethics committees. The chapter concludes with a discussion of a relevant case in which legal and ethical issues overlapped.

- Additional key concepts for nurse managers include the following:
  - Privacy and confidentiality
  - Reporting statutes

- Staffing concerns
- Informed consent issues, including rights of research participants
- Decision-making models
- Resource availability
- Guidelines for encouraging a professional and satisfying work setting

TIPS FOR INCORPORATING LEGAL AND ETHICAL ISSUES IN PRACTICE SETTINGS

- Read the state nurse practice act, ensuring compliance with the allowable scope of practice.
- Apply legal principles in all healthcare settings.

- Understand and follow federal employment laws.
- Follow the *Code of Ethics for Nurses* (ANA, 2001) in all aspects of healthcare delivery.

REFERENCES

Age Discrimination in Employment Act of 1967, P.L. 90-202, December 15, 1967.

American Nurses Association (ANA). (1988). *Standards for nurse administrators*. Kansas City, Mo: Author.

American Nurses Association (ANA). (2001). *Code of ethics for nurses with interpretive statements*. Washington, DC: Author.

American Nurses Association (ANA). (2008). *Principles for delegation*. Washington, DC: Author.

American Nurses Association (ANA). (2009). *Nurse staffing plans and ratios*. Washington, DC: Author. Retrieved October 1, 2009, from www.safestaffingsaveslives.org//WhatisANADoing/StateLegislation/StaffingPlansandRatios.aspx.

Americans with Disabilities Act (ADA) of 1990. (1990). 42 U.S.C. § 12101 *et seq.*

Andrus, M. R., & Roth, M. T. (2002). Health literacy: A review. *Pharmacotherapy*, 22(3), 282-302.

Bunn-Penn v. Southern Regional Medical Corporation, 488 S.E. 2d. 747 (Ga. App., 1997).

Christus Spohn v. De La Fuente, WL 2323989 (Tex. App., August 16, 2007).

Civil Rights Act of 1964, § 703 et seq. (1978).

Civil Rights Act of 1991, P.L. 102-166, November 21, 1991.

Cody v. Cigna Healthcare of St. Louis, Inc., 139 F.3d 595 (8th Cir., 1998).

Cummings, G. G., Olson, K., Hayduk, L., Bakker, D., Fitch, M., Green, E., Butler, L., & Conlon, M. (2008). The relationship between nursing leadership and nurses' job satisfaction in Canadian oncology work environments. *Journal of Nursing Management*, 16, 508-518.

Dovenmuehler v. St. Cloud Hospital, WL 4233160 (8th Cir., December 4, 2007).

Equal Employment Opportunity Commission v. Catholic Healthcare West, WL 141917 (C.D. Cal., January 3, 2008).

Equal Pay Act of 1963, P.L. 88-38, June 10, 1963.

Failla, K. R., & Stichler, J. F. (2008). Manager and staff perceptions of the manager's leadership style. *Journal of Nursing Administration*, 38(11), 480-487.

Fairfax Nursing Home, Inc. v. Department of Health and Human Services, 123 S. Ct. 901, 71 USLW 3471, 2003 WL 98478 (United States, January 13, 2003).

Family and Medical Leave Act of 1993, P.L. 103-103, February 5, 1993.

Family and Medical Leave Amended Act of 2008, P.L. 110-181, January 28, 2008.

Code of Federal Regulations (CFR), Sec. 46.111, 46.101(b), 46.110, and 46.116 (1991).

Code of Federal Regulations (CFR), Sec. 46.401 et seq. (1998).

Garrett v. University of Alabama, 2007 WL 3378398 (11th Cir., November 16, 2007).

Health Insurance Portability and Accountability Act (HIPAA) of 1996. P.L. 104-191, 1996.

Hill, K. (2006). Collaboration is a competency! *Journal of Nursing Administration*, 36(9), 390-392.

Howard v. North Mississippi Medical Center, 939 F. Supp. 505 (N.D. Miss., 1996).

Jones v. Kerrville State Hospital, 142 F. 3rd 263 (5th Cir., 1998).

Laurin v. Providence Hospital and Massachusetts Nurses Association, 150 F.3d 52 (1st Cir., 1998).

Maniaci, M. J., Heckman, M. G., & Dawson, N. L. (2008). Functional health literacy and understanding of medications at discharge. *Mayo Clinical Proceedings*, 83(5), 554-558.

Mauro v. Borgess Medical Center, 4:94 CV 05 (Mich., 1995).

Nicholson v. West Penn Allegheny Health System, WL 4863910 (W.D. Penn., October 23, 2007).

Occupational Safety and Health Act of 1970, *Code of Federal Regulations*, Title 29, Chapter XVII, Part 1910, 1970.

O'Shea v. State of New York, WL 1516492 (N.Y. Ct. Cl., January 22, 2007).

Pender v. Natchitoches Parish Hospital, WL 21017235 (La. App., May 7, 2003).

Piper, L. E. (2007). Ethics: The evidence of leadership. *Health Care Manager, 26*(3), 249-254.

Potter, P., & Grant, E. (2004). Understanding RN and unlicensed assistive personnel working relationships in designing care delivery strategies. *Journal of Nursing Administration, 34*(1), 19-25.

Safe Nurse Staffing Legislation, Washington State HB 3123 (March, 2008).

Sabol v. Richmond Heights General Hospital, 676 N. E.2d 958 (Ohio App. 1996).

Squibb v. Memorial Medical Center, WL 23256173 (7th Cir., August 16, 2007).

Storkamp v. Geren, WL 360991 (E.D. N.C., February 8, 2008).

Timmons, L. (2009). Creating a no-lift, no-transfer environment in the OR. *AORN Journal, 89*(4), 733-736.

Trombley v. Southwestern Vermont Medical Center, 738 A. 2d 103 (Vt., 1999).

Vierra v. Wayne Memorial Hospital, WL 288665 (3rd Cir., February 8, 2006).

Watkins v. Unemployment Compensation Board of Review, 689 A.2d 1019 (Pa. Commonwealth, 1997).

Wellstar Health System, Inc. v. Green, WL 31324127 (Ga. App., October 18, 2002).

Wendeln v. Beatrice Manor, Inc., WL 903598 (Neb., April 7, 2006).

Wolfson, J. (2005). Erring on the side of Theresa Schiavo: Reflections of the special guardian ad Litem. *The Hastings Center Report, 35*(3), 16-19.

Zamudio v. Patia, 956 F. Supp. 803 (N.D. Ill., 1997).

SUGGESTED READINGS

Baum, N. M., Gollust, S. E., Goold, S. D., & Jacobson, P. D. (2009). Ethical issues in public health practice in Michigan. *American Journal of Public Health, 99*(2), 369-371.

Cohen, J. S., & Erickson, J. M. Ethical dilemmas and moral distress in oncology nursing practice. *Clinical Journal of Oncology Nursing, 10*(6), 775-780.

Dembe, A. E. (2009). Ethical issues relating to the health effects of long working hours. *Journal of Business Ethics, 84*(Suppl. 1), 151-165.

Locke, A. (2008). Developmental coaching: A bridge to organizational success. *Creative Nursing, 14*(3), 102-110.

Randolph, S. A. (2006). Developing policies and procedures. *AAOHN Journal: Official Journal of the American Association of Occupational Health Nurses, 5*(11), 501-504.

Watters, S. (2009). Shared leadership: Taking flight. *The Journal of Nursing Administration, 39*(1), 26-29.

Wlody, G. S. (2007). Nursing management and organizational ethics in the intensive care unit. *Critical Care Medicine, 35*(Suppl. 2), S29-S35.

6

Making Decisions and Solving Problems

Rose Aguilar Welch

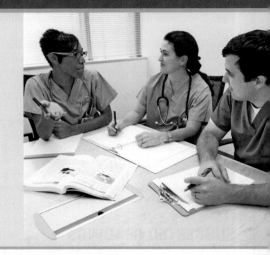

This chapter describes the key concepts related to problem solving and decision making. The primary steps of the problem-solving and decision-making processes, as well as analytical tools used for these processes, are explored. Moreover, strategies for individual or group problem solving and decision making are presented.

OBJECTIVES

- Apply a decision-making format to list options to solve a problem, identify the pros and cons of each option, rank the options, and select the best option.
- Evaluate the effect of faulty information gathering on a decision-making experience.
- Analyze the decision-making style of a nurse leader/manager.
- Critique resources on the Internet that focus on critical thinking, problem solving, and decision making.

TERMS TO KNOW

autocratic	decision making	participative
creativity	democratic	problem solving
critical thinking	optimizing decision	satisficing decision

THE CHALLENGE

Vickie Lemmon, RN, MSN
Director of Clinical Strategies and Operations, WellPoint, Inc.,
Ventura, California

Healthcare managers today are faced with numerous and complex issues that pertain to providing quality services for patients within a resource-scarce environment. Stress levels among staff can escalate when problems are not resolved, leading to a decrease in morale, productivity, and quality service. This was the situation I encountered in my previous job as administrator for California Children Services (CCS). When I began my tenure as the new CCS administrator, staff expressed frustration and dissatisfaction with staffing, workload, and team communications. This was evidenced by high staff turnover, lack of teamwork, customer complaints, unmet deadlines for referral and enrollment cycle times, and poor documentation. The team was in crisis, characterized by in-fighting, blaming, lack of respectful communication, and lack of commitment to program goals and objectives. I had not worked as a case manager in this program. It was hard for me to determine how to address the problems the staff presented to me. I wanted to be fair but thought that I did not have enough information to make immediate changes. My challenge was to lead this team to greater compliance with state-mandated performance measures.

What do you think you would do if you were this nurse?

INTRODUCTION

Problem solving and decision making are essential skills for effective nursing practice. Carol Huston (2008) identified "expert decision-making skills" as one of the eight vital leadership competencies for 2020. These processes not only are involved in managing and delivering care but also are essential for engaging in planned change. Myriad technologic, social, political, and economic changes have dramatically affected health care and nursing. Increased patient acuity, shorter hospital stays, shortage of healthcare providers, increased technology, greater emphasis on quality and patient safety, and the continuing shift from inpatient to ambulatory and home health care are some of the changes that require nurses to make rational and valid decisions. Moreover, increased diversity in patient populations, employment settings, and types of healthcare providers demands efficient and effective decision making and problem solving. More emphasis is now placed on involving patients in decision making and problem solving and using multidisciplinary teams to achieve results.

Nurses must possess the basic knowledge and skills required for effective problem solving and decision making. These competencies are especially important for nurses with leadership and management responsibilities.

DEFINITIONS

Problem solving and *decision making* are not synonymous terms. However, the processes for engaging in both processes are similar. Both skills require critical thinking, which is a high-level cognitive process, and both can be improved with practice.

Decision making is a purposeful and goal-directed effort that uses a systematic process to choose among options. Not all decision making begins with a problem situation. Instead, the hallmark of decision making is the identification and selection of options or alternatives.

Problem solving, which includes a decision-making step, is focused on trying to solve an immediate problem, which can be viewed as a gap between "what is" and "what should be."

Effective problem solving and decision making are predicated on an individual's ability to think critically. Although critical thinking has been defined in numerous ways, Scriven and Paul (2007) refer to it as " the intellectually disciplined process of actively and skillfully conceptualizing, applying, analyzing, synthesizing, and/or evaluating information gathered from, or generated by, observation, experience, reflection, reasoning, or communication, as a guide to belief and action." Effective critical thinkers are self-aware individuals who strive to improve their reasoning abilities by asking "why," "what," or "how." A nurse who questions why a patient is restless is thinking critically. Compare the analytical abilities of a nurse who assumes a patient is restless because of anxiety related to an upcoming procedure with those of a nurse who asks if there could be another explanation and proceeds to investigate possible causes. It is important for nurse leaders and managers to assess staff members' ability to think critically and enhance their knowledge and skills through staff-development programs, coaching, and role modeling. Establishing a positive and motivating work environment can enhance attitudes and dispositions to think critically.

Creativity is essential for the generation of options or solutions. Creative individuals can conceptualize new and innovative approaches to a problem or issue by being more flexible and independent in their thinking. It takes just one person to plant a seed for new ideas to generate.

The model depicted in Figure 6-1 demonstrates the relationship among related concepts such as professional judgment, decision making, problem solving, creativity, and critical thinking. Sound clinical judgment requires critical or reflective thinking. Critical thinking is the concept that interweaves and links the others. An individual, through the application of critical-thinking skills, engages in problem solving and decision making in an environment that can promote or inhibit these skills. It is the nurse leader's and manager's task to model these skills and promote them in others.

DECISION MAKING

This section presents an overview of concepts related to decision models, decision-making styles, factors affecting decision making, group decision making (advantages and challenges), and strategies and tools.

The phases of the decision-making process include defining objectives, generating options, identifying advantages and disadvantages of each option, ranking the options, selecting the option most likely to achieve the predefined objectives, implementing the option, and evaluating the result. Box 6-1 contains a form that can be used to complete these steps.

A poor-quality decision is likely if the objectives are not clearly identified or if they are inconsistent with the values of the individual or organization. Lewis Carroll illustrates the essential step of defining the goal, purpose, or objectives in the following excerpt from *Alice's Adventures in Wonderland:*

> One day Alice came to a fork in the road and saw a Cheshire Cat in a tree. "Which road do I take?" she asked. His response was a question: "Where do you want to go?" "I don't know," Alice answered. "Then," said the cat, "it doesn't matter."

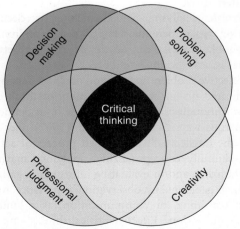

FiGURE 6-1 Problem-solving and decision-making model.

BOX 6-1   DECISION-MAKING FORMAT

Objective: _____

Options	Advantages	Disadvantages	Ranking

Add more rows as necessary. Rank priority of options, with "1" being most preferred. Select the best option.

Implementation plan: _____
_____

Evaluation plan: _____
_____

Decision Models

The decision model that a nurse uses depends on the circumstances. Is the situation routine and predictable or complex and uncertain? Is the goal of the decision to make a decision conservatively that is just good enough or one that is optimal?

If the situation is fairly routine, nurse leaders and managers can use a normative or prescriptive approach. Agency policy, standard procedures, and analytical tools can be applied to situations that are structured and in which options are known.

If the situation is subjective, non-routine, and unstructured or if outcomes are unknown or unpredictable, the nurse leader and manager may need to take a different approach. In this case, a descriptive or behavioral approach is required. More information will need to be gathered to address the situation effectively. Creativity, experience, and group process are useful in dealing with the unknown. In the business world, Camillus described complex problems that are difficult to describe or resolve as "wicked" (as cited in Huston, 2008). This term is apt in describing the issues that nurse leaders face. In these situations, it is especially important for nurse leaders to seek expert opinion and involve key stakeholders.

Another strategy is satisficing. In this approach, the decision maker selects the solution that minimally meets the objective or standard for a decision. It allows for quick decisions and may be the most appropriate when time is an issue.

Optimizing is a decision style in which the decision maker selects the option that is best, based on an analysis of the pros and cons associated with each option. A better decision is more likely using this approach, although it does take longer to arrive at a decision.

For example, a nursing student approaching graduation is contemplating seeking employment in one of three acute care hospitals located within a 40-mile radius of home. The choices are a medium-size, not-for-profit community hospital; a large, corporate-owned hospital; and a county facility. A satisficing decision might result if the student nurse picked the hospital that offered a decent salary and benefit packet or the one closest to home. However, an optimizing decision is more likely to occur if the student nurse lists the pros and cons of each acute care hospital being considered such as salary, benefits, opportunities for advancement, staff development, and mentorship programs.

Decision-Making Styles

The decision-making style of a nurse manager is similar to the leadership style that the manager is likely to use. A manager who leans toward an autocratic style may choose to make decisions independent of the input or participation of others. This has been referred to as the "decide and announce" approach, an authoritative style. On the other hand, a manager who uses a democratic or participative approach to management involves the appropriate personnel in the decision-making process. It is imperative for managers to involve nursing personnel in making decisions that affect patient care. One mechanism for doing so is by seeking nursing representation on various committees or task forces. Participative management has been shown to increase work performance and productivity, decrease employee turnover, and enhance employee satisfaction.

Any decision style can be used appropriately or inappropriately. Like the tenets of situational leadership theory, the situation and circumstances should dictate which decision-making style is most appropriate. A Code Blue is not the time for managers to democratically solicit volunteers for chest compressions!

The autocratic method results in more rapid decision making and is appropriate in crisis situations or when groups are likely to accept this type of decision style. However, followers are generally more supportive of consultative and group approaches. Although these approaches take more time, they are more appropriate when conflict is likely to occur, when the problem is unstructured, or when the manager does not have the knowledge or skills to solve the problem.

EXERCISE 6-1

Interview colleagues about their most preferred decision-making model and style. What barriers or obstacles to effective decision making have your colleagues encountered? What strategies are used to increase the effectiveness of the decisions made? Based on your interview, is the style effective? Why or why not?

Factors Affecting Decision Making

Numerous factors affect individuals and groups in the decision-making process. Tanner (2006) conducted an extensive review of the literature to develop a Clinical Judgment Model. Out of the research, she concluded that five principle factors influence decision making. (See the Literature Perspective below.)

Internal and external factors can influence how the situation is perceived. Internal factors include variables such as the decision maker's physical and emotional state, personal philosophy, biases, values, interests, experience, knowledge, attitudes, and risk-seeking or risk-avoiding behaviors. External factors include environmental conditions, time, and resources. Decision-making options are externally limited when time is short or when the environment is characterized by a "we've always done it this way" attitude.

 LITERATURE PERSPECTIVE

Resource: Tanner, C. A. (2006). Thinking like a nurse: A research-based model of clinical judgment in nursing. *Journal of Nursing Education, 45*(6), 204-211.

Tanner engaged in an extensive review of 200 studies focusing on clinical judgment and clinical decision making to derive a model of clinical judgment that can be used as a framework for instruction. The first review summarized 120 articles and was published in 1998. The 2006 article reviewed an additional 71 studies published since 1998. Based on an analysis of the entire set of articles, Tanner proposed five conclusions which are listed below. The reader is referred to the article for detailed explanation of each of the five conclusions.

The author considers clinical judgment as a "problem-solving activity." She notes that the terms "clinical judgment," "problem solving," "decision making," and "critical thinking" are often used interchangeably. For the purpose of aiding in the development of the model, Tanner defined clinical judgment as actions taken based on the assessment of the patient's needs. Clinical reasoning is the process by which nurses make their judgments (e.g., the decision-making process of selecting the most appropriate option) (Tanner, 2006, p. 204):

1. Clinical judgments are more influenced by what nurses bring to the situation than the objective data about the situation at hand.
2. Sound clinical judgment rests to some degree on knowing the patient and his or her typical pattern of responses, as well as an engagement with the patient and his or her concerns.
3. Clinical judgments are influenced by the context in which the situation occurs and the culture of the nursing care unit.
4. Nurses use a variety of reasoning patterns alone or in combination.
5. Reflection on practice is often triggered by a breakdown in clinical judgment and is critical for the development of clinical knowledge and improvement in clinical reasoning.

The Clinical Judgment Model developed through the review of the literature involves four steps that are similar to problem-solving and decision-making steps described in this chapter. The model starts with a phase called "Noticing." In this phase, the nurse comes to expect certain responses resulting from knowledge gleaned from similar patient situations, experiences, and knowledge. External factors influence nurses in this phase such as the complexity of the environment and values and typical practices within the unit culture.

The second phase of the model is "Interpreting," during which the nurse understands the situation that requires a response. The nurse employs various reasoning patterns to make sense of the issue and to derive an appropriate action plan.

The third phase is "Responding," during which the nurse decides on the best option for handling the situation. This is followed by the fourth phase, "Reflecting," during which the nurse assesses the patient's responses to the actions taken.

Tanner emphasized that "reflection-in-action" and "reflection-on-action" are major processes required in the model. Reflection-in-action is real-time reflection on the patient's responses to nursing action with modifications to the plan based on the ongoing assessment. On the other hand, reflection-on-action is a review of the experience, which promotes learning for future similar experiences.

Nurse educators and managers can employ this model with new and experienced nurses to aid in understanding thought processes involved in decision making. As Tanner (2006) so eloquently concludes, "If we, as nurse educators, help our students understand and develop as moral agents, advance their clinical knowledge through expert guidance and coaching, and become habitual in reflection-on-practice, they will have learned to think like a nurse" (p. 210).

Implications for Practice

Nurse educators and managers can employ this model with new and experienced nurses to aid in understanding thought processes involved in decision making. For example, students and practicing nurses can be encouraged to maintain reflective journals to record observations and impressions from clinical experiences. In clinical post-conferences or staff development meetings, the nurse educator and manager can engage them in applying to their lived experiences the five conclusions Tanner proposed. The ultimate goal of analyzing their decisions and decision-making processes is to improve clinical judgment, problem-solving, decision-making, and critical-thinking skills.

Values affect all aspects of decision making, from the statement of the problem/issue through the evaluation. Values, determined by one's cultural, social, and philosophical background, provide the foundation for one's ethical stance. The steps for engaging in ethical decision making are similar to the steps described earlier; however, alternatives or options identified in the decision-making process are evaluated with the use of ethical resources. Resources that can facilitate ethical decision making include institutional policy; principles such as autonomy, nonmaleficence, beneficence, veracity, paternalism, respect, justice, and fidelity; personal judgment; trusted coworkers; institutional ethics committees; and legal precedent.

Certain personality factors, such as self-esteem and self-confidence, affect whether one is willing to take risks in solving problems or making decisions. Keynes (2008) asserts that individuals may be influenced based on social pressures. For example, are you inclined to make decisions to satisfy people to whom you are accountable or from whom you feel social pressure?

Characteristics of an effective decision maker include courage, a willingness to take risks, self-awareness, energy, creativity, sensitivity, and flexibility. Ask yourself, "Do I prefer to let others make the decisions? Am I more comfortable in the role of 'follower' than leader? If so, why?"

EXERCISE 6-2

Identify a current or past situation that involved resource allocation, end-of-life issues, conflict among healthcare providers or patient/family/significant others, or some other ethical dilemma. Describe how the internal and external factors previously described influenced the decision options, the option selected, and the outcome.

Group Decision Making

There are two primary criteria for effective decision making. First, the decision must be of a high quality; that is, it achieves the predefined goals, objectives, and outcomes. Second, those who are responsible for its implementation must accept the decision.

Higher-quality decisions are more likely to result if groups are involved in the problem-solving and decision-making process. In reality, with the increased focus on quality and safety, decisions cannot be made alone. When individuals are allowed input into the process, they tend to function more productively and the quality of the decision is generally superior. Taking ownership of the process and outcome provides a smoother transition. Multidisciplinary teams should be used in the decision-making process, especially if the issue, options, or outcome involves other disciplines.

Research findings suggest that groups are more likely to be effective if members are actively involved, the group is cohesive, communication is encouraged, and members demonstrate some understanding of the group process. In deciding to use the group process for decision making, it is important to consider group size and composition. If the group is too small, a limited number of options will be generated and fewer points of view expressed. Conversely, if the group is too large, it may lack structure, and consensus becomes more difficult. Homogeneous groups may be more compatible; however, heterogeneous groups may be more successful in problem solving. Research has demonstrated that the most productive groups are those that are moderately cohesive. In other words, divergent thinking is useful to create the best decision.

For groups to be able to work effectively, the group facilitator or leader should carefully select members on the basis of their knowledge and skills in decision making and problem solving. Individuals who are aggressive, are authoritarian, or manifest self-oriented behaviors tend to decrease the effectiveness of groups.

The nurse leader or manager should provide a nonthreatening and positive environment in which group members are encouraged to participate actively. Using tact and diplomacy, the facilitator can control aggressive individuals who tend to monopolize the discussion and can encourage more passive individuals to contribute by asking direct, open-ended questions. Providing positive feedback such as "You raised a good point," protecting members and their suggestions from attack, and keeping the group focused on the task are strategies that create an environment conducive to problem solving.

Advantages of Group Decision Making

The advantages of group decision making are numerous. The adage "two heads are better than one" illustrates that when individuals with different knowledge, skills, and resources collaborate to solve a problem or make a decision, the likelihood of a quality outcome is increased. More ideas can be generated by groups than by individuals functioning alone. In addition, when followers are directly involved in this process, they are more apt to accept the decision, because they have an increased sense of ownership or commitment to the decision. Implementing solutions becomes easier when individuals have been actively involved in the decision-making process. Involvement can be enhanced by making information readily available to the appropriate personnel, requesting input, establishing committees and task forces with broad representation, and using group decision-making techniques.

The group leader must establish with the participants what decision rule will be followed. Will the group strive to achieve consensus, or will the majority rule? In determining which decision rule to use, the group leader should consider the necessity for quality and acceptance of the decision. Achieving both a high-quality and an acceptable decision is possible, but it requires more involvement and approval from individuals affected by the decision.

Groups will be more committed to an idea if it is derived by consensus rather than as an outcome of individual decision making or majority rule. Consensus requires that all participants agree to go along with the decision. Although achieving consensus requires considerable time, it results in both high-quality and high-acceptance decisions and reduces the risk of sabotage.

Majority rule can be used to compromise when 100% agreement cannot be achieved. This method saves time, but the solution may only partially achieve the goals of quality and acceptance. In addition, majority rule carries certain risks. First, if the informal group leaders happen to fall in the minority opinion, they may not support the decision of the majority. Certain members may go so far as to build coalitions to gain support for their position and block the majority choice. After all, the majority may represent only 51% of the group. In addition, group members may support the position of the formal leader, although they do not agree with the decision, because they fear reprisal or they wish to obtain the leader's approval. In general, as the importance of the decision increases, so does the percentage of group members required to approve it.

To secure the support of the group, the leader should maintain open communication with those affected by the decision and be honest about the advantages and disadvantages of the decision. The leader should also demonstrate how the advantages outweigh the disadvantages, suggest ways the unwanted outcomes can be minimized, and be available to assist when necessary.

Challenges of Group Decision Making

Although group problem solving and decision making have distinct advantages, involving groups also carries certain disadvantages and may not be appropriate in all situations. As previously stated, group decision making requires more time. In some situations, this may not be appropriate, especially in a crisis situation requiring prompt decisions.

Another disadvantage of group decision making relates to unequal power among group members. Dominant personality types may influence the more passive or powerless group members to conform to their points of view. Furthermore, individuals may expend considerable time and energy defending their positions, resulting in the primary objective of the group effort being lost.

Groups may be more concerned with maintaining group harmony than engaging in active discussion on the issue and generating creative ideas to address it. Group members who manifest a "groupthink" mentality are so concerned with avoiding conflict and supporting their leader and other members that important issues or concerns are not raised. Failure to bring up options, explore conflict, or challenge the status quo results in ineffective group functioning and decision outcomes.

Strategies

Strategies to minimize the problems encountered with group problem solving and decision making include decision-making techniques, such as brainstorming, nominal group techniques, focus groups, and the Delphi technique.

Brainstorming can be an effective method for generating a large volume of creative options. Often, the premature critiquing of ideas stifles creativity and idea generation. When members use inflammatory statements, euphemistically referred to as *killer phrases,* the usual response is for members to stop contributing. Some killer phrases are "It will never work," "Administration won't go for it," "What a dumb idea," "It's not in the budget," "If it ain't broke, don't fix it," and "We tried that before."

The hallmark of brainstorming is to list all ideas as stated without critique or discussion. The group leader or facilitator should encourage people to tag onto or spin off ideas from those already suggested. One idea may be piggybacked on others. Ideas should not be judged, nor should the relative merits or disadvantages of the ideas be discussed at this time. The goal is to generate ideas, no matter how seemingly unrealistic or absurd. It is important for the group leader or facilitator to cut off criticism and be alert for nonverbal behaviors signaling disapproval. Because the emphasis is on the volume of ideas generated, not necessarily the quality, solutions may be superficial and fail to solve the problem. Group brainstorming also takes longer, and the logistics of getting people together may pose a problem. If the facilitator allows the group to establish the rules for discussion, the aspects that stymie an open discussion often are eliminated by the group's norms or rules of participation.

The nominal group technique allows group members the opportunity to provide input into the decision-making process. Participants are asked to not talk to each other as they write down their ideas to solve a predefined problem or issue. After a period of silent generation of ideas, generally no more than 10 minutes, each member is asked to share an idea, which is displayed on a chalkboard or flip chart. Comments and elaboration are not allowed during this phase. Each member takes a turn sharing an idea until all ideas are presented, after which, discussion is allowed. Members may "pass" if they have exhausted their list of ideas. During the next step, ideas are clarified and the merits of each idea are discussed. In the third and final step, each member privately assigns a priority rank to each option. The solution chosen is the option that receives the highest ranking by the majority of participants. The advantage of this technique is that it allows equal participation among members and minimizes the influence of dominant personalities. The disadvantages of this method are that it is time-consuming and requires advance prep-

aration. A similar process can be facilitated via the use of web conferencing technologies.

The purpose of focus groups is to explore issues and generate information. Focus groups can be used to identify problems or to evaluate the effects of an intervention. The groups meet face-to-face to discuss issues. Under the direction of a moderator or facilitator, the participants are able to validate or disagree with ideas expressed. Depending on the purpose of a focus group, it may be helpful for an objective individual to facilitate the discussion (e.g., someone other than the manager). Because the interaction is face-to-face, potential disadvantages include the logistics of getting people together, time, and issues revolving around group dynamics already mentioned. Nevertheless, if managed effectively, the experience can yield valuable information.

Another group decision-making strategy is the Delphi technique. It involves systematically collecting and summarizing opinions and judgments from respondents, such as expert panels, on a particular issue through interviews, surveys, or questionnaires. Opinions of the respondents are repeatedly fed back to them with a request to provide more refined opinions and rationales on the issue or matter under consideration. Between rounds, the results are tabulated and analyzed so that the findings can be reported to the participants. This allows the participants to reconsider their responses. The goal is to achieve a consensus.

There are different variations on the Delphi technique. Nevertheless, the procedure generally calls for anonymous feedback, multiple rounds, and statistical analyses. One advantage of this technique is the ability to involve a large number of respondents, because the participants do not need to assemble together. Indeed, participants may be located throughout the country or world. Also, the questionnaire or survey requires little time commitment on the part of the participant. This technique may actually save time because it eliminates the "off-the-subject" digressions typically encountered in face-to-face meetings. In addition, the Delphi technique avoids the negative or unproductive verbal and nonverbal interactions that can occur when groups work together. Although the Delphi technique has its advantages, using it may result in a lower sense of accomplishment and involvement because the participants are detached from the overall process and do not communicate with each other.

Nursing lore places value on actions based on intangible and invisible "gut feeling" responses referred to as *nursing intuition*. What is nursing intuition? Like critical thinking, there is no one definition, but the themes that emerge from the definitions relate to "knowing or understanding" (Smith, 2007). The author asserts that intuition can be enhanced through decision-making strategies like brainstorming and group discussion. For more information, refer to the summary of Smith's article in the Literature Perspective at left.

Decision-Making Tools

Nurse leaders and managers can use a variety of decision-making tools such as decision grids and SWOT analyses in the decision-making process. These tools are most appropriately used when information is available and options are known.

Decision grids facilitate the visualization of the options under consideration and allow comparison of options using common criteria. Criteria, which are determined by the decision makers, may include time required, ethical or legal considerations, equipment needs, and cost (Figure 6-2). The relative advantages and disadvantages should be listed for each option. For example, the manager of a hospital education department is assessing whether it is better to retain

---

📖 LITERATURE PERSPECTIVE

Resource: Smith, A. J. (2007). Embracing intuition in nursing practice. *The Alabama Nurse, 34*(3), 16-17.

Intuition has been referred to as the "affective component of critical thinking" (Smith, 2007, p. 16). Ask a nurse for an example of intuition in practice and the usual response is, "I had a bad feeling about my patient." Physical and emotional responses result when intuition emerges.

Smith (2007) suggests that although the experienced nurse can claim using intuition and has confidence in using it, even nursing students and novice nurses have reported that they have experienced the gut-level and chill-type feelings associated with intuition.

Intuition is generally connected with experience which, as cited in Smith, is consistent with Patricia Benner's definition of an expert nurse. Intuitive nurses are said to possess certain characteristics such as confidence in their intuitive abilities, willingness to approach problem solving in unconventional ways, abstract thinking skills, and an awareness of spirituality in practice.

Implications for Practice
Smith recommends that, instead of discounting intuition, it should be fostered through a variety of strategies, such as mind-quieting exercises such as meditation, progressive relaxation, exercise, visualization, and guided imagery; sharing examples of intuition in practice; promoting creativity; and journal writing, group brainstorming, and small-group discussion. Although nurse educators and managers should acknowledge that intuition is not a strong indicator of "evidence," they can encourage these techniques to foster "out-of-the-box" thinking.

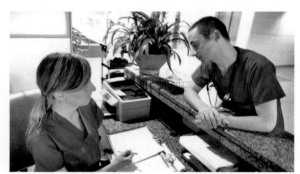

To be part of the solution, followers must be a part of making the decisions.

Options Under Consideration	Time	Cost	Legal/Ethical Considerations	Equipment Needed

FIGURE 6-2 Decision grid.

the services of an outside consultant to coordinate an advanced cardiac life support (ACLS) course in the hospital, pay the per-person fees to send the staff to another hospital for the training, or train staff in the agency as ACLS instructors to be able to provide the training in-house. The type of information this manager might compile includes a breakdown of the costs for the three options, equipment needs, benefits of each option, the number of nurses needing the course, future training needs, and feasibility of training hospital staff to conduct the course.

A SWOT analysis is commonly used in strategic planning or marketing efforts but can also be used by individuals and groups in decision making. Using the SWOT analysis, the individual or team lists the **S**trengths, **W**eaknesses, **O**pportunities, and **T**hreats related to the situation under consideration. Strengths and weaknesses are internal to the individual, group, or organization, whereas the opportunities and threats are external factors (Pearce, 2007). For example, Estella has worked in a medical-surgical unit for 5 years and is contemplating requesting to be transferred to the intensive care unit (ICU). Box 6-2 is a SWOT analysis outlining potential or actual strengths, weaknesses, opportunities, and threats for this example.

Examples of decision-making tools can be viewed in the Internet Resources section on p. 117. One of the Internet resources, *Mindtools.com*—a commercial website—provides links to software and other resources. Many of the tools are free to download. Click on the links to "Decision Making" and/or "Problem Solving."

EXERCISE 6-3

Design a decision grid for a current situation you are experiencing. Identify the components you need to explore in the decision-making process, such as cost, time, resources, advantages, and disadvantages, for the various options you are considering.

PROBLEM SOLVING

"The ability to solve problems effectively comes from experience facing and overcoming obstacles" (Maxwell, 1999, p. 101). The effective leader can anticipate problems and develops methods for dealing with them.

Problem solving includes the decision-making processes. However, in this case, the trigger for action is the existence of a "problem" or issue. Before attempting to solve a problem, a nurse must ask certain key questions:

1. Is it important?
2. Do I want to do something about it? (e.g., Do I "own" the problem?)
3. Am I qualified to handle it?
4. Do I have the authority to do anything?
5. Do I have the knowledge, interest, time, and resources to deal with it?
6. Can I delegate it to someone else?
7. What benefits will be derived from solving it?

If the answers to questions 1 through 5 are "no," why waste time, resources, and personal energy? At this juncture, a conscious decision is made to ignore the problem, refer or delegate it to others, or consult or collaborate with others to solve it. On the other hand,

---

BOX 6-2	SWOT ANALYSIS

Strengths
- Familiar with the healthcare system
- Clinically competent and has received favorable performance appraisals
- Good communication skills; well liked by her peers
- Recently completed 12-lead electrocardiogram (ECG) interpretation class

Weaknesses
- Has not attended the critical care class
- Has had a prior unresolved conflict with one of the surgeons who frequently admits to the intensive care unit (ICU)
- Is uncertain whether she wants to work full time, 12-hour shifts

Opportunities
- Anticipated staff openings in the ICU in the next several months
- Critical care course will be offered in 1 month
- Advanced cardiac life support (ACLS) course is offered four time a year
- A friend who already works in ICU has offered to mentor her

Threats
- Possible bed closures in another critical care unit may result in staff transfers, thus eliminating open positions
- Another medical-surgical nurse is also interested in transferring

if the answers are "yes," the nurse chooses to accept the problem and thus assume responsibility for it.

After identifying the problem, nurses must decide whether it is significant enough to require intervention and whether it is even within their control to do anything about. Sometimes individuals believe they need to "solve" every problem brought to their attention. Some situations, such as some interpersonal conflicts, are best resolved by the individuals who own the problem. Known as *purposeful inaction,* a "do nothing" approach might be indicated when other persons should resolve problems or when the problem is beyond one's control. Consider the following scenario:

Mary complains to the nurse manager that Sam, a fellow nurse, was rude and abrupt with her when passing in the hall. How should the nurse manager handle Mary's complaint? Should the manager discuss the problem with Sam? Should Mary be present during the discussion? What are the possible risks or benefits of such an approach? Alternatively, should the manager assist Mary in developing her communication skills so that Mary can address the problem herself?

EXERCISE 6-4

Using the decision-making format presented in Box 6-1 on p. 102, list other options for this scenario and the advantages and disadvantages of each approach. Rank the options in order of most desirable to least desirable, and select the best option. Determine how you would implement and evaluate the chosen option.

Some decisions are "givens" because they are based on firmly established criteria in the institution, which may be based on the traditions, values, doctrines, culture, or policy of the organization. Every manager has to live with mandates from persons higher in the organizational structure. Although managers may not

have the authority to control certain situations, they may be able to influence the outcome. For example, because of losses in revenue, administration has decided to eliminate the clinical educator positions in a home health agency and place the responsibility for clinical education with the senior home health nurses. It is beyond the manager's control to reverse this decision. Nevertheless, the manager can explore the nurses' fear and concerns regarding this change and facilitate the transition by preparing them for the new role.

In these examples, it is a misnomer to refer to the approach as *do nothing,* because there is deliberate action on the part of the manager. This approach should not be confused with the laissez-faire (hands off) approach taken by a manager who chooses to do nothing when intervention is indicated.

Problem-Solving Process

Several models or approaches to problem solving exist. The traditional process for problem solving is illustrated in Figure 6-3. This figure gives the appearance of a sequential and linear process. However, the problem-solving process is a dynamic one. Although individuals can certainly follow the problem-solving steps, a team approach is more likely to succeed. For example, Van Horn and Freed (2008) determined that when students engaged in reflective journaling in pairs, specific benefits were achieved. (See the Research Perspective on p. 111.)

Define the Problem, Issue, or Situation

The main principles for diagnosing a problem are (1) know the facts, (2) separate the facts from interpretation, (3) be objective and descriptive, and (4) determine the scope of the problem. Nurses also need to determine how to establish priorities for solving problems. For example, do you tend to work on problems that are encountered first, that appear to be the

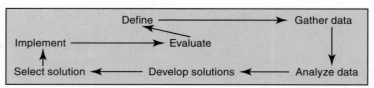

FIGURE 6-3 The problem-solving process.

easiest, that take the shortest amount of time to solve, or that may have the greatest urgency?

The most common cause for failure to resolve problems is the improper identification of the problem/issue; therefore problem recognition and identification are considered the most vital steps. The quality of the outcome depends on accurate identification of the problem, which is likely to recur if the true underlying causes are not targeted. Problem identification is influenced by the information available; by the values, attitudes, and experiences of those involved; and by time. Sufficient time should be allowed for the collection and organization of data. Too often, an inadequate amount of time is allocated for this essential step, resulting in unsatisfactory outcomes. Nurse leaders and managers should use the "5 Why" approach (Institute for Healthcare Improvement): after answering the first question as to why a problem occurred, ask why again, and so on, so on, and so on. This is particularly helpful for problems that keep resurfacing over time because it gets to the actual root causes of problems.

Girard (2005) asserted, "One of the most important one-word sentences that exists is 'Why?'" (p. 961). She claims that because of increased reliance on unit protocols, algorithms, and policy and when "habits take over thinking" (p. 962), nurses forget to ask why they are doing something. She illustrated the value in asking "why" when a problem with operating room staff using broken stretchers was noted. The

 RESEARCH PERSPECTIVE

Resource: Van Horn, R., & Freed, S. (2008). Journaling and dialogue pairs to promote reflection in clinical nursing education. *Nursing Education Perspectives, 29*(4), 220-225.

Van Horn and Freed (2008) sought to explore whether working in pairs would enhance students' knowledge and problem-solving skills. The researchers separated students enrolled in an associate's degree nursing program into two groups; half the group worked in pairs while the other half were unpaired. Students were instructed to maintain a weekly journal describing their clinical experiences over a 9-week period. The paired and unpaired students answered specific questions in the journals, but the paired students were encouraged to discuss the questions before recording their responses in the journal.

The questions posed related to the nursing and problem-solving processes. They were as follows:

1. Looking back, do you think that the problems that you identified were the most important ones for the patients? What additional problems do you now identify as the result of caring for the patients?
2. Identify a problem or a need that arose during the shift. Explain the circumstances of this problem including who, what, when, where, and how urgent the problem was.
3. What knowledge was required for you to solve the problem?
4. What resources helped you solve the problem?
5. What steps did you take to help solve the problem?
6. What influenced your thinking about this problem?
7. What were your strengths for this clinical experience?
8. What were your weaknesses, and how will you strengthen these weaknesses in the next clinical experience?
9. What were other thoughts and feelings about your clinical experience today? (p. 222)

Three themes emerged from analysis of the students' journals: emotions, connections, and learning. Journal entries demonstrated that the paired students were able to support each other in the clinical setting, thus relieving anxiety and stress. Students who were unpaired experienced a higher degree of anxiety, fear, and doubt.

One of the purposes of journaling was to help students apply theoretical knowledge in the clinical setting. Both groups demonstrated the ability to make this connection. In addition, both groups demonstrated that learning took place as a result of the reflective practice of journaling. However, in the unpaired students, the learning was primarily psychomotor skills (e.g., describing procedures that were accomplished). Students who were paired described learning that was of a social nature (e.g., learning from each other).

Van Horn and Freed (2008) assert that having students work in pairs helps students in "finding their professional voice, learning to negotiate, checking one another for accuracy, and recognizing each other as a source of knowledge" (p. 224). They recommend that instructors model their thinking processes and how they solve problems.

Implications for Practice
Expert clinicians such as clinical nurse specialists, clinical nurse leaders, unit-based nurse managers, and clinical educators can adapt this approach in mentoring new staff on a unit. Reviewing the novice nurses' responses to the questions can yield valuable information about their critical-thinking, problem-solving, and decision-making skills and serve as a foundation for ongoing staff development, mentoring, and support.

postanesthesia care nurses wanted a policy written to address sending patients to the recovery area. Instead, by asking five "why" questions to different department personnel, Girard learned that the stretchers being used were not reparable because of obsolete parts. Instead, the solution was to make a case for ordering new stretchers. In this example, it is clear that writing a new policy would not have addressed the root cause of the problem.

Kritek (2002) asserted that there are two primary phases in solving a problem: (1) identifying the problem and (2) selecting the best solution to resolve it. However, she believes that a common error is to skip the first step and proceed directly to the second one. As a result, too few options may be determined or solutions may be implemented for an unrelated problem. Why does this happen? Kritek holds that the likely explanation is that people may avoid the step that requires the problem to be understood because it can reveal negative aspects about themselves that they may not want to address.

It is important to differentiate between the actual problem and the symptoms of a problem. Consider the problem of an inadequately stocked emergency cart from which emergency medications often are missing and equipment often fails to function properly. Individuals charged with resolving this problem may discover that this is symptomatic of the underlying problem, perhaps inadequate staffing or staffing mix. Based on the proper identification of the problem in this scenario, a possible solution might be to assign the task of checking and stocking the emergency cart to the unlicensed personnel in the unit.

In work settings, problems often fall under certain categories that have been described as the *four M's: m*anpower, *m*ethods, *m*achines, and *m*aterials. Manpower issues might include inadequate staffing or staffing mix and knowledge or skills deficits. Methods issues could include communication problems or lack of protocols. Machine issues could include lack of equipment or malfunctioning equipment. Last, problems with materials could include inadequate supplies or defective materials. A fishbone diagram, also known as a *cause-and-effect diagram,* is a useful model for categorizing the possible causes of a problem. The diagram graphically displays, in increasing detail, all of the possible causes related to a problem to try to discover its root causes. This tool encourages problem

solvers to focus on the content of the problem and not be sidetracked by personal interests, issues, or agendas of team members. It also collects a snapshot of the collective knowledge of the team and helps build consensus around the problem. The "effect" is generally the problem statement, such as decreased morale, and is placed at the right end of the figure (the "head" of the fish). The major categories of causes are the main bones, and these are supported by smaller bones, which represent issues that contribute to the main causes. An example of a fishbone diagram appears in Figure 6-4.

EXERCISE 6-5

Using a fishbone diagram, identify all the factors (causes) that are at the root of a problem you are currently facing in the workplace. After you have listed as many issues as possible, share the diagram with a work colleague. Are there other issues you did not consider? Where do most of the factors influencing the problem fit: manpower, methods, machines, or materials?

Gather Data

After the general nature of the problem is identified, individuals can focus on gathering and analyzing data to resolve the issue. Assessment, through the collection of data and information, is done continuously throughout this dynamic process. The data gathered consist of objective (facts) and subjective (feelings) information. Information gathered should be valid, accurate, relevant to the issue, and timely. Moreover, individuals involved in the process must have access to information and adequate resources to make cogent decisions.

Analyze Data

Data are analyzed to further refine the problem statement and identify possible solutions or options. It is important to differentiate a problem from the symptoms of a problem. For example, a nurse manager is dismayed by the latest quality improvement (QI) report indicating nurses are not documenting patient teaching. Is this evidence that patient teaching is not being done? Is lack of documentation the actual problem? Perhaps it is a symptom of the actual problem. On further analysis, the manager

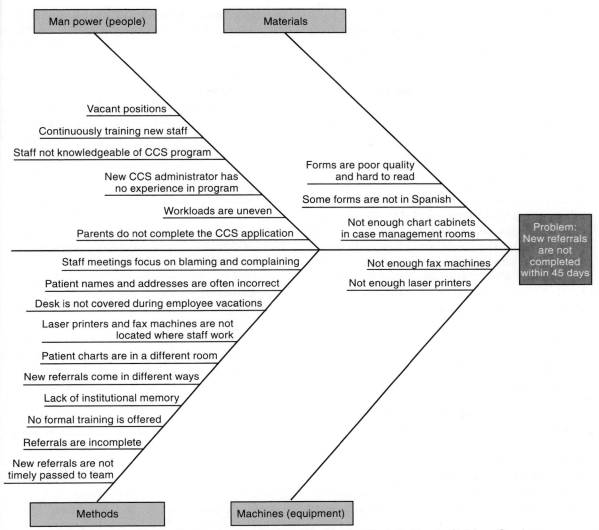

FIGURE 6-4 Analysis of root causes of referral problems. *CCS*, California Children Services.

may discover that the new computerized documentation system is not user-friendly. By distinguishing the problem from the symptoms of the problem, a more appropriate solution can be identified and implemented.

Develop Solutions

The goal of generating options is to identify as many choices as possible. Occasionally, rigid "black and white" thinking hampers the quality of outcomes. A nurse who is unhappy with his or her work situation

and can think of only two options—stay or quit—is displaying this type of thinking.

Being flexible, open-minded, and creative—attributes of a critical thinker—is critical to being able to consider a range of possible options. Everyone has preconceived notions and ideas when confronted with certain situations. Although putting these notions on hold and considering other ideas is beneficial, it is difficult to do. However, asking questions such as the following can allow a person to consider other viewpoints:

- Am I jumping to conclusions?
- If I were (insert name of role model), how would I approach it?
- How are my beliefs and values affecting my decision?

Select a Solution

The decision maker should then objectively weigh each option according to its possible risks and consequences as well as positive outcomes that may be derived. Criteria for evaluation might include variables such as cost-effectiveness, time, and legal or ethical considerations. The options should be ranked in the order in which they are likely to result in the desired goals or objectives. The solution selected should be the one that is most feasible and satisfactory and has the fewest undesirable consequences. Nurses must consider whether they are picking the solution because it is the best solution or because it is the most expedient. Being able to make cogent decisions based on thorough assessment of a situation is an important yardstick of a nurse's effectiveness.

Implement the Solution

The implementation phase should include a contingency plan to deal with negative consequences if they arise. In essence, the decision maker should be prepared to institute "plan B" as necessary.

Evaluate the Result

Considerable time and energy are usually spent on identifying the problem or issue, generating possible solutions, selecting the best solution, and implement-ing the solution. However, not enough time is typically allocated for evaluation and follow-up. It is important to establish early in the process how evaluation and monitoring will take place, who will be responsible for it, when it will take place, and what the desired outcome is. Be prepared to make mistakes and take responsibility for them. The key is to learn from mistakes and use the experiences to help guide future actions, or, as Henry Ford said, "Failure is only the opportunity to begin again more intelligently."

Individuals and groups may not adopt a structured problem-solving approach because it takes too much time, the process may be boring, people are too busy to get involved, and participants may perceive there is little or no recognition for their participation. Leaders should be cognizant of these potential barriers to prevent or minimize them.

Maxwell (1999) proposes a T-E-A-C-H method for approaching problem solving:

Time: Take the time to discover the real issue (e.g., root cause analysis).

Exposure: Learn what others have done.

Assistance: Have members of the team investigate all aspects of the issue.

Creativity: Brainstorm to identify multiple possible solutions.

Hit it: Implement with best solution.

Regardless of the model or approach taken, using a systematic approach helps address issues in an organized and focused manner. All nurses, whether they are managers, leaders, or followers, need adequate problem-solving and decision-making skills to be effective in their roles.

THE SOLUTION

In a previous job, I had used multidisciplinary process improvement teams (PITs), which consisted of key stakeholders, to initiate process improvement. I chose to try this concept in this setting. Our team consisted of the public health nurse (PHN) case managers, the CCS case workers, the billing and claims staff, the CCS medical director, clerical and support staff, and me. I believed that a group approach to these problems would yield the most information and gain the greatest support for any changes that would be made. The team met weekly for an hour. We began by identifying our custom-ers and key stakeholders and their expectations. This was extensive and took a few months to complete. Key stakeholders included the patient (children) and their parents, the providers (physicians and hospitals), pharmacies, vendors, schools, other insurance plans, the taxpayers (state and county), our own team members, and other agencies. The expectations for each stakeholder were listed, discussed for clarity, and recorded. During this exercise, the team learned a great deal about each person's job duties (there were a few surprises) and about the effect each person's job had on other team members' ability to do their job. As the team began under-standing each person's job and issues, they focused less on blaming and more on how to change our processes.

Next, the team brainstormed (divergent thinking) a list of issues. The numerous issues were then grouped according to similarity, and duplicates were eliminated. Multi-voting was then used to deter-mine the three highest-priority issues. Our number-one problem related to cycle time. When a client is referred to CCS, determina-tion of eligibility, opening (or denying) the case, and authorizing care are key cycles. Patient care is often coordinated based on the cli-ent's eligibility, and delays in service can result when the process is not completed in a timely manner. The reasons for our failure to meet these deadlines seemed overwhelming and confusing. We needed a method to find the root-causes to improve our perfor-mance. We chose to use a fishbone diagram, also known as a *cause-and-effect diagram* (see Figure 6-4). Our problem was "New referrals are not completed within 45 days." We categorized our known barriers on the four "bones" of the fish, manpower, methods, machines, and materials. Once we had identified the factors con-tributing to our problem, we prioritized them and generated action plans for each major factor. These action plans were extensive and involved implementing training and education programs, re-design-ing work space for greater efficiency, purchasing more equipment, revising job descriptions, increasing provider outreach activities, and more. Performance data did not improve during the initial year of our PIT, and I chose not to share it with staff to avoid demoralizing them. My management team and I were taking a leap of faith that

our process would eventually result in the desired outcome of meeting the performance metrics.

It took 18 months for CCS to "turn the curve," but once improve-ment started, it was exponential. The cycle time measure for "refer-ral to case open" was initially 57 days. Two years later, it was 30 days. The cycle time "referral to deny" began at 97 days, and 2 years later was down to 39 days. Most important, the cycle time "referral to first authorization" decreased from an initial 189 days to just 49 days! It was at this time that I shared the outcome data with the team. They were ecstatic! I asked the team to list the problems they believed we had solved through our PIT's efforts. They listed (1) improved staffing, (2) increased staff morale and decreased turnover (all the positions were now filled), (3) better understanding of the job expectations and the rationale behind those expectations, (4) improved teamwork, and (5) more efficient and effective work space. They have maintained enthusiastic support of the PIT, and participation remains high. The team is still highly focused on problem solving. I have learned that when assuming leadership of a department in which one has no experience, a structured team approach to information gathering, assessment of data, identifica-tion of problems, and implementation of action plans can be highly effective in the resolution of priority problems.

—*Vickie Lemmon*

Would this be a suitable approach for you? Why?

THE EVIDENCE

Porter-O'Grady and Malloch, authors of *Quantum Leadership* (2007), propose that the three essential components to effective problem solving within orga-nizations are tactical methods, strategic approaches, and cultural changes. Too often, nurse leaders and managers use a "firefighting" approach to problems, which is ineffective and generally causes more prob-lems than it resolves.

Tactical methods for dealing with problems include getting assistance from someone with a fresh perspective. This may require sharing some "dirty laundry" outside of the unit or organization, but a new point of view is helpful to bring clarity to a situ-ation. Second, the authors suggest trying something new. As stated earlier, we sometimes rely on practices out of habit. Last, triage problems by tackling the more urgent problems first.

Strategic approaches include strategies like priori-tizing problems to deal with critical issues first and developing learning scenarios to develop staff to take ownership of problems and skills to deal with them independently. This will address the tendency of staff to go to "mamma" to fix everything for them.

Cultural changes within the organization are nec-essary to make all of this work. The organization needs to avoid "patching" as a problem-solving approach. Porter-O'Grady and Malloch refer to this as focusing on the symptoms of a problem instead of the actual issue. They hold that deadlines are irrele-vant if the methodology used to solve problems is effective. Last, the authors also emphasized that fire-fighting should not be rewarded within the organization.

NEED TO KNOW NOW

- Decision making is challenging and crucial.
- Knowing how to find evidence can make decision making easier.
- Being able to cite sources increases your credibility.

- Many organizations use some kind of mentor/coach/preceptor strategy to support new employees in their initial decision-making situations.

CHAPTER CHECKLIST

The ability to make good decisions and encourage effective decision making in others is a hallmark of nursing leadership and management. A nurse manager or leader is in a good position to facilitate effective decision making by individuals and groups. This requires good communication skills, conflict resolution and mediation skills, knowledge of the vagaries of group dynamics, and the ability to foster an environment conducive to effective problem solving, decision making, and creative thinking.

- A decision-making format involves the following:
  - Listing options
  - Identifying the pros and cons of each option
  - Ranking the options in order of preference
  - Selecting the best option
- The main steps of the traditional problem-solving process are as follows:
  - Define the problem, issue, or situation
  - Gather data
  - Analyze data
  - Develop solutions and options
  - Select a solution with a desired outcome
  - Implement the solution
  - Evaluate the result
- If you want to make sound decisions or solve problems effectively, information gathered must be as follows:
  - Accurate
  - Relevant
  - Valid
  - Timely
- The situation and circumstances should dictate the leadership style used by managers to solve problems and make decisions. Analytical tools are helpful in planning and illustrating decision-making activities.

TIPS FOR DECISION MAKING AND PROBLEM SOLVING

- Seek additional information from other sources, even if they do not support the preferred action.
- Learn how other people approach problem situations.
- Talk to colleagues and superiors who you believe are effective problem solvers and decision makers. Observe positive role models in action such as

clinical nurse specialists, clinical nurse leaders, educators, and managers.
- Research journal articles and relevant sections of textbooks to increase your knowledge base.
- Risk using new approaches to problem resolution through experimentation, and calculate the risk to self and others.

REFERENCES

Girard, N. J. (2005). Never underestimate the importance of asking "why?" *Association of Operating Room Nurses, 82*(6), 961-962.

Huston, C. (2008). Preparing nurse leaders for 2020. *Journal of Nursing Management, 16*(8), 905-911.

Keynes, M. (2008). Making good decisions, Part 1. *Nursing Management, 14*(9), 32-34.

Kritek, P. (2002). *Negotiating at an uneven table: Developing moral courage in resolving our conflicts.* San Francisco: John Wiley & Sons.

Maxwell, J. C. (1999). *The 21 indispensible qualities of a leader.* Nashville, TN: Thomas Nelson.

Pearce, C. (2007). Ten steps to carrying out a SWOT analysis. *Nursing Management, 14*(2), 25.

Porter-O'Grady, T., & Malloch, K. (2007). *Quantum leadership.* Boston: Jones & Bartlett.

Scriven, M., & Paul, R. (2007). *Defining critical thinking.* Foundation for Critical Thinking. Retrieved October 6, 2009, from www.criticalthinking.org/aboutCT/definingCT.cfm.

Smith, A. J. (2007). Embracing intuition in nursing practice. *Alabama Nurse, 34*(3), 16-17.

Tanner, C. A. (2006). Thinking like a nurse: A research-based model of clinical judgment in nursing. *Journal of Nursing Education, 45*(6), 204-211.

Van Horn, R., & Freed, S. (2008). Journaling and dialogue pairs to promote reflection in clinical nursing education. *Nursing Education Perspectives, 29*(4), 220-225.

INTERNET RESOURCES

Institute for Healthcare Improvement. www.ihi.org/IHI/ Programs/StrategicInitiatives/ TransformingCareAtTheBedside.htm.

Institute for Healthcare Improvement. www.ihi.org/IHI/Topics/ Improvement/ImprovementMethods/Tools/.

Mind Tools. www.mindtools.com/.

Robert Wood Johnson Foundation. www.rwjf.org (search on transforming care at the bedside).

The Joint Commission. Framework for conducting a root cause analysis and action plan: www.jointcommission.org/ SentinelEvents/Forms/.

SUGGESTED READINGS

Billings D. M., & Kowalski, K. (2008). Appreciative inquiry. *The Journal of Continuing Education in Nursing, 39*(3), 104.

Billings, D. M., & Kowalski, K. (2008). Argument mapping. *The Journal of Continuing Education in Nursing, 39*(6), 246-247.

Cleary-Holdforth, J., & Leufer, T. (2008). Essential elements in developing evidence-based practice. *Nursing Standard, 23*(2), 42-46.

Ireland, M. (2008). Assisting students to use evidence as part of reflection on practice. *Nursing Education Perspectives, 29*(2), 90-93.

Lahaie, U. D. (2008). Is nursing ready for webquests? *Journal of Nursing Education, 47*(12), 567-570.

Reavy, K., & Taverneir, S. (2008). Nurses reclaiming ownership of their practice: Implementation of an evidence-based

practice model and process. *The Journal of Continuing Education in Nursing, 39*(4), 166-172.

Smith, A. J. (2007). Embracing intuition in nursing practice. *The Alabama Nurse, 34*(3), 16-17.

Smith-Strom, H., & Nortvedt, M. W. (2008). Evaluation of evidence-based methods used to teach nursing students to critically appraise evidence. *Journal of Nursing Education, 47*(8), 372-375.

Tanner, C. A. (2006). Thinking like a nurse: A research-based model of clinical judgment in nursing. *Journal of Nursing Education, 45*(6), 204-211.

Van Horn, R., & Freed, S. (2008). Journaling and dialogue pairs to promote reflection in clinical nursing education. *Nursing Education Perspectives, 29*(4), 220-225.

Healthcare Organizations

Mary E. Mancini

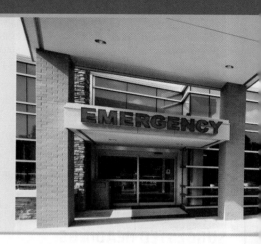

This chapter presents an overview of existing and emerging healthcare organizations, their characteristics, and their designs. Economic, social, and demographic factors that influence organizational development are discussed. A major emphasis is placed on management and leadership responses that professional nurses must consider in planning the delivery of nursing care in the changing environment. Leaders, managers, followers, and nursing students engaged in active practice must be aware of the changing dynamics if they are to be effective healthcare professionals and advocate for patients, families, and community.

OBJECTIVES

- Identify and compare characteristics that are used to differentiate healthcare organizations.
- Classify healthcare organizations by major types.
- Analyze economic, social, and demographic forces that drive the development of healthcare organizations.
- Describe the impact of the evolution of healthcare organizations on nursing leadership and management roles.

TERMS TO KNOW

accreditation
consolidated systems
deeming authority
fee-for-service
for-profit organization
horizontal integration

managed care
networks
primary care
private non-profit (or not-for-profit) organization
public institution

secondary care
teaching institution
tertiary care
third-party payers
vertical integration

INTRODUCTION

Organizations are collections of individuals brought together in a defined environment to achieve a set of predetermined objectives. Economic, social, and demographic factors affect the purpose and structuring of the system, which in turn interact with the mission, philosophy, and structure of healthcare organizations.

Healthcare organizations provide two general types of services: illness care (restorative) and wellness care (preventive). Illness care services help the sick and injured. Wellness care services promote better health as well as illness and accident prevention. In the past, most organizations (e.g., hospitals, clinics, public health departments, community-based organizations, and physicians' offices) focused their attention on illness services. Recent economic, social, and demographic changes have placed emphasis on the development of organizations that focus on the full spectrum of health, especially wellness and prevention, to meet consumers' needs in more effective ways. Emphasis is being placed on the role of the nurse as both a designer of these restructured organizations and a healthcare leader and manager within the organizations. For example, the manner in which chronic and acute illnesses are managed is dramatically different from such a decade ago. Nurses take a much more active and independent role in providing these services. Similarly, as population numbers increase and the demand for nurses exceeds the supply, we can anticipate more changes in how nurses function within the healthcare system. An increased focus on continuous performance improvement

and benchmarking demands that organizations constantly consider their own practices and make appropriate changes, including those related to the organization's culture and the role of nurses within the organization.

Nurses practice in many different types of healthcare organizations. Nursing roles develop in response to the same social, cultural, economic, legislative, and demographic factors that shape the organizations in which they work. As the largest group of healthcare professionals providing direct and indirect care services to consumers, nurses have an obligation to be involved in the development of health care, social, and economic policies that shape healthcare organizations.

CHARACTERISTICS AND TYPES OF ORGANIZATIONS

Responding to the rapidly changing nature of the economic, social, and demographic environment at the national, state, and local level, the United States healthcare system is in a continual state of flux as are the organizations within this system. Organizations either anticipate or respond to these environmental changes.

Institutional Providers

Acute care hospitals, long-term care facilities, and rehabilitation facilities have traditionally been classified as institutional providers. Major characteristics that differentiate institutional providers as well as other healthcare organizations are (1) types of services provided, (2) length of direct care services provided, (3) ownership, (4) teaching status, and (5) accreditation status.

Types of Services Provided

The type of services offered is a characteristic used to differentiate institutional providers. Services can be classified as either general or special care. Facilities that provide specialty care offer a limited scope of services, such as those targeted to specific disease entities or patient populations. Examples of special care facilities are those providing psychiatric care, burn care, children's care, women's and infants' care, and oncology care. Alternatively, facilities such as general hospitals provide a wide range of services to multiple segments of the population.

Length of Direct Care Services Provided

Another characteristic that is used to differentiate healthcare organizations is the duration of the care provided. According to the American Hospital Association (AHA) (2009), most hospitals are acute care facilities giving short-term, episodic care. The AHA defined an acute care hospital as a facility in which the average length of stay is less than 30 days. Chronic care or long-term facilities provide services for patients who require care for extended periods in excess of 30 days. In acute care institutions, patients

are discharged as soon as their conditions are stabilized. An example of a long-term care facility is a geriatric organization that provides care services from onset of impairment until death. Many institutions have components of both short-term and long-term services. They may provide acute care, home care, hospice care, ambulatory clinic care, day surgery, and an increasing number of other services, such as day care for dependent children and adults or focused services such as Meals-on-Wheels. The term *healthcare network* refers to interconnected units that either are owned by the institution or have cooperative agreements with other institutions to provide a full spectrum of wellness and illness services. The spectrum of care services provided are typically described as **primary care** (first-access care), **secondary care** (disease-restorative care), and **tertiary care** (rehabilitative or long-term care). Table 7-1 describes the continuum of care and the units of healthcare organizations that provide services in the three phases of the continuum.

EXERCISE 7-1

Using the local telephone directory, determine the types and numbers of primary care, secondary care, and tertiary care services available. Table 7-2 provides an example of a format for collecting data.

TABLE 7-1 CONTINUUM OF HEALTHCARE ORGANIZATIONS

TYPE OF CARE	PURPOSE	ORGANIZATION OR UNIT PROVIDING SERVICES
Primary	• Entry into system • Health maintenance • Long-term care • Chronic care • Treatment of temporary nonincapacitating malfunction	• Ambulatory care centers • Physicians' offices • Preferred provider organizations • Nursing centers • Independent provider organizations • Health maintenance organizations • School health clinics
Secondary	• Prevention of disease complications	• Home health care • Ambulatory care centers • Nursing centers
Tertiary	• Rehabilitation • Long-term care	• Home health care • Long-term care facilities • Rehabilitation centers • Skilled nursing facilities • Assisted living programs/retirement centers

Ownership

Ownership is another characteristic used to classify healthcare organizations. Ownership establishes the organization's legal, business, and mission-related imperative. Healthcare organizations have three basic ownership forms: public, private non-profit, and for-profit. **Public institutions** provide health services to individuals under the support and/or direction of local, state, or federal government. These organizations must answer directly to the sponsoring government agency or boards and are indirectly responsible to elected officials and taxpayers who support them. Examples of these service recipients at the federal level are veterans, members of the military, Native Americans and prisoner healthcare organizations. State-supported organizations may be health service teaching facilities, chronic care facilities, and prisoner facilities. Locally supported facilities include county-supported and city-supported facilities. Table 7-2 shows how several common healthcare organizations are classified.

Private non-profit (or not-for-profit) organizations—often referred to as *voluntary agencies*—are controlled by voluntary boards or trustees and provide care to a mix of paying and charity patients. In these organizations, excess revenue over expenses is redirected into the organization for maintenance and growth rather than returned as dividends to stockholders. These organizations are required to serve people regardless of their ability to pay. Non-profit organizations located in impoverished urban and rural areas are often economically disadvantaged by the amount of uncompensated care that they provide. In 2007, roughly 60% of uncompensated care in the United States was provided by 14% of hospitals (United States Department of the Treasury, 2009). Some states, such as New York, have created charity pools to which all non-profit organizations in the state are required to contribute to offset financial problems of the disadvantaged institutions. Historically, non-profit organizations have been exempt from paying taxes as they commit to providing an important community service. The owners of such organizations include churches, communities, industries, and special interest groups such as the Shriners. It is important for nurses to understand the impact of ownership on how organizations are structured, the services they provide, and the patients they serve.

For-profit organizations are also referred to as *proprietary* or *investor-owned organizations*. These organizations operate with the specific intent of earning a profit by providing healthcare services to individuals who can afford to pay for these services. Organizations such as private or public insurers who provide healthcare insurance coverage are known as **third-party payers.** Owners may be individuals, partnerships, corporations, or multisystems. Many for-profit organizations, like the not-for-profit ones, receive supplementary funds through private and public sources to provide special services and research. This funding allows them to provide financial assis-

TABLE 7-2 CHARACTERISTICS AND TYPES OF HEALTHCARE ORGANIZATIONS

HEALTHCARE ORGANIZATION	TYPE	SERVICES	OWN	FIN	TCHG	MULTI
Veterans Administration	Institution	General	Federal	NP	Y	Y
Academic Medical Center	Institution	General	Private	NP	Y	Y
Community General	Institution	General	Private	NP	N	Y
Public Hospital	Institution	General	County	NP	Y	N
Shriners Burn Hospitals	Institution	Specialty	Private	NP	N	N
Prepaid Health Plan	HMO	General	Private	NP-P	N	N
Public Health Department	Community	General	State	NP	N	N
Women's and Infants' Project	Community	Specialty	State	NP	N	N
Geriatric Corporation	Institution	Long term	Private	NP	N	Y
Visiting Nurses Association	Community	Specialty	Private	NP	N	N

Fin, Financing; *HMO*, health maintenance organization; *Multi*, multiunit; *N*, no; *NP*, non-profit; *Own*, ownership; *P*, profit; *Tchg*, teaching status; *Y*, yes.

tance to patients who can afford ordinary care but are not in a position to finance catastrophic occurrences such as vital organ failure, birth of premature or sick infants, or transplant operations.

Multihospital systems, which are defined as two or more institutional providers having common owners, represent a significant development that has taken place in the past two decades. Investor-owned, multihospital systems are becoming increasingly popular. Nursing homes, home care, psychiatric services, and health maintenance organizations (HMOs) are commonly units in such systems.

Research has shown that ownership can impact efficiency and quality. Although hospital ownership is defined legally, there are significant differences within the three sectors related to teaching status, location, bed size, and corporate affiliation. For-profit hospitals, which represent approximately 15% of the beds in short-term acute care hospitals, are typically nonteaching, suburban facilities with small to medium bed capacity and have the ability to access group purchasing cooperatives that lower non-salary expenses. For-profit hospitals tend to have higher hospital charges and lower wage and salary costs that most likely represent an aggressive approach to maximizing return on investment.

Ownership results in differential treatment relative to regulatory requirements. Public and non-profit hospitals are tax exempt and have a concomitant responsibility to provide mandated community service such as delivering care to the poor and indigent. Thus one can expect operational differences between and among the three ownership sectors. Ownership impacts the organization's level of effort in regard to the provision of uncompensated care. Those organizations with taxing authority or direct support from local or state government have a clear mandate to care for indigent patients and receive at least some level of dedicated funds to do so. For-profit hospitals offer fewer unprofitable services and actively seek to avoid providing uncompensated care and are required to pay taxes that can have an impact on their bottom line. To keep their non-profit status, these facilities must make a good-faith effort to provide community service and charity care. Unfortunately, the literature provides conflicting and inconclusive evidence in regard to the impact of ownership on hospital financial performance.

Teaching Status

Teaching status is a characteristic that can differentiate healthcare organizations. The term teaching institution is applied to academic health centers (those directly affiliated with a school of medicine and at least one other health profession school) and affiliated teaching hospitals (those that provide only the clinical portion of a medical school teaching program). Studies have shown that although care is usually more costly at teaching hospitals than at non-teaching hospitals (estimates range from 12% more expensive in Canada to 27% in the United States), teaching hospitals generally offer better care because of their access to state-of-the-art technology and researchers. The higher costs of teaching hospitals have been attributed to the unique missions these institutions tend to pursue, including graduate medical education, biomedical research, and the maintenance of stand-by capacity for highly specialized patient care (Flatt & Rahal, 2006).

Traditionally, teaching hospitals have received government reimbursement to cover these additional costs. There are, however, intrinsic costs of providing a medical training program that are not fully reimbursed by the government. Maintaining a teaching program places a financial burden on hospitals relative to the direct cost of the program and the indirect cost of the inefficiencies surrounding the training process. These inefficiencies include (1) salaries of physicians who supervise students' care delivery and participate in educational programs such as teaching rounds and seminars; (2) duplicated tests or procedures; and (3) delays in processing patients related to the teaching process. Currently, these expenses are reimbursed based on a formula that considers the cost of caring for the low-income and uninsured patients who populate most academic teaching programs. This reimbursement is being revised as states reduce subsidies for the education of physicians. Hospitals make strategic decisions about their level of participation in physician training. Because of the additional costs, few for-profit hospitals sponsor teaching programs. Teaching hospitals are usually located close to their affiliated medical school. They tend to be larger and located in more urban and economically depressed inner-city areas than their non-teaching counterparts. Teaching hospitals, therefore, tend to exhibit weaker economic performance compared with non-teaching hospitals.

EXERCISE 7-2

Return to the data you started in the first exercise and add financial and teaching status information.

Accreditation Status

Whether or not a healthcare organization has been accredited by an external body as having the structure and process necessary to provide high quality care is another characteristic that can be used to distinguish one organization from another. Private organizations play significant roles in establishing standards and ensuring care delivery compliance with standards by accrediting healthcare organizations. Examples of these organizations are The Joint Commission and The National Committee for Quality Assurance (NCQA). The Joint Commission provides accreditation programs for ambulatory care, behavioral health care, acute care and critical access hospitals, laboratory services, long-term care, and hospital-based surgery. The NCQA is a non-profit organization that accredits, certifies, and recognizes a wide variety of healthcare organizations, services, and providers. More information on accrediting organizations is provided in the "Accrediting Bodies" section on pp. 127-128.

Consolidated Systems and Networks

Healthcare organizations are being organized into consolidated systems through both the formation of for-profit or not-for-profit multihospital systems and the development of networks of independently owned and operated healthcare organizations.

Consolidated Systems

Consolidated systems tend to be organized along five levels. The first level includes the large national hospital companies, most of which are investor owned. The second level involves large voluntary affiliated systems, which provide members with access to capital, political power, management expertise, joint venture opportunities, and links to health insurance services or, as in Canada, to a national healthcare coverage program. The third level involves regional hospital systems that cover a defined geographic area, such as an area of a state. The fourth level involves metropolitan-based systems. The fifth level is composed of the special interest groups that own and operate units organized along religious lines, teaching interests, or related special interests that drive their activities. This level often crosses over the regional, metropolitan, and national levels already described. Through the creation of multiunit systems, an organization has greater marketing, policy, and contracting potentials.

Networks

Healthcare markets with 100,000 or more residents are generally served by one to three health networks. The networks usually follow one of three organizational models: public utilities, for-profit businesses, or loose alliances. Public utility models are organized and governed just like today's public utilities (e.g., the county water department). Their aim is serving large regional populations. In most markets, two or three competing markets have emerged that require significant capital, causing many traditional not-for-profit providers to shift to for-profit status. Loose alliances take the shape of loosely connected "virtual" networks that emulate integrated health systems through contracts and linked computer systems.

Ambulatory-Based Organizations

Many health services are provided on an ambulatory basis. The organizational setting for much of this care has been the group practice or private physician's office. Prepaid group practice plans, referred to as *managed care systems,* combine care delivery with financing and provide comprehensive services for a fixed prepaid fee. A goal of these services is to reduce the cost of expensive acute hospital care by focusing on out-of-hospital preventive care and illness follow-up care. Group practice plans take various forms. One form has a centralized administration that directs and pays salaries for physician practice (e.g., HMOs).

The HMO is a configuration of healthcare agencies that provide basic and supplemental health maintenance and treatment services to voluntary enrollees who prepay a fixed periodic fee without regard to the amount of services used. To be federally qualified, an HMO company must offer inpatient and outpatient services, treatment and referral for drug and alcohol problems, laboratory and radiology services, preventive dental services for children younger than 12 years, and preventive healthcare services in addition to physician services.

Independent practice associations (IPAs) (or professional associations [PAs]) are a form of group practice in which physicians in private offices are paid on a fee-for-service basis by a prepaid plan to deliver care to enrolled members. Preferred provider organizations (PPOs) operate similarly to IPAs; contracts are developed with private practice physicians, but fees are discounted from their usual and customary charges. In return, physicians are guaranteed prompt payment.

Nurse practitioners' leadership in managing patients in group practices has contributed greatly to their success. Examples of this can be found by reviewing literature related to nurses' activities at Kaiser Permanente HMO, the Harvard Community Health Plan, and Minute Clinics.

There is increasing evidence that nurse-run clinics as well as ambulatory care centers can succeed whether they are integrated within a larger medical complex or physically and administratively separate organizations. Examples of freestanding organizations include surgicenters, urgent care centers, primary care centers, and imaging centers. Benefits and risks are associated with geographic and administrative separation between organizations. For example, when an ambulatory surgery center is located separate from an acute care facility, there is a need to address emergency response teams and seamless transfer of patients in need of a higher level of care. On the other hand, having the ambulatory surgery center apart from the acute care hospital typically provides the opportunity for more patient-focused amenities such as parking and family waiting. It is often the nurse manager in these facilities who is charged with identifying the strategies to maximize the benefits and minimize the risks or challenges inherent in the characteristics of the facility and organization.

> **EXERCISE 7-3**
> Again return to the data started in the first exercise and add information about the status of the multiunit systems that are in place.

Other Organizations

Although hospitals, nursing homes, health departments, visiting nurse services, and private physicians'

offices have made up the traditional primary service delivery organizations, it is important to recognize the critical role being played by other organizations that may be freestanding or units of hospitals or other community organizations. These include community service organizations, subacute facilities, and a proliferating number of home health agencies, long-term care facilities, and hospices. In addition, nurse-owned/nurse-organized services and self-help voluntary organizations contribute to the overall service provision. Growth in these organizations was spurred by the implementation of the prospective payment system, which resulted in early discharge of many patients from acute care facilities. These patients require highly technical continuing nursing care to maintain a stable status. The focus of these organizations is on the care of individuals and their family and significant others rather than on the community as a whole. Many of these organizations are functioning as PPOs, and this is expected to be a continuing pattern in the future.

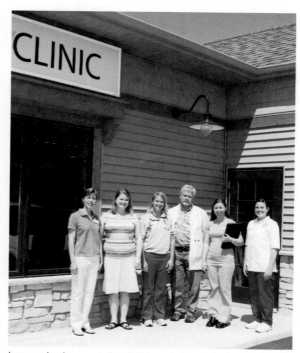

Increasingly, care is delivered through freestanding clinics or community or hospital-affiliated services.

Community Services

Community services, including public health departments, are focused on the treatment of the community rather than that of the individual. The historical focus of these organizations has been on control of infectious agents and provision of preventive services under the auspices of public health departments. Local, state, and federal governments allocate funds to health departments to provide a variety of necessary services. These funds provide personal health services that include maternal and child care, care for communicable diseases such as acquired immunodeficiency syndrome (AIDS) and tuberculosis, services for children with birth defects, mental health care, and investigation of epidemiology and treatment of bioterrorism threats and attacks such as anthrax. Monies are allocated also for environmental services (e.g., ensuring that food services meet established standards) and for health resources (e.g., control of reproduction, promotion of safer sex, and breast cancer screening programs). Local health departments have been provided some autonomy in determining how to use funds that are not assigned to categorical programs.

School health programs whose funds are also allocated to them by local, state, and federal governments traditionally have been organized to control infectious disease outbreaks; to detect and refer problems that interfere with learning; to treat on-site injuries and illnesses; and to provide basic health education programs. Increasingly, schools are being seen as primary care sites for children.

Visiting nurse associations, which are voluntary organizations, have provided a large amount of the follow-up care for patients after hospitalization and for newborns and their mothers. Some are organized by cities, and others serve entire regions. Some operate for profit; others do not.

Subacute Facilities

As hospitals began to discharge patients earlier in their recuperation, the subacute facility emerged as a healthcare organization. Initially, many of these facilities were old-style nursing homes refurbished with the high-tech equipment necessary to deal with patients who have just come out of surgery or who are still acutely ill and have complex medical needs. Today, many are newly built centers or new businesses that have taken over existing clinical facilities.

Home Health Organizations

Home health organizations have numerous configurations; they may be freestanding or owned by a hospital and may be for-profit or not-for-profit organizations. Professional nurses with expert skills in assessing patients' self-care competencies and in building structures to overcome patients' and families' social and emotional deficits in providing sick and palliative care are needed to meet home care needs. Home care agencies staffed appropriately with adequate numbers of professional nurses have the potential to keep older adults, those with disabilities, and persons with chronic illnesses comfortable and safe at home. An increasing number of restrictions on home care by managed care companies, as well as changing financial reimbursement strategies, are threatening the adequate performance of this function.

Home care is the fastest growing segment in health care. The organizational design will likely change to the integration of a functional and divisional structure because the home health service industry is becoming more complex and is changing rapidly. For example, reimbursement for home care is primarily an arrangement of contract pricing and capitation. The integration of clinical, financial, human resources, and patient outcome information will influence the organizational design of the home care agency in the future.

Long-Term Care and Residential Facilities

Long-term care (LTC) facilities may also be known as *skilled nursing facilities*. These organizations provide long-term rehabilitation and professional nursing services. In residential facilities, no skilled care is provided but residents who have special needs are offered safe, sheltered environments in which to live.

Hospice

Hospices can be located on inpatient nursing units, such as the kind commonly found in Canada, the United Kingdom, and Australia, or in the home or residential centers in the community. The concept of hospice or palliative care was launched at St. Christopher Hospice in London. Hospices focus on confirming rather than denying the reality of death and thus provide care that ensures dignity and comfort.

Nurse-Owned and Nurse-Organized Services

Nursing centers, which are nurse-owned and nurse-operated places where care is provided by nurses, are another form of community-based organization. Many nursing centers are administered by schools of nursing and serve as a base for faculty practice and research and clinical experience for students. Others are owned and operated by groups of nurses. These centers have a variety of missions. Some focus on care for specific populations, such as the homeless, or on care for people with AIDS. Others have taken responsibility for university health services. Some have assumed responsibility for school health programs in the community, and others operate employee wellness programs, hospices, and home care services. Some are freestanding, and others are units within hospitals. Church-affiliated organizations, sometimes operating as parish or shul (a service of synagogues) nursing facilities, are also examples of nurse-based organizations.

Self-Help Voluntary Organizations

Other organizations are the self-help/self-care organizations. These organizations also come in various forms. They are often composed of and directed by peers who are consumers of healthcare services. Their purpose is most often to enable patients to provide support to each other and raise community consciousness about the nature of a specific physical or emotional disease. AIDS support groups and Alcoholics Anonymous are two examples. Community geriatric organizations, frequently sponsored by healthcare organizations and offering multiple services for promoting wellness and rehabilitation, are increasing rapidly.

Supportive and Ancillary Organizations

Organizations involved in the direct provision of health care are supported by a number of other organizations whose operations have a significant effect on provider organizations, as well as on the overall performance of the health system. These organizations include regulatory organizations, accrediting bodies, third-party financing organizations, pharma-ceutical and medical equipment supply corporations, and various professional, educational, and training organizations.

EXERCISE 7-4

Identify supportive and ancillary organizations operating in your community. Can you determine whether nurses are playing leadership or staff roles in those organizations and what functions are incorporated into existing nursing roles?

Regulatory Organizations

Regulatory organizations set standards for the operation of healthcare organizations, ensure compliance with federal and state regulations developed by governmental administrative agencies, and investigate and make judgments regarding complaints brought by consumers of the services and the public. They approve organizations for licensure as providers of health care. Healthcare organizations are regulated by a number of different federal, state, and local agencies to protect the health and safety of the patients and communities they serve. A number of different regulatory agencies monitor functions in healthcare organizations. These include the Centers for Medicare & Medicaid Services (CMS), the U.S. Food and Drug Administration, the Occupational Health and Safety Administration, the Equal Employment Opportunity Commission, and state licensing boards for various health professions. Regardless of the type of organization in which they work, nurses are often involved in these processes. Therefore all nurses need to be familiar with the regulations that impact their organization.

Established in 1965, Medicare is the country's largest and most influential health insurance program, providing healthcare funding for more than 40 million individuals. This makes the federal government the primary payer of healthcare costs in the United States. The Medicare program is not limited to individuals age 65 years or older. Persons with certain permanent illnesses, such as end-stage renal disease, also receive Medicare health benefits. Because of the size of the Medicare market, the federal government serves as the leading regulator of healthcare services in this country.

The CMS administers the Medicare and Medicaid programs. Participation in these programs is regulated by a complex set of rules outlined in a lengthy set of guidelines—the Conditions of Participation (CoP). These guidelines are established to improve quality and protect the health and safety of Medicare and Medicaid beneficiaries by specifying the requirements that organizations must meet to be eligible to receive Medicare and Medicaid reimbursement.

To be in compliance with the CoP, hospitals must meet certain quality assessment and performance improvement requirements. Through its Quality Improvement Organization program (formerly called *Peer Review*), CMS contracts with one organization in each state to work with healthcare organizations to improve the quality, efficiency, and effectiveness of care provided in that state to Medicare beneficiaries. CMS provides a financial incentive for hospitals to report quality data. These data will be used to establish minimum quality standards for healthcare facilities and by patients to help them make decisions about hospital care. The program is designed to ensure that hospitals systematically examine the quality of care provided and that they use the data obtained to develop and implement projects that improve quality, enhance patient safety, and reduce medical errors. To help reach these quality goals, CMS sponsors the Medicare Quality Improvement Community (MedQIC). The MedQIC website contains information and tools to support healthcare providers and organizations in creating community-based approaches to quality improvement.

Nurses are actively involved in CMS quality improvement processes. The level of their participation may be as participants in facility-based quality or utilization management activities, or they may be involved as case managers. Nurse case managers can serve in a number of different roles, but they frequently serve as the organization's interface with the physician. In this role, these case managers routinely monitor for appropriate physician documentation of medical necessity and other required CoP elements. In the ambulatory or acute care setting, the case managers typically work with physician advisors to ensure that care follows the recognized standards and facilitates patient flow to the appropriate setting for care.

Nurses also play key roles in developing, implementing, and evaluating the review processes of these regulatory agencies. As members of healthcare organizations providing both direct and indirect services to patients and as members of or advisors to regulatory agencies, nursing leaders have active roles in establishing standards and ensuring that organizations comply with standards

Accrediting Bodies

Accreditation refers to the approval, recognition, or certification by an official review board that an organization has met certain standards. CMS is responsible for the enforcement of its standards through its certification activities. For a healthcare organization to participate in and receive payment from either Medicare or Medicaid, the organization must be certified as complying with the CoP. One manner that an organization can be recognized as complying with the CoP is through a survey process conducted by a state agency on behalf of CMS. Alternatively, an organization can be surveyed and accredited by a national accrediting body holding "deeming authority" for CMS. To obtain deeming authority, an accreditation organization must undergo a comprehensive evaluation by CMS to ensure that the standards of the accrediting organization are at least as rigorous as CMS standards. Healthcare organizations accredited by an organization with CMS deeming authority are therefore "deemed" as meeting Medicare and Medicaid certification requirements. A number of states accept national accreditation by an approved accrediting agency in lieu of other types of regulatory activity. For these reasons, healthcare organizations often seek accreditation by an accrediting body with deeming authority rather than through a multiple survey process conducted by state agencies and CMS. There are multiple deeming accreditations.

Healthcare organizations commonly seek accreditation by either The American Osteopathic Association (AOA) or The Joint Commission (formally known as the *Joint Commission on Accreditation of Healthcare Organizations or JCAHO*). Both of these organizations have been granted "deeming" authority by CMS. The AOA is a professional association specifically for osteopathic healthcare organizations. It accredits osteopathic acute care hospitals, mental health facilities, substance abuse centers, and physical rehabilitation centers. The Joint Commission is an independent, not-for-profit organization that currently accredits more than 15,000 healthcare organizations in the United States and internationally. The explicit mission of The Joint Commission is to continuously improve the safety and quality of care provided to the public through the provision of healthcare accreditation and related services that support improvement of performance in healthcare organizations. The Joint Commission accredits approximately 80% of acute care hospitals in the United States, as well as numerous ambulatory surgicenters, clinical laboratories, critical access hospitals, HMOs, PPOs, home healthcare agencies, hospices, and acute care hospitals.

In the late 2000s, a new group called the DNV (Det Norske Veritas) was granted deeming status. This international group accredits disparate fields (e.g., auto manufacturing and health care) and uses ISO (International Organization for Standardization) standards as a basis for these accreditations. Some hospitals hold both TJC and DNV, and others remain with TJC or are transitioning to DNV. The influence of DNV is likely to grow but to what extent is currently unknown.

Third-Party Financing Organizations

Organizations that provide financing for health care comprise another subset of supportive and ancillary organizations. As noted earlier, the government, through CMS, finances a large portion of the population and represents the largest third-party organization involved in healthcare provision. Private health insurance carriers, who account for most of the remaining financing, are composed of not-for-profit and for-profit components. Blue Cross/Blue Shield is an example of a not-for-profit insurance company. The Blues, as they are often called, have led the move of insurers from fee-for-service insurance to managed care. This has been both a cost-reduction mechanism and a marketing response to the managed care concept introduced by HMOs and the arrangements discussed previously in relation to physician practice agreements. Commercial insurance companies represent the private sector.

Third-party financing organizations have a major effect on the actual delivery of health care. They do so by identifying those procedures, tests, services, or drugs that will be covered under their healthcare insurance programs. In addition, they indirectly affect the configuration of the healthcare delivery system through the use of their significant political influence. As the cost of health care increases and the number of medically uninsured and underinsured grows, pressure increases for significant changes in healthcare reimbursement. Reconfiguration of the current system is certain to bring with it restructuring of the organizations responsible for delivery of healthcare services. An understanding of the interrelated changes in healthcare organizations can be gained by examining the results of the 1982 enactment by Congress of the Tax Equity and Fiscal Reimbursement Act (TEFRA), which introduced the prospective payment system for Medicare reimbursement.

Pharmaceutical and Medical Equipment Supply Organizations

About one tenth of all healthcare expenditures is allocated to drugs and medical equipment, and this is increasing. When other healthcare supply organizations, such as healthcare information system corporations, are considered, the estimated percentage may rapidly escalate toward the one-quarter mark. Nurses, as primary users of these products, play a significant role in healthcare organizations in setting standards for safe and efficient products that meet both consumers' and organizations' needs in a cost-effective manner. Supply organizations often seek nurses as customers and as participants in market surveys for the design of new products, services, and marketing techniques. Nurses are employed by these organizations as designers of new products, marketing representatives, and members of the sales and research staffs. Examples of the roles nurses play can be seen by studying organizations that employ nurses to design new products and market them through production and distribution of a newsletter and ongoing continuing-education presentations.

Professional, Educational, and Training Organizations

Professional organizations have as their primary goal the protection and enhancement of the interests of the service delivery organizations and their disciplines. Because of their direct impact on the healthcare delivery system as well as their tremen-dous political influence, professional healthcare organizations must be considered in any discussion of health care in this country. Professional organizations operate at the local, state, and national levels and perform a number of functions, including protection and support through political lobbying; education; and the development and maintenance of standards for caregivers, resources, environment, and care. Examples of these are the American Nurses Association, the American Medical Association, the American Pharmacists Association, and the American Hospital Association. In addition to the professional organizations, labor organizations representing healthcare organization employees play an increasing role in healthcare organization development. Educational and training organizations, such as the American Heart Association, contribute to the development of healthcare organizations through the creation and dissemination of practice standards.

Organizational Relationships

Organizational relationships are complex. In addition, as in business, most healthcare organizations have experienced (or will experience) acquisitions or mergers.

Integration

As the healthcare industry faces continuing and increasing pressure to be both efficient and effective, healthcare organizations are entering into a number of different organizational relationships. Organizations can come together to form affiliations, consortiums, and consolidations that result in multihospital systems and/or multi-organizational arrangements. When organizations that provide similar services come together, the arrangement is referred to as horizontal integration. An example of horizontal integration is a group of acute care facilities that come together to provide coverage for an expanded region. When organizations align to provide a full array or continuum of services, the arrangement is referred to as vertical integration. Organizations brought together in a vertical integration might include an acute care facility, a rehabilitation facility, a home care agency, an ambulatory clinic, and a hospice. Benefits attributed to vertical integration include enhanced coordination of services, efficiency, and customer services.

Acquisitions and Mergers

The economic forces of capitated payments and managed care are causing healthcare organizations to reorganize, restructure, and reengineer to decrease waste and economic inefficiency. Many organizations are forming multi-institutional alliances that integrate healthcare systems under a common organizational infrastructure. These alliances are accomplished through acquisitions or mergers. Acquisitions involve one organization directly buying another. Mergers involve combining two or more organizations and their assets to form a new entity. Mergers can also happen within organizations as departments or patient care units come together. People, structure, culture, and political issues or organizational change can be very traumatic and lead to dysfunctional outcomes if it is not managed well.

FORCES THAT INFLUENCE HEALTHCARE ORGANIZATIONS

Economic, social, and demographic factors provide the input for future development and act as major forces driving the evolution of healthcare organizations.

Economic Factors

During the past two decades, overall economic conditions as well as decisions surrounding the financing of health care have shaped the supply, configuration, and distribution of healthcare organizations and substantially changed the provision of health care in the United States. Although the overall number of hospitals has decreased, the demand for health services has grown (AHA, 2009). This increase has been particularly notable in the ranks of the needy and uninsured. According to the Kaiser Commission (2009), the majority of non-elderly Americans still receive health insurance coverage through their employers but the percentage of individuals with employment-based insurance is decreasing. In 2007, only 62% of non-elderly Americans received their health insurance coverage through their employers. This is the lowest level in more than a decade. Medicare covers almost all older adults at some level. Still, millions of individuals lack health insurance because either their employers do not offer it or they simply cannot afford to pay for it. In August 2008, the Census Bureau reported that in 2007, nearly 46 million people—18% of the population younger than 65 years—were without health insurance coverage (DeNavas-Walt, Proctor, & Smith, 2008).

An increase in the number of persons without health insurance has a significant impact on the communities in which they live and the healthcare organizations where they seek care. In an ongoing series of reports on the impact of the lack of health insurance on individuals, families, and communities, the Institute of Medicine consistently notes that the presence of a large number of uninsured people in a community could affect the availability of medical care for everyone (Institute of Medicine, 2003a, 2003b, 2004, 2009). The uninsured strain the resources of hospitals and divert tax dollars away from other necessary public health programs. The financial strain impacts the financial performance of local governments and healthcare providers alike. The report goes on to say that it is misguided, even dangerous, to assume that lack of health insurance harms only those who are uninsured. It hurts everyone when immunizations are missed and infectious diseases flourish or when chronic care is missed and an acute exacerbation occurs. Higher uninsurance rates are a significant predictor of the level of uncompensated care incurred by hospitals. In 2007, hospitals in the United States provided $34 billion of uncompensated care, threatening the economic viability of many of these organizations (AHA, 2009). The radical restructuring of the healthcare system that is required to reduce the continuing escalation of economic resources into the system and to make health care accessible to all citizens will necessitate ongoing changes in healthcare organizations. As the impact of healthcare reform legislation unfolds, more people will be covered by insurance, and more services will be needed.

In addition to struggling to respond to the increasing numbers of uninsured patients and the concomitant increase in the amounts of uncompensated care, healthcare organizations are being confronted daily with the financial pressures associated with rapidly escalating drug costs, expensive new technology, and spiraling personnel costs associated with healthcare labor shortages (Henry J. Kaiser Foundation, 2006; Kaiser Commission, 2009). The CMS reported that in 2008, healthcare spending reached 16.6% of the gross domestic product (Centers for Medicare & Medicaid Services [CMS], 2009). With costs escalating for legitimate reasons, one could reasonably expect that reimbursement would be increasing as well. This is, unfortunately, not the case.

Contemporaneous with cost inflation, payments by all payer groups are being reduced. The Kaiser Commission (2009) reports that both state and local governments are facing increasing financial pressure from the growing numbers of uninsured persons who are seeking health care at public expense as a result of losing their healthcare coverage because of unemployment. Beyond the higher cost associated with the increased enrollment because of layoffs, as the economy contracts, state and local governments face declining revenues that result in fewer resources to pay for the expanding programs. With the majority of state budgets in financial crisis, the common response has been massive state reductions, including major cutbacks in Medicaid eligibility levels, covered services, and payments to physicians and hospitals.

Compounding the impact of the direct reduction in governmental payments and subsidies on healthcare organizations is the expansion of managed care as a healthcare insurance product. During the past decade, the U.S. healthcare system has become increasingly competitive. As managed care plans compete for business primarily on their rate structures, these plans emphasize controlling patient access to care and lowering payments to providers while increasing patient co-pays and deductibles. As payments to hospitals are reduced, access to care for the uninsured is eroded because these hospitals have less financial capacity to provide charity care.

The complexity of controlling costs remains a major issue driving changes in the healthcare system. Perhaps the most significant changes will come from the discussions surrounding universal access to health coverage and control of healthcare costs. Beyond coverage and cost issues, revised Medicare rules related to implementation of electronic medical records (EMR) and other health information technology (HIT) requirements are expected to drive substantial change in the organization of healthcare services. Many hope that a significant infusion of capital for HIT will rapidly transform health care in the United States. However, experiences to date with HIT implementation have encountered many difficulties and therefore many individuals predict mixed results. Adoptions of EMR and HIT are typically long-term journeys toward improvement as opposed to quick fixes to endemic problems (Brokel & Harrison, 2009). Despite the challenges associated with acquiring and implementing these complex information systems, reflecting upon the importance of informatics to patient safety, in 2003 the IOM identified that using information technology is one of the five core competencies for all health professions.

Another concept associated with maximizing quality and minimizing costs is regionalization of services in which local coalitions consisting of community health providers, consumers, and corporations act to unify business initiatives in healthcare cost containment and to provide consumers with input into health planning and policy development. Wellness programs designed to modify consumers' use of and demand for services (e.g., health-promotion campaigns, ergonomic programs to reduce work-related injuries such as carpal tunnel syndrome, and fitness and exercise programs) are other industrial corporate initiatives being introduced to reduce costs. Again, nurses are assuming key roles in managed care and in organizing and directing wellness programs.

Nurses have a major role to play in demonstrating that access to care and quality management are essential components of cost control. With the increasing involvement of industry, business management techniques will assume greater emphasis in healthcare organizations. Nurses will need to lead efforts to redesign roles and restructure healthcare organizations. Nurse leaders and managers will need to go beyond obtaining education in business techniques to gaining skill in adapting that knowledge to meet the specific needs of delivery of cost-effective, quality care. The increasing focus on preparing registered nurses at the level of clinical nurse leader (CNL) and doctor of nursing practice (DNP) reflects the clear need for practicing nurses, nurse managers, and nurse administrators to be able to work efficiently and effectively in a constantly changing healthcare environment. The Evidence section on p. 135 describes the role and impact of the CNL.

Social Factors

Increasing consumer attention to disease prevention and promotion of healthful lifestyles is redefining relationships of healthcare organizations and their patients. Patients are becoming increasingly active in care planning, implementation, and evaluations and are seeking increased participation with their providers. Demands will be made of healthcare organizations for more personal, responsive, and coordinated care. As such, development of strategies that allow patients to become empowered controllers of their own health status is essential. Responsive structural changes in service delivery will be needed to maintain congruence with new missions and philosophies developed in response to cultural demands and social changes. Continuous evaluation will be needed to assess cost and quality outcomes related to these changes. Maintaining focus on the quality of care provided as well as access to care will be required so that bottom-line costs do not overshadow quality care provisions. Nursing's history of work with the development of patient-centered interactive strategies places nurses in a position to assume leadership roles in this area of organizational development.

Demographic Factors

Geographic dispersion, regional access to care, incomes of the population, aging of the population, and immigration trends are among the demographic factors influencing the design of healthcare organizations. Changing economic and demographic characteristics of many communities are resulting in a larger number of uninsured and underinsured individuals. Geographic isolation often limits access to necessary health services and impedes recruitment of healthcare personnel. Community-based rural health networks that provide primary care links to urban health centers for teaching, consultation, personnel sharing, and the provision of high-tech services are one solution for meeting needs in rural areas. Federal and state funding, which includes incentives for healthcare personnel to work in rural areas, is another approach. Strategic planning by nursing is critical to address community needs.

A major influence exerted on healthcare organizations comes from the aging of the population. By the year 2025, more than 18% of the population is expected to be older than 65 years. The number of "the old-old," those older than 80 years, is increasing dramatically. In response to this demographic shift, the CMS provides the Program of All-inclusive Care for the Elderly (PACE) to ensure that quality care is provided to impaired and frail elderly who are nursing home eligible. PACE aims to keep this population out of nursing homes by providing access to a full continuum of comprehensive community-based care. Although this segment of the population does not necessarily have dependency needs, a need exists for more long-term beds, supportive housing, and community programs. To meet these emerging needs of older adults, new healthcare organizations will continue to evolve, be evaluated, and be restructured based on findings. New roles for nurses as leaders and managers of the care of older adults are evolving, such as the role of advanced nurse practitioners to direct the care of patients who have become members of geriatric care organizations such as retirement centers.

Another significant effect on the system will come from the increasing number of individuals and families who cannot afford care to meet even their most basic needs. These individuals may be truly indigent or may be the working poor who are but one paycheck or illness from being hungry or homeless. Without a broad array of basic healthcare services affordable and available to these individuals, failure to treat a minor problem such as high blood pressure can result in a high-cost illness such as a cerebrovascular accident. This lack of healthcare provision is compounded by the number of people excluded from coverage because of preexisting health conditions, job loss, or immigration status.

A THEORETICAL PERSPECTIVE

Systems Theory

Systems theory attempts to explain productivity in terms of a unifying whole as opposed to a series of unrelated parts (Thompson, 1967). Systems can be either closed (self-contained) or open (interacting with both internal and external forces). In systems theory, a system is described as comprising four elements: structure, technology, people, and their environment. Systems theorists focus on the interplay among these elements in a framework of (1) inputs—resources such as people, money, or materials; (2) throughputs—the processes that produce a product from the inputs; and (3) outputs—the product of inputs and throughputs.

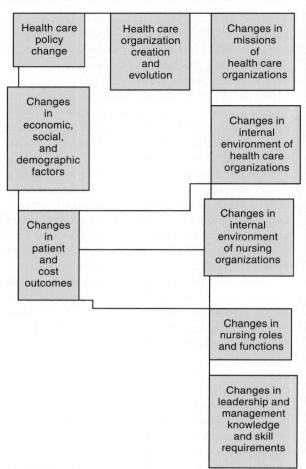

FIGURE 7-1 Healthcare organizations as open systems.

The theoretical concepts of systems theory have been applied to nursing and to organizations. Systems theory presents an explanation of organizational evolution that is similar to biological evolution. Systems theory produces a model that explains the process of healthcare organization evolution (Figure 7-1). The survival of the organization, as portrayed throughout this chapter, depends on its evolutionary response to changing environmental forces; it is seen as an open system. The response to environmental changes brings about internal changes, which produce changes that alter environmental conditions. The changes in the environment, in turn, act to bring about changes in the internal operating conditions of the organization.

A very simplified example of this can be seen by again studying the implementation of the prospective payment system that was caused by the economic driving force of escalating healthcare costs in the 1990s. Ambulatory surgery, same-day admissions, and hospital- and community-based home care organizations are some of the internal healthcare organization changes that resulted from an environmentally driven policy change—the cap that was placed on reimbursing expenses incurred by hospitalized patients. These internal organizational developments placed pressure on the external environment to create mechanisms to respond to increasing percentages of the population with self-care deficits who were returning to the community.

This open systems approach to organizational development and effectiveness emphasizes a continual process of adaptation of healthcare organizations to external driving forces and a response to the adaptations by the external environment, which generates continuing inputs for further healthcare organization development. This open system is in contrast to a closed system approach that views a system as being sufficient unto itself and thus is untouched by that which happens around it. (The effects of external forces on internal structures of healthcare organizations are discussed in Chapter 8.)

Chaos Theory

Unfortunately, health care as an industry is not always as predictable and orderly as systems theorists would have us believe. In contrast to the somewhat orderly universe described in systems theory, in which an organization can be viewed in terms of a linear, cause-and-effect model, chaos theory sees the universe as filled with unpredictable and random events (Hawking, 1998). According to the proponents of chaos theory, organizations must be self-organizing and adapt readily to change in order to survive. Organizations, therefore, must accept that change is inevitable and unrelenting. When one embraces the tenets of chaos theory, one gives up on any attempt to create a permanent organizational structure. Using creativity and flexibility, successful managers will be those who can tolerate ambiguity, take risks, and experiment with new ideas that respond to each day's unique situation or environment. They will not rest upon a successful transition or organizational model

---

THEORY BOX

Systems and Chaos Theories

Systems Theory	• Definition: A system comprises four elements (structure, technology, people, and environment) forming a unified whole • Viewed as inputs, throughputs, and outputs • Closed systems—self-contained • Open systems—interacting with internal and external forces
Chaos Theory	• Definition: The universe is chaotic and requires organizations to be self-organizing and adaptive to survive • Viewed as unpredictable and random events • Constant change resulting in little long-term stability

---

because they know the environment within which it flourished is fleeting. The successful nurse leaders will be those individuals who are committed to life-long learning and problem solving. The Theory Box above notes key elements of systems and chaos theories.

EXERCISE 7-5

Think about the economic, social, and demographic changes you can identify in your community. How will they influence healthcare organizations and the provision of health care in your community? How can systems theory and chaos theory help provide a context for discussing these trends?

NURSING ROLE AND FUNCTION CHANGES

Leadership and management roles for nurses are proliferating in healthcare organizations that are developing or evolving in response to environmental driving forces. The proportion of nursing jobs in the community is increasing. Nurses need new knowledge and skills to coordinate the care of patients or communities with the many other disciplines and organizational units that are providing the continuum of care. Our society needs nurses who can engage in the political process of policy development, coor-

RESEARCH PERSPECTIVE

Resource: Bogue, R. J., Joseph, M. L., & Sieloff, C. L. (2009). Shared governance as vertical alignment of nursing group power and nurse practice council effectiveness. *Journal of Nursing Management, 17*(1), 4-14.

If healthcare organizations are to survive the continuous assault of rapid economic, social, and demographic shifts, they must find ways to be responsive to the ever-changing demands at the front line of patient care. Nurse empowerment has been demonstrated to be associated with improved nurse satisfaction, increased job engagement, and enhanced patient outcomes. The authors note that empowerment of nurses occurs with the vertical alignment of nursing group power and the actual practices of the nursing unit. The lack of a tool for measuring the effectiveness of activities within a nursing practice council was seen as a limiting factor in understanding and thus maximizing organizational support for nurse empowerment. The purpose of this study was to develop and validate a tool—The Nursing Practice Council Effectiveness Scale (NPCes)—to measure the effectiveness of nurse practice councils.

The authors found that NPCes in combination with the Sieloff-King Assessment of Group Power can be used to better understand the dynamics of shared governance at the department and unit levels.

Implications for Practice

These findings provide nursing leadership with specific tools that can be used to examine group power and unit level practices. Using these tools, nursing and organizational leadership can obtain a more complete view of the barriers to nurse empowerment and thus can construct specific strategies to improve nurses' power competencies, communication competencies, power capacity, and resources to exercise power. Increasing these competencies will serve to establish healthy work environments in which employee engagement is maximized and job satisfaction, as well as positive patient outcomes, is increased. These factors are related to overall organizational effectiveness and sustainability, especially in difficult economic times.

dinate care across disciplines and settings, use conflict management techniques to create win-win situations for patients and providers in resolving the healthcare system's delivery problems, and use business savvy to market and prepare financial and organizational plans for the delivery of cost-effective care.

Remember that economic, social, and demographic changes are not limited to patients and communities. These shifts are affecting the workplace as well. Farag, Tullai-McGuinness, and Anthony (2009) note that nurses in various age cohorts perceive the same manager and unit culture in distinctly different ways. To be effective, nurse leaders need to consider how this phenomenon affects the workplace in the same way they consider it when seeking to address the needs of their patients and the communities they serve. To be efficient and effective, nurse leaders must be not only patient-centered but also employee-centered. The Research Perspective above suggests how nurse leaders can use measurement tools to assess the dynamics of shared governance at the department and unit level. These results can be used to increase nurses' power competencies, thus establishing healthy work environments in which employee engagement

is maximized and job satisfaction and positive patient outcomes are increased. (Shared governance as an organizing structure is discussed in Chapter 8.)

Whether influenced by systems or chaos theory, today's healthcare organizations are in a dynamic state. Nurses must be continuously alert to assessing both the internal and external environment for forces that act as inputs to changes needed in their healthcare organization and for the effects of changes that are made. Awareness of the changing status of healthcare organizations and the ability to play a leading role in creating and evaluating adaptation in response to changing forces will be central functions of nurse leaders and managers in healthcare organizations. Nurses need to develop a foundation of leadership and management knowledge that they can build on through a planned program of continuing education. Even in tumultuous times within the healthcare industry, nursing leaders have demonstrated their ability to strengthen the quality of both their organizations and the practice of nursing. As healthcare organizations continue to undergo transformation, tomorrow's nurses—whether leaders, managers, or followers—need to carry these lessons forward.

THE SOLUTION

I contacted the hospital case manager, who arranged for this patient to have access to special programs in the hospital to fund the medications and support the case management expenses. We arranged for the patient to be seen by a state agency that provides emergency funds for utilities and phone service and assisted him with a Medicaid application with a request for a retroactive initiation date. Finally, we contacted hospice and the American Cancer Society to support the tube-feeding expenses and worked with other agencies to delay billings until Medicaid was available. Clearly, today's nurse manager has to be connected with the extended resources in the community to ensure care for patients who require assistance.

—*Beth A. Smith*

Would this be a suitable approach for you? Why?

THE EVIDENCE

The American Association of Colleges of Nursing introduced the role of the master's-prepared clinical nurse leader (CNL) in 2004. Through the presentation of three case studies, Stanley et al. (2008) describe the impact of the role of the CNL on patient care outcomes and cost. Impact was described in terms of innovation (as described in journals kept by CNLs), quality (as measured by rates of falls, falls with injury, and the percentage of patients reporting "excellent" in pain management), and patient satisfaction (in terms of patients reporting "excellent" in nurses' response to calls and overall nursing care). Analysis of the three case studies demonstrated significant cost savings and increased satisfaction over short periods following implementation of the role.

The evidence supports the positive impact of CNLs on patients (quality of care measures and patient satisfaction), employee engagement (nursing turnover and vacancy rate), and organizations (customer loyalty and cost).

NEED TO KNOW NOW

- Know the economic and demographic characteristics of the patients and communities you serve.
- Identify and stay abreast of the resources available within your community.
- Actively seek educational opportunities related to leadership development.
- Become involved in the development and implementation of public policy related to healthcare issues.

CHAPTER CHECKLIST

Knowledge of types of healthcare organizations and characteristics used to differentiate healthcare organizations provides a foundation for examining the operation of the healthcare system. Understanding the economic, social, and demographic forces driving changes in healthcare organizations identifies needs that organizations must be designed to fit. Recognizing that alterations in the environment and in healthcare organizations are mutually interactive is necessary to determine the effects of change and the steps that need to be taken in response to the constant changes.

Changes in nursing roles as well as in the settings in which services are provided require that nurses expand their knowledge and skills. These changes are part of a continual evolution that demands a foundation in leadership and management knowledge that serves as a basis for future development.

- Key characteristics that differentiate types of healthcare organizations are as follows:
  - Types of services provided
  - Length of services provided
  - Ownership

- Teaching status
- Accreditation status
- Major types of healthcare organizations are as follows:
  - Institutional providers
  - Acute care facilities
  - Long-term facilities
  - Rehabilitation facilities
  - Consolidated systems and networks
  - Ambulatory-based organizations
  - Other organizations
    - Community services
    - Subacute care facilities
    - Home health organizations
    - Long-term care and residential facilities
    - Hospice
    - Nurse-owned/nurse-organized services
    - Self-help voluntary organizations
  - Supportive and ancillary organizations
    - Regulatory organizations
    - Accrediting bodies
    - Third-party financing organizations (insurers)
    - Pharmaceutical and medical equipment supply corporations
    - Professional, educational, and training organizations
- Economic forces driving the development of healthcare organizations are numerous and are continually evolving, escalating the percentage of the GNP comprising healthcare costs.
  - An increasing number of uninsured patients threaten the health of the community.
  - Decreasing reimbursement threatens the economic viability of healthcare organizations.
  - Social forces driving development of healthcare organizations include the following:
    - A focus of society that is changing from illness to health (wellness)
    - An increasing demand by individuals that they participate in designing their own customized care plans
- Demographic forces driving development of healthcare organizations include the following:
  - The increasing percentage of society who are older adults. An increasing percentage of poor people who do not have the financial resources to have access to care
  - The inability of communities to provide ready and economical access to needed health services
- Implications of healthcare organization evolution for leadership and management role functions of professional nurses include the following:
  - An increased ability to attune to the altered environmental driving forces that predict and direct necessary changes in healthcare organizations
  - An increased ability to attune to the healthcare organization's internal environment to predict and direct changes required in both the internal and external environment
  - Knowledge and skill both in influencing the development of and in developing healthcare policy at the federal, state, local, and organizational levels
  - Knowledge and skill in coordinating and collaborating with peers and other disciplines providing services within a point of service and in networks created by the interconnection of many points of service
  - Skill in using business knowledge in planning and evaluating delivery of health care in healthcare organizations that must market cost and outcome effectiveness to survive
  - Knowledge and skill in planning and directing group work, which promotes optimal health statuses with minimal use of personnel and material resources

TIPS FOR HEALTHCARE ORGANIZATIONS

- Knowledge of economic, social, and demographic changes is essential to redesigning healthcare organizations to meet society's needs.

- Increasing consolidation of healthcare services that provide all levels of care necessitates the development of communication systems that provide

information on patients receiving services at the various points of care in the network.
- Diversified positions will be available for professional nurses in the various organizations that are developing to enhance the provision of care.

- New configurations of healthcare delivery will demand that professional nurses continually acquire new knowledge and skills in leadership and management.

REFERENCES

American Hospital Association (AHA). (2009). *The 2009 AHA environmental scan.* Chicago: Author.

Bogue, R. J., Joseph, M. L., & Sieloff, C. L. (2009). Shared governance as vertical alignment of nursing group power and nurse practice council effectiveness. *Journal of Nursing Management, 17*(1), 4-14.

Brokel, J. M., & Harrison, M. I. (2009). Redesigning care processes using an electronic health record: A system's experience. *Joint Commission Journal on Quality and Patient Safety, 35*(2), 82-92.

Centers for Medicare & Medicaid Services (CMS). (2009). *Highlights: National health expenditures, 2007.* Retrieved October 22, 2009, from www.cms.hhs.gov/ NationalHealthExpendData/downloads/highlights.pdf.

DeNavas-Walt, B., Proctor, C. B., & Smith, J. (2008). *Income, poverty, and health insurance coverage in the United States: 2007.* Washington, DC: U.S. Census Bureau.

Farag, A. A., Tullai-McGuinness, S., & Anthony, M. K. (2009). Nurses' perception of their manager's leadership style and unit climate: Are there generational differences? *Journal of Nursing Management, 17*(1), 26-34.

Flatt, A., & Rahal, R. (2006). *A study of the impact of clinical education on academic hospital expenses.* Ontario, Canada: Council of Academic Hospitals of Ontario.

Hawking, S. (1998). *A brief history of time.* London: Bantam Press.

Henry J. Kaiser Family Foundation. (2006). *The uninsured: A primer, key facts about Americans without health insurance.* Washington, DC: Author.

Institute of Medicine. (2003a). *A shared destiny: Effects of uninsurance on individuals, families, and communities.* Washington, DC: National Academies Press.

Institute of Medicine. (2003b). *Health professions education: A bridge to quality.* Washington, DC: National Academies Press.

Institute of Medicine. (2004). *Insuring America's health: Principles and recommendations.* Washington, DC: National Academies Press.

Institute of Medicine. (2009). *America's uninsurance crisis: Consequences for health and healthcare.* Washington, DC: National Academies Press.

Kaiser Commission on Medicaid and the Uninsured. (2009). *Rising unemployment, Medicaid and the uninsured.* Washington, DC: Henry J. Kaiser Family Foundation.

Stanley, J. M., Gannon, J., Gabaut, S., Adams, N., Mayes, C., Shouse, G. M., Edwards, B. A., & Burch, D. (2008). The clinical nurse leader: A catalyst for improving quality and patient safety. *Journal of Nursing Management, 16*(5), 612-622.

Thompson, J. D. (1967). *Organization in action.* New York: McGraw-Hill.

United States Department of the Treasury. (2009). Exempt organizations compliance project: Final report. Washington, DC: Author.

SUGGESTED READINGS

Etheridge, P. (1997). The Carondelet experience. *Nursing Management, 28*(3), 26-28.

Institute of Medicine. (2007). *The learning healthcare system.* Washington, DC: National Academies Press.

Institute of Medicine. (2008). *Knowing what works in healthcare: A roadmap for the nation.* Washington, DC: National Academies Press.

Kaiser Commission on Medicaid and the Uninsured. (2004). *Health care coverage in America.* Washington, DC: Henry J. Kaiser Family Foundation.

Kast, F. E., & Rosenweiz, J. E. (1991). General systems theory: Applications for organizations and management. In M. J. Ward & S. A. Price (Eds.), *Issues in nursing administration: Selected readings* (pp. 60-73). St. Louis: Mosby.

Naswall, K., Hellgren, J., & Sverke, M. (2008). *The individual in the changing worklife.* Cambridge, UK: Cambridge University Press.

Porter-O'Grady, T. (1996). The seven basic rules for successful redesign. *Journal of Nursing Administration, 26*(1), 46-55.

Ruger, J. P. (2008). Ethics in American health: An ethical framework for health system reform. *American Journal of Public Health, 98*(10), 1756-1763.

Running, A., & Sheppard, K. (2005). Minute clinics: Are they a solution for the current times? *The Journal for Nurse Practitioners, 2*(4), 254-255.

Sisko, A., Truffer, C., Smith, S., Keehan, S., Cylus, J., Poisal, J. A., Clemens, M. K., & Lizonitz, J. (2009). Health spending projections through 2018: Recession effects add uncertainty to the outlook. *Health Affairs, 28*(2), 346-357.

Surakka, T. (2008). The nurse manager's work in the hospital environment during the 1990's and 2000's: Responsibility, accountability and expertise in nursing leadership. *Journal of Nursing Management, 16*(5), 525-534.

INTERNET RESOURCES

Centers for Medicare & Medicaid Services (CMS): www.cms.gov
Community Health Assessment Program (CHAP):
    www.chapinc.org
Government Accountability Office (GAO): www.gao.gov
Institute for Healthcare Improvement (IHI): www.ihs.gov
Kaiser Family Foundation—Kaiser Commission on Medicaid and
    the Uninsured: www.kff.org/

Medicare Quality Improvement Community (MedQIC):
    www.qualitynet.org
National Committee on Quality Assurance (NCQA):
    www.ncqa.org
National PACE Association (NPA): www.npaonline.org
The Joint Commission: www.jointcommission.org

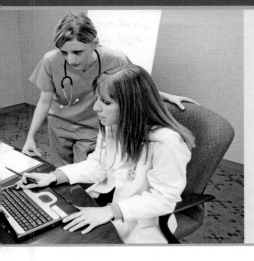

Understanding and Designing Organizational Structures

Mary E. Mancini

This chapter explains key concepts related to organizational structures and provides information on designing effective structures. This information can be used to help new managers function in an organization and to design structures that support work processes. An underlying theme is designing organizational structures that will respond to the continuous changes taking place in the healthcare environment.

OBJECTIVES

- Analyze the relationships among mission, vision, and philosophy statements and organizational structure.
- Analyze factors that influence the design of an organizational structure.
- Compare and contrast the major types of organizational structures.
- Evaluate the forces that are necessitating reengineering of organizational systems.

TERMS TO KNOW

bureaucracy	organization	service-line structures
chain of command	organizational chart	shared governance
flat organizational structure	organizational culture	span of control
functional structure	organizational structure	staff function
hierarchy	organizational theory	system
hybrid	philosophy	systems theory
line function	redesign	vision
matrix structure	reengineering	
mission	restructuring	

INTRODUCTION

Since time began, people have organized themselves into groups. The term organization has multiple meanings. It can refer to a business structure designed to support specific business goals and processes, or it can refer to a group of individuals working together to achieve a common purpose. Regardless of how the term is used, learning to determine how an organization accomplishes its work, how to operate productively within an organization, and how to influence organizational processes is essential to a successful professional nursing practice.

Organizational theory (sometimes called *organizational studies*) is the systematic analysis of how organizations and their component parts act and interact. Organizational theory is based largely on the systematic investigation of the effectiveness of specific organizational designs in achieving their purpose. Organizational theory development is a process of creating knowledge to understand the effect of identified factors, such as (1) organizational culture; (2) organizational technology, which is defined as all the work being carried out; and (3) organizational structure or organizational development. A purpose of such work is to determine how organizational effectiveness might be predicted or controlled through the design of the organizational structure.

Specific organizational theories provide insight into areas such as effective organizational structures, motivation of employees, decision making, and leadership. A common framework in health care for analysis and application of organizational theory is systems theory. A system is an interacting collection of components or parts that together make up an integrated whole. The basic tenet of systems theory is that the individual components of any system interact with each other and with their environment. To be effective, professional nurses need to understand the specific part—role and function—they play within a system and how they interact, influence, and are influenced by other parts of the system.

An organization's mission, vision, and philosophy form the foundation for its structure and performance as well as the development of the professional practice models it uses. An organization's mission, or reason for the organization's existence, influences the design of the structure (e.g., to meet the healthcare needs of a designated population, to provide supportive and stabilizing care to an acute care population, or to prepare patients for a peaceful death). The vision is the articulated goal to which the organization aspires. A vision statement conveys an inspirational view of how the organization wishes to be described at some future time. It suggests how far to strive in all endeavors. Another key factor influencing structure is the organization's philosophy. A philosophy expresses the values and beliefs that members of the organization hold about the nature of their work, about the people to whom they provide service, and about themselves and others providing the services.

EXERCISE 8-1

Consider how you might use the information in the Introduction (1) to analyze an organization that you are considering joining to determine whether it fits your professional development plans, (2) to assess the functioning of an organization of which you are already a member, or (3) to make a plan to reengineer the structure or philosophy to better accomplish the mission of an organization you are considering joining or of which you are already a member.

MISSION

The mission statement defines the organization's reason or purpose for being. The mission statement identifies the organization's customers and the types of services offered, such as education, supportive nursing care, rehabilitation, acute care, and home care. It enacts the vision statement.

The mission statement sets the stage by defining the services to be offered, which, in turn, identify the kinds of technologies and human resources to be employed. The mission statement of healthcare systems typically refers to the larger community the organizations serve as well as the specific patient pop-ulations to whom they provide care. An example of a mission statement appears in Box 8-1. Hospitals' missions are primarily treatment-oriented; the missions of ambulatory care group practices combine treatment, prevention, and diagnosis-oriented services; long-term care facilities' missions are primarily maintenance and social support–oriented; and the missions of nursing centers are oriented toward promoting optimal health status for a defined group of people. The definition of services to be provided and its implications for technologies and human resources greatly influence the design of the organizational structure, the arrangement of the work group.

BOX 8-1   MISSION, VISION, AND PHILOSOPHY FOR A NEUROSURGICAL UNIT

Mission Statement

This unit's purpose is to provide high-quality nursing care for neurosurgical patients during the acute phase of their illness that facilitates their progression to the rehabilitation phase. We strive to cultivate a multidisciplinary approach to the care of the neurosurgical patient and provide multiple educational opportunities for the professional development of neurosurgical nurses.

Vision Statement

To be the premier neurosurgical nursing unit in the state.

Philosophy

The philosophy is based on Roy's Adaptation Model and on the American Association of Neurosurgical Nursing conceptual framework.

Patients

We believe

- It is the right of the patients to make informed choices concerning their treatment.
- Patients have a right to high-quality nursing care and opportunities for improving their quality of life, regardless of the potential outcomes of their illness.
- The patient/family/significant other has a right to exercise personal options to participate in care to the extent of individual abilities and needs.

Nursing

We believe

- Neuroscience nursing is a unique area of nursing practice because neurosurgical interventions and/or neurological dysfunction affect all levels of human existence.
- The goal of the neuroscience nurse is to engage in a therapeutic relationship with his or her patients to facilitate adaptation to changes in physiological, self-concept, role performance, and interdependent modes.

- The ultimate goal for the neuroscience nurse is to foster internal and external unity of patients to achieve optimal health potentials.

Nurse

We believe

- The nurse is the integral element who coordinates nursing care for the neurosurgical patient using valuable input from all members of the patient care team.
- The nurse has an obligation to assume accountability for maintaining excellence in practice.
- The nurse has three basic rights: human rights, legal rights, and professional rights.
- The nurse has a right to autonomy in providing nursing care based on sound nursing judgment.

Nursing Practice

We believe

- Nursing practice must support and be supported by activities in practice, education, research, and management.
- Insofar as possible, patients must be assigned one nurse who is responsible and accountable for their care throughout their stay on the neurosurgical unit.
- The primary nurse is responsible for consulting and collaborating with other healthcare professionals in planning and delivering patient care.
- The contributions of all members of the nursing team are valuable, and an environment must be created that allows each member to participate fully in the delivery of care in accord with his or her abilities and qualifications.
- The nursing process is the vehicle used by nurses to operationalize nursing practice.
- Data generated in nursing practices must be continually and consistently collected and analyzed for the purpose of managing the quality of nursing practice.

Courtesy Upstate Medical University, University Hospital, Syracuse, NY (W. Painter, J. Van Nest-Kinne).

Nursing, as a profession providing a service within a healthcare agency, formulates its own mission statement that describes its contributions to achieve the agency's mission. One of the purposes of the nursing profession is to provide nursing care to patients. The statement should define nursing based on theories that form the basis for the model of nursing to be used in guiding the process of nursing care delivery. Nursing's mission statement tells why nursing exists within the context of the organization. It is written so that others within the organization can know and understand nursing's role in achieving the agency's mission. The mission should be the guiding framework for decision making. It should be known and understood by other healthcare professionals, by patients and their families, and by the community. It indicates the relationships among nurses and patients, agency personnel, the community, and health and illness. This statement provides direction for the evolving statement of philosophy and the organizational structure. It should be reviewed for accuracy and updated routinely by professional nurses providing care. Units that provide specific services such as intensive care, cardiac services, or maternity services also formulate mission statements that detail their specific contributions to the overall mission.

VISION

Vision statements are future-oriented, purposeful statements designed to identify the desired future of an organization. They serve to unify all subsequent statements toward the view of the future and to convey the core message of the mission statement. Typically, vision statements are brief, consisting of only one or two phrases or sentences. An example of a vision statement is provided in Box 8-1.

PHILOSOPHY

A philosophy is a written statement that articulates the values and beliefs held about the nature of the work required to accomplish the mission and the nature and rights of both the people being served and those providing the service. It states the nurse managers' and practitioners' vision of what they believe nursing management and practice are and sets the stage for developing goals to make that vision a reality.

It states the beliefs of nurse managers and staff as to how the mission or purpose will be achieved. For example, the mission statement may incorporate the provision of individualized care as an organizational purpose. The philosophy statement would then support this purpose through an expression of a belief in the responsibility of nursing staff to act as patient advocates and to provide quality care according to the wishes of the patient, family, and significant others.

Philosophies are evolutionary in that they are shaped both by the social environment and by the stage of development of professionals delivering the service. Nursing staff reflect the values of their time. The values acquired through education are reflected in the nursing philosophy. Technology developments can also help shape philosophy. For example, information systems can provide people with data that allow them greater control over their work; workers are consequently able to make more decisions and take more autonomous action. Philosophies require updating to reflect the extension of rights brought about by such changes. Box 8-1 shows an example of a philosophy developed for a neurosurgical unit with the leadership of a nurse manager and clinical instructor.

EXERCISE 8-2

Obtain a copy of the philosophy of a nursing department and identify behaviors that you observe on a unit of the department that relate or do not relate to the beliefs and values expressed in the document.

ORGANIZATIONAL CULTURE

An organization's mission, vision, and philosophy both shape and reflect organizational culture. Organizational culture is the reflection of the norms or traditions of the organization and is exemplified by behaviors that illustrate values and beliefs. Examples include rituals and customary forms of practice, such as celebrations of promotions, publications, degree attainment, professional performance, weddings, and retirements. Other examples of norms that reflect organizational culture are the characteristics of the people who are recognized as heroes by the organization and the behaviors—either positive or negative—that are accepted or tolerated within the organization.

In organizations, culture is demonstrated in two ways that can be either mutually reinforcing or conflict-producing. Organizational culture is typically expressed in a formal manner via written mission, vision, and philosophy statements; job descriptions; and policies and procedures. Beyond formal documents and verbal descriptions given by administrators and managers, organizational culture is also represented in the day-to-day experience of staff and patients. To many, it is the lived experience that reflects the true organizational culture. Do the decisions that are made within the organization consistently demonstrate that the organization values its patients and keeps their needs at the forefront? Are the employees treated with trust and respect, or are the words used in recruitment ads simply empty promises with little evidence to back them up? When there is a lack of congruity between the expressed organizational culture and the experienced organizational culture, confusion, frustration, and poor morale often result (Casida, 2008; Melnick, Ulaszek, Lin, & Wexler, 2009).

Organizational culture can be effective and promote success and positive outcomes, or it can be ineffective and result in disharmony, dissatisfaction, and poor outcomes for patients, staff, and the organization. A number of workplace variables are influenced by organizational culture (Chen, 2008). When seeking employment or advancement, nurses need to assess the organization's culture and develop a clear understanding of existing expectations as well as the formal and informal communication patterns. Various techniques and tools are available to assist the nurse in performing a cultural assessment of an organization (Casida, 2008). With a solid understanding of organizational culture, nurses will be better able to be effective change agents and help transform the organizations in which they work. The Research Perspective at left presents a study on the relationship between leadership and organizational culture in acute care hospitals.

 RESEARCH PERSPECTIVE

Resource: Casida, J., & Pinto-Zipp, G. (2008). Leadership-organizational culture relationship in nursing units of acute care hospitals. *Nursing Economic$, 26*(1), 7-15.

The concepts of leadership and organizational culture are well described in the literature. Using a convenience sample of managers and staff nurses from four hospitals in a large New Jersey healthcare system, this study attempts to explicate the relationship between the two concepts in terms of nurse managers in acute care hospitals. Descriptive and explanatory correlational designs were used to describe the leadership styles of the nurse managers as well as the organizational culture on the managers' units. Data from 37 nurse managers and 278 staff nurses support the notion that transformational and transactional contingent reward leadership styles are likely to create an effective organizational culture characterized by a focus on mission, adaptability, involvement, and consistency. A laissez-faire leadership approach was not shown to influence organizational culture in a positive manner. These findings were attributed to the purposeful interactions between staff and managers who demonstrated transformational leadership and the lack of purposeful interactions when the manager demonstrated a laissez-faire style.

Implications for Practice
This study supports the belief that well-prepared nurse managers who demonstrate transformational and transactional contingent reward leadership styles have a positive impact on unit culture and staff. Nurse administrators can use the results from this study to guide their efforts to develop robust selection and development programs for future nurse managers. Staff nurses and nurse managers can use this study to help identify their own leadership style. In addition, staff nurses can use the information to help them identify work units where they are likely to find a supportive organizational culture.

FACTORS INFLUENCING ORGANIZATIONAL DEVELOPMENT

To be most effective, organizational structures must reflect the organization's mission, vision, philosophy, goals, and objectives. Organizational structure defines how work is organized, where decisions are made, and the authority and responsibility of workers. It provides a map for communication and outlines decision-making paths. As organizations change through acquisitions and mergers, it is essential that structure changes to accomplish revised missions.

Probably the best theory to explain today's nursing organizational development is chaos (complexity, nonlinear, quantum) theory. (See Chapter 7 and the Index.) In essence, chaos theory suggests that lives—and organizations—are really weblike. Pulling on one small segment rearranges the web, a new pattern emerges, and yet the whole remains. This theory, applied to nursing organizations, suggests that differences logically exist between and among various organizations and that the constant environmental forces continue to affect the structure, its functioning, and the services. Brafman and Beckstrom (2008), in their aptly named book, *The Starfish and the Spider,* identified how organizations differ and yet are successful. Spider organizations are built like a spider, and when the head is destroyed, the spider dies. The starfish, on the other hand, can lose an appendage, and it just grows another one. In fact, a starfish, when cut in half, creates two starfish. Organizations that are controlled in a heavily centralized way can diminish quickly without the strong, central figure. Organizations that are self-generating quickly share leadership as needed and often continue to thrive. The important point for any organization is to find what is known as the "sweet spot," the point of balance between centralization and decentralization.

The issues in healthcare delivery, with their concomitant changes such as reimbursement regulation and the development of networks for delivery of health care, have profound effects on organizational structure designs. Consumerism, the consumer demand that care be customized to meet individual needs, necessitates that decision making be done where the care is delivered. Increased consumer knowledge and greater responsibility for selecting healthcare providers and options have resulted in consumers who demand immediate access to customized care. Information from Internet sources and direct-to-consumer advertising are significantly altering the expectation and behaviors of healthcare consumers. For example, *Hospital Compare (www. hospitalcompare.hhs.gov)* is a tool that consumers can use to access a searchable database of information describing how well hospitals care for patients with certain medical and surgical conditions. Access to this information allows consumers to make informed decisions about where they seek their health care. In response to consumer expectations, facilities concentrate on consumer satisfaction and delivery of patient-focused care. Changes in both facility design and care delivery systems are likely to continue as efforts are made to reduce cost while still striving to meet or exceed consumer expectations and improve patient outcomes.

Competition for patients is another factor influencing structure design. These three factors—consumerism, change, and competition—necessitate reengineering healthcare structures. Whereas redesign is a technique to analyze tasks to improve efficiency (e.g., identifying the most efficient flow of supplies to a nursing unit) and restructuring is a technique to enhance organizational productivity (e.g., identifying the most appropriate type and number of staff members for a particular nursing unit), reengineering involves a total overhaul of an organizational structure. It is a radical reorganization of the totality of an organization's structure and work processes. In reengineering, fundamentally new organizational expectations and relationships are created. An example of where reengineering is required is technologic change, particularly in information services, that provides a means of customizing care. Its potential for making all information concerning a patient immediately accessible to direct care givers has the potential for a profound positive impact on healthcare decision making.

The Transforming Care at the Bedside (TCAB) initiative is an example of redesigning the work environment from the bottom up. The initiative, funded by the Robert Wood Johnson Foundation and the Institute for Healthcare Improvement, was started in 2003 to develop and validate an evidence-based process for transforming care in acute care facilities. Reports from TCAB facilities demonstrate the value of nurse involvement in the process as well as the value to nurses in terms of their participation (Martin et al., 2007; Upenieks et al., 2008).

Regardless of the level of changes made within an organization—redesign, restructuring, or reengineering—staff and patients alike feel the impact. Some of the changes result in improvements, whereas others may not; some of the impacts are expected, whereas others are not. It is critical, therefore, that nurse managers as well as staff nurses are vigilant for both anticipated and unanticipated results of these changes. Nurses need to position themselves to participate in change discussions and evaluations. Ultimately, it is their day-to-day work with their patients that is affected by the decisions made in response to a rapidly changing environment (Martin et al., 2007; Murphy & Roberts, 2008). The Evidence section on p. 155 describes the impact of organizational restructuring on nurses.

EXERCISE 8-3
Arrange to interview a nurse employed in a healthcare agency or use your own experience to identify examples of changes taking place that necessitate reengineering. These may include changes associated with implementation of new reimbursement strategies, development of policies to carry out legislative regulations related to patient confidentiality, or development of chest pain centers. Identify examples of how previous systems of communication and decision making were either adequate or inadequate to cope with these changes.

CHARACTERISTICS OF ORGANIZATIONAL STRUCTURES

The characteristics of different types of organizational structures provide a catalog of options to consider in designing structures that fit specific situations. Knowledge of these characteristics also help managers understand the structures in which they currently function.

Organizational designs are often classified by their characteristics of complexity, formalization, and centralization. *Complexity* concerns the division of labor in an organization, the specialization of that labor, the number of hierarchical levels, and the geographic dispersion of organizational units. *Division of labor* and *specialization* refer to the separation of processes into tasks that are performed by designated people. The horizontal dimension of an organizational chart, the graphic representation of work units and reporting relationships, relates to the division and specialization of labor functions attended by specialists. Hierarchy connotes lines of authority and responsibility. Chain of command is a term used to refer to the hierarchy and is depicted in vertical dimensions of organizational charts. Hierarchy vests authority in positions on an ascending line away from where work is performed and allows control of work. Staff members are often placed on a bottom level of the organization, and those in authority, who provide control, are placed in higher levels. Span of control refers to the number of subordinates a supervisor manages. For budgetary reasons, span of control is often a major focus for organizational restructuring. Although there are cost implications when a span of control is too narrow, when a span of control becomes too large, supervision can become less effective. The Literature Perspective at right describes the effect of

LITERATURE PERSPECTIVE

Resource: Lucas, V., Laschinger, H. K., & Wong, C. A. (2008). The impact of emotional intelligent leadership on staff nurse empowerment: The moderating effect of span of control. *International Journal of Nursing Management, 16*(8), 964-973.

Multiple studies have shown that managers are critical to creating environments that empower nurses for professional practice. Still, efforts to improve efficiency and decrease costs often result in a reduction in the number of frontline managers. Using a descriptive correlational survey design, Lucas, Laschinger, and Wong tested a model to evaluate staff nurses' perceptions of their manager's emotionally intelligent leadership style and the impact of the manager's number of direct reports (span of control).

The hypothesized model was tested with staff nurses in two community hospitals in Ontario, Canada. Sixty-eight percent (n=230) of nurses surveyed returned usable questionnaires. Analysis of the data demonstrated that span of control was a significant moderator of the relationship between the nurses' feeling of empowerment and their perception of their manager's emotionally intelligent behaviors.

Implications for Practice
During times of restructuring, administrators need to be aware of the correlation between a manager's span of control and their staff nurses' perceptions of empowerment and support. If an empowered nursing workforce is valued, efforts must be made to maintain a reasonable span of control for managers. Staff at all levels must be aware of this effect and actively develop plans with this correlation in mind.

span of control on perceived empowerment of staff nurses.

Geographic dispersion refers to the physical location of units. Units of work may be in one building; in several buildings in one location; spread throughout a city; or in different counties, states, or countries. The more dispersed an organization is, the greater are the demands for creative designs that place decision making related to patient care close to the patient and, consequently, far from corporate headquarters. A similar type of complexity exists in organizations that deliver care at multiple sites in the community; for example, the care delivery sites of school health programs are in schools that usually are at great distances from the corporate office that has overall responsibility for the programs.

Formalization is the degree to which an organization has rules, stated in terms of policies that define a member's function. The amount of formalization varies among institutions. It is often inversely related to the degree of specialization and the number of professionals within the organization.

Centralization refers to the location where a decision is made. Decisions are made at the top of a centralized organization. In a decentralized organization, decisions are made at or close to the patient-care level. Highly centralized organizations often delegate *responsibility* (the obligation to perform the task) without the *authority* (the right to act, which is necessary to carry out the responsibility). For example, some hospitals have delegated both the responsibility and the authority for admission decisions to the charge nurse (decentralized), whereas others require the nurse supervisor or chief nurse executive to make such decisions (centralization).

BUREAUCRACY

Many organizational theories in use today find their basis in the works of early twenty-first century theorists Max Weber, a German sociologist who developed the basic tenets of bureaucracy (Weber, 1947), and Henri Fayol, a French industrialist who crafted 14 principles of management (Fayol, 1949). Initially, bureaucracy referred to the centralization of authority in administrative bureaus or government departments. The term has come to refer to an inflexible approach to decision making or an agency encumbered by "red tape" that adds little value to organizational processes.

Bureaucracy is an administrative concept imbedded in how organizations are structured. It arose at a time of societal development when services were in short supply, workers' and clients' knowledge bases were limited, and technologies for sharing information were undeveloped. Characteristics of bureaucracy arose out of a need to control workers and were centered on the division of processes into discrete tasks. Weber proposed that organizations could achieve high levels of productivity and efficiency only by adherence to what he called "bureaucracy." Weber believed that bureaucracy, based on the sociological concept of rationalization of collective activities, provided the idealized organizational structure. Bureaucratic structures are formal and have a centralized and hierarchical command structure (chain of command). In bureaucratic structures, there is a clear division of labor and well-articulated and commonly accepted expectations for performance. Rules, standards, and protocols ensure uniform actions and limit individualization of services and variance in workers' performance. In bureaucratic organizations, as shown in Figure 8-1, communication and decisions flow from top to bottom. Although it enhances consistency, bureaucracy, by nature, limits employees' autonomy.

In developing his 14 principles of management, Fayol outlined structures and processes that guide how work is accomplished within an organization. Consistent with theories of bureaucracy, his principles of management include division of labor or specialization, clear lines of authority, appropriate levels of discipline, unity of direction, equitable treatment of staff, the fostering of individual initiative, and the promotion of a sense of teamwork and group pride. More than 60 years after they were described, these principles remain the basis of most organizations. Therefore, to be effective organizational leaders, nurses need to be familiar with the theory and concepts of bureaucracy.

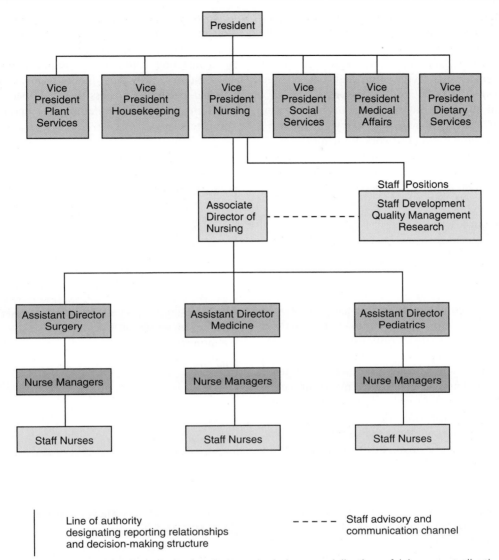

Figure 8-1 A bureaucratic organizational chart depicting specialization of labor, centralization, hierarchical authority, and line and staff responsibilities.

At the time that bureaucracies were developed, these characteristics promoted efficiency and production. As the knowledge base of the general population and employees grew and technologies developed, the bureaucratic structure no longer fit the evolving situation. Increasingly, employees and consumers functioning in bureaucratic situations complain of red tape, procedural delays, and general frustration.

The characteristics of bureaucracy can be present in varying degrees. An organization can demonstrate bureaucratic characteristics in some areas and not in others. For example, nursing staff in intensive care units may be granted autonomy in making and carrying out direct patient care decisions, but they may not be granted a voice in determining work schedules or financial reimbursement systems for hours worked.

One method to determine the extent to which bureaucratic tendencies exist in organizations is to assess the organizational characteristics of the following:

- Labor specialization (the degree to which patient care is divided into highly specialized tasks)
- Centralization (the level of the organization on which decisions regarding carrying out work and remuneration for work are made)
- Formalization (the percentage of actions required to deliver patient care that is governed by written policy and procedures)

EXERCISE 8-7

Analyze the decisions identified in Exercise 8-6 from a manager's perspective. Is that perspective similar to or different from the original perspective you identified?

Decision making and authority can be described in terms of line and staff functions. **Line functions** are those that involve direct responsibility for accomplishing the objectives of a nursing department, service, or unit. Line positions may include registered nurses, licensed practical/vocational nurses, and unlicensed assistive (or nursing) personnel who have the responsibility for carrying out all aspects of direct care. **Staff functions** are those that assist those in line positions in accomplishing the primary objectives. In this context, the term "staff positions" should not be confused with specific jobs that include "staff" in their names such as "staff nurse" or "staff physician." Staff positions include individuals such as staff development personnel, researchers, and special clinical consultants who are responsible for supporting line positions through activities of consultation, education, role modeling, and knowledge development, with limited or no direct authority for decision making. Line personnel have authority for decision making, whereas personnel in staff positions provide support, advice, and counsel. Organizational charts usually indicate line positions through the use of solid lines and staff positions through broken lines (reminder: in this context, the term "staff position" does not reference staff nurses). Line structures have a vertical line, designating reporting and decision-making responsibility. The vertical line connects all positions to a centralized authority (see Figure 8-1).

To make line and staff functions effective, decision-making authority is clearly spelled out in position descriptions. Effectiveness is further ensured by delineating competencies required for the responsibilities, providing methods for determining whether personnel possess these competencies, and providing means of maintaining and developing the competencies.

EXERCISE 8-8

Organizational structures vary in the extent to which they have bureaucratic characteristics. Using observations from your current situations, place a check mark (✓) in the "Present" column beside the bureaucratic characteristics that you believe apply to the agency. What does this analysis indicate about the bureaucratic tendency of the agency? Do the environment and technologies fit the identified bureaucratic tendency? (Consider the state of development of information systems, method of care delivery, patients' characteristics, workers' characteristics, regulatory status, and competition.)

CHARACTERISTIC	PRESENT
Hierarchy of authority	———
Division of labor	———
Written procedures for work	———
Limited authority for workers	———
Emphasis on written communication related to work performance and workers' behaviors	———
Impersonality of personal contact	———

TYPES OF ORGANIZATIONAL STRUCTURES

In healthcare organizations, there are several common types of organizational structures: functional, service line, matrix, or flat. Nursing organizations often combine characteristics of several of these structures to form a hybrid structure. Shared governance is an organizing structure designed to meet the changing needs of professional nursing organizations.

Functional Structures

Functional structures arrange departments and services according to specialty. This approach to organizational structure is common in healthcare organizations. Departments providing similar functions

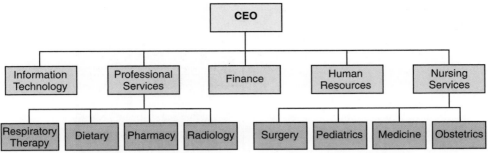

Figure 8-2 Functional structure. *CEO,* Chief executive officer.

report to a common manager or executive (Figure 8-2). For example, a healthcare organization with a functional structure would have vice presidents for each major function: nursing, finance, human resources, and information technology.

This organizational structure tends to support professional expertise and encourage advancement. It may, however, result in discontinuity of patient care services. Delays in decision making can occur if a silo mentality develops within groups. In fact, Lencioni (2006) points out the pitfalls of silos. That is, issues that require communication across functional groups typically must be raised to a senior management level before a decision can be made.

Service-Line Structures

In service-line structures (sometimes called *product lines*), the functions necessary to produce a specific service or product are brought together into an integrated organizational unit under the control of a single manager or executive (Figure 8-3). For example, a cardiology service line at an acute care hospital might include all professional, technical, and support personnel providing services to the cardiac patient population. The manager or executive in this service line would be responsible for the chest pain evaluation center situated within the emergency department, the coronary care unit, the cardiovascular surgery intensive care unit, the telemetry unit, the cardiac catheterization lab, and the cardiac rehabilitation center. In addition to managing the budget and the facilities for these areas, the manager typically would be responsible for coordinating services for the physicians and other providers who admit and care for these patients.

The benefits of a service-line approach to organizational structure include coordination of services, expedited decision-making process, and clarity of purpose. The limitations of this model can include increased expense associated with duplication of services, loss of professional or technical affiliation, and lack of standardization.

Matrix Structures

Matrix structures are complex and designed to reflect both function and service in an integrated organizational structure. In a matrix organization, the manager of a unit responsible for a service reports to both a functional manager and a service or product line manager. For example, a director of pediatric nursing could report to both a vice president for pediatric services (the service-line manager) and a vice president of nursing (the functional manager) (Figure 8-4).

Matrix structures can be effective in the current healthcare environment. The matrix design enables timely response to the forces in the external environment that demand continual programming, and it facilitates internal efficiency and effectiveness through the promotion of cooperation among disciplines.

A matrix structure combines both a bureaucratic structure and a flat structure; teams are used to carry out specific programs or projects. A matrix structure superimposes a horizontal program management over the traditional vertical hierarchy. Personnel from various functional departments are assigned to a specific program or project and become responsible to two supervisors—their functional department head and a program manager. This creates an interdisciplinary team.

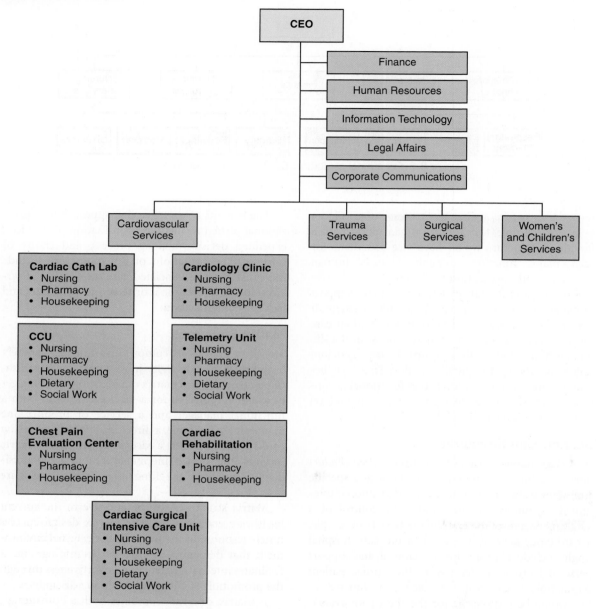

Figure 8-3 Service-line structure. *CCU,* Coronary care unit; *CEO,* chief executive officer.

A line manager and a project manager must function collaboratively in a matrix organization. For example, in nursing, there may be a chief nursing executive, a nurse manager, and staff nurses in the line of authority to accomplish nursing care. In the matrix structure, some of the nurse's time is allocated to project or committee work. Nursing care is delivered in a teamwork setting or within a collaborative model. The nurse is responsible to a nurse manager for nursing care and to a program or project manager when working within the matrix overlay. Well-developed collaboration and coordination skills

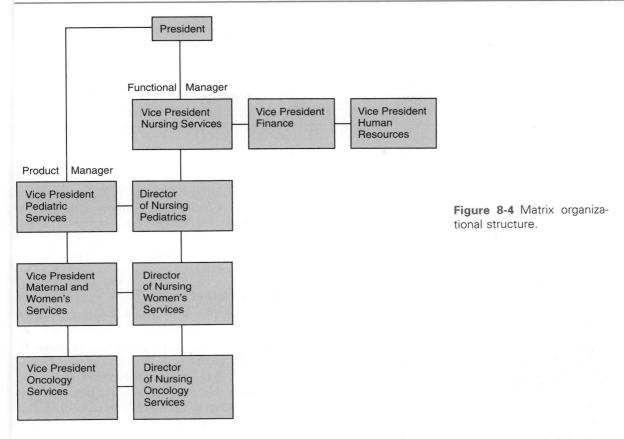

Figure 8-4 Matrix organizational structure.

are essential to effective functioning in a matrix structure. The nature of a matrix organization with its complex interrelationships requires workers with knowledge and skill in interpersonal relationships and teamwork.

One example of the matrix structure is the patient-focused care delivery model that is being implemented in some facilities. Another example is the program focused on specialty services such as geriatric services, women's services, and cardiovascular services. A matrix model can be designed to cover both a patient-focused care delivery model and a specialty service. Other examples are special healthcare facility programs such as discharge planning, total quality management, and cardiopulmonary resuscitation.

Flat Structures

The primary organizational characteristic of a flat structure is the delegation of decision making to the professionals doing the work. The term *flat* signifies the removal of hierarchical layers, thereby granting authority to act and placing authority at the action level (Figure 8-5). Decisions regarding work methods, nursing care of individual patients, and conditions under which employees work are made where the work is carried out. In a **flat organizational structure,** decentralized decision making replaces the centralized decision making typical of functional structures. Providing staff with authority to make decisions at the place of interaction with patients is the hallmark of a flat organizational structure. Magnet™ hospitals have recognized the benefits of decentralized decision making and its impact on both nursing satisfaction and patient outcomes (Aiken, Buchan, Ball, & Rafferty, 2008; Manojlovich, 2005).

Flat organizational structures are less formalized than hierarchical organizations. A decrease in strict adherence to rules and policies allows individualized decisions that fit specific situations and meet the needs created by the increasing demands associated

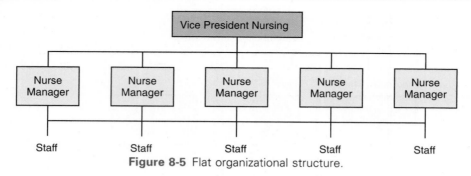

Figure 8-5 Flat organizational structure.

with consumerism, change, and competition. Work supported by the Institute for Healthcare Improvement *(www.ihi.org/IHI/)*, as an example, capitalizes on decisions being made at the unit level. The focus of this work is to improve patient safety. Therefore nurses on a clinical unit can make changes in real time rather than use the traditional organizational hierarchy that includes committees and administrative channels.

Decentralized structures are not without their challenges, however. These include the potential for inconsistent decision making, loss of growth opportunities, and the need to educate managers to communicate effectively and demonstrate creativity in working within these nontraditional structures (Mathews, Spence, Laschinger, & Johnstone, 2006).

The degree of flattening varies from organization to organization. Organizations that are decentralizing often retain some bureaucratic characteristics. They may at the same time have units that are operating as matrix structures. A hybrid structure is one that has characteristics of several different types of structures.

As organizational structures change, some managers are hesitant to relinquish their traditional role in a centralized decision-making process. This reluctance, when combined with recognition of the need to move to a more facilitative role, is partially responsible for the development of hybrid structures. Managers are unsure of what needs to be controlled, how much control is needed, and which mechanisms can replace control. Fear of chaos without control predominates. Education that prepares managers to use leadership techniques that empower nursing staff to take responsibility for their work is one method of minimizing managers' fears. These fears stem from loss of centralized control as authority with

its concomitant responsibilities moves to the place of interaction. The evolutionary development of shared-governance structures in nursing departments demonstrates a type of flat structure being used to replace hierarchical control.

Shared Governance

Shared governance goes beyond participatory management through the creation of organizational structures that facilitate nursing staff more autonomy to govern their practice. Accountability forms the foundation for designing professional governance models. To be accountable, authority to make decisions concerning all aspects of responsibilities is essential. This need for authority and accountability is particularly important for nurses who treat the wide range of human responses to wellness states and illnesses. Organizations in which professional autonomy is encouraged have demonstrated higher levels of staff satisfaction, enhanced productivity, and improved retention (Moore & Hutchinson, 2007; Ulrich, Beurhaus, Donelan, Norman, & Dittus, 2007).

A major cause of nurses' dissatisfaction with their work revolves around the absence of professional autonomy and accountability. The early Magnet™ hospital study (McClure, Poulin, Sovie, & Wandelt, 1983), which identified characteristics of hospitals successful in recruiting and retaining nurses, found that the major contributing characteristic to success was a nursing department structured to provide nurses the opportunity to be accountable for their own practice. Studies of Magnet™ hospitals demonstrate that governance structures provide nurses with accountability that will be effective in recruiting and retaining nursing staff while also meeting consumers' demands and remaining competitive. These findings continue to be validated and expanded upon (Bogue,

Joseph, & Sieloff, 2009; Schmalenberg & Kramer, 2007). Magnet™ characteristics are now accepted as affecting not only the quality of the work environment but also the quality of patient care (Aiken et al, 2008; McGillis-Hall & Doran, 2007). The Research Perspective on p. 143 presents a study on leadership and organizational culture.

Shared or self-governance structures, sometimes referred to as *professional practice models,* go beyond decentralizing and diminishing hierarchies. In an organization that embraces shared governance, the structure's foundation is the professional workplace rather than the organizational hierarchy. Shared governance vests the necessary levels of authority and accountability for all aspects of the nursing practice in the nurses responsible for the delivery of care. The management and administrative level serves to coordinate and facilitate the work of the practicing nurses. Mechanisms are designed outside of the traditional hierarchy to provide for the functional areas needed to support professional practice. These functions include areas such as quality management, competency definition and evaluation, and continuing education. Changing nurses' positions from dependent employees to independent, accountable professionals is a prerequisite for the radical redesign of healthcare organizations that is required to create value for patients. It requires administrators, managers, and staff to abandon traditional notions regarding the division of labor in healthcare organizations. Structures of shared governance organizations vary. Box 8-2 shows three governance structures in progressive stages of evolution. As shown, evolution is moving structure beyond committees imposed on hierarchical structures to governance structures at the unit level.

Shared governance structures require new behaviors of all staff, not just new assignments of accountability. The areas of interpersonal relationship development, conflict resolution, and personal acceptance of responsibility for action are of particular importance. Education, experience in group work, and conflict management are essential for successful transitions.

ANALYZING ORGANIZATIONS

When an organization is analyzed, it is important to scrutinize the various systems that exist to accomplish

---

BOX 8-2 SHARED-GOVERNANCE STRUCTURE EVOLUTION

Phase One

Representative staff nurses are members of clinical forums, which have authority for designated practice issues and some authority for determining roles, functions, and processes. Managers are members of the management forums, which are responsible for the facilitation of practice through resource management and location. Recommendations for action go to the executive committee, which has administrative and staff membership that may or may not be in equal proportion. The nurse executive retains decision-making authority.

Phase Two

Representative staff nurses belong to nursing committees that are designated for specific management and/or clinical functions. These committees are chaired by staff nurses or administrators appointed by the vice president of nursing. The nursing committee chairs and nurse administrators make up the nursing cabinet, which makes the final decision on recommendations from the committees.

Phase Three

Representative staff nurses belong to councils with authority for specific functions. Council chairs make up the management committee charged with making all final operational organizational decisions.

---

the work of the enterprise. This includes delineating the processes or procedures that have been developed to coordinate the work to be done. To conceptualize how the organization functions, it is imperative to know the recruitment procedures, the method of selecting individuals for positions, the reporting relationships, the information network, and the governance structure for nurses. A positive organization reflects a fit of the mission, vision, and philosophy with the structure and practices. Understanding the criteria for Magnet™ facilities (American Nurses Credentialing Center, 2009), irrespective of structure, could form the basis for evaluating nursing services.

EMERGING FLUID RELATIONSHIPS

As the continuum of care moves health services outside of institutional parameters, different skill sets, relationships, and behavioral patterns will be required. Organizations are beginning to lose their traditional boundaries. Old boundaries of hierarchy, function, and geography are disappearing. Vertical integration aligns dissimilar but related entities such as hospital, home care agency, rehabilitation center, long-term care facility, insurance provider, and medical office/clinic. New technologies, fast-changing markets, and global competition are revolutionizing relationships in health care, and the roles that people play and the tasks that they perform have become blurred and ambiguous.

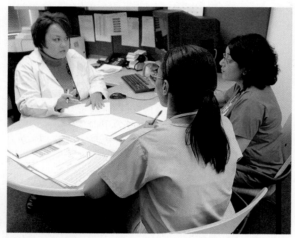

Nurses must have the ability to work with other members of the organization to design organizational models for care delivery that meet patient/customer needs and priorities.

In the future, nurses will no longer practice in geographically limited settings but, rather, in systems of care that have extended boundaries. Reframing or changing current static organizations into vibrant learning organizations will require significant effort (Garvin, Edmondson, & Gino, 2008). To be successful in the future, nurses need to be able to participate as active members in these living-learning organizations. Nurses, whether leaders, managers, or staff, must have the ability to work with other members of the organization and with society at large to design organizational models for care delivery that meet patient/customer needs and priorities. It is essential to take a new look at the nature of the work of nursing and propose innovative models for nursing practice that consider emerging labor-saving assistive technologies and rapidly changing healthcare needs. Employee participation and learning environments go hand in hand, and work redesign needs to be regarded as a continuous process. It is essential that nurses value their and others' autonomy to deal successfully in these new structures.

THE SOLUTION

Immediately, I established what the management structure would be. For example, I changed the scope of responsibility for the individual managers. I then actively recruited for those positions and put in place specific retention strategies to ensure that those who were already a part of the team were engaged in the new direction. I also created a staff development position to fulfill my strategy of clinical management.

After I created the management team, I created core competencies for the clinical staff. Obviously, staff representatives participated in the establishment and design of the initial set of competencies. Now we are working on the design and implementation of the second set of competencies that are more unit-specific. It really is exciting to see how the nurses here have focused their energy in meeting this challenge. I am very fortunate, also, because the staff development educator has had experience in a university, and therefore has connections for recruitment, and she is acutely aware of standards and consistency.

—*Rebecca M. Patton*

Would this be a suitable approach for you? Why?

THE EVIDENCE

Restructuring of healthcare organizations is a common occurrence. This study provides evidence of the impact of organizational change on the psychological well-being of nurses and makes recommendations for how managers might reduce the negative impact of restructuring activities.

Using a quasi-experimental design, this study from the United Kingdom (Brown, Zijlstra, & Lyons, 2006) compared responses from nurses affected by a restructuring event (at least one of the following: management changes, relocation of unit, dispersion of existing work group) with those from nurses who had not been affected. Nurses were surveyed relative to restructuring initiatives; information and participation; coping actions including union activity and morale boosting; and coping effectiveness including job insecurity, job satisfaction, high stress/lack of support, physical well-being, and intention to quit.

The authors reported statistically significant differences between nurses who were affected and those not affected by restructuring events. Compared with non-affected nurses, affected nurses reported higher levels of stress, lower levels of information and participation, and lower coping effectiveness (higher job insecurity and stress; lower job satisfaction and lower physical, psychological, and environmental quality of life). There was no difference noted between affected and non-affected nurses in terms of coping actions. The authors note that managers need to be cognizant of the potential for restructuring to represent a personal threat to personnel and respond by increasing opportunities to share information, provide a vision for how individual nurses might fit within the organization's future state, and avoid an authoritarian management style.

NEED TO KNOW NOW

- Know the mission, vision, and philosophy of your organization and work unit.
- Identify the expected lines of communication as presented on the formal organizational chart.
- Analyze actual workplace practices for opportunities to streamline decision making.

CHAPTER CHECKLIST

The mission, vision, and philosophy of the organization determine how nursing care is delivered in a healthcare organization. Changes occurring in the organization's mission affect both the culture of the workplace and the philosophies regarding the work required to accomplish the mission. Actualizing new missions and philosophies requires reengineered organizational structures that place decision-making authority and responsibility where care is delivered. Decision-making responsibility requires staff to understand the organization's mission and to participate in the development of mission and philosophy statements.

- Five factors influencing design of an organization structure are the following:

  - The types of service performed or the product produced
  - The characteristics of the employees performing the service or producing the product
  - The beliefs and values held by the people responsible for delivering the service concerning the work, the people receiving the services, and the employees
  - The technologies used to perform the service and produce the product
  - The needs, desires, and characteristics of the consumers using the product or service
- Reengineering, the complete overhaul of an organization's structures, is driven by forces of the following:

- Change
- Consumerism
- Competition
- Bureaucratic structures are characterized by the following:
  - A high degree of formalization
  - Centralization of decision making at the top of the organization
  - A hierarchy of authority
  - Structures can be organized along the following lines:
    - Functional
    - Service
    - Matrix
    - Flat
- Functional structures are characterized by the following:
  - Departments and services organized according to specialty
  - Discontinuity of patient services because of silo mentality, even when structure supports professional expertise and encourages advancement
- Service structures are characterized by the following:
  - Functions necessary to provide a specific service brought together under a single line of authority
- Matrix structures are characterized by the following:
  - Dual authority for product and function
  - Mechanisms such as committees to coordinate actions of product and function managers
  - Success that depends on recognition and appreciation of each others' missions and philosophies and commitment to the organization's mission and philosophy
- Flat organizations are characterized by the following:
  - Decision making concerning work performed, decentralized to the level where the work is done
  - Authority, accountability, and autonomy, as well as responsibility, provided to staff performing care
  - Low level of formalization in relation to rules, with processes tailored to meet individual consumer's needs
- Mission, vision, and philosophy determine the characteristics of the organizational structure by doing the following:
  - Describing the consumers and services as a prescription for the technologies and human resources needed to accomplish the defined purpose (mission)
  - Creating an ultimate state of existence (vision)
  - Citing values and beliefs that shape and are shaped by the nature of the work and the rights and responsibilities of workers and consumers (philosophy)
  - Designing characteristics that support the service implementation to fulfill the mission and philosophy (structure)
- Shared governance is characterized by the following:
  - The creation of organizational structures that allow nursing staff more autonomy to govern their practice
  - Recruitment and retention of nursing staff while meeting patient needs in an effective and efficient manner

TIPS FOR UNDERSTANDING ORGANIZATIONAL STRUCTURES

- Professional nurses in staff or followership positions need to understand the mission, vision, philosophy, and structure at the organization and unit level to maximize their contributions to patient care.
- The overall mission of the organization and the mission of the specific unit in which a professional nurse is employed or is seeking employment provide information concerning the major focus of the work to be accomplished and the manner in which it will be accomplished.
- Understanding the philosophy of the organization and/or unit where work occurs provides knowledge of the behaviors that are valued in the delivery

of patient care and in interactions with persons employed by the organization.
- Formal organizational structures describe the expected channels of communication and decision making.
- Matrix organizations usually have two persons responsible for the work, and therefore it is impor-

tant to know to whom you are responsible for what.
- For a shared-governance structure to function effectively, the professionals providing the care must put mechanisms in place to promote decision making about patient care.

REFERENCES

Aiken, L. H., Buchan, J., Ball, J., & Rafferty, A. M. (2008). Transformative impact of Magnet designation: England case study. *Journal of Clinical Nursing, 17*(24), 3330-3337.

Aiken, L. H., Clarke, S. P., Sloane, D. M., Lake, E. T., & Chaney, T. (2008). Effects of hospital environment on patient mortality and nurse outcomes. *Journal of Nursing Administration, 38*(5), 223-229.

American Nurses Credentialing Center. (2009). *Health care organization instructions and application process manual.* Washington, DC: Author.

Bogue, R. J., Joseph, M. L., & Sieloff, C. L. (2009). Shared governance as vertical alignment of nursing group power and nurse practice council effectiveness. *Journal of Nursing Management, 17*(1), 4-14.

Brafman, O., & Beckstrom, R. A. (2008). *The starfish and the spider: The unstoppable power of leaderless organizations.* New York: Penguin Books.

Brown, H., Zijlstra, F., & Lyons, E. (2006). The psychological effects of organizational restructuring on nurses. *Journal of Advanced Nursing, 53*(3), 344-357.

Casida, J. (2008). Linking nursing unit's culture to organizational effectiveness: A measurement tool. *Nursing Economic$, 26*(2), 106-110.

Casida, J., & Pinto-Zipp, G. (2008). Leadership-organizational culture relationship in nursing units of acute care hospitals. *Nursing Economic$, 26*(1), 7-15.

Chen, Y. C. (2008). Restructuring the organizational culture of medical institutions: A study of a community hospital in the I-Lan area. *Journal of Nursing Research, 16*(3), 211-219.

Fayol, H. (1949). *General and industrial management.* London: Pitman.

Garvin, D. A., Edmondson A. C., & Gino, F. (2008). Is yours a learning organization? *Harvard Business Review, 86*(3), 109-116.

Lencioni, P. (2006). *Silos, politics and turf wars: A leadership fable.* San Fransisco, CA: Jossey-Bass.

Lucas, V., Laschinger, H. K., & Wong, C. A. (2008). The impact of emotional intelligent leadership on staff nurse empowerment: The moderating effect of span of control. *International Journal of Nursing Management, 16*(8), 964-973.

Manojlovich M. (2005). The effect of nursing leadership on hospital nurses' professional practice behaviors. *Journal of Nursing Administration, 35*(7-8):366-374.

Martin, S. C., Greenhouse, P. K., Merryman, T., Shovel, J., Liberi, C. A., & Konzier, J. (2007). Transforming care at the bedside: Implementation and spread model for single-hospital and multihospital systems. *Journal of Nursing Administration, 37*(10), 444-451.

Mathews, S., Spence Laschinger, H. K., & Johnstone, L. (2006). Staff nurse empowerment in line and staff organizational structures for chief nurse executives. *Journal of Nursing Administration, 36*(11), 526-533.

McClure, M. L., Poulin, M. A., Sovie, M. D., & Wandelt, M. A. (1983). *Magnet hospitals, attrition and retention of professional nurses.* Kansas City, MO: American Nurses Association.

McGillis-Hall, L., & Doran, D. (2007). Nurses' perceptions of hospital work environments. *Journal of Nursing Management, 15*(3), 264-273.

Melnick, G., Ulaszek, W. R., Lin, H. J., & Wexler, H. K. (2009). When goals diverge: Staff consensus and the organizational culture. *Drug and Alcohol Dependence, 103*(Suppl 1), S17-22.

Moore, S. C., & Hutchinson, S. A. (2007). Developing leaders at every level: Accountability and empowerment actualized through shared governance. *Journal of Nursing Administration, 37*(12), 556-558.

Murphy, N., & Roberts, D. (2008). Nurse leaders as stewards at the point of service. *Nursing Ethics, 15*(2), 243-253.

Schmalenberg, C., & Kramer, M. (2007). Types of intensive care units with the healthiest, most productive work environments. *American Journal of Critical Care, 16*(5), 458-468.

Ulrich, B. T., Beurhaus, P. I., Donelan, K., Norman, L., & Dittus, R. (2007). Magnet status and registered nurse views of the work environment and nursing as a career. *Journal of Nursing Administration, 37*(5), 212-220.

Upenieks, V. V., Needleman, J., Soban, L., Pearson, M. L., Parkerton, P., & Yee, T. (2008). The relationship between the volume and type of transforming care at the bedside innovations and changes in nurse vitality. *Journal of Nursing Administration, 38*(9), 386-394.

Weber, M. (1947). *The theory of social and economic organization.* Parsons, NY: Free Press.

SUGGESTED READINGS

Aiken, L. H., Clarke, S. P., & Sloane, D. M. (2000). Hospital restructuring: Does it adversely affect care and outcomes? *Journal of Nursing Administration, 30*(10), 457-465.

Armstrong, K., Laschinger, H., & Wong, C. (2009). Workplace empowerment and Magnet hospital characteristics as predictors of patient safety climate. *Journal of Nursing Care Quality, 24*(1), 55-62.

Brown, H., Zijlstra, E., & Lyons, E. (2006). The psychological effects of organizational restructuring on nurses. *Journal of Advanced Nursing, 53*(3), 344-357.

Dixon, J. F. (2008). The American Association of Critical Care Nurses standards for establishing and sustaining healthy work environments: Off the printed page and into practice. *Critical Care Nursing Clinics of North America, 20*(4), 393-401.

Kennedy, S. H. (1996). Effects of shared governance on perceptions of work and work environment. *Nursing Economic$, 14*(2), 111-116.

Porter-O'Grady, T. (1996). The seven basic rules for re-design. *Journal of Nursing Administration, 26*(1), 46-53.

Poteet, G., & Hill, A. (1988). Identifying the components of a nursing service philosophy. *Journal of Nursing Administration, 18*(10), 29-35.

Robertson-Malt, S., & Chapman, Y. (2008). Finding the right direction: The importance of open communication in a governance model of nurse management. *Contemporary Nurse, 29*(1), 60-66.

Smythe, W. E., Malloy, D. C., Hadjistavropoulas, T., Martin, R. R., & Bardutz, H. A. (2006). An analysis of the ethical and linguistic content of hospital mission statements. *Health Care Management Review, 31*(2), 92-98.

White, K. R., & Dandi, R. (2009). Intrasectoral variation in mission and values: The case of the Catholic health system. *Health Care Management Review, 34*(1), 68-79.

Wilson, B., Squires, M., Widger, K., Cranley, L., & Tourangeau, A. (2008). Job satisfaction among a multigenerational nursing workforce. *Journal of Nursing Management, 16*(6), 716-723.

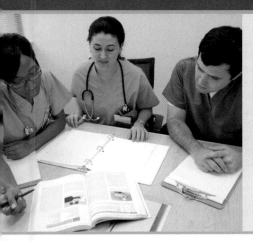

Cultural Diversity in Health Care

Karen A. Esquibel and Dorothy A. Otto

This chapter focuses on the importance of cultural considerations for patients and staff. Although it does not address comprehensive details about any specific culture, it does provide guidelines for actively incorporating cultural aspects into the roles of leading and managing. Diverse workforces are discussed, as well as how to capitalize on their diverse traits and how to support differences to work more efficiently. The chapter presents concepts and principles of transculturalism, describes techniques for managing a culturally diverse workforce, emphasizes the importance of respecting different lifestyles, and discusses the effects of diversity on staff performance. Scenarios and exercises to promote an appreciation of cultural richness are also included.

OBJECTIVES

- Evaluate the use of concepts and principles of acculturation, culture, cultural diversity, and cultural sensitivity in leading and managing situations.
- Analyze differences between cross-cultural, transcultural, multicultural, and intracultural concepts and cultural marginality.
- Describe common characteristics of any culture.
- Evaluate individual and societal factors involved with cultural diversity.
- Compare values and beliefs about illness that affect management of nursing care interventions involving patients from specific cultures.

TERMS TO KNOW

acculturation	cultural imposition	ethnicity
cross-culturalism	cultural marginality	ethnocentrism
cultural competence	cultural sensitivity	multiculturalism
cultural diversity	culture	transculturalism

Sally C. Fernandez, RN, MSN, ANP
Nurse Manager, Emergency Center, University of Texas M.D.
Anderson Cancer Center, Houston, Texas

I work with a large staff of men and women from several cultures, and they have different perspectives about their assignments. Hispanics, Asians, Asian Indians, and Nigerians provide a challenge for me. If I try to address a work issue, such as assignments, some become defensive. Some men feel that they are superior to me. It might be because I am a woman. In contrast, I have noticed that some Asians are more submissive and do better with female-to-

female interactions. We frequently have a high patient census in the emergency department. There are times when either the charge nurse or I tell staff members to complete a task more quickly within their assignment because of the number of patients waiting to be seen in the emergency department. This does not set well with some staff, who tend to become defensive. For example, a male staff member of one culture felt he was being "overpowered" by the charge nurse from another culture.

What do you think you would do if you were this nurse?

INTRODUCTION

Nurse leaders and managers are concerned with cultural diversity from two perspectives: (1) the care of a diverse patient population and (2) positive work experiences in a culturally diverse workforce. In its report to the Secretary of Health & Human Resources and Congress, the National Advisory Council on Nurse Education and Practice (NACNEP) (2000) addressed the need for a culturally diverse workforce to meet the healthcare needs of our nation. The Council defined that a national action-oriented agenda is needed to address the underrepresentation of racial-ethnic minorities in the workforce. To this end, the NACNEP solicited, through the Division of Nursing, an Expert Workgroup on Diversity to advise them on the development of the National Agenda. The Workgroup based its recommendations on the following four overarching goals:

1. Enhancing efforts to increase the recruitment, retention, and subsequent graduation of minority nurses
2. Promoting leadership development for minority nurses
3. Developing a practice environment that promotes diversity
4. Promoting the preparation of all nurses so that culturally competent care can be provided

If the aim of nursing is to reflect the population we serve, then we have a long way to go.

Effective leaders can shape the culture of their organization to be accepting of persons from all races, ethnicities, religions, ages, and genders. These interactions of acceptance should involve a minimum of

misunderstandings. Multicultural phenomena are cogent for each person, place, and time. Connerley and Pedersen (2005) provided 10 examples for leading from a complicated culture-centered perspective. For example, "3. Explain the action of employees from their own cultural perspective; 6. Reflect culturally appropriate feelings in specific and accurate feedback" (p. 29). Therefore culture-centered leadership provides organizational leaders, such as nurse managers, the opportunity to influence cultural differences and similarities among their unit staff.

The American Nurses Association (ANA) has a long and vital history related to ethics, human rights, and numerous efforts to eliminate discriminatory practices against nurses as well as patients. The ANA *Code of Ethics for Nurses with Interpretive Statements*, Provision 8 states, "The nurse collaborates with other health professionals and the public in promoting community, national, and international efforts to meet health needs" (2008, p. 23). This provision helps the nurse recognize that health care must be provided to culturally diverse populations in the United States and on all continents of the world. Although a nurse may be inclined to impose his or her own cultural values on others, whether patients or staff, avoiding this imposition affirms the respect and sensitivity for the values and healthcare practices associated with different cultures.

According to Noone (2008):

Nursing leaders at all levels are calling for a nursing workforce able to provide culturally competent care. Our commitment to social justice and the practical demands of the workplace call for nursing to take strong, sustained, and measurable actions to produce a workforce that closely parallels the population it serves. Minority nurses are underrepresented in today's nursing workforce as compared to United States ethnicity demographics. (p. 133)

This author identified barriers reported from several studies that involved interviews with students of ethnically diverse backgrounds. The barriers related to "financial needs, academic needs, feeling isolated, and experiences with discrimination from faculty, peers and patients" (p. 135). One particular example cited by Noone was the different modes of communication, such as lack of assertiveness, difficulty with languages, and different customs. If this occurred with nursing students in an academic setting, do these barriers continue or do they change based on action strategies to modify them? The results will have either a positive or a negative impact on the future employment of these prospective members of the nursing workforce.

Health care in the United States has consistently focused on individuals and their health problems but has failed to recognize the cultural differences, beliefs, symbolisms, and interpretations of illness of some people as a group. Commonly, the patients for whom healthcare practitioners provide care are newcomers to health care in the United States. Similarly, new staff are neither acculturated nor assimilated into the cultural values of the dominant culture.

Currently, accessibility to health care in the United States is linked to specific social strata. This challenges nurse leaders, managers, and followers who strive for worth, recognition, and individuality for patients and staff regardless of their ascribed economic and social standing. Beginning nurse leaders, managers, and followers may sense that the knowledge they bring to their job lacks "real-life" experiences that provide the springboard to address staff and patient needs. In reality, although lack of experience may be slightly hampering, it is by no means an obstacle to addressing individualized attention to staff and patients. The key is that if the nurse manager and staff respect people and their needs, economic and social standings become moot points. Nurse managers must be cognizant of divergent views about health care as a right for all people rather than a privilege for a few.

Resources are a must for nurses to use to learn about working with culturally diverse staff and patients. D'Avanzo (2008) wrote a fitting resource

book about a variety of cultural groups, their differences in worldwide views and concepts of reality, and their variety of social, political, economic, and religious values and many concepts of health and illness. They noted that diversity exists both within and between groups, which may lead to intragroup and intergroup conflict. Lipson and Dibble (2005) indicated that culture is influenced by intersections of forces larger than the individual and by shared values of what constitutes ethical, professional practice. They provide an excellent set of general guidelines to alert nurses in the hospital or community settings to the similarities and differences within and among the cultural and ethnic groups. They have expanded the types of cultural and ethnic groups to include Roma (gypsies), former Yugoslavians, Russians, and other former Soviet Union people. All the cultural groups were selected based on their size according to the U.S. Census (each numbering at least 100,000) and/or on the lack of readily obtainable information elsewhere about a particular group (Lipson & Dibble, 2005). *Caring for Women Cross-Culturally* (St. Hill, Lipson, & Meleis, 2003) is a rich, comprehensive resource of culturally relevant information about immigrant and minority women. Interspersed through each chapter are "notes to health providers." These notes purport to alert the provider to potential problems the nurse may encounter at certain developmental stages or when dealing with a particularly sensitive topic. The authors suggest helpful ways to approach these issues.

The International Classification for Nursing Practice (ICNP) (International Council of Nurses, 2008) is a unified nursing language system that should be considered by nurse clinicians in the workplace and by nurse educators:

Globalization is a reality and global visibility of healthcare needs, delivery and quality is changing the face of health care around the world…there is a need to communicate about nursing worldwide, across many languages and cultures….Standardized nursing terminologies are needed to document nursing practice with its unique features and multiple variations. The consistent and valid data from the documentation of nursing practice can then be used to articulate and evaluate nursing practice nationally, regionally, and internationally….Clinical nursing data can also be used to assess and assure quality, promote changes in nursing practice, and advance nursing science through research. (p. 5)

Translating a message in one language to another language to ensure equivalence includes maintaining the same meaning of the word or concept. Equivalency is accomplished through interpretation, which extends beyond "word-for-word" translation to explain the meaning of concepts. When providing care to a culturally diverse patient, the nurse must realize that the process of translation of illness/disease conditions and treatment is complex and requires certain tasks. Two important tasks are "(a) transferring data from the source language to the target language and (b) maintaining or establishing cross-cultural semantic equivalence" (International Council of Nurses, 2008, p. 5).

MEANING OF DIVERSITY IN THE ORGANIZATION

Nursing as a profession has historically lagged the general demographics related to ethnic and gender diversity. These data can be tracked through a quadrennial survey by the Division of Nursing. The 2008 National Sample Survey of Registered Nurses (NSSRN), distributed by the Health Resources and Services Administration (HRSA) (2008), represents about 2% of all registered nurses. These data cover the number and characteristics of employment status and practice settings, racial/ethnic background, age-group, and education and training.

Recent data from the 2008 National Sample Survey of Registered Nurses (HRSA, 2010) show an estimated 3,063,163 licensed registered nurses in the United States. This number reflects an overall increase of about 5.3%, which is logical based on the significant increases in enrollments in schools of nursing and subsequent graduations over the past several years. Slightly less than 85% of the RN population is actively employed in nursing, with the majority employed full-time and in hospital settings. According to the 2008 data, approximately 84% of the RN population was white and non-Hispanic compared with 65.6% of the general U.S. population. The RN population comprising "Hispanic/Latino, any race" was 3.6%, whereas the percentage for the U.S. population was 15.4%. The RN population of "Black/African American, non-Hispanic" was 5.4% compared with 12.2% for the general U.S. population.

| TABLE 9-1 | COMPARISON OF ETHNICITIES OF THE US POPULATION AND NURSING POPULATION (2008, 2004 DATA) |

	UNITED STATES	RNs
White, non Hispanic	65.6%	84%
Hispanic/Latino, any race	15.4%	3.6%
Black/African-American, non-Hispanic	12.2%	5.4%
Asian or Native Hawaiian or Pacific Islander, non-Hispanic	4.5%	5.8%

Data from US Bureau of Labor Statistics, Bulletin 2307, Retrieved June 20, 2010, from *www.bls.gov/cps/home.htm;* and Health Resources and Services Administration. (2008). Division of Nursing's 2008 *National Sample Survey of Registered Nurses.* Retrieved June 20, 2010, from *http://bhpr.hrsa.gov/healthworkforce/rnsurvey04/appendixa.htm.*

Only those individuals identified as "Asian or Native Hawaiian or Pacific Islander, non-Hispanic" (5.8% of RNs) exceeded the percentage of the U.S. population in that category (4.5%) (Table 9-1). As these data show, the profession of nursing is not reflective of the population it serves. These facts have many implications from recruitment into the profession, such as programs to enrich the majority members' understanding of diversity, as well as support of ethnic minorities in the workplace.

The numbers of men recruited into the profession have risen but not to the point of creating gender equality. Although stereotypes (e.g., "not smart enough for medical school") have diminished over the years, the numbers of men in nursing still do not approach the proportional numbers of men in the United States.

Because nursing is not a particularly diverse profession, it is critical to provide support in employment settings for RNs in minority categories and to enhance the appreciation of the majority for culturally diverse workforces and care.

EXERCISE 9-1
Access the 2008 NSSRN and find other diversities in nursing such as place of employment, position, and education.

Health disparities between majority and racial ethnic minority populations are not new issues and

RESEARCH PERSPECTIVE

Resource: Seago, J. A., & Spetz, J. (2008). Minority nurses' experiences on the job. *Journal of Cultural Diversity, 15*(1), 16-23. Retrieved February 27, 2009, from ProQuest Nursing & Allied Health Source database (Document ID: 14336481).

Seago and Spetz's study described the work environment, job advancement, and promotion experiences of registered nurses in California who self-identify an ethnic affiliation. They posed the question, Do minority nurses face more and/or different barriers to career advancement and promotion experiences in their workplace?

The overall results of this correlational and cross-sectional study found that minority nurses have positive views of their opportunities and workplaces. In addition, the sample of minority nurses was more likely than white nurses to agree that they have opportunities to advance in their workplace and to learn new skills at work. They believed their job assignments to be analogous to their skills performance. The study participants came from a convenience sample. A mailed survey was used for data collection. The subjects comprised a variety of ethnic and racial backgrounds: African American, Asian Pacific American, Latino, Filipino, and Caucasian. The study sample did not mirror the racial and ethnic composition of the state's population, because African Americans, non-Filipino Asians, and Latinos were underrepresented in the nursing workforce. When identifying gender, 8.6% were males and 91.4% were females. The average age of the study sample was 45.7 years, which was lower than the average age (49.1 years) of the employed California registered nurses. This study identified situations that employers need to consider to increase satisfaction of the nursing workforce and to remove problems of racial/ethnic inequities.

Implications for Practice

Nurses are at a vantage point to advocate for their culturally diverse colleagues in the workplace to learn new skills and to seek opportunities for advancement.

Nurses need to assess and use their capabilities to determine the challenges that will help them function at their fullest potential in the workplace.

---

continue to be problematic as they exist for multiple and complex reasons. Causes of disparities in health care include poor education, health behaviors of the minority group, inadequate financial resources, and environmental factors. Disparities in health care that relate to quality of care include provider/patient relationships, provider bias and discrimination, and patient variables of mistrust of the healthcare system and refusal of treatment (Baldwin, 2003). Health disparities in ethnic and racial groups are observed in cardiovascular disease, which has a 40% higher incidence in U.S. blacks than in U.S. whites; cancer, which has a 30% higher death rate for all cancers in U.S. blacks than in U.S. whites; and Hispanics with diabetes, who are twice as likely to die from this disease than non-Hispanic whites. In 2000, Native Americans had a life expectancy that was 5 years less than the national average, whereas Asians and Pacific Islanders were considered among the healthiest population groups. However, within the Asian and Pacific Islander population, health outcomes were more diverse. Solutions to health and healthcare disparities among ethnic and racial populations must be accomplished through research to improve care. Such research could include preventive services, health education and interventions, treatment services, and health outcomes (Baldwin, 2003). Consider how these disparities in disease and in healthcare services might affect the healthcare providers in the workplace in relationship to their ethnic or racial group. What should you know about the sick-leave policy based on acute or chronic disease/illness in your institution? Portillo (2003) wrote that "our leadership efforts will have to move beyond the beginning to reduce health disparities. A better understanding of the strengths and limitations of the concepts of race and ethnicity is a priority of nursing" (p. 5). It is necessary to increase healthcare providers' knowledge so that they can more effectively manage and treat diseases related to ethnic and racial minorities, which might include themselves.

Leading and managing cultural diversity in an organization means managing personal thinking and helping others to think in new ways. Managing issues that involve culture—whether institutional, ethnic, gender, religious, or any other kind—requires patience, persistence, and much understanding. One way to promote this understanding is through shared stories that have symbolic power.

EXERCISE 9-2
Think of a recent event in your workplace, such as a project, task force, celebration, or something similar. What meaning did people give the event? Was it viewed as being a symbol of some quality of the workplace, such as its effectiveness, its values and beliefs, or its innovations?

BOX 9-1 **TECHNIQUES FOR MANAGING A CULTURALLY DIVERSE WORKFORCE**

- Have patience. Treat all questions as equally important even though they may be common, everyday knowledge to you.
- Be cognizant that international or minority staff may not consider themselves deprived or of lesser socioeconomic status than the majority.
- Do not treat gender bias or those with different lifestyles as needing intervening techniques to change behaviors. Assume they are happy with their choice.
- Do not assume emotional outbursts represent anger. This may be a natural communication style for different groups. Consider, however, how these outbursts fit with The Joint Commission expectations regarding disruptive behaviors.
- Treat compliments from your staff with respect. Avoid feeling that they are trying to request a special favor from you. In some cultures, compliments are used quite often to demonstrate respect.
- Do not assume that physical features denote a specific race or ethnic identity. Some Hispanics demonstrate Asian features, whereas some Puerto Ricans or Jamaicans may be mistaken for African blacks.
- Take the time to know your colleagues. Make time for conversational chats that will facilitate learning about each other.
- Always remember that the less you know about your staff, the more difficult your job will be as an effective manager.
- Be aware that people in your workforce may at one time or another have actually felt a part of an oppressed group. Give them a feeling of value and dignity.

Staff who know what is valuable to patients and to themselves can act accordingly and feel good about work. Having a clear mission, goals, rewards, and acknowledgment of efforts leads to a greater productivity and work effort from a culturally diverse staff who aspires to unity and uniqueness (see the Research Perspective on p. 163). When assessing staff diversity, the nurse leader or manager can ask these two questions:

- What is the cultural representation of the workforce?
- What kind of team-building activities are needed to create a cohesive workforce for effective healthcare delivery?

Box 9-1 lists some of the techniques that may be effective when managing a culturally diverse workforce.

CONCEPTS AND PRINCIPLES

What is *culture?* Does it exhibit certain characteristics? What is *cultural diversity,* and what do we think of when we refer to *cultural sensitivity?* Are *culture* and *ethnicity* the same? Various authors have different views. Cultural background stems from one's ethnic background, socio-economic status, and family rituals, to name three key factors. Ethnicity, according to *The Merriam Webster Dictionary* (Merriam-Webster Inc., 2005), is defined as related to groups of people who are "classified" according to common racial, tribal, national, religious, linguistic, or cultural backgrounds. This description differs from what is commonly used to identify racial groups. This broader definition encourages people to think about how diverse the populations in the United States are.

Inherent characteristics of culture are often identified with the following four factors:

1. It develops over time and is responsive to its members and their familial and social environments.
2. Its members learn it and share it.
3. It is essential for survival and acceptance.
4. It changes with difficulty.

For the nurse leader or manager, the characteristics of ethnicity and culture are important to keep in mind because the underlying thread in all of them is that staff's and patients' culture and ethnicity have been with them their entire lives. They view their cultural background as normal; the diversity challenge is for others to view it as normal also and to assimilate it into the existing workforce. Cultural diversity is the term currently used to describe a vast range of cultural differences among individuals or groups, whereas cultural sensitivity describes the affective behaviors in individuals—the capacity to feel, convey, or react to ideas, habits, customs, or traditions unique to a group of people.

Spector (2009) addressed three themes involved with acculturation:

socialization…being raised within a culture and acquiring the characteristics of that group; acculturation, becoming a competent participant in the dominant culture…process is involuntary…forced to learn the new culture to survive; and assimilation

...developing a new cultural identity becoming in all ways like the members of the dominant culture. (p. 19)

The overall process of acculturation into a new society is extremely difficult. According to Spector (2009):

In the United States, people assume that the usual course of acculturation takes three generations; hence, the adult grandchild of an immigrant is considered fully Americanized. (p. 19)

Consider how you might adapt to a new country and its society.

Based on the *Code of Ethics for Nurses* (ANA, 2008), nurses believe that they must care for all patients regardless of differences—whether it be cultural, economic status, or gender. Providing care for a person or people from a culture other than one's own is a dynamic and complex experience. The experience according to Spence (2004) might involve "prejudice, paradox and possibility" (p. 140). Using hermeneutic interpretation, her study consisted of accounts from 17 New Zealand nurses who delivered nursing care to patients in acute medical and surgical wards, public health centers, mental health settings, and midwifery specialties. Spence used *prejudice* as conditions that enabled or constrained interpretation based on one's values, attitudes, and actions. By talking with people outside one's "circle of familiarity," one can enhance one's understanding of personally held prejudices.

The lack of mutual understanding between healthcare providers and immigrants, particularly children and adolescents, was addressed as early as 2001 by Choi. She explored the concept of cultural marginality, which she defined as "situations and feelings of passive betweenness when people exist between two different cultures and do not yet perceive themselves as centrally belonging to either one" (p. 193). A model cultural marginality case of a 15-year-old high school student who moved to the United States from Korea when she was 14 years old is described by Choi.

EXERCISE 9-4

Reflect on your experiences with immigrant adolescents in which cultural marginality—the betweenness—was an existing challenge to them, as well as to their family members or peers. In what ways did values change as new generations of a culture group adopt the new country's views over time? Consider that first-generation groups very often have stronger ties to traditions and customs from their country of origin than do second and third generations.

How do leaders, managers, or followers take all of the expanding information on the diversity of healthcare beliefs and practices and give it some organizing structure to provide culturally competent and culturally sensitive care to patients or clients? Purnell and Paulanka (2008), Campinha-Bacote (1999, 2002), Giger and Davidhizar (2002), and Leininger (2002a) provide an overview of each of their theoretical models to guide healthcare providers for delivering culturally competent and culturally sensitive care in the workplace.

Purnell and Paulanka's (2008) Model for Cultural Competence provides an organizing framework. The model uses a circle with the outer zone representing global society, the second zone representing community, the third zone representing family, and the inner zone representing the person. The interior of the circle is divided into 12 pie-shaped wedges delineating cultural domains and their concepts (e.g., workplace issues, family roles and organization, spirituality, and healthcare practices). The innermost center circle is black, representing unknown phenomena. Cultural consciousness is expressed in behaviors from "unconsciously incompetent—consciously incompetent—consciously competent to unconsciously competent" (p. 10). The usefulness of this model is derived from

---

EXERCISE 9-3

In a group, discuss the values and beliefs of justice and equality. As a nurse, you may have strong values and beliefs but you may never have observed their application in health care. Consider language, skin color, dress, and gestures of patients and staff from other cultures. How will you learn and value what differences exist? Prejudices "enable us to make sense of the situations in which we find ourselves, yet they also constrain understanding and limit the capacity to come to new or different ways of understanding. It is this contradiction that makes prejudice paradoxical" (Spence, 2004, p. 163). Paradox, although it may seem incongruent with prejudice, describes the dynamic interplay of tensions between individuals or groups. It is our responsibility to acknowledge the "possibility of tension" as a potential for new and different understandings derived from our communication and interpretation. Possibility, therefore, presumes a condition for openness with a person from another culture (Spence, 2004).

its concise structure, applicability to any setting, and wide range of experiences that can foster inductive and deductive thinking when assessing cultural domains. The Literature Perspective below describes the importance of being culturally congruent with the population an organization serves.

Purnell (2009) described the dominant cultural characteristics of selected ethnocultural groups and a guide for assessing their beliefs and practices. The Purnell Model for Cultural Competence serves as an organizing framework for providing cultural care, which is based on 20 major assumptions.

Campinha-Bacote's (1999, 2002) culturally competent model of care identifies five constructs: (1)

📖 LITERATURE PERSPECTIVE

Resource: Schim, S. M., Doorenbos, A., Benkert, R., & Miller, J. (2007). Culturally congruent care: Putting the puzzle together. *Journal of Transcultural Nursing, 18*(2), 103-110.

A growing need to develop cultural awareness and provide cultural diversity to all healthcare employees at all levels has rapidly developed over the past 5 years. This steady development is in the wake of the 1991 U.S. Department of Health and Human Services Office of Minority Health Culturally and Linguistically Appropriate Service (CLAS) standards and the 1994 Joint Commission on Accreditation of Healthcare Organizations (now The Joint Commission) mandates. The authors present the 3-D puzzle model of culturally congruent care, which builds on Leininger's pioneering work in transcultural nursing. This model draws heavily from prior work and synthesizes concepts and processes in a new and refreshing way.

The four basic constructs, the pieces of the 3-D puzzle model at the healthcare provider level, are (1) cultural diversity, (2) cultural awareness, (3) cultural sensitivity, and (4) cultural competence. Each construct is conceptualized as well as the relationships among the constructs. The model suggests that there are two levels, the provider level and the client level, coming together to create culturally congruent care.

Implications for Practice

The 3-D model extends Leininger's work, which specifically focuses on the use of qualitative methods to understand the ways in which culture influences nursing care from an emic perspective. The 3-D model extension, and implication for practice, includes concrete articulations of constructs relevant to design and implementation of intervention strategies for teaching and measuring competency among nurses and other healthcare providers. The 3-D puzzle model, as it evolves, presents promise as a way of conceptualizing the concepts, constructs, and relationships that form all aspects of culturally congruent health care.

awareness, (2) knowledge, (3) skill, (4) encounters, and (5) desire. She defined cultural competence as "the process in which the healthcare provider continuously strives to achieve the ability to effectively work within the cultural context of a client (individual, family, or community)" (Campinha-Bacote, 1999, p. 203). Cultural awareness is the self-examination and in-depth exploration of one's own cultural and professional background. It involves the recognition of one's bias, prejudices, and assumptions about the individuals who are different (Campinha-Bacote, 2002). "One's world view can be considered a paradigm or way of viewing the world and phenomena in it" (Campinha-Bacote, 1999, p. 204). Cultural knowledge is the process of seeking and obtaining a sound educational foundation about diverse cultural and ethnic groups. Obtaining cultural information about the patient's health-related beliefs and values will help explain how he or she interprets his or her illness and how it guides his or her thinking, doing, and being (Campinha-Bacote, 2002). The skill of conducting a cultural assessment is learned while assessing one's values, beliefs, and practices to provide culturally competent services. The process of cultural encounters encourages direct engagement in cross-cultural interactions with individuals from other cultures. This process allows the person to validate, negate, or modify his or her existing cultural knowledge. It provides culturally specific knowledge bases from which the individual can develop culturally relevant interventions. Cultural desire requires the intrinsic qualities of motivation and genuine caring of the healthcare provider to "want to" engage in becoming culturally competent (Campinha-Bacote, 1999).

The Giger and Davidhizar Transcultural Assessment Model identifies phenomena to assess provision of care for patients who are of different cultures (2002). Their model includes six cultural phenomena: communication, time, space, social organization, environmental control, and biological variations. Each one is described based on several premises (e.g., culture is a patterned behavioral response that develops over time; is shaped by values, beliefs, norms, and practices; guides our thinking, doing, and being; and implies a dynamic, ever-changing, active or passive process).

Leininger's (2002a) central purpose in her theory of transcultural nursing care is "to discover and explain diverse and universal culturally based care factors influencing the health, well-being, illness, or death of individuals or groups" (p. 190). She uses her classic "Sunrise Model" to identify the multifaceted theory and provides five enablers beneficial to "teasing out vague ideas," two of which are The Observation, Participation, and Reflection Enabler and the Researcher's Domain of Inquiry. Nurses can use Leininger's model to provide culturally congruent, safe, and meaningful care to patients or clients of diverse or similar cultures.

Nurse leaders and managers who ascribe to a positive view of culture and its characteristics effectively acknowledge cultural diversity among patients and staff. This includes providing culturally sensitive care to patients while simultaneously balancing a culturally diverse staff. For example, cultural diversity might mean being sensitive to or being able to embrace the emotions of a large multicultural group comprising staff and patients. Unless we understand the differences, we cannot come together and make decisions that are in the best interest of the patient.

Transculturalism sometimes has been considered in a narrow sense as a comparison of health beliefs and practices of people from different countries or geographic regions. However, culture can be construed more broadly to include differences in health beliefs and practices by gender, race, ethnicity, economic status, sexual preference, age, and disability or physical challenge. Thus, when concepts of transcultural care are discussed, we should consider differences in health beliefs and practices not only between and among countries but also between genders and among, for example, races, ethnic groups, and different economic strata. This requires us to consider multiple factors about all individuals.

The range of attitudes toward culturally diverse groups can be viewed along a continuum of intensity (Lenburg et al., 1995, p. 4): hate → contempt → tolerance → respect → celebration/affirmation. Managers need to be aware of this continuum so that they can apply these strategies appropriately to the workforce—for example, contempt versus affirmation.

Two questions that are addressed by Lenburg et al. (1995, p. 10) regarding becoming culturally competent should be considered by practicing nurses:

1. What has more influence on health and illness behavior—a group's cultural characteristics or the political and economic context in which it exists?
2. Is it the cultural characteristics of patients that affect their behavior in the healthcare system or the knowledge and behavior of providers?

Variables that may influence the nurse's response may include how the illness is perceived by the culture and the cultural competency of the healthcare provider. Leininger (2002a) identified several major theoretical premises relating to transcultural nursing theory that nurse managers and staff can follow (see the Theory Box below).

Shannon (2008) described her concern that refusal of nursing care and/or end-of-life care tends to be ignored particularly with some culturally diverse groups. For example, two groups were cited: African-Americans and those groups with greater religiosity. It is her premise that we should focus on communication solutions and not treat patients and families as strangers. "More recently clinicians have been challenged by patients and families who want more aggressive treatment at end-of-life than many clinicians believe to be effective, cost-efficient, or humane" (Shannon, 2008, p. 97). Thus circumstances such as

---

THEORY BOX

Cultural Care Theory

THEORY/CONTRIBUTOR	KEY IDEAS	APPLICATION TO PRACTICE
Leininger (2002a) is credited with developing and advancing a theory of transcultural nursing care since the mid-1950s.	The theory is explicitly focused on the close relationships of culture and care on well-being, health, illness, and death; it is holistic and multidimensional, generic (emic, folk) and professional (etic) care and has a specifically designed research method (ethnonursing).	Care is the essence of nursing, and culturally based care is essential for well-being, health, growth, and survival and for facing handicaps or death.

interprofessional communication might create workplace issues for staff discussion among the nursing staff and physicians. Consider "how does communication, healthcare professionals, nursing, justice and ethics fit together?"—a significant question posed by Shannon (2008, p. 97).

To understand, value, and use diversity, nurse managers need to approach every staff person as an individual. Although staff of different cultural groups may be diverse in appearance, values, beliefs, communication patterns, and mannerisms, they have many things in common. Staff members want to be accepted by others and to succeed in their jobs. With fairness and respect, nurse managers should openly support the competencies and contributions of staff members from all cultural groups with a goal of achieving quality patient care. Nurse managers hold the key to allowing the full potential of each person on the staff.

Sullivan and Decker (2009) described the importance of communication and how cultural attitudes, beliefs, and behavior affect communication. Body movements, gestures, verbal tone, and physical closeness when communicating are all part of a person's culture. For the nurse manager, understanding these cultural behaviors is imperative in accomplishing effective communication within the diverse workforce population. Tappen (2001) addressed differences across cultures that the nurse leader/manager needs to monitor. These differences include relationships to people in authority, spatial differences, eye contact, expressions of feelings, meaning of different language versions, thinking modes, evidence-based decision making, and preferred leadership/management style. Nurses need to ensure that ineffective communication by staff with patients and others does not lead to misunderstandings and eventual alienation.

Failure to address cultural diversity leads to negative effects on performance and staff interactions. Nurse managers can find many ways to address this issue. For example, in relation to performance, a nurse manager can make sure messages about patient care are received. This might be accomplished by sitting down with a staff nurse and analyzing the situation to ensure that understanding has occurred. In addition, the nurse manager might use a communication notebook that allows the nurse to slowly "digest" information by writing down communication areas that may be unclear. For effective staff interaction, the nurse manager also can make a special effort to pair mentors and mentees who have different ethnic backgrounds. The use of a bilingual health professional interpreter can be an effective strategy when caring for non–English-speaking or limited–English-speaking proficiency patients.

The current practice seems to be one of using interpreters rather than translators when speaking with non–English-speaking patients and clients. Why? Purnell and Paulanka (2008) advocate that trained healthcare providers as interpreters can decode words and provide the right meaning of the message. However, the authors also suggest being aware that interpreters might affect the reporting of symptoms, using their own ideas or omitting information. It is important to allow time for translation and interpretation and to clarify information as needed. Purnell and Paulanka provided 21 guidelines for communicating with those who are non–English-speaking.

EXERCISE 9-5

During one of your group meetings, have everyone share one or two slang words that may have a different meaning for different groups of people. After this meeting, have one in your group post a list of the words and meanings discussed in the meeting. Allow everyone to continue to add slang words that staff members use that may create confusion or misunderstanding. Reviewing the list regularly allows staff to understand phrases and, in some instances, to gain a cultural perspective connected to the phrase.

INDIVIDUAL AND SOCIETAL FACTORS

Nurse managers must work with staff to foster respect of different lifestyles. To do this, nurse managers need to accept three key principles: multiculturalism, which refers to maintaining several different cultures; cross-culturalism, which means mediating between/among cultures; and transculturalism, which denotes bridging significant differences in cultural practices.

Cultural differences among groups should not be taken in the context that all members of a certain group or subgroup are indistinguishable. Tappen (2001) described this "indistinguishable" phenomenon and recommended that cultural differences be viewed as group tendencies. For example, regarding gender differences, women are perceived to have a more participative management style; however, this does not mean that all male managers use an authoritative management model. Likewise, female managers may use multiple sources of information to make decisions, and this does not mean that all male managers make decisions on limited data. Thus the norm for gender recognition should be that women and men be hired, promoted, rewarded, and respected for how successfully they do the job, not for who they are, where they come from, or whom they know.

EXERCISE 9-6

Consider doing a group exercise to enhance cultural sensitivity. Ask each group member to write down four to six cultural beliefs that he or she values. When everyone has finished writing, have the group members exchange their lists and discuss why these beliefs are valued. When everyone has had a chance to share lists, have a volunteer compile an all-encompassing list that reflects the values of your workforce. (The key to this exercise is that many of the values are similar or perhaps even identical.)

In today's workplace, female-male collaboration should provide efficacious models for the future. Gender does not determine response in any given situation. However, men reportedly seem to be better at deciphering what needs to be done, whereas women are better at collaborating and getting others to collaborate in accomplishing a task. Men tend to take neutral, logical, and objective stands on problems, whereas women become involved in how the problems affect people. It is important to recognize that women and men bring separate perspectives to resolving problems, which can help them function more effectively as a team on the nursing unit. Men and women must learn to work together and value the contributions of the other and the differences they bring to any situation. Similar kinds of comparisons can be made related to other elements of diversity. Nurses have embraced information related to generational differences and have used religious and ethnic contexts as ways to begin dialogs about values and beliefs.

Social capital was described by Carlson and Chamberlain (2003). Their study was done to synthesize empirical findings using PubMed, CINAHL, and applicable journals that link the concept of social capital to health outcomes and to identify implications for health disparities. The question that arises with this concept is, Is it an attribute of an individual, a social network, or a geographic space? People within geographic areas interact and develop social norms of behavior that can be transferred into the workplace by the healthcare providers. The rationale that social capital might be associated with racial and ethnic health disparities has remained relatively unexplored according to the authors.

EXERCISE 9-7

Read Carlson and Chamberlain's article (2003) about social capital, which is defined as "the quality and quantity of the social relations embedded within community norms of interaction" (p. 325). Do a self-analysis using the following questions, and decide whether you might have prejudices or biases toward people (staff) of color or of your own ethnic or racial group. The attributes of social capital include trust and reciprocity. For trust, ask yourself these questions: "Do you think most people [staff] would try to take advantage of you if they got a chance, or would they try to be fair?" and "Generally speaking, would you say that most people [staff] can be trusted or that you can't be too careful in dealing with people?" (Carlson & Chamberlain, 2003, p. 326). For reciprocity, ask yourself this question: "Would you say that most of the time people [staff] try to be helpful, or are they mostly looking out for themselves?" (Carlson & Chamberlain, 2003, p. 326). Review the researchers' findings and conclusions. Consider their importance to your practice specialty.

Ethnocentrism "refers to the belief that one's own ways are the best, most superior, or preferred ways to act, believe, or behave" (Leininger, 2002b, p. 50), whereas cultural imposition is defined as "the tendency of an individual or group to impose their values, beliefs, and practices on another culture for varied reasons" (Leininger, 2002b, p. 51). Such practices constitute a major concern in nursing and "a largely unrecognized problem as a result of cultural ignorance, blindness, ethnocentric tendencies, biases, racism or other factors" (Leininger, 2002b, p. 51).

Although the literature has addressed multicultural needs of patients, it is sparse in identifying effective methods for nurse managers to use when dealing with multicultural staff. Differences in education and culture can impede patient care, and uncomfortable situations may emerge from such differences. For example, staff members may be reluctant to admit language problems that hamper their written communication. They may also be reluctant to admit their lack of understanding when interpreting directions. Psychosocial skills may be problematic as well, because non-Westernized countries encourage emotional restraint. Staff may have difficulty addressing issues that relate to private family matters. Non-Asian nurses may have difficulty accepting the intensified family involvement of Asian cultures. The lack of assertiveness and the subservient physician-nurse relationships of some cultures are other issues that provide challenges for nurse managers. Unit-oriented workshops arranged by the nurse manager to address effective assertive techniques and family involvement as it relates to cultural differences are two ways of assisting staff with cultural work situations.

Giddens' (2008) described the concept of "multi-contextuality" and provided an exemplar of this concept, a virtual community known as the "The Neighborhood." It is designed to promote a conceptual-based learning environment and to offer an alternative approach of learning for diverse learners in current undergraduate nursing programs. According to Giddens, this student-oriented learning environment presents nursing concepts in a rich personal and community context through stories and supplemental multimedia. Given a diverse nursing work-

force, use of this innovative teaching strategy provides an opportunity for a nurse manager to expand the understanding of staff members' knowledge. In addition, such activity would address the Institute of Medicine's (2004) reported evidence that lack of diversity in represented minority groups in the nursing workforce affects the quality of healthcare delivery.

Providing quality of life and human care is difficult to accomplish if the nurse does not have knowledge of the recipient's culture as it relates to care. Leininger believes that "culture reflects shared values, beliefs, ideas, and meanings that are learned and that guide human thoughts, decisions, and actions. Cultures have *manifest* (readily recognized) and *implicit* (covert and ideal) rules of behavior and expectations. Human cultures have material items or symbols such as artifacts, objects, dress, and actions that have special meaning in a culture" (Leininger, 2002b, p. 48). Leininger (2002b) states that her views of cultural care are "a synthesized construct that is the foundational basis to understanding and helping people of different cultures in transcultural nursing practices" (p. 48). Accordingly, "quality of life" must be addressed from an emic (inside) cultural viewpoint and compared with an etic (outsider) professional's perspective. By comparing these two viewpoints, more meaningful nursing practice interventions will evolve. This comparative analysis will require nurses to include global views in their cultural studies that consider the social and environmental context of different cultures.

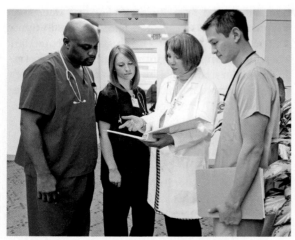

Respecting cultural diversity in the team fosters cooperation and supports sound decision making.

EXERCISE 9-8

As a small group activity, assess several clinical settings. Do these settings have programs related to cultural diversity? Why? What are the programs like? If there are no programs, why do you think they have not been implemented?

DEALING EFFECTIVELY WITH CULTURAL DIVERSITY

Doing an annual personal cultural audit helps an individual identify opportunities for developing skills that promote productivity and efficiency (Wallace, 2004). Answering questions related to tolerance for different views helps individuals perceive their personal perspective of diversity.

The first individuals in the organizational structure who have to address cultural diversity are the leaders and managers. They have to give "unwavering" support to embracing diversity in the workplace rather than using a standard "cookie cutter" approach. Creating a culturally sensitive work environment involves a long-term vision and financial and healthcare-provider commitment. Leaders and managers need to make the strategic decision to design services and programs especially to meet the needs of diverse cultural, ethnic, and racial differences of staff and patients. They need to focus first on building a knowledge base whereby employees are required to attend educational sessions to become familiar with cultural practices and to achieve a culture-friendly environment (Biggerstaff & Hamby, 2004).

Nurse managers hold the key to making the best use of cultural diversity. Managers have positions of power to begin programs that enrich the diversity among staff. For example, capitalizing on the knowledge that all staff bring to the patient is possible for better quality care outcomes. One method that can be used is to allow staff to verbalize their feelings about particular cultures in relationship to personal beliefs. Another is to have two or three staff members of different ethnic origins present a patient-care conference, giving their views on how they would care for a specific patient's needs based on their own ethnic values.

Mentorship programs should be established so that all staff can expand their knowledge about cultural diversity. Mentors have specific relationships with their mentees. The more closely aligned a mentor is with the mentee (e.g., same gender, age-group, ethnicity, and primary language), the more effective the relationship. Programs that address the staff's cultural diversity should not try to make people of different cultures pattern their behavior after the prevailing culture. Nurse managers must carefully select those mentors who ascribe to transcultural, rather than ethnocentric, values and beliefs. A much richer staff exists when nurse managers build on the valuable culture of all staff members and when diversity is rewarded. The pacesetter for the cultural norm of the unit is the nurse manager. For example, to demonstrate commitment to cultural diversity, a nurse manager might make a special effort to ensure that U.S. black, Asian-American, and Hispanic holidays or other cultural representations on the unit are recognized by the staff. Staff members who are active participants in these programs can then be given positive reinforcement by the nurse manager. These activities promote a better understanding and appreciation of individuals' cultural heritage.

Nurse managers are aware of the increasing shortage of nurses, demanding work environment with its surrounding influences, and statistics indicating that almost 50% of all new nurses leave their first professional nursing position by the first year because of job dissatisfaction and level of stress. This period may be even more challenging for individuals whose culture differs from the predominant unit culture.

The National Quality Forum (NQF) (2009) has in place a project that seeks to endorse a comprehensive national framework/core competencies for evaluating cultural competency across all healthcare settings, as well as a minimum set of preferred practices based on the framework. The framework identifies four "Guiding Principles" and six "Domains and Subdomains." It behooves nursing leaders and their staff to read and take action as appropriate to enhance their practice of delivering culturally competent patient care within the setting.

Continuing-education programs should help nurses learn about the care of different ethnic groups. For example, professional organizations related to cultural groups (National Hispanic Nurses Association, Philippine Nurses Association of America, National Black Nurses Association) and institutions might develop or sponsor a workshop or conference on cross-cultural nursing for nursing service staff and faculty in schools of nursing who have had limited preparation in cultural care or cultural beliefs in healing.

EXERCISE 9-9

Identify a situation in which working with culturally diverse staff had positive or negative outcomes. If a negative outcome resulted, what could you have done to make it a positive one?

Muslims are one of the fastest growing populations in the United States and worldwide. El Gindy

(2004b) addressed the need for showing respect for accommodating Muslim nurses' dress requirements and understanding the role of Islam in their lives. For example, one Muslim nurse wore her hijab and became frustrated because the infection control staff consistently asked her to wear short sleeves or to roll up the sleeves. El Gindy stated the importance of the Islamic dress code as a way of life to obey Allah; therefore it was mandatory. Healthcare providers should be made aware of this religious belief and respond to it in a positive way.

Sensitive or controversial issues are often addressed by behaviors that represent avoidance or coercion. The similarities or differences about the issue or person are not acknowledged, either subconsciously or consciously. Avoidance precludes any opportunities for open discussion and potential for change. Avoidance can be a powerful and controlling strategy, but situations do not vanish because they are avoided. Aspects of the situations may eventually resurface. If the situation becomes intolerable, frustration and anger probably will occur. Various responses are possible, and insistence that the issue is no longer visible in the setting does not imply its resolution.

Coercion is acted out through the use of power or status to persuade people to act in specific ways. Although coercion is not a negative behavior, it can lead to negative consequences through the inequity of power. Coercive tactics limit choices and may result in powerlessness, although the importance of the outcome varies greatly. For example, the use of coercion in a situation may result in anger, which is a normal response to feelings of powerlessness that result from being or feeling controlled. Passivity and aggression often perpetuate the situation, and individuals may not recognize the effect of their actions.

Choices, decisions, and behaviors reflect learned beliefs, values, ideals, and preferences. The goal of communication is maintenance or restoration of personal integrity and recognition of worth and respect of individuals or groups.

The two scenarios described in Box 9-2 illustrate how problem-solving communication can promote mutual understanding and respect. The first scenario involves a compromise between staff members and a patient's family, and the second involves a nurse manager and a staff member from a different culture.

EXERCISE 9-10

Identify a situation involving a staff member requesting additional days of leave that required a culturally sensitive decision. What religious or ethnic practices did you learn about in regard to this request and decision?

Passages of life that culminate in happy events also can challenge the nurse manager, for example, the quinceanera observed by Hispanic families. This event is the celebration for 15-year-old girls to be introduced into society. The nurse whose daughter is celebrating this event must have time to make plans for this festive celebration. Because of the significance of the celebration and the pride that the parents take in their daughter, inviting "key" staff to the quinceanera is common. Nurse managers who understand and value cultural rituals can help individuals meet their needs and help staff, in general, learn and accept various cultural practices and perspectives.

EXERCISE 9-11

Holiday celebrations have cultural significance. Select a specific holiday such as Chinese Lunar New Year (China and Chinatowns) or Araw ng mga Patay (Philippines) or Diwali (India). What is the cultural meaning of the specific holiday? How do staff members of the respective culture celebrate the festive day? Does the nursing unit engage in recognition of special holidays? Table 9-2 provides examples of holiday celebrations.

IMPLICATIONS IN THE WORKPLACE

Considering culture from a healthcare staff person and the nursing workforce perspective is a daunting task, one that can lead to a more solidly aligned service-community relationship. Even if the workforce is not as diverse as one might desire, learning about the cultures of the groups within the workforce is important. Making clear that diversity is valued, in fact celebrated, attracts others to engage in the complexity of care. One way is to make clear how staff are valued as people, not as representatives of some group. Showing respect to all patients irrespective of their cultural differences tells the staff that their differences also can be valued. The key is for managers and leaders to attend to the workforce issues with the same zest as they do the patient issues. Cultural differences enrich all of us when we make deliberate efforts to include them in our daily values.

BOX 9-2 PROBLEM-SOLVING COMMUNICATION: HONORING CULTURAL ATTITUDES TOWARD DEATH AND DYING

Scenario 1: Staff and a Patient's Family

What nurses often call *interference with the care of a patient* commonly reflects family attitudes toward death and dying. Often, Hispanic families rush to the hospital as soon as they hear of a relative's illness. Because most Hispanics believe that death is the passing of an individual to a life that offers tranquility and everlasting happiness, being at the bedside offering prayers and encouragement is the norm rather than the unusual exception. The nurse manager in this situation, herself a non–American-educated nurse manager, had worked extensively at helping her staff understand different cultures. A consensus compromise was worked out between the staff and one such Hispanic family. The family, consisting of three generations, was given the authority to decide what family members could stay at the loved one's side and for how long. By doing this, the family felt they had control of the environment and quickly developed a priority list of family members who could stay no more than 5 minutes at the patient's side. As the family member left the bedside, his or her task was to report the condition of the patient to other family members "camping" in the visitors' lounge. Although their loved one did not survive a massive intracranial hemorrhage, all of the family felt that they were a part of their loved one's "passage of life."

Scenario 2: A Nurse Manager and Another Staff Member

Eastern World cultures that profess Catholicism as their faith celebrate the death of a loved one 40 days after the death. The nurse manager needs to recognize that time off for the nurse involved in this celebration is imperative. Such an occurrence had to be addressed by a nurse manager of Asian descent. The nurse manager quickly realized that the nurse, whose mother died in India, did not ask for any time off to make the necessary burial arrangements but, rather, waited 40 days to celebrate his mother's death. The celebration included formal invitations to a church service, as well as a dinner after the service. One day during early morning rounds, the nurse explained how death is celebrated by Eastern World Catholics. The Bible's description of the Ascension of the Lord into heaven 40 days after his death served as the conceptual framework for the loved one's death. The grieving family believed their loved one's spirit would stay on earth for 40 days. During these 40 days, the family held prayer sessions meant to assist the "spirit" to prepare for its ascension into heaven. When the 40 days have passed, the celebration previously described marks the ascension of the loved one's spirit into heaven.

Because this particular unit truly espoused a multicultural concept, the nurses had no difficulty in allowing the Indian nurse 2 weeks of unplanned vacation so that his mother's "passage of life" celebration could be accomplished in a respectful, dignified manner.

TABLE 9-2 EXAMPLES OF HOLIDAY CELEBRATIONS OF CULTURAL SIGNIFICANCE

TERM	COUNTRY	DATE
Araw ng mga Patay	All Saints Day, Philippines	November 1
Chinese Lunar New Year	China, Chinatowns	January or February (varies with Chinese Calendar)
Cinco de Mayo	Independence Day, Mexico	May 5
Ramadan	Muslim/Islamic festival, India	Ninth month of Muslim year
Deepavali/Diwali	Hindu festival of lights, India	October-November
Hanukkah/Chanukah	Jewish festival of lights, United States	December
Christmas	Many nations with Christian populations	December 25 (United States)
Kwanzaa	U.S. Blacks	Between Christmas and New Year's Day, 7 days
Boxing Day	Worker's Recognition, Canada, Australia, Great Britain	December 26
Martin Luther King, Jr.	Civil rights, United States	January 20
Eid ul-Adha	Feast of Sacrifice, Muslim	January, 3-day feast
Day of Mourning for all manifestations of racism; ethnic discrimination (1969)	Various countries; holiday for Buddhists (Tibetan, Zen, Pure Land, and Theravada)	January 4

THE SOLUTION

As a nurse manager, I prefer to talk on a one-to-one basis. I had a meeting with the male staff member to learn from him, "What made you upset with the charge nurse when she made your assignment?" In our discussion, he told me, "The charge nurse used words [slang] for which I did not know the meaning .... I did not understand why she said it ...she was trying to overpower me ... I didn't like it ... so I was defensive about it." We talked about being sensitive to cultural communication and the need to understand meanings of words and to ask for immediate clarification when such situations arise with members of two different cultures.

—*Sally C. Fernandez*

Would this be a suitable approach for you? Why?

THE EVIDENCE

1. Acknowledging cultural diversity in patients and staff requires leaders to be proactive.
2. Working with minority nursing organizations enhances opportunities for successful recruitment and retention.
3. Taking deliberate actions to acknowledge and celebrate culturally related events helps employees from various groups feel valued.

NEED TO KNOW NOW

- Determine what the dominant cultural groups are in your community and know what the implications for care are.
- Be alert for opportunities to learn about co-workers' cultural backgrounds and practices.
- Know how to retrieve literature and research related to best practice and evidence for cultural topics in health care.

CHAPTER CHECKLIST

All potential or current nurse leaders or managers must acknowledge and address cultural diversity among staff and patients. Culture lives in each of us. It determines how we think, what we value, how we behave, and how we communicate with each other. In everyday work activities, the nurse manager must be able to do the following:

- Assess staff diversity and use techniques to manage a culturally diverse workforce and recognize staff members' diverse strengths. Use the strengths to benefit the unit and patients.
- Lead staff with a clear understanding of principles that embrace culture, cultural diversity, and cultural sensitivity.
- Be able to communicate effectively with staff and patients from diverse cultural backgrounds:
  - Recognize slang terms that have different meanings in different cultures.
  - Understand that nonverbal behaviors also carry different connotations depending on one's culture.
- Select basic characteristics of any culture.
- Appraise factors, both individual and societal, inherent in cultural diversity:
  - Three key principles relate to respect for different lifestyles:
    - *Multiculturalism* refers to maintaining several different cultures simultaneously.
    - *Cross-culturalism* refers to mediating between two cultures (one's own and another).
    - *Transculturalism* denotes bridging significant differences in cultural practices.

- Remember that sexual orientation and gender recognition are important factors to consider in dealing fairly with all patients and staff members.
- Use tools that clarify staff cultural diversity effectively:
  - Mentoring programs can help staff expand their knowledge of cultural diversity and recognize their own biases while integrating them with diverse colleagues.

- Continuing education programs can help nurses learn about caring for different ethnic groups in ways that honor their beliefs.
- Internet websites can assist nurses to quickly and effectively obtain information on cultural topics.
- Appreciate the cultural richness found among staff and patients.

TIPS FOR DEALING WITH CULTURAL DIVERSITY

Being a nurse manager in a country that views its strength in its population's cultural diversity requires special skills. The nurse manager needs to do the following:

- Ascribe to effective techniques for managing a culturally diverse workforce.
- Appreciate and encourage programs that address cultural diversity of staff.

- Assist staff in problem solving special cultural needs of colleagues.
- Embrace three key principles relating to culture: multiculturalism, cross-culturalism, and transculturalism.
- Commit to lifelong learning about culture for self and staff.

REFERENCES

American Nurses Association (ANA). (2008). *Code of ethics for nurses with interpretative statements.* Washington, DC: American Nurses Publishing.

Baldwin, D. (2003). Disparities in health and health care: Focusing efforts to eliminate unequal burdens. *Online Journal of Issues in Nursing, 8*(1). Retrieved October 22, 2009, from www.nursingworld.org/MainMenuCategories/ANAMarketplace/ANAPeriodicals/OJIN/TableofContents/Volume82003/No1Jan2003/DisparitiesinHealthandHealthCare.aspx.

Biggerstaff, G., & Hamby, L. (2004). Diversity—An evolving leadership initiative. *Nurse Leader, 2*(4), 30. St. Louis: Elsevier.

Campinha-Bacote, J. (1999). A model and instrument for addressing cultural competence in health care. *Journal of Nursing Education, 38*(5), 203-207.

Campinha-Bacote, J. (2002). The process of cultural competence in a delivery of healthcare services: A model of care. *Journal of Transcultural Nursing, 13*(3), 181-184.

Carlson, E. D., & Chamberlain, R. M. (2003). Social capital, health, and health disparities. *Journal of Nursing Scholarship, 35*(4), 325-331.

Choi, H. (2001). Cultural marginality: A concept analysis with implications for immigrant adolescents. *Issues in Comprehensive Pediatric Nursing, 24*, 193-206.

Connerley, M. L., & Pedersen, R. B. (2005). *Leadership in a diverse and multicultural environment: Developing awareness, knowledge and skills.* Los Angeles: Sage Publications.

D'Avanzo, C. E. (2008). *Pocket guide to cultural health assessment* (4th ed.). St. Louis: Mosby.

El Gindy, G. (Winter 2004b). Treating Muslims with cultural sensitivity in a post-9/11 world. *Minority Nurse*, 44-46.

Giddens, J. F. (2008). Online content: Achieving diversity in nursing through multicontextual learning environments. *Nursing Outlook, 56*, 78-83.

Giger, J. N., & Davidhizar, R. (2002). The Giger and Davidhizar transcultural assessment model. *Journal of Transcultural Nursing, 13*(3), 185-188.

Health Resources and Services Administration (HRSA). (2008). *Division of Nursing's 2008 National Sample Survey of Registered Nurses (NSSRN).* Retrieved February 4, 2009, from http://bhpr.hrsa.gov/healthworkforce/rnsurvey04/appendixa.htm.

Institute of Medicine. (2004). *In the nation's compelling interest: Ensuring diversity in the health-care workforce.* Washington, DC: National Academies Press.

International Council of Nurses. (2008). Translation guidelines for International Classification for Nursing Practice (ICNP). Geneva, Switzerland. Retrieved April 1, 2009, from www.icn.ch.

Leininger, M. (2002a). Cultural care theory: A major contribution to advance transcultural nursing knowledge and practice. *Journal of Transcultural Nursing, 13*(3), 189-192.

Leininger, M. (2002b). Essential transcultural nursing care concepts, principles, examples, and policy statements. Cited in M. Leininger, & M. R. McFarland (Eds.), *Transcultural nursing: Concepts, theories, research & practice* (3rd ed.). New York: McGraw-Hill Medical Publishing Division.

Lenburg, C. B., Lipson, J. G., Demi, A. S., Blaney, D. R., Stern, P. N., Schultz, P. R., & Gage, L. (1995). *Promoting cultural competence in and through nursing education: A critical review and comprehensive plan for action*. Washington, DC: American Academy of Nursing.

Lipson, J. G., & Dibble, S. L. (2005). *Culture & clinical care*. San Francisco: UCSF Nursing Press.

Merriam-Webster Inc. (2005). *The Merriam-Webster Dictionary*. Springfield, Mass: Merriam-Webster.

National Advisory Council on Nurse Education and Practice (NACNEP). (2000). *A national agenda for nursing workforce, racial/ethnic diversity*. Washington, DC: U.S. Department of Health and Human Services, Health Resources & Service Administration, Bureau of Health Professions.

National Quality Forum. (2009). Endorsing a framework and preferred practices for measuring and reporting cultural competency. (Pre-publication draft manuscript) (Retrieved March 12, 2009, from www.qualityforum.org/projects/cultural_competency.aspx.

Noone, J. (2008). The diversity imperative: Strategies to address a diverse nursing workforce. *Nursing Forum, 43*(3), 133-143.

Portillo, C. J. (2003). Health disparities and culture—Moving beyond the beginning. *Journal of Transcultural Nursing, 14*(1), 5.

Purnell, L. D., & Paulanka, B. J. (2008). *Transcultural health care: A culturally competent approach* (3rd ed.). Philadelphia: FA Davis.

Purnell, L. D. (2009). *Guide to culturally competent health care* (2nd ed.). Philadelphia: FA Davis.

Seago, J. A., & Spetz, J. (2008). Minority nurses' experiences on the job. *Journal of Cultural Diversity, 15*(1), 16-23. Retrieved February 27, 2009, from ProQuest Nursing & Allied Health Source database (Document ID: 14336481).

Shannon, S. E. (2008). Ethics for neighbors. Cited in W. J. Ellenchild Pinch & A. M. Haddad (Eds.), *Nursing and health care ethics: A legacy and a vision*. American Nurses Association: Nursebooks.org. Chap. 9, 91-101.

Schim, S. M., Doorenbos, A., Benkert, R., & Miller, J. (2007). Culturally congruent care: Putting the puzzle together. *Journal of Transcultural Nursing, 18*(2), 103-110.

Spector, R. E. (2009). *Cultural diversity in health and illness* (7th ed.). Upper Saddle River, NJ: Pearson Prentice Hall.

Spence, D. (2004). Prejudice, paradox and possibility: The experience of nursing people from cultures other than one's own. In K. H. Kavanaugh & V. Knowlden (Eds.), *Many voices: Toward caring culture in healthcare and healing*. Madison, WI: The University of Wisconsin Press.

St. Hill, P., Lipson, J. G., & Meleis, A. I. (2003). *Caring for women cross-culturally*. Philadelphia: FA Davis.

Sullivan, E. J., & Decker, P. J. (2009). *Effective leadership and management in nursing* (5th ed.). Upper Saddle River, NJ: Prentice Hall.

Tappen, R. (2001). *Nursing leadership and management: Concepts and practice* (4th ed.). Philadelphia: FA Davis.

U.S. Bureau of Labor Statistics, Bulletin 2307. (n.d.) Retrieved October 28, 2009, from www.bls.gov/cps/home.htm.

U.S. Census. (2004). Retrieved November 17, 2008 from www.census.gov/prod/2004pub/04statab/labor.pdf

U.S. Census. (2010). Retrieved October 28, 2009, from http://2010.census.gov/2010census/.

Wallace, L.S. (December 12, 2004). The cultural coach: Honesty is essential in personal cultural audit. *Houston Chronicle*, E2.

SUGGESTED READINGS

American Association of Colleges of Nursing. (2008). *Cultural competency in baccalaureate nursing education*. Website: www.aacn.nche.edu/Education/cultural.htm.

Bonder, B., Martin, L., & Miracle, A. (2002). *Culture in clinical care*. Thorofare, NJ: Slack.

Corlese, I. B., Nicholas, P. K., & Nokes, K. M. (2001). Issues in cross-cultural quality-life research. *Journal of Nursing Scholarship, 33*(1), 15-20.

Engebretson, J., Mahoney, J., & Carlson, E. D. (2008). Cultural competence in the era of evidence-based practice. *Journal of Professional Nursing, 24*(3), 172-178.

Hagman, L. W. (2006). Cultural self-efficacy of licensed registered nurses in New Mexico. *Journal of Cultural Diversity, 13*(2), 105-112.

National Quality Forum. (2009). *A comprehensive framework and preferred practices for measuring and reporting cultural competence: A consensus report*. Washington, DC. Website: www.qualityforum.org/Search.aspx?keyword=A+comprehensive+framework+and+preferred+practices+for+measuring+and+reporting+cultural+competence%3a+A+concensus+report.

Singleton, K., & Krause, E. M. S. (September 30, 2009). Understanding cultural and linguistic barriers to health literacy. *The Online Journal of Issues in Nursing*, pp. 1-13. Retrieved October 28, 2009, from www.nursingworld.org/MainMenuCategories?ANAMarketplace/ANAPeriodicals/OJIN/TableofCo …

University of Washington Medical Center Patient and Family Education services (n.d.). *Culture clues. Tip sheets regarding diverse cultures*. Website: http://depts.washington.edu/pfes/CultureClues.htm.

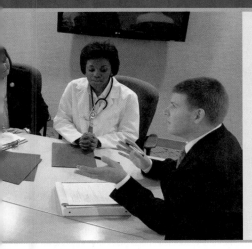

Power, Politics, and Influence

Karen Kelly

This chapter describes how power and politics influence the roles of leaders and managers and how leaders and managers use power and politics to be influential. Contemporary concepts of power, empowerment, types of power exercised by nurses, key factors in developing a powerful image, personal and organizational strategies for exercising power, and the power of nurses to shape health policy by taking action in the arena of legislative politics are explored. Engaging in the politics of the workplace is critical for effective nursing leadership and management.

OBJECTIVES

- Explore the concepts of professional and legislative politics related to nursing.
- Value the concept of power as it relates to leadership and management in nursing.
- Use different types of power in the exercise of nursing leadership.
- Develop a power image for effective nursing leadership.
- Choose appropriate strategies for exercising power to influence the politics of the work setting, professional organizations, legislators, and the development of health policy.

TERMS TO KNOW

coalitions	negotiating	politics
empowerment	policy	power
influence		

Anonymous, a retired emergency department staff nurse

Our hospital was trying hard to improve customer service. The emergency department (ED) had been receiving frequent calls that were not relevant to the work of the ED, such as asking how long to cook a turkey and where the closest 24-hour veterinary clinic is. In some cases, in efforts to provide good customer service, the ED staff provided phone numbers (e.g., the Butterball turkey hotline; the phone number for a 24-hour animal hospital). Often we had to tell callers we could not provide them with the information requested; these responses were met with hostile and even obscene reactions from some callers. Other calls (e.g., calls to determine how much a 20-minute late-night visit to the ED or an X-ray would cost) were also met with hostility at times. Staff requested an in-service on how to handle such calls while providing good customer service. Our director provided us with such a program. We learned to deal with verbal hostility with assertive communication.

Shortly after the in-service, late on a Friday morning, I took a call from a woman who wanted to know how to treat an infected wound on her cat's back. I gave her the name and phone number of the 24-hour animal clinic. The woman responded by screaming obscenities at me, indicating she had taken the cat to a veterinarian and wasn't going to go back. She screamed so loudly that the ED's medical director and other staff heard the woman's tirade. Feeling

empowered, I used my new skills to assertively end the conversation. A secretary paged our nursing director to come to the ED while the call was in progress. She arrived just as the call ended. I was debriefed by the director. The others who overheard the call gave her the same account of the call. I began to write an incident report on the event before my director was paged to go to the office of the vice president (VP) of nursing.

The VP had just gotten off the phone with the chief executive officer (CEO) of the hospital. The woman with the cat called him to accuse me of calling her obscene names and refusing to help her. The director told my VP what I had told her. She emphasized that the caller was the one using obscenities, not me. The VP directed her to suspend me immediately to placate the CEO; my director insisted that I had done nothing wrong and refused to suspend me, based on the information the others had given her. The VP came to the ED after the director left her office. She then confronted me, threatening to fire me unless I called the woman and apologized. The VP left only when the medical director of the ED insisted that I had used no obscenities and had not responded to the call inappropriately. Badly shaken, I paged the director to come back to the ED as soon as the VP left.

What do you think you would do if you were this nurse?

INTRODUCTION

The profession of nursing developed in the United States at a time when women had limited legal rights (e.g., most were prohibited from voting, and many could not own property). Women were viewed as neither powerful nor political; in the late nineteenth century, *feminine* and *powerful* were practically contradictory terms. During the twentieth century, as the status and role of women changed, so did the status and role of nurses. As the economic and social power of women evolved, so did the power of nurses. This is significant because nursing historically has been and continues to be a discipline comprising primarily women.

Now in the twenty-first century, nurses must exercise their power to create a strong voice for nursing in shaping an evolving healthcare environment. This is an era of rapid and often unplanned change with a dramatic nursing shortage like none before. Nurses must use their collective power and flex their political

muscles to create a preferred future for the healthcare system, healthcare consumers, and the profession of nursing.

HISTORY

The word *power* comes from the Latin word *potere*, meaning "to be able." Simply defined, power is the ability to influence others in an effort to achieve goals. Power was once considered almost a taboo in nursing. In nursing's formative years, the exercise of power was considered inappropriate, unladylike, and unprofessional. During nursing's earliest decades in America, many decisions about nursing education and practice were made by persons outside of nursing (Ashley, 1976). Nurses began to exercise their collective power with the rise of early nursing leaders such as Lillian Wald, Isabel Stewart, Annie Goodrich, Lavinia Dock, M. Adelaide Nutting, Mary Eliza Mahoney, and Isabel Hampton Robb and the development of organizations that evolved into the American Nurses Association (ANA) and the National League for Nursing (NLN).

Many social, technologic, scientific, and economic trends have shaped nursing and nurses and nursing's ability to exercise power during the twentieth century. The American Medical Association (AMA), in 1988, proposed a new category of healthcare worker (the registered care technologist or RCT) to replace nurses during a time of nursing shortage. Nurses and nursing organizations responded powerfully. Nursing leaders came together in "summit meetings" to formulate powerful responses to the AMA and implemented a range of actions, including public education and the education of legislators. The new healthcare worker did not materialize from this proposal. Today, in an era of expanding nursing roles (e.g., advanced practice nurses, clinical nurse leaders, and new roles for graduates of doctor of nursing practice [DNP] programs), nurses must continue to exercise their power to shape the continuing development of the profession of nursing and the future of the healthcare system.

Sadly, the media, politicians, organized medicine, some healthcare executives, and some nurses have traditionally viewed nurses and nursing as powerless. That view began to change dramatically in the 1990s as nurses began to appear more often on local and national news and on talk shows as experts on health care, the changes occurring in the healthcare system, and the effect of these changes on the public. Nurses have become increasingly visible in political campaigns on the local, state, and national levels, both as candidates and as political influentials. For example, Congresswoman Lois Capps, MA, BSN, RN, represents a California congressional district; she assumed the office held by her husband upon his death. A former school nurse, Congresswoman Capps has since been re-elected by her constituents to the House seat. Nurses and nursing have gained new respect in the political arena in recent years. Sheila Burke, MPA, RN, FAAN, served as Chief of Staff for Senator Robert Dole while he was Senate Majority Leader in the United States Congress, making her one of the most powerful congressional staff people in Washington. During the Clinton administration, nurse leaders were prominent: two former ANA presidents, Virginia Trotter Betts, MSN, JD, RN, FAAN, and Beverly

Malone, PhD, RN, FAAN, served in roles that helped shape health policy for the nation. Diana J. Mason, PhD, RN, FAAN, editor emerita of the *American Journal of Nursing*, has long hosted a radio talk show in New York City on healthcare issues. Mary Wakefield, PhD, RN, FAAN, serves as the administrator of the Health Resources and Services Administration (HRSA) under President Barack Obama. She served in the 1990s as chief of staff to North Dakota senators Kent Conrad and Quentin Burdick.

As we experience a new and different era of nursing shortage, there are still some nurses who see themselves as powerless and oppressed, demonstrating aspects of oppressed group behavior. Roberts (1983) addressed the historical evidence of oppressed group behavior among nurses, based on models developed from the study of politically and economically oppressed populations. Oppressed group behavior is apparent when a population is dominated by another group. This subordinate or oppressed group begins to take on the characteristics of the dominant group and reject the characteristics of their own group, although this behavior fails to create a balance of power with the dominant group (Roberts 1983). Matheson and Bobay (2007) conducted a review of the literature to validate oppressed group behavior in nursing. They noted that nurses continue to demonstrate some of the behaviors characteristic of oppressed groups, but they could not validate that these behaviors occur directly as a result of oppression by outside groups. Among nurses, oppressed group behavior is manifested in low self-esteem (e.g., "I'm just a nurse"), passive aggressiveness (e.g., nurse-on-nurse bullying), distancing oneself from other nurses (e.g., the failure of nurses to join professional organizations), and engaging in intragroup conflicts (e.g., "infighting" or horizontal violence) (Matheson & Bobay, 2007; Roberts, 1983).

Schools of nursing too often fail to socialize students to be activists. Students need to be exposed to the concepts of political action and public policy. Students need to recognize that policy is just a plan for action related to an issue that affects a group's well-being. All nurses need to continue to expand their understanding of the concept of power and to develop their skills in exercising power. Avoiding involvement in the politics of nursing in the workplace, in the profession at large, or in the area of public policy limits the power of the individual nurse and the profession as a whole.

Some nurses are still uncomfortable with politics and the use of power, treating "politics" as if it were a dirty word. Historically, politics has been viewed with some disdain. Writer Robert Louis Stevenson noted, "Politics is perhaps the only profession for which no preparation is thought necessary." But contemporary nursing's need to thrive within a healthcare system demands that nursing education prepare nurses to engage in professional, workplace, and legislative politics.

Politics can be defined in many ways. One simple definition of politics that this author uses when teaching health policy and politics in nursing is "a process of human interaction within organizations." Politics permeates all organizations, including workplaces, legislatures, professions, and even families. Young children often learn that one parent is more likely to readily give permission for special activities or more likely to buy toys and other desired items. They quickly learn to ask permission or ask for a desired item from that parent before asking the other. This is an unwritten political rule in many families. Political activism should be an unwritten rule in nursing (see the Literature Perspective at right).

The model of political activism, noted below, is based on elements from models of political activism (Leavitt, Chaffee, & Vance, 2007). This model can be applied to the political development and activism of individual nurses related to both professional and legislative political arenas (Kelly, 2007):

1. Apathy: no membership in professional organizations; little or no interest in legislative politics as they relate to nursing and health care
2. Buy-in: recognition of the importance of activism within professional organizations (without active participation) and legislative politics related to critical nursing issues
3. Self-interest: involvement in professional organizations to further one's own career; the development and use of political expertise to further the profession's self-interests
4. Political sophistication: high level of professional organization activism (e.g., holding office at the local and state level) moving beyond self-interests; recognition of the need

 LITERATURE PERSPECTIVE

Resource: Kelly, K. (2007). From apathy to savvy to activism: Becoming a politically active nurse. *American Nurse Today, 2*(8), 55-56.

Politics in nursing can refer to both legislative and professional politics. Legislative politics deals with law and public policy. Professional politics focuses on the workplace and professional nursing organizations. Too often, nurses view politics as irrelevant to their daily practice. Yet public policy and politics shape what we do as nurses, from the nurse practice acts that allow for the licensure of nurses to policies that drive reimbursement for healthcare services. Nursing exists because public policy acknowledges that nursing meets a need to provide for the health care of the public.

Nurses can move from political apathy to activism by learning the requisite skills through (1) holding an active membership in professional organizations that provide information and opportunities for networking; (2) attending workshops, conferences, and academic courses that support the development of political skills and expansion of political/policy knowledge; (3) engaging with legislators through lobbying and campaign work; and (4) moving into leadership roles in nursing organizations.

Implications for Practice

If all nurses became actively engaged in professional nursing organizations, the entire profession could move ahead in a dramatic manner. Activism involves being politically active on behalf of patients and the profession.

for activism on behalf of the public and the profession

5. Leading the way: serving in elected or appointed positions in professional organizations at the state and national levels; providing true leadership on broad healthcare interests within legislative politics, including seeking appointment to policy-making bodies and election to political positions

FOCUS ON POWER

Some nurses, including both new graduates and seasoned veterans, have too often viewed power as if it were something immoral, corrupting, and totally contradictory to the caring nature of nursing. However, the definition on p. 178 (the ability to influence others in an effort to achieve goals) demonstrates the essential nature of power to nursing. Nurses routinely influence patients to improve their health status, an essential element of nursing practice. When nurses provide health teaching to patients and their families, the goal is to change patient/family behavior to promote optimal health. That is an exercise of power in nursing practice. Changing the behavior of one's colleagues by instructing them about a new policy being implemented on the nursing unit is another example of how nurses exercise power. Coaching nurses to improve their performances is an exercise of power. Serving as the chief nursing officer of a hospital, managing a multimillion-dollar budget, demonstrates another exercise of power.

EXERCISE 10-1

Recall a recent opportunity in which you observed the work of an expert nurse. Think about that nurse's interactions with patients, family members, nursing colleagues, and other professionals. What kinds of power did you observe this nurse using? What did the nurse do that told you, "This is a powerful person"?

Social scientists have studied the use and abuse of power in human organizations. They have analyzed and categorized the sources and applications of power in human experience. Hersey, Blanchard, and Natemeyer (1979) offer a classic formulation on the basis of social power. Sullivan (2004, p. 33) offers a revised view of types of power that readily apply to the efforts of nurses in the workplace, in professional organizations, and in politics (see the Theory Box on p. 182). These types of power are not mutually exclusive. They are often used in concert to exert influence on individuals or groups.

Nurses commonly use all of these types of power while implementing a wide range of nursing activities. Nurses who teach patients use expert and information power by virtue of the information they share with patients; they also exercise position power because they are registered nurses and therefore are accorded a certain status by society. Members of a state nurses' association who lobby members of the state legislature use expert, perceived, personal, and position power when trying to gain legislators' support for healthcare legislation. New graduates, employed on probationary status until they demonstrate the initial clinical competencies of a position, may view the nurse manager as exercising both position and expert power related to their evaluation for continued employment. Nursing faculty and skilled clinicians exercise expert and perceived power as students emulate their behavior. Connection power is evident at any social gathering in the workplace. People of high status (e.g., vice presidents, directors, deans) within an organization may be sought out for conversation by those who want to move up the organizational hierarchy.

Having a high-status position in an organization immediately provides stature, but power depends on the ability to accomplish goals from that position. Although some may think that "knowledge is power," acting on that knowledge is where the real power lies. Sharing knowledge expands one's power and, in turn, empowers others, including colleagues and patients, by giving them information or skills that they need to take action in a situation.

Nursing's early history in the United States was marked by powerlessness (Ashley, 1976). Nurses were absent from the decision-making processes about their education, practice, and employment. As the social, political, and economic status of women and nurses changed, so did the exercise of power by nursing as a profession and nurses as individuals. Powerlessness, a behavior still exhibited by some nurses, results in negative emotions such as apathy and anger. This can result in a workplace culture that is marked by conflict, anger, and other dysfunctional behaviors. Sharing power and facilitating the empowerment of colleagues so that they exercise their power are strong forces in creating vibrant workplace cultures.

Influence is the process of using power. Influence can range from the punitive power of coercion to the interactive power of collaboration. Coaching a new graduate nurse to complete a complicated nursing procedure successfully vividly demonstrates the ability of the experienced nurse to influence that orientee. The coach uses expert, position, perceived, and information power to influence the orientee not only at that moment but also perhaps over the span of a career. A nurse who lobbies legislators uses expertise, information, and perceived power to encourage support for a bill to expand healthcare services to the children of the working poor. Nurses can use personal, expert, and perceived power while working on the campaigns of legislators who support nursing and healthcare issues.

THEORY BOX

Types of Power*

KEY CONTRIBUTORS	KEY IDEAS	APPLICATION TO PRACTICE
Types or bases of social power were formulated by Hersey, Blanchard, and Natemeyer (1979) to explain the personal use of power. Sullivan (2004) reorganized these types, eliminating much of the overlap in the original categories.	**Personal power:** Based on one's reputation and credibility.	The leader of a state nurses' association (SNA) may have access to the leaders of the state legislature based on the leader's personal power, which is based on years of work with members of the legislature. The SNA president has always delivered on promises of support and provided useful information to legislators on matters of health policy.
	Expert power: Results from the knowledge and skills one possesses that are needed by others.	An advanced practice nurse is viewed as the clinical expert on a nursing unit and as a powerful person.
	Position power: Possessed by virtue of one's position within an organization or status within a group.	The dean of a college of nursing is viewed on campus as powerful because this dean leads the fastest growing academic unit on campus.
	Perceived power: Results from one's reputation as a powerful person.	A nursing student seeks a certain nurse manager as a preceptor during a senior clinical practicum because of the manager's reputation as an effective manager within the organization.
	Information power: Stems from one's possession of selected information that is needed by others.	A staff nurse demonstrates great skill in teaching patients difficult self-care activities and is sought out by colleagues to help them teach their patients.
	Connection power: Gained by association with people who have links to powerful people.	At a Nurses' Week celebration, nurses take advantage of the opportunity to have extended, informal conversations with those who report to the chief nursing officer.

*These categories help explain how we use power to influence others. The categories are not mutually exclusive and usually are used in concert with one another.

EMPOWERMENT

Empowerment is a term that has come into common usage in nursing in recent years. It has been used extensively in the nursing literature related to administration and management; it is also highly relevant to the domain of clinical practice. Empowerment is the process of exercising one's own power. It is also the process by which we facilitate the participation of others in decision making and taking action so they are free to exercise power (Ozimek, 2007). Empowerment is consistent with the contemporary view of leadership, a paradigm that is exemplified by behaviors characteristic of all nurse leaders: facilitator, coach, teacher, and collaborator. Nursing leaders, whether in their employment settings or in profes-sional organizations, exercise power in making professional judgments in their daily work.

These leadership skills are also essential to effective followers. Powerful nurse managers enable nurses to exercise power, influencing them to grow professionally. Powerful nurses support their patients and families so they can participate actively in their own care. Hence these leadership skills can be viewed as an essential component of professional nursing practice whether one is a clinician, an educator, a researcher, or an executive/manager.

Empowerment is the process by which power is shared with colleagues and patients as part of the nurse's exercise of power. This is in sharp contrast to traditional conceptualizations of power, a patriarchal model of power that relies on coercion, hierarchy, authority, control, and force. Viewed with a feminist perspective, empowerment is supported through collaboration, not competition and power plays (Sullivan, 2004).

Nurses sometimes view power as a finite quantity: "If I give you some of my power, I will have less." Empowerment emphasizes the notion that power grows when shared. Envision the exercise of shared power along a spectrum from low to high levels of sharing. The opposing ends of the spectrum can be characterized by two very different groups of nurses:

- Nurses who view power as finite will avoid cooperation with their colleagues and refuse to share their expertise.
- Nurses who view power as infinite are strong collaborators who gain satisfaction by helping their colleagues expand their expertise and their power base.

Empowered nurses make professional practice possible, the kind of professional practice that is satisfying to all nurses. Empowered clinicians are essential for effective nursing management, just as empowered managers set the stage for excellence in clinical practice. Encouraging a reticent colleague to be an active participant in committee meetings serves to empower that nurse and to shape practice policy with the institution. Guiding a novice nurse in exercising professional judgment empowers both the senior nurse and the novice clinician. Coaching a patient on how to be more assertive with a physician who is reluctant to answer the patient's questions is another form of empowerment.

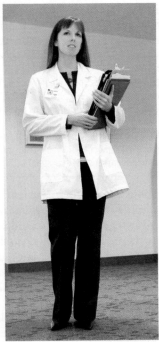

A sense of self-confidence is essential for successful political efforts in the workplace, within the profession, and within the public policy arena.

> **EXERCISE 10-2**
> Think about a recent clinical experience in which you empowered a patient. What did you do for and/or with the patient (and family) that was empowering? How did you feel about your own actions in this situation? How did the patient (or family) respond to your efforts?

Strategies for Developing a Powerful Image

Consider the words of Lady Margaret Thatcher, former prime minister of Great Britain: "Being powerful is like being a lady. If you have to tell people you are, you aren't." You don't have to wear a sign around your neck to show that you are powerful!

The most basic power strategy is the development of a powerful image. If nurses think they are powerful, others will view them as powerful (perceived power); if they view themselves as powerless, so will others. A sense of self-confidence is a strong foundation in developing one's "power image," and it is essential for successful political efforts in the workplace, within the profession, and within the public policy arena. Several key factors contribute to one's power image:

- Self-image: thinking of oneself as powerful and effective
- Grooming and dress: ensuring that clothing, hair, and general appearance are neat, clean, and appropriate to the situation
- Good manners: treating people with courtesy and respect
- Body language: maintaining good posture, using gestures that avoid too much drama, maintaining good eye contact, and being confident in movement

- Speech: using a firm, confident voice; good grammar and diction; an appropriate vocabulary; and strong communication skills.

EXERCISE 10-3

Think about a powerful public figure whom you admire. What key factors contribute to this person's powerful image? Think about a powerful nurse you have met. Identify this person's key image factors. Think about nurses who work in wrinkled scrubs, whose hair is pulled back haphazardly into ponytails, and who fail to make eye contact with patients or their family members. What kind of power image message do they send?

Concern about a powerful image may seem superficial. However, the impressions we make on people influence the way they view us now and in the future, as well as how they value what we do and say. We get only one chance to make a first impression. Given similar educational and experiential backgrounds, who is more likely to be hired for a nursing position: the candidate who comes dressed in a suit or the candidate who arrives in jeans and sandals? Who will be seen as the more competent professional by a patient: the nurse in wrinkled scrubs or the nurse in neat street clothes and a freshly laundered lab coat? Who will have a greater positive impact on a member of the state legislature: the nurse who visits in a sweatshirt and shorts or the nurse in a suit? Who will be perceived by the patient as the more competent caregiver: a nurse with multiple body piercings and 4-inch bright red acrylic nails or the nurse with a single pair of stud earring and neatly trimmed fingernails? While tattoos and body piercing may be socially acceptable among post–baby boomer generations, some healthcare organizations may prohibit the display of either or both during work hours. The display of tattoos by nurses may not be acceptable to some patients, thus limiting the power of those nurses. A powerful image signals to others that one is professionally competent, influential, powerful, and capable of exercising appropriate judgments.

Attitudes and beliefs are other important aspects of a powerful image; they reflect one's values. Believing that power is a positive force in nursing is essential to one's powerful image. A firm belief in nursing's value to society and the centrality of nursing's contribution to the healthcare delivery system is also important. Powerful nurses do not allow the phrase "I'm just a nurse" in their vocabulary. Behavior reflects one's pride in the profession of nursing. This not only increases a nurse's own power but also helps empower nursing colleagues.

Make a Commitment to Nursing as a Career

Nursing is a profession; professions offer careers, not just a series of jobs. Decades ago, nursing marketed itself to recruits as the perfect preparation for marriage and family. Some people still view nurses only as members of an occupation who drop in and out of employment, not as members of a profession with a long-term career commitment. Having a career commitment does not preclude leaving employment temporarily for family, education, or other demands. Having a career commitment means that nurses view themselves first and foremost as members of the discipline of nursing with an obligation to make a contribution to the profession. Status as an employee of a particular hospital, home health agency, long-term care facility, or other venue is secondary to one's status as a member of the profession of nursing.

Value Continuing Nursing Education

Valuing education is one of the hallmarks of a profession. The continuing development of one's nursing skills and knowledge is an empowering experience, preparing nurses to make decisions with the support of an expanding body of evidence. Seminars, workshops, and conferences offer opportunities for continued professional growth and empowerment. Seeking advanced nursing degrees or post-baccalaureate/post-graduate certificates is also a powerful growth experience and reflects commitment to the profession. At one time, some nurses thought the best way to get ahead in nursing was to seek education outside of nursing at the baccalaureate and graduate level. To develop expertise in the science and art of nursing, one must be educated in the discipline of nursing.

Change will continue in the healthcare system, necessitating continuing education to empower nurses to be proactive, not just reactive. A well-educated nursing workforce is essential if nursing is to have a strong voice in shaping the changes in health care. An additional advantage of participating in educational experiences is that it creates opportunities for networking, a strategy that is discussed in the "Networking" section on pp. 185-187.

PERSONAL POWER STRATEGIES

Developing a collection of power strategies or tools is a critical aspect of personal empowerment. These strategies are used in situations that demand the exercise of leadership. Such strategies support building a professional power base and developing political skills within an organization (Boxes 10-1 and 10-2). They also indicate to others that one is a powerful nurse and a leader. These boxes identify personal power strategies beyond those discussed in this section. These "power tools" have been developed and collected by this author during nearly 30 years of nursing experience and observation of successful, effective, powerful nurses.

Communication Skills

The most basic tool is effective verbal communication skills. These are the same communication skills nurses learn to ensure effective interaction with patients and families. Listening skills are essential leadership skills. Just as the clinician listens to the patient to collect assessment data, the manager uses listening skills to assess and evaluate. Managers and other leaders who are good listeners develop reputations for being fair and consistent. Listening for recurring themes related to minor issues of staff dissatisfaction in informal conversations can enable a manager to take action before a staff crisis occurs.

Verbal and nonverbal skills are important personal power strategies; the ability to assess these messages is a critical power strategy. Experts in communication estimate that 90% of the messages we communicate to others are nonverbal. When nonverbal and verbal messages are in conflict, the nonverbal message is always more powerful. The basic lessons on the power of nonverbal communication that most nurses learn in an introductory psychiatric course are relevant in all areas of nursing!

BOX 10-1   POWER STRATEGIES FOR NURSING LEADERS AND ASPIRING LEADERS

Developing a Powerful Image
- Self-confidence
- Body language
- Self-image, including grooming, dress, and speech
- Career commitment and continuing professional education
- Attitudes, beliefs, and values

Additional Personal Power Strategies
- Be honest.
- Be courteous; it makes other people feel good!
- Smile when appropriate; it puts people at ease.
- Accept responsibility for your own mistakes, and then learn from them.
- Be a risk taker.
- Win and lose gracefully.
- Learn to be comfortable with conflict and ambiguity; they are both normal states of the human condition.
- Give credit to others where credit is due.
- Develop the ability to take constructive criticism gracefully; learn to let destructive criticism "roll off your back."
- Use business cards when introducing yourself to new contacts, and collect the business cards of those you meet when networking.
- Follow through on promises.

EXERCISE 10-4

You encounter an old friend at a nursing conference. You greet one another warmly, each stating how good it is to see the other. Yet your friend visibly backs away when you extend your arms to embrace. What is your immediate reaction? Despite the warm words of greeting, do you question your old friend's sincerity because of the strong nonverbal message regarding physical contact? Consider other situations you have experienced recently when words and actions contradict one another. Which message, the verbal or the nonverbal, did you accept as the person's "real" communication to you? Practice with a friend: Pretend you are greeting a visitor to your home. In trial #1, state your greeting warmly, extend your hand to shake the other person's hand, smile, and make eye contact. In trial #2, use the same words of greeting, but in an angry tone of voice, avoid eye contact, and fold your arms across your chest while moving one step back from the other person. Observe the physical actions and listen carefully, especially to the tone of voice. Repeat the exercise, switching roles. Discuss your response to these interactions.

Networking

Networking is an important power strategy and political skill. A network is the result of identifying, valuing, and maintaining relationships with a system of individuals who are sources of information, advice, and support. Networking supports the empowerment of participants through interaction and the refinement of their interpersonal skills. Many nurses have

BOX 10-2   POLITICAL ASTUTENESS INVENTORY

Place a check mark (✓) next to those items for which your answer is "yes." Then give yourself one point for each "yes." After completing the inventory, compare your total score with the scoring criteria at the end of the inventory.

1. I am registered to vote.
2. I know where my voting precinct is located.
3. I voted in the last general election.
4. I voted in the last two elections.
5. I recognized the names of the majority of the candidates on the ballot and was acquainted with the majority of issues in the last election.
6. I stay abreast of current health issues.
7. I belong to the state professional or student nurse organization.
8. I participate (e.g., as a committee member, officer) in this organization.
9. I attended the most recent meeting of my district nurses' association.
10. I attended the last state or national convention held by my organization.
11. I am aware of at least two issues discussed and the stands taken at this convention.
12. I read literature published by my state nurses' association, a professional journal/magazine/newsletter, or other literature on a regular basis to stay abreast of current health issues.
13. I know the names of my senators in Washington.
14. I know the name of my representative in Washington.
15. I know the name of the state senator from my district.
16. I know the name of the state representative from my district.
17. I am acquainted with the voting record of at least one of the above in relation to a specific health issue.
18. I am aware of the stand taken by at least one of the above in relation to a specific health issue.
19. I know whom to contact for information about health-related issues at the state or federal level.
20. I know whether my professional organization employs lobbyists at the state or federal level.
21. I know how to contact these lobbyists.
22. I contribute financially to my state and national professional organization's political action committee (PAC).
23. I give information about effectiveness of elected officials to assist the PAC's endorsement process.
24. I actively supported a senator or representative during the last election.
25. I have written to one of my state or national representatives in the last year regarding a health issue.
26. I am personally acquainted with a senator or representative or member of his or her staff.
27. I serve as a resource person for one of my representatives or his or her staff.
28. I know the process by which a bill is introduced in my state legislature.
29. I know which senators or representatives are supportive of nursing.
30. I know which house and senate committees usually deal with health-related issues.
31. I know the committees of which my representatives are members.
32. I know of at least two health issues related to my profession that are currently under discussion.
33. I know of at least two health-related issues that are currently under discussion at the state or national level.
34. I am aware of the composition of the state board that regulates my profession.
35. I know the process whereby one becomes a member of the state board that regulates my profession.
36. I know what DHHS stands for.
37. I have at least a vague notion of the purpose of the DHHS.
38. I am a member of a health board or advisory group to a health organization or agency.
39. I attend public hearings related to health issues.
40. I find myself more interested in political issues now than in the past.

Scoring:

0-9: Totally unaware politically/apathetic
10-19: Slightly more aware of the implications of the politics of nursing/buy-in
20-29: Beginning political astuteness/self-interest to political sophistication
30-40: Politically astute, an asset to nursing/leading the way

From Goldwater, M., & Zusy, M.J.L. (1990). *Prescription for nurses: Effective political action.* St. Louis: Mosby; with permission by M. Goldwater.

relatively limited networks within the organizations where they are employed. They tend to have lunch or coffee with the people with whom they work most closely. One strategy to expand a workplace network is to have lunch or coffee with someone from another department, including managers from non-nursing departments, at least two or three times a month.

Active participation in nursing organizations is the most effective method of establishing a professional network outside one's place of employment. Although only a minority of nurses actively participate in professional organizations, such participation can propel a nurse into the politics of nursing, including involvement in shaping health policy. State and district nurses' associations offer excellent opportunities to develop a network that includes nurses from various clinical and functional areas. Membership in specialty organizations, especially organizations for nurse managers and executives, provides the opportunity to network with nurses with similar expertise and interests. In addition, membership in civic, volunteer, and special interest groups and participation in educational programs (e.g., formal academic programs and conferences) also provide networking opportunities.

The successful networker identifies a core of networking partners who are particularly skilled, insightful, and eager to support the development of colleagues. These partners need to be nurtured through such strategies as sharing information with them that relates to their interests; introducing them to persons who have comparable interests or who are connected with others of influence; staying connected through notes, e-mail, calls, or instant messages; and meeting them at important events. Successful networkers are not a burden to others in making requests for support, and they do not refuse the support that is provided.

Mentoring

Mentoring has become an important force in nursing. Mentors are competent, experienced professionals who develop a relationship with a less experienced nurse for the purpose of providing advice, support, information, and feedback to encourage the development of that person. Mentoring has been an important element in the career development of men in business, academia, and selected professions. Mentoring has become a significant power strategy for women in general and for nurses in particular during the past 30 years. Mentoring provides expanded access to information, power, and career opportunities. Mentors have historically been a critical asset to novice nurses trying to negotiate workplace and professional politics.

Effective mentoring in nursing benefits both the mentor and the mentee. Mentors benefit by expanding their own professional development and that of their colleagues, improving their own self-awareness, experiencing the intrinsic benefits of teaching another, nurturing their own interpersonal skills, and expanding their political savvy. Mentees receive one-on-one

nurturing and coaching from the men or savvy about the political rules of th and learn about organizational cult insider, can expand their self-confiden portive relationship, receive career d advice, profit from the mentor's profession and have a unique opportunity for individualized professional development.

Mentoring is an empowering experience for both mentors and protégés. The process of seeking out mentors is an exercise in growth for protégés. Mentors often come from one's professional networks. Mentors sometimes select their protégés; at other times, the reverse is true.

Protégés learn new skills from influential mentors and gain self-confidence. Mentors share their influence through the influence of those they mentor and gain satisfaction by experiencing the evolution of those nurses into experienced nurses.

Goal-Setting

Goal-setting is another power strategy. Every nurse knows about setting goals. Students learn to devise patient care goals or patient outcomes as part of the care-planning process. Nurses may be expected to write annual goals for performance reviews at work. Even a project at home (e.g., painting the bedrooms) may necessitate setting goals (e.g., painting a room each day of one's vacation). Goals help one know if what was planned was actually accomplished. Likewise, a successful nursing career needs goals to define what one wants to achieve as a nurse. Without such goals, one can wander endlessly through a series of jobs without a real sense of satisfaction. To paraphrase what the Cheshire Cat told Alice during her trip through Wonderland: Any road will take you there if you don't know where you are going.

Well-defined, long-term goals may be hard to formulate early in a career. For example, few new graduates know specifically that they want to be chief nurse executives, deans, managers, or researchers, yet, eventually, some will choose those career paths. However, developing such a vision early in a career is an important personal power strategy. Once this career vision is developed, one must create opportunities to move toward that vision. Such planning is empowering—putting the nurse in charge rather than letting a career unfold by chance. Having this sense of vision is con-

...nt with a commitment to a career in nursing, part of developing a power image. This vision is always subject to revision as new opportunities are encountered and new interests, knowledge, and skills are gained. Education and work experiences are tools for achieving the vision of one's career.

Developing Expertise

As noted earlier in this chapter, expertise is one of the bases of power. Developing expertise in nursing is an important power strategy. Nursing expertise must not be limited to clinical knowledge. Leadership and communication skills, for example, are essential to the effective exercise of power in a range of nursing roles. Education and practice provide the means for developing such expertise in any domain of nursing—clinical practice, education, research, and management. Developing expertise expands one's power among nursing colleagues, other professional colleagues, and patients. A high level of expertise can make one nearly indispensable within an organization. This is a powerful position to have within any organization, whether it is the workplace or a professional association. A high level of expertise can also lead to a high level of visibility within an organization.

High Visibility

The strategy of high visibility within an organization can begin with volunteering to serve as a member or the chairperson of committees and task forces. High visibility can be nurtured by attending open meetings in the workplace, professional associations, or the community. Even if you are not a member and if meetings deal with local health issues, you can be visible. Review the agendas of these meetings if they are circulated or posted online ahead of time. Use opportunities both before and after meetings to share your expertise and provide valuable information and ideas to members and leaders of such groups. Share your expertise at open meetings when appropriate. Speak up confidently, but have something relevant to say. Be concise and precise; members of the committee will ask for more information if they need it. Create your own business cards using a computer and sheets of business card stock (purchased in any office supply store). Give members of these committees your personal card so that they can contact you later for information.

EXERCISING POWER AND INFLUENCE IN THE WORKPLACE AND OTHER ORGANIZATIONS: SHAPING POLICY

To use influence effectively in any organization, one must understand how the system works and develop organizational strategies. Developing organizational savvy includes identifying the real decision makers and those persons who have a high level of influence with the decision makers. Recognize the informal leaders within any organization. An influential senior staff nurse may have more decision-making power related to direct patient care than the nurse manager. The senior staff nurse may have more clinical expertise and a greater knowledge about the history of the unit and its personnel than a nurse manager with excellent management and leadership skills who is new to the unit.

For example, the executive assistants of chief nursing officers (CNOs) are usually very powerful people, although they are not always recognized as such. The CNO's assistant has control over information, making decisions about who gets to meet with the nurse executive and when, screening incoming and outgoing mail, letting the CNO know when a document needs immediate attention, or placing a memo under a stack of mail for review at a later time.

Collegiality and Collaboration

Nursing does not exist in a vacuum, nor do nurses work in isolation from one another, other professionals, or support personnel. Nurses function within a wide range of organizations, such as schools, hospitals, community health organizations, government agencies, insurance companies, professional associations, and universities. Nurses have been too long divided over the appropriate educational level for entry into practice. Nurses are also noted for their failure to join nursing organizations.

Developing a sense of unity requires each nurse to act collaboratively and collegially in the workplace and in other organizations (e.g., professional associations). Collegiality demands that nurses value the accomplishments of nursing colleagues and express a sincere interest in their efforts. Turning to one's colleagues for advice and support empowers them and expands one's own power base at the same time. Unity of purpose does not contradict diversity of thought. One does not have to be a friend to everyone who is a colleague. Collegiality demands mutual respect, not friendship.

Collaboration and collegiality require that nurses work collectively to ensure that the voice of nursing is heard in the workplace and the legislature. Volunteer to serve on committees and task forces in the workplace, not only within the nursing department but also on organization-wide committees. Become an active member of nursing organizations, especially one's state nursing organization (affiliates of the ANA) and a specialty organization consistent with one's clinical specialty (e.g., American Association of Critical Care Nurses [AACN]) or functional role (e.g., American Organization of Nurse Executives [AONE]). If eligible, become a member of a chapter of Sigma Theta Tau International, Honor Society of Nursing. Get involved in the politics of organizations, in the workplace, and in professional associations. If the workplace uses shared governance or other participatory models, get involved in these councils, committees, task forces, and work groups to share your energy, ideas, and expertise. Many organizations have instituted interdisciplinary committees that bring together nurses, physicians, and other healthcare professionals to improve the quality of professional collaboration and, in turn, the quality of patient care. Become an active, productive member of such groups within the workplace and in the professional associations and community groups dealing with healthcare issues and problems.

An Empowering Attitude

Demonstrate a positive and professional attitude about being a nurse to nursing colleagues, patients and their families, other colleagues in the workplace, and the public, including legislators. This attitude facilitates the exercise of power among colleagues while educating others about nurses and nursing. A powerful image is an important aspect of demonstrating this positive professional attitude. The current practice of nurses to identify themselves by first name may only decrease their power image in the eyes of physicians, patients, and others. Physicians are always addressed as "Doctor"; when they address others by their first names, inequality of power and status is evident. The use of first names among colleagues is not inappropriate so long as everyone is playing by the same rules. Managers may want to enhance the empowerment of their staff members by encouraging them to introduce themselves as "Dr.," "Ms.," or "Mr." Arriving at work, appointments, or meetings on time; looking neat and appropriately attired for the work setting or other professional situation; and speaking positively about one's work are examples of how easy it is to demonstrate a positive, powerful, and professional attitude.

Magnet™ institutions, as recognized by the American Nurses Credentialing Center (ANCC), are characterized by work environments that empower nurses (ANCC, 2009). Leadership activities have been identified as a critical element of the work culture in Magnet™ hospitals; and quality of leadership is one of the "forces of magnetism."

EXERCISE 10-5

How do you routinely introduce yourself to patients, families, physicians, and other colleagues? A powerful and positive approach involves making eye contact with each individual, shaking hands, and introducing yourself by saying, "I'm Terry Jones, a registered nurse [or nursing student]." If you do not currently use this technique, try it out. Note any difference in the responses of people whom you meet using this technique in comparison with a less formal approach.

Developing Coalitions

The exercise of power is often directed at creating change. Although an individual can often be effective at exercising power and creating change, creating certain changes within most organizations requires collective action. Coalition building is an effective political strategy for collective action. Coalitions are groups of individuals or organizations that join together temporarily around a common goal. This goal often focuses on an effort to effect change. The networking among organizations that results in coalition building requires members of one group to reach out to members of other groups. This often occurs at the leadership level and may come through formal mechanisms such as letters that identify an issue or problem—a shared interest—around which a coalition could be built. For example, a state nurses' association may invite the leaders of organizations interested in child health (e.g., organizations of pediatric nurses, public health nurses and physicians, elementary school teachers, daycare providers) and consumers (e.g., parents) to discuss collaborative support for a legislative initiative to improve access to immunization programs in urban and rural areas. Such coalitions of professionals and consumers are powerful in influencing public policy related to health care.

Collaboration among groups and individuals with common interests and goals often results in greater success in effecting change and exercising power in the workplace and within other organizations, including legislative bodies. For example, in Illinois, a coalition of nursing organizations and individuals concerned about the nursing shortage was created. In its early years, the Illinois Coalition for Nursing Resources (n.d.) brought together a diverse group of nursing and healthcare organizations and individuals to address the nursing shortage crisis and to maximize nursing resources in the state. It now serves as a forum for discussion of urgent nursing issues. Expanding networks in the workplace, as suggested earlier in this chapter, facilitates creating a coalition by developing a pool of candidates for coalition building before they are needed. Invite people with common goals to lunch or coffee to begin building a coalition around an issue. Discuss this shared interest, and gain the commitment of the individuals. Meet informally with members of the committee or task force that is working on this issue. Attend the open meetings of professional groups that share the same interests as the organization to which you belong. Share ideas on how to create the desired change most effectively while building coalitions.

Coalition building is an important skill for involvement in legislative politics. Nursing organizations often use coalition building, such as the development of the Illinois Coalition for Nursing Resources, when dealing with state legislatures and Congress. Changes in nurse practice acts to expand opportunities for advanced nursing practice have been accomplished in many states through coalition building. State medical societies or the state agencies that license physicians often oppose such changes. Efforts by a single nursing organization (e.g., a state nurses' association or a nurse practitioners' organization), representing a limited nursing constituency, often lack the clout to overcome opposition by the unified voice of the state's physicians. However, the unified effort of a coalition of nursing organizations, other healthcare organizations, and consumer groups can be powerful in effecting change through legislation.

Negotiating

Negotiating, or bargaining, is a critically important skill for organizational and political power. It is a process of making trade-offs. Children are natural negotiators. Often, they will initially ask their parents for more than what they are willing to accept in the way of privileges, toys, or activities. The logic is simple to children: Ask for more than is reasonable and negotiate down to what you really want!

Negotiating often works the same way within organizations. People will sometimes ask for more than they want and be willing to accept less. In other situations, both sides will enter negotiations asking for radically different things but each may be willing to settle for a position that differs markedly from its original position. In the simplest forms of bargaining, each participant has something that the other party values: goods, services, or information. At the "bargaining table," each party presents an opening position. The process moves on until they reach a mutually agreeable result or until one or both parties walk away from a failed negotiation.

Bargaining may take many forms. Individuals may negotiate with a supervisor for a more desirable work schedule or with a peer to effect a schedule change so that one can attend an out-of-town conference. A nurse manager may sit at the bargaining table with the department director during budget planning to expand education hours for the nursing unit in the next year's budget. Representatives of a coalition of nursing organizations meeting with a legislator may negotiate with the legislator over sections of a proposed healthcare-related bill in an effort to eliminate or modify those sections not viewed by the nursing coalition as in the best interests of nurses, patients, or the healthcare system. Nurses may bargain with nursing and hospital administration over wages, staffing levels, other working conditions, and the conditions and policies that govern clinical practice. This is called *collective bargaining,* a specific type of negotiating that is regulated by both state and federal labor laws and that usually involves representation by a state nurses' association or a nursing or non-nursing labor union (see Collective Action in Chapter 19).

Successful negotiators are well informed about not only their own positions but also those of the opposing side. Negotiators must be able to discuss the pros and cons of both positions. They can assist the other party in recognizing the costs versus the benefits of each position. These skills are also essential to exercising power effectively with the arenas of professional and legislative politics. When lobbying a member of the legislature to support a bill that is desired by nurses, one must understand the position of those opposed to the bill to respond effectively to questions that the legislator may ask.

EXERCISE 10-6

Consider a situation in which you engaged in bargaining or negotiating. Have you ever bought a car? Negotiating the price of the car is a great American tradition. Few people enter into the purchase of a car intending to pay the sticker price. The manufacturer sets most sticker prices at a level that gives the dealer room to negotiate the price down; a few manufacturers of automobiles have firm sticker prices with no room for negotiation. Have you ever negotiated a schedule change at work or school? Have you ever negotiated a raise in your salary? What was the trade-off you made in the process? How far did the other person move from his or her original position? What factors led to your success or failure in this negotiation?

Taking Political Action to Influence Policy

In the 1990s, Carolyn McCarthy was a licensed practical nurse (LPN) from New York when a tragedy turned her life around. Her husband was killed and her son injured by a gunman on the Long Island Railroad. She sought the support of her congressman on gun control legislation as a result of her personal tragedy. He refused to support such legislation. She took extraordinary action, changing her party affiliation from Republican to Democrat and then running against the incumbent for his seat in Congress. She is still an LPN, and she has also become Congresswoman Carolyn McCarthy (D-NY). Taking action may include such simple acts as working in a legislative campaign or volunteering to work on a church committee to establish a parish health ministry. Extraordinary actions like those taken by Carolyn McCarthy are also essential for nursing's voice to be heard loudly and clearly in the uncertain future.

Gaining political skills, like any other skill set, is a developmental process. Some suggested strategies for developing political skills are presented in Box 10-3.

The personal power strategies mentioned earlier in this chapter are also important for building one's political power. Nurses can no longer be passive observers of the political world. Political involvement is a professional responsibility, not just a privilege; political advocacy is a mandate (Abood, 2007).

BOX 10-3 DEVELOPING POLITICAL SKILLS

- Build a working relationship with a legislator, such as one's state senator or representative or member of the U.S. Congress and the legislative staff members.
- Join and be an active member of your state nurses' association affiliate of the ANA.
- Invite a legislator to a professional organization meeting.
- Invite a legislator or staff person from the legislator's office to spend a day with you at work.
- Register to vote, and vote in every election.
- Join your state nurses' association's government relations or legislative committee and political action committee (PAC); join ANA's political action committee.
- Be in touch with your federal and state legislators on nursing and healthcare issues, especially related to specific bills, by letter writing, telephone calls, or e-mails.
- Participate in Nurse Lobby Day and meet with your state legislators.
- Work on a federal or state legislative campaign.
- Visit your U.S. senators and member of congress if visiting in the Washington, DC, area to discuss federal legislation related to nursing and health care, or visit their local offices.
- Get involved in the local group of your political party.
- Run for office at the local, county, state, or congressional level.
- Enhance the image of nursing in all your policy efforts.
- Communicate your message effectively and clearly.
- Develop your expertise in shaping policy.
- Seek appointive positions or elective office to shape policy more effectively.

RESEARCH PERSPECTIVE

Resource: Buerhaus, P.I., Ulrich, B., Donelan, K., & DesRoches, C. (2008). Registered nurses' perspectives on health care and the 2008 presidential election. *Nursing Economic$, 26*, 227-235, 257.

The 2008 National Survey of Registered Nurses (NSRN) included questions related to RNs' attitudes about healthcare policy and the presidential election. Nurses' attitudes are compared with those of the general public (from other data sources). The NSRN was conducted by mail from March 4 to June 3, 2008, using a random sample of RNs. Funding was provided by Johnson & Johnson and the Gannett Healthcare Group. Harris Interactive also supported the research through fieldwork. An eight-page survey was mailed out to 3500 RNs in a sample drawn from Gannett Healthcare Group's database of RNs. RNs who did not respond were sent up to five reminders to encourage their participation in the study.

Incentives for participation were included in the materials sent to the sample of RNs: two hours of continuing education valued at $35 and an opportunity to participate in a drawing for a voucher to use for travel to a professional conference. Nine RNs responded that they declined to participate; 75 addresses were invalid and correct addresses could not be identified; and 17 RNs were deemed to be ineligible. A total of 903 RNs responded with usable surveys.

The respondents were 94% female and 5% male; 72% were married; 84% Caucasian, 4% African American, 3% Hispanic, and 3% Asian or Pacific Islander. Thirty-three percent were ages 45 to 54 years, and 37% were 55 years or older. Eighty-seven percent were working in nursing within the past year. Acute care settings were the place of employment for 52% of the respondents. Level of nursing education (listing all education) included the following: 25% with diplomas, 43% with associate degrees, 49% with baccalaureate degrees; and 15% with master's/doctoral degrees. Respondents reported that 67% of them worked in direct care positions, with an additional 7% in advanced practice, 16% in management/administration, and 10% in clinical or academic education. Party affiliation was reported as 35% Democrat, 29% Republican, 17% Independent, and 19% all others or no affiliation. Ideology was identified as the following: 34% conservative/very conservative, 41% moderate, and 22% liberal or very liberal. The percentage did not always add up to 100% because of rounding or nonresponses.

The responses of RNs were compared with polling data of the registered voters from the general public during the same time frame. When asked about the most important problems facing the nation during the 2008 presidential campaign, 32% of the RNs identified health care as the most important issue versus 6% of the public; 24% of RNs identified the economy as most important versus 37% of the public. When asked which of three choices they would prefer to see in a candidate's healthcare reform proposal, RNs indicated the following:

- A new health plan to provide insurance to all or nearly all of the uninsured, but with a major increase in spending, 47% (vs. 43% of registered voters)
- A more limited health plan to cover some of the uninsured but with less new spending, 28% (vs. 31% of registered voters)
- Keep things basically as they are, 15% (vs. 5% of registered voters)
- Don't know, 10% (vs. 18% of registered voters)

When asked "if all nurses could join together to address one of the following healthcare problems (racial/ethnic disparities in health care; number of Americans who are uninsured; violence in America; drug/alcohol abuse; obesity in children and adults; chronic illnesses; and other), which do you think is the most important to address?" (p. 231), 51% selected the number of uninsured Americans, with 16% selecting obesity, and 9% indicating chronic illness.

When asked how much confidence these RNs had in a variety of government groups, private agencies, and other organizations to make the right decisions related to the cost and quality of health care (p. 232), 57% indicated they had confidence in nursing organizations, 31% in physician organizations, and 19% in The Joint Commission. Among government entities, RNs reported hardly any confidence in Medicare/Medicaid agencies (36%) and Congress (38%). Pharmaceutical companies (69%) and insurance companies (72%) also rated "hardly any confidence."

Ninety-three percent of the RNs indicated they were registered voters, and 86% indicated they intended to vote in the 2008 November election. This compares with 82% of the public reporting that they were registered voters, according to a 2008 Kaiser Family Foundation study.

Implications for Practice
The authors of the study stated that the results of the survey could "be used to increase the effectiveness of nurses' political involvement and raise interest among the candidates and their parties in winning the vote of RNs" (p. 235).

Nurses' perspectives of the issues that are critical to improving the healthcare system can shape the policy agenda of the nation's political leadership (Buerhaus, Ulrich, Donelan, & DesRoches, 2008) (see the Research Perspective above).

The Political Astuteness Inventory (Goldwater & Zusy, 1990) is a helpful tool in determining how well prepared you are to influence legislative politics and public policy, especially public policy related to health care (see Box 10-2).

THE SOLUTION

The director gave me the rest of the shift off with pay. I decided to use the weekend off to consider whether I should resign. My director went back to the VP's office with my incident report about the phone call and presented it to the VP. She indicated that this was a true and accurate report of the event, now known as the "cat lady call." All the witnesses had signed the report, including the medical director. She calmly told the VP that she understood how the VP was being pressured by the CEO to take some immediate action. But she restated her belief that I handled the situation appropriately and that the caller was not honest with the CEO. She asserted that there would be no apology issued by her or by me. The VP said she would talk to us on Monday, after consulting with the hospital's legal counsel. From experience, we all knew that this meant the VP was considering firing both of us.

On Monday morning, the director received a new incident report. The report noted that the local police had brought an elderly woman into the ED on Saturday night. She was covered with scratches, many of which were infected. She was an animal hoarder and had created a disturbance in her neighborhood that resulted in the police bringing her into the hospital and removing dozens of cats from her home. She kept telling the ED staff that she didn't want to be cared for by the nurse she talked to on Friday. She was our "cat lady caller." She was verbally and physically abusive to the ED staff and the police. She was treated and released to family.

The director gave the VP this incident report, which vindicated me. She asked the VP how she would like to proceed with this issue. The VP's face reddened with embarrassment, and she told the director to apologize to me for her. I had already heard from the night staff about the woman's visit to the ED over the weekend by the time my director came to the ED. She was disappointed that the VP would not apologize to me in person. Because of my director's powerful response to the VP, I remained a hospital employee until my retirement a few years later. The VP's misuse of positional power was blocked by my director's use of personal and informational power. Her support empowered me.

—*Anonymous*

Would this be a suitable approach for you? Why?

THE EVIDENCE

Manojlovich (2005) surveyed five hundred members of the Michigan Nurses Association to examine the effect of unit level nursing leadership on the professional practice behaviors of registered nurses. A total of 365 nurses responded to the survey, with 251 usable surveys included in the data analysis, which excluded respondents who were nurse managers, in other administrative positions, and nursing faculty. Each respondent included in the survey completed four surveys that assessed structural empowerment, self-efficacy, professional autonomy and practice, and nursing leadership. Demographic information was also collected. The surveys assessed the nurses' level of empowerment and their beliefs about their own abilities to express and demonstrate caring in their relationships with patients and to demonstrate critical elements of professional nursing practice. The respondents were also asked to assess the leadership abilities and skills of their unit level managers.

The data analysis indicated that nurses whose managers demonstrated strong nursing leadership practiced more professionally. Although direct relationships could not be established, the findings indicated that "structural empowerment contributes to more professional practice behaviors through self-efficacy, especially in the presence of strong nursing leadership" (Manojlovich, 2005, p. 373). The need for more research to establish the relationship between strong nursing leadership and professional practice behaviors is identified. The value of investing in leadership training for nurse managers is also noted as important in strengthening the professional practice behaviors of nurses who work with these managers.

NEED TO KNOW NOW

- Remember that *power* is not a "dirty word," nor is it an undesirable professional characteristic for nurses; it is the ability to influence others effectively.
- Empower patients, families, and colleagues to accomplish their goals by exercising your own power in the workplace and other professional activities.
- Believe in your own ability to create change (i.e., exercise power), value the exercise of power, and project a powerful image (e.g., grooming, manners, body language, communication skills).
- Participate in networking and mentoring, set clear career goals, and develop your expertise.

CHAPTER CHECKLIST

Power was once a taboo issue in nursing. The exercise of power in nursing conflicted sharply with the historical feminine stereotypes that surrounded nursing. The evolving social and political status of women has also opened nursing to the exercise of power. Power is essential to the effective implementation of both the clinical and the managerial roles of nurses.

- Contemporary concepts of power focus on power as influence and a force for collaboration rather than coercion; an infinite quality rather than a finite quantity.
- Empowerment is a feminine-feminist process of power-sharing and leadership.
- Contemporary views of leadership in social systems are consistent with the concept of empowerment.
- Six types of power exercised by nurses are the following:
  - Position
  - Perceived
  - Expert
  - Personal
  - Information
  - Connection

- Key factors in developing a powerful image include the following:
  - Self-confidence
  - Body language
  - Self-image, including grooming, dress, and speech
  - Career commitment and continuing professional education
  - Attitudes, beliefs, and values
- Key personal and organizational strategies for exercising power include the following:
  - Communication skills
  - High visibility
  - A sense of unity
  - Coalition building and networking, collaboration and collegiality
  - Demonstrating expertise
  - Organizational savvy
  - Negotiation skills
  - Mentoring
  - An empowering attitude

TIPS FOR USING INFLUENCE

- Become an active member of selected nursing organizations, especially one's state nurses' association and a specialty organization (e.g., special role organization or clinical specialty organization).
- Develop a powerful personal/professional self-image.
- Invest in your nursing career by continuing your education.
- Make nursing your career, not just a job.
- Develop networking skills.
- Be visible and competent in the organizations in which you work and network.

REFERENCES

Abood, S. (2007). Influencing health care in the legislative arena. *The Online Journal of Issues in Nursing, 12*(1). Retrieved October 1, 2009, from www.nursingworld.org/MainMenuCategories/ANAMarketplace/ANAPeriodicals/OJIN/TableofContents/Volume122007/No1Jan07/tpc32_216091.aspx.

American Nurses Credentialing Center (ANCC). (2009). *Program overview.* Retrieved September 23, 2009, from www.nursecredentialing.org/Magnet.aspx.

Ashley, J.A. (1976). *Hospitals, paternalism, and the role of the nurse.* New York: Teachers College Press.

Buerhaus, P. I., Ulrich, B., Donelan, K., & DesRoches, C. (2008). Registered nurses' perspectives on health care and the 2008 presidential election. *Nursing Economic$, 26,* 227-235, 257.

Goldwater, M., & Zusy, M. J. L. (1990). *Prescription for nurses: Effective political action.* St. Louis: Mosby.

Hersey, P., Blanchard, K., & Natemeyer, W. (1979). Situational leadership, perception and impact of power. *Group and Organizational Studies, 4,* 418-428.

Illinois Coalition for Nursing Resources. (n.d.). *About us.* Retrieved September 23, 2009, from www.ic4nr.org.

Kelly, K. (2007). From apathy to savvy to activism: Becoming a politically active nurse. *American Nurse Today, 2*(8), 55-56.

Leavitt, J. K., Chaffee, M. W., & Vance, C. (2007). Learning the ropes of policy and politics. In D. J. Mason, J. K. Leavitt, & M. W. Chaffee (Eds.), *Policy & politics in nursing and health care* (5th ed., pp. 34-46). St. Louis: Saunders.

Manojlovich, M. (2005). The effect of nursing leadership on hospital nurses' professional practice behavior. *Journal of Nursing Administration, 35,* 366-374.

Matheson, L. K., & Bobay, K. (2007). Validation of oppressed group behaviors in nursing. *Journal of Professional Nursing, 23,* 226-234.

Ozimek, R. W. (2007). Taking action: Distributed campaigns—Using the Internet to empower activism. In D. J. Mason, J. K. Leavitt, & M. W. Chaffee (Eds.), *Policy & politics in nursing and health care* (5th ed., pp. 171-176). St. Louis: Saunders.

Roberts, S. J. (1983). Oppressed group behavior: Implications for nursing. *Advances in Nursing Sciences, 5,* 21-30.

Sullivan, E. J. (2004). *Becoming influential: A guide for nurses.* Upper Saddle River, NJ: Pearson Education.

SUGGESTED READINGS

Ashley, J. A. (1980). Power in structured misogyny: Implications for the politics of care. *Advances in Nursing Science, 2,* 3-22.

Borman, J., & Biordi, D. (1992). Female nurse executive: Finally, at an advantage? *Journal of Nursing Administration, 22*(9), 37-41.

Campbell-Heider, N., & Hart, C. A. (1993). Updating the nurse's bedside manner. *Image: Journal of Nursing Scholarship, 25,* 133-139.

Cohen, S. S., Mason, D. J., Kovner, C., Leavitt, J. K., Pulcini, J., & Sochalski, J. (1996). Stages of nursing political development: Where we've been and where we ought to go. *Nursing Outlook, 44,* 259-266.

Cunningham, M. P. (2000). Breaking the mold: The many legacies of nurses in progressive movements. *American Journal of Nursing, 100*(10), 121-136 (passim).

Gebbie, K. M., Wakefield, M., & Kerfoot, K. (2000). Nursing and health policy. *Journal of Nursing Scholarship, 32,* 307-315.

Greene, R. (2000). *The 48 Laws of Power.* New York: Penguin Books.

Heim, P., & Goliant, S. K. (2005). *Hardball for women: Winning at the game of business.* Los Angeles: Plume Books.

Kovach, C. R., & Morgan, S. W. (2003). Doctor's orders: Rethinking language and intent. *Journal of Nursing Administration, 33,* 563-564.

Kramer, M., & Schmalenberg, C. (2004). Development and evaluation of an essentials of magnetism tool. *Journal of Nursing Administration, 34,* 365-378.

Kritek, P. B. (2002). *Negotiating at an uneven table: A practical approach to working with differences and diversity* (2nd ed.). San Francisco: Jossey-Bass.

Mason, D. J., Leavitt, J. K., & Chaffee, M. W. (2007). *Policy & politics in nursing and health care* (5th ed.). St. Louis: Saunders.

Wakefield, M. (1999). Nursing future in health care policy. In E. J. Sullivan (Ed.), *Creating nursing's future: Issues, opportunities, and challenges.* St. Louis: Mosby.

PART 2

Managing Resources

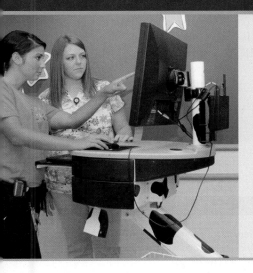

Caring, Communicating, and Managing with Technology

Janis B. Smith and Cheri Hunt

This chapter describes current biomedical technology, with an emphasis on information technology that allows nurses to use data gathered at the point of care effectively and efficiently. It discusses nurses as knowledge workers who use biomedical and information technology to care for patients. It includes sections on biomedical, information, and knowledge technology with subsections that discuss informatics competencies, standardized terminologies, information systems hardware, the science of informatics, evidence-based practice, and patient care safety and quality. Nurses build knowledge for practice by comparing and contrasting not only current patient data with previous data for the same patient but also data across patients with the same diagnosis. Information tools and skills are essential for these decision-making processes now and in the future.

OBJECTIVES

- Articulate the role of several new technologies in patient safety.
- Describe the core components of informatics: data, information, and knowledge.
- Evaluate a model to change accepted practice into evidence-based practice.
- Describe three types of healthcare information technology trends.
- Apply one structured nursing terminology to a nursing scenario.
- Analyze three types of technology for capturing data at the point of care.
- Discuss decision support systems and their impact on patient care.
- Explore the issues of patient safety, ethics, and information security and privacy within information technology.
- Value the use of the Internet for healthcare information.

TERMS TO KNOW

bar-code technology	database	Nursing Minimum Data Set
biomedical technology	electronic health record (EHR)	(NMDS)
blog	electronic medical record (EMR)	smart card
clinical decision support	evidence-based practice	speech recognition (SR)
clinical decision support systems	informatics	structured nursing terminology
communication technology	information	telehealth
computerized provider order	information technology	weblog
entry (CPOE)	knowledge technology	
data	knowledge worker	

THE CHALLENGE

Cheri Hunt, RN, MHA, NEA-BC
Vice President and Chief Nursing Officer, Children's Mercy
Hospitals and Clinics, Kansas City, Missouri

The nursing leadership team in my hospital is collaborating with the hospital's medical staff, information systems leadership, and allied health professionals to evaluate information technology solutions and select a clinical information system that will support patient care work processes, clinical decision making, communication, outcomes, and financial and administrative processes. Our team has several questions to consider:

1. Can information technology support our patient safety initiatives?

2. Do we replicate our current paper forms and computer screens/functions, or do we take this opportunity to transform work processes?
3. What types of hardware are most appropriate in our various care settings?
4. How can direct care nurses be involved in answering these questions?

We need to make prudent and futuristic decisions.

What do you think you would do if you were this nurse?

INTRODUCTION

Technology surrounds us! Intravenous pumps are "smart," biomedical monitoring is no longer exclusively an intensive care practice, and computers are used at the bank, at the grocery checkout, in our cars, and in almost every other aspect of daily living, including the provision of health care. Health care is both a technology and an information intensive business; therefore the success of nurses using biomedical technology, information technology, and knowledge technology will contribute to their personal and professional development and career achievement.

In the hospital of the future, technology will be the foundation of patient care planning, organization, and delivery (Parker, 2005). Poor resource use is widespread in the U.S. healthcare system, as cited in the Institute of Medicine (IOM) report, "Crossing the Quality Chasm" (IOM, 2001). Many leaders in health

care see technology as a means to facilitate decision making, improve efficacy and efficiency, enhance patient safety and quality, and decrease healthcare costs (Ball, Weaver, & Abbot, 2003; IOM, 2000, 2001, 2004). If appropriately implemented and fully integrated, technology has the potential to improve the practice environment for nurses, as well as for patients and their families. However, we are also cautioned by patient safety and quality experts that technology is not a panacea (IOM, 2004).

Good decision making for patient care requires good information. Nurses are knowledge workers, who need data and information to provide effective and efficient patient care. Knowledge work is not routine or repetitive but, instead, requires considerable cognitive activity and critical thinking (Drucker, 1993). Data and information must be accurate, reliable, and presented in an actionable form. Technology can facilitate and extend nurses' decision-making abilities and support nurses in the following areas: (1) storing clinical data, (2) translating clinical data into information, (3) linking clinical data and domain knowledge, and (4) aggregating clinical data (Snyder-Halpern, Corcoran-Perry, & Narayan, 2001).

TYPES OF TECHNOLOGIES

As nurses, we commonly use and manage three types of technologies: biomedical technology, information technology, and knowledge technology. **Biomedical technology** involves the use of equipment in the clinical setting for diagnosis, physiologic monitoring, testing, or administering therapies to patients. **Information technology** entails recording, processing, and using data and information for the purpose of delivering and documenting patient care. **Knowledge technology** is the use of expert systems to assist clinicians to make decisions about patient care. In nursing, these systems are designed to mimic the reasoning of nurse experts in making patient care decisions.

Biomedical Technology

Biomedical technology is used for (1) physiologic monitoring, (2) diagnostic testing, (3) intravenous fluid and medication dispensing and administration, and (4) therapeutic treatments.

Physiologic Monitoring

Physiologic monitoring systems measure heart rate, blood pressure, and other vital signs. They also monitor cardiac rhythm; measure and record central venous, pulmonary wedge, intracranial, and intra-abdominal pressures; and analyze oxygen and carbon dioxide levels in the blood.

Data about adverse events in hospitalized patients indicate that a majority of physiologic abnormalities are not detected early enough to prevent the event, even when some of the abnormalities are present for hours before the event occurs (Considine & Botti, 2004; Liewelyn, Martin, Shekleton, & Firlet, 1998). Patient surveillance systems are designed to provide early warning of a possible impending adverse event. One example is a system that provides wireless monitoring of heart rate, respiratory rate, and attempts by a patient at risk for falling to get out of bed unassisted; this monitoring is via a mattress coverlet and bedside monitor. Nurses at one hospital decreased the rate of patient falls by 60% with the use of surveillance monitoring (Matsuo et al., 2008).

Innovative technology permits physiologic monitoring and patient surveillance by expert clinicians who may be distant from the patient. The remote or virtual intensive care unit (vICU) is staffed by a dedicated team of experienced critical care nurses, physicians, and pharmacists who use state-of-the-art technology to leverage their expertise and knowledge over a large group of patients in multiple intensive care units (Breslow, 2007; Myers & Reed, 2008).

Intracranial pressure (ICP) monitoring systems monitor the cranial pressure in critically ill patients with closed head injuries or postoperative craniotomy patients. The ICP, along with the mean arterial blood pressure, can be used to calculate perfusion pressure. This allows assessment and early therapy as changes occur. When the ICP exceeds a set pressure, some systems allow ventricular drainage. Similarly, monitoring pressure within the bladder has recently been demonstrated to accurately detect intra-abdominal hypertension as measures of maximal and mean intra-abdominal pressures and abdominal perfusion pressure are made. Intra-abdominal hypertension occurs with abdominal compartment syndrome and other acute abdominal illnesses and has been demonstrated to be independently associated with mortality in these patients (Malbrain et al., 2005; Vidal et al., 2008).

Continuous dysrhythmia monitors and electrocardiograms (ECGs) provide visual representation of electrical activity in the heart and can be used for surveillance and detection of dysrhythmias and for interpretation and diagnosis of the abnormal rhythm. Although not a new technology, these systems have grown increasingly sophisticated. More important, integration with wireless communication technology permits new approaches to triaging alerts to nurses about cardiac rhythm abnormalities. Voice technology and integrated telemetry and nurse paging systems have both been demonstrated to close the communication loop and dramatically decrease response time to dysrhythmia alarms (Bonzheim, 2006).

Biomedical devices for physiologic monitoring can be interfaced with clinical information systems. Monitored vital signs and invasive pressure readings are downloaded directly into the patient's electronic medical record, where the nurse confirms their accuracy and affirms the data entry.

Diagnostic Testing

Dysrhythmia systems can also be diagnostic. The computer, after processing and analyzing the ECG, generates a report that is confirmed by a trained professional. ECG tracings can be transmitted over telephone lines from remote sites, such as the patient's home, to the physician's office or clinic. Patients with implantable pacemakers can have their cardiac activity monitored without leaving home.

Other systems for diagnostic testing include blood gas analyzers, pulmonary function systems, and intracranial pressure monitors. Contemporary laboratory medicine is virtually all automated. In addition, point-of-care testing devices extend the laboratory's testing capabilities to the patient's bedside or care area. In critical care areas, for example, blood gas, ionized calcium, hemoglobin, and hematocrit values often are measured from unit-based "stat labs." Point-of-care blood glucose monitors can download results of bedside testing into an automated laboratory results system and the patient's electronic record. Results can be communicated quickly and trends analyzed throughout patients' hospital stays and at ongoing ambulatory care visits. Results can calculate the necessary insulin doses based on evidence for tight blood glucose control and evoke electronic orders for administration. This is an example of integrating a diagnostic test result with the appropriate orders-based intervention.

Intravenous Fluid and Medication Administration

Intravenous (IV) fluid and medication distribution and dispensing via Automated Dispensing Cabinets (ADCs) were introduced in the 1980s and are used in a majority of hospitals today. ADCs can decrease the amount of time before a medication is available on patient care units for administration, ensure greater protection of medications (especially controlled substances), and efficiently and accurately capture drug charges. Most important, ADCs can reduce the risk of medication errors but only when safeguards are available and used. The Institute for Safe Medication Practices (ISMP) has developed guidelines for safest use of ADCs (ISMP, 2008). The guidelines contain 12

core practices associated with safe ADC use and are available on the ISMP website (*www.ismp.org/Tools/guidelines/labelFormats/comments/default.asp*).

IV smart pumps are used to deliver fluids, blood and blood products, and medications either continuously or intermittently at rates between 0.1 and 999 mL per hour. Twenty-first century pumps offer safety features, accuracy, advanced pressure monitoring, ease of use, and versatility. These pumps have rate-dependent pressure detection systems, designed to provide an early alert to IV cannula occlusion with real-time display of the patient-side pressure reading in the system. Smart pumps can be programmed to calculate drug doses and medication infusion rates, as well as determine the volume and duration of an infusion. Smart syringe pumps can be used in environments such as the intensive care unit and in anesthesia where precise delivery of concentrated medications is required. Infusion rates as small as 0.01 mL per hour can be delivered.

Therapeutic Treatments

Treatments may be administered via implantable infusion pumps that administer medications at a prescribed rate and can be programmed to provide boluses or change doses at set points in time. These pumps are commonly used for hormone regulation, treatment of hypertension, chronic intractable pain, diabetes, venous thrombosis, and cancer chemotherapy.

Therapeutic treatment systems may be used to regulate intake and output, regulate breathing, and assist with the care of the newborn. Intake and output systems are linked to infusion pumps that control arterial pressure, drug therapy, fluid resuscitation, and serum glucose levels. These systems calculate and regulate the IV drip rate.

Increasingly sophisticated mechanical ventilators are used to deliver a prescribed percentage of oxygen and volume of air to the patient's lungs and to provide a set flow rate, inspiratory-to-expiratory time ratio, and various other complex functions with less trauma to lung tissue than was previously possible. Computer-assisted ventilators are electromechanically controlled by a closed-loop feedback system to analyze and control lung volumes and alveolar gases. Ventilators also provide sophisticated, sensitive alarm systems for patient safety.

In the newborn and intensive care nursery, computers monitor the heart and respiratory rates of the babies there. In addition, newborn nursery systems can regulate the temperature of the infant's environment by sensing his or her temperature and the air of the surrounding environment. Alarms can be set to notify the nurse when preset physiologic parameters are exceeded. Computerized systems monitor fetal activity before delivery, linking the ECGs of the mother and baby and the pulse oximetry, blood pressure, and respirations of the mother.

Biomedical technology affects nursing as nurses provide direct care to patients treated with new technologies: monitoring data from new devices, administering therapy with new techniques, and evaluating patients' responses to care and treatment. Nurses must be aware of the latest technologies for monitoring patients' physiologic status, diagnostic testing, drug administration, and therapeutic treatments. It is important to identify the data to be collected, the information that might be gained, and the many ways that these data might be used to provide new knowledge. More important, nurses must remember that biomedical technology supplements but does not replace the skilled observation, assessment, and evaluation of the patient.

Nursing leaders must be aware of how these technologies fit into the delivery of patient care and the strategic plan of the organization in which they work. They must have a vision for the future and be ready to suggest solutions that will assist nurses across specialties and settings to improve patient care safety and quality.

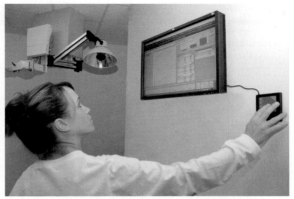

Patient data displayed with computerized systems to provide meaningful information and trends.

Information Technology

Health care is an information-intensive and knowledge-intensive enterprise. Information technology can help healthcare providers acquire, manage, analyze, and disseminate both information and knowledge. Health care in the twenty-first century should be safe, effective, patient-centered, timely, efficient, and equitable (IOM, 2001). Comprehensive data on patients' conditions, treatments, and outcomes are at the foundation of such care (Stead & Lin, 2009).

Computers offer the advantage of storing, organizing, retrieving, and communicating digital data with accuracy and speed. Patient care data can be entered once, stored in a database, and then quickly and accurately retrieved many times and in many combinations by healthcare providers and others. A database is a collection of data elements organized and stored together. Data processing is the structuring, organizing, and presenting of data for interpretation as information. For example, vital signs for one patient can be entered into the computer and communicated on a graph; many patients' blood pressure measurements can be compared with the number of doses of anti-hypertension medication. Vital signs for male patients between the ages of 40 and 50 years can be correlated and used to show relationships with age, ethnicity, weight, presence of co-morbid conditions, and so on.

THEORY BOX

Information Theory

KEY CONTRIBUTOR	KEY IDEAS	APPLICATION TO PRACTICE
Tan (1995) describes the elements of information theory as the following: • Source • Transmitter • Channel • Receiver • Destination	The information *source* selects the message or information to be conveyed. An underlying code or set of characters represents the message to be processed by the computer. The *transmitter* has an encoding function that converts the message to be sent. The communication *channel* (cable, air waves) provides the medium necessary for the information to be transmitted. The *receiver* converts the information from its transmitted form. The *destination* is the final stage of reception, at which point the message is decoded to be understandable.	The physician enters an order for laboratory tests *(source, message)*. The computer program converts the message *(transmitter)*. The converted order is sent over the computer network (communication *channel*) to the laboratory *(receiver)*. The order is converted and read by the computer system in the laboratory *(destination)*.

BOX 11-1   DEVELOPMENT OF INFORMATION MANAGEMENT SKILLS: NOVICE TO EXPERT PRACTICE

Novice nurses focus on learning what data to collect, the process of collecting and documenting the data, and how to use this information. They learn what clinical applications are available for use and how to use them. Computer and informatics skills focus on applying concrete concepts.

As nurses grow in expertise, they look for patterns in the data and information. They aggregate data across patient populations to look for similarities and differences in response to interventions. Expert nurses integrate theoretical knowledge with practical knowledge gained from experience.

Expert nurses know the value of personal professional reflection on knowledge and synthesize and evaluate information for discovery and decision making.

Humans process data continuously, but in an analog form. Computers process data in a digital form, process data faster and more accurately than humans, and provide a method of storage so that data can be retrieved as needed. The Theory Box above provides key concepts of information processing, and Box 11-1 describes the development of information management skills from novice to expert.

Structured Terminologies

Collecting a set of basic data from every patient at every healthcare encounter makes sense because comparisons can be made among many patients, institutions, or countries, almost in any combination imaginable, as well as for individual patients and patient groups across time. The uniform minimum health data set (UMHDS) is a minimum set of information items with standard definitions and categories that meets the needs of multiple data users.

Since the mid-1980s, nursing has recognized the importance of demonstrating its distinct contributions to patient care. Clark and Lang (1992, p. 109) stated, "If we cannot name it (nursing), we cannot control it, practice it, research it, teach it, finance it or put it into public policy." Werley and Lang (1988) convened a work group to define essential data elements to be collected on all patients, defining the Nursing Minimum Data Set (NMDS). Four elements in the NMDS are unique to nursing: nursing diagnosis, nursing intervention, nursing outcome, and intensity of nursing care. Box 11-2 lists the elements of the NMDS. The purposes of the NMDS are the following:

1. To establish the comparability of patient care data across clinical populations, settings, geographic areas, and time

2. To describe the care of patients and families in various settings
3. To provide a means to mark the trends in the care provided and the allocation of nursing resources based on health problems or nursing diagnosis
4. To stimulate nursing research through links to existing data
5. To provide data about nursing care to influence and facilitate healthcare policy decision making

Some NMDS elements (e.g., interventions and outcomes) are not collected as easily as the demographic and service elements, which are often captured at patient registration or discharge. This is because we lack uniform or unified structured nursing terminology. Significant efforts have been made to bridge this gap. Thirteen classification systems have been recognized by the American Nurses Association (ANA) (Elfrink, Bakken, Coenen, McNeil, & Bick-ford, 2001). These recognized classification systems differ. Some contain vocabularies for diagnosis, interventions, and outcomes, whereas others focus on only one or two of these groups. Some terminologies are specialty specific, such as the perioperative nursing data set.

During the 1990s, a few nursing terminology leaders began to recognize the importance of nursing terminologies being computerized and connected (interoperable) with one another and with other terminologies in health care. Since 1999, terminology leaders have worked together in a series of nursing terminology summit conferences to develop a united, global, standardized reference terminology for nurses (Ozbolt & Saba, 2008). At the end of the first decade of the twenty-first century, nursing has the data and terminology tools to create patient care records that reflect what nurses have contributed and permit comparison of nursing interventions and patient outcomes. However, many challenges remain. Nurses need education to appreciate the importance and power of standard terminologies compared with locally used terms (Ozbolt & Saba, 2008).

- Nursing records must be integrated with other records so that patient information is integrated and can be communicated among the healthcare team.
- Clinical nursing experts are needed to work with terminology experts to develop standard language in areas of nursing not yet adequately developed.
- Nursing leaders must advocate for use of structured nursing terminologies with the creators and vendors of information systems.

Standardized, computerized nursing terminology will allow us to collect, aggregate, and analyze patient data for decision support, quality improvement, and research. Data from within and across patient populations are needed to build evidence from practice and to use evidence in practice. These data are also needed to quantify and describe nursing practice and its impact on the quality of care provided and on patient outcomes.

INFORMATION SYSTEMS

A patient information system can be manual or computerized—in fact, we have collected and recorded information about patients and patient care since the dawn of health care. Computer information systems manage large volumes of data, examine data patterns and trends, solve problems, and answer questions. In other words, computers can help translate data into information. Ideally, data are recorded at the point in the care process where they are gathered and are available to healthcare providers when and where they are needed. This is accomplished, in part, by networking computers both within and among organizations to form larger systems. These networked systems might link inpatient care units and other departments, hospitals, clinics, hospice centers, home health agencies, and/or physician practices. Data from all patient encounters with the healthcare system are stored in a central data repository, where they are accessible to authorized users located anywhere in the world. These provide the potential for automated patient records, which contain health data from birth to death.

Adopting the technology necessary to computerize patient care information systems is complex and must be accomplished in stages. The Health Information and Management Systems Society (HIMSS) has described seven stages of adoption—the seventh of which marks achievement of a fully electronic healthcare record. The seven stages of adoption are listed and described in Table 11-1. It is important to note that only 1% of U.S. hospitals have achieved stage 6 and that fewer than 0.1% have achieved stage 7 (HIMSS Analytics, 2008).

Nurses care for patients in acute care, ambulatory, and community settings, as well as in patients' homes. In all settings, nurses focus not only on managing acute illnesses but also on health promotion, maintenance, and education; care coordination and continuity; and monitoring chronic conditions. Ideally, information systems support the work of nurses in all settings.

Communication networks are used to transmit data entered at one computer and received by others in the network. These networks can reduce the clerical functions of nursing. They can provide patient demographic and census data, results from tests, and lists of medications. Nursing policies and procedures can be linked to the network and accessed, when needed, at the point of care. Links can be provided between the patient's home, hospital, and/or physician office with computers, handheld technologies, and point-of-care devices. Day-to-day events can be recorded and downloaded into the patient record remotely in community nursing settings or at the point of care in the hospital or clinic.

EXERCISE 11-3

Select a healthcare setting with which you are familiar. What information systems are used? Make a list of the names of these systems and the information they provide. How do they help you in caring for patients or in making management decisions? Think about the communication of data and information among departments. Do the systems communicate with each other? If you do not have computerized systems, think about how data and information are communicated. How might a computer system help you be more efficient?

As an example, assume that an abdominal magnetic resonance imaging (MRI) with contrast has been ordered. In a paper-based system, handwritten requisitions are sent to nutrition services, pharmacy, and the radiology department. With a computerized system, the MRI is ordered and the requests for dietary changes, bowel preparation medications, and the diagnostic study itself are automatically sent to the appropriate departments. Radiology would compare its schedule openings with the patient's schedule and automatically place the date and time for the MRI on the patient's automated plan of care. The images and results of the diagnostic procedure are available online.

Nurses caring for patients in home health care and hospice must complete documentation necessary to meet government and insurance requirements. Computers assist with direct entry of all required data in the correct format. Portable computers are used to

STAGE	DESCRIPTION
TABLE 11-1	**ELECTRONIC MEDICAL RECORD ADOPTION MODEL***
7	• The healthcare organization has a paperless electronic medical record (EMR) environment. • Clinical information can be shared via electronic transactions with all entities within the health information network (i.e., other hospitals, clinics, subacute settings, employers, payers, and patients). • The healthcare organization can share and use health and wellness information with consumers and providers. • Data warehousing and mining technologies are used to capture and analyze care data and improve care via decision support.
6	• Full physician documentation using structured templates is implemented for at least one patient care service area. • A full complement of all radiology images (digital and film) is available to providers via an intranet or other secure network.
5	• Closed-loop medication administration is fully implemented in at least one patient care service area. • The electronic medication administration record (e-MAR) and bar coding or other auto-identification technology (e.g., radio frequency identification [RFID]) are implemented and integrated with computerized order entry and pharmacy to maximize patient safety for medication administration.
4	• Computerized provider order entry (CPOE) is implemented. • Clinical decision support at the second level (related to evidence-based protocols) is implemented.
3	• Clinical documentation (e.g., vital signs, flow sheets, nursing notes, care planning, and the e-MAR) is implemented and integrated for at least one service in the organization. • First-level clinical decision support for error checking with order entry (e.g., drug/drug, drug/allergy, drug/food, drug/lab conflict checking) is implemented. • Some radiology images can be accessed from picture archive and communication systems (PACSs) via a secure network.
2	• Major ancillary clinical systems feed data to a clinical data repository that permits clinicians access for retrieving and reviewing results. • The data repository contains a controlled vocabulary and the rules and clinical decision support for rudimentary conflict checking.
1	• Major ancillary (laboratory, radiology, and pharmacy) clinical systems are installed.
0	• Some clinical automation may exist. • Laboratory and/or pharmacy and/or radiology clinical systems are not installed.

*From HIMSS Analytics, Health Information Management Systems Society. (2008). *EMR Adoption Model*. Retrieved from www.himssanalytics.org/hc_ providers/emr_adoption.asp.

download files of the patients to be seen during the day from a main database. During each visit, the computer prompts the nurse for vital signs, assessments, diagnosis, interventions, long-term and short-term goals, and medications based on previous entries in the medical record. Nurses enter any new data, modifications, or nursing information directly. Entries can be transmitted by telephone line to the main computer at the office or downloaded from the device at the end of the day. This action automatically updates the patient record and any verbal order entry records, home visit reports, federally mandated treatment plans, productivity and quality improvement reports, and other documents for review and signature. Portable and wireless computers have made recording

patient care information more efficient and have improved personnel productivity and compliance with necessary documentation.

Placing computers or handheld devices "patient-side" permits nurses to enter data once, at the point of care. Documentation of patient assessments and care provided patient-side saves time, gives others more timely access to the data, and decreases the likelihood of forgetting to document vital information. Point-of-care devices and systems that fit with nurses' workflow, personalize patient assessments, and simplify care planning are available. Patient care areas with point-of-care computers have improved the quality of patient care by decreasing errors of omission, providing greater accuracy and completeness of

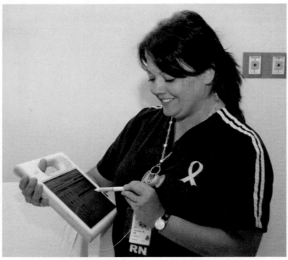

A handheld computer permits "point-of-care" documentation.

care outlines what patient care needs to occur, orders are entered to prescribe needed care, and documentation confirms that the care was provided. Computers can capture and aggregate data to demonstrate both the processes of care and the patient outcomes achieved.

The Joint Commission (TJC), an independent, not-for-profit organization, evaluates and provides accreditation and certification to more than 15,000 healthcare organizations and programs in the United States. Accreditation and certification by TJC are recognized nationwide as symbols of an organization's commitment to meeting performance standards focused on improving the quality and safety of patient care.

The *Comprehensive Accreditation Manual for Hospitals* and the manuals for other healthcare programs include a chapter of standards for information management. Planning for information management is the initial focus of the chapter, since a well-planned system meets the internal and external information needs of an organization with efficiency and accuracy. The goals of effective information management are to obtain, manage, and use information to improve patient care processes and patient outcomes, as well as to improve other organizational processes. Planning is also necessary to provide care continuity should an organization's information systems be disrupted or fail. Planning also is necessary to ensure privacy, security, confidentiality, and integrity of data and information.

A second chapter in the 2009 accreditation manuals is "The Record of Care, Treatment and Services." This chapter provides standards and recommendations for the components of a complete medical record. It details documentation requirements that include accuracy, authentication, and thorough, timely documentation. Other standards address the requirements for auditing and retaining records (The Joint Commission [TJC], 2009).

All nurses, including nurse leaders, share responsibility to ensure that cost-effective, high-quality patient care is provided. Nursing administrative databases, containing both clinical and management data, support decision making for these purposes. Administrative databases assist in the development of the organization's information infrastructure, which ultimately allows for links between management deci-

documentation, reducing medication errors, providing more timely responses to patient needs, and improving discharge planning and teaching. These systems can eliminate redundant charting and facilitate patient handoffs from shift to shift or between care areas.

EXERCISE 11-4

Think about the data you gather as you care for a patient through the day. How do you communicate information and knowledge about your patient to others? Does the information system support the way you need this information organized, stored, retrieved, and presented to other healthcare providers? For example, if a patient's pain medication order is about to expire and you want to assess the patient's use and response to the pain medication during the past 24 hours, can the information system generate a graph for this patient comparing the time, dose, and pain score for this period? If your assessment is that the medication order needs to be renewed, how do you communicate that message to the prescriber?

Information Systems Quality and Accreditation

Quality management and measuring patient care efficiency, effectiveness, and outcomes are necessary for accreditation and licensing of healthcare organizations. This is demonstrated by documentation of patient care processes and outcomes. The plan of

sions (e.g., staffing or nurse : patient ratios), costs, and clinical outcomes.

Selection of a clinical information system and software partner may be one of the most important decisions of a chief nursing officer and the nursing leadership team (Simpson, 2003). Nurse leaders and direct care nurses must be members of the selection team, participate actively, and have a voice in the selection decision. Remember, nurses are knowledge workers who require data, information, and knowledge to deliver effective patient care. The information system must make sense to the people who use it and fit effectively with the processes for providing patient care. Box 11-3 identifies key elements of an ideal clinical information system that can guide the decision making necessary for selecting or developing health information software. It is imperative to make site visits at organizations already using the software being considered for selection. Discussions at site visits include both the utility and performance of the software and the customer service and responsiveness of the vendor.

Information Systems Hardware

Placing the power of computers for both entering and retrieving data at the point of patient care is a major thrust in the move toward increased adoption of clinical information systems. Many hospitals and clinics are using a number of computing devices in the clinical setting—desktop, laptop, or tablet computers , and personal digital assistants (PDAs)—as we learn about both the possibilities and limitations of different hardware solutions. Theoretically, nurses may work best with robust mobile technology. Installing computers on mobile carts, also known as *Computers on Wheels* or *COWs,* may create work efficiency and timesavings. However, if the cart is cumbersome to move around or if concern about infection risk is associated with moving the cart from one room to another, some organizations favor keeping one cart stationed in each patient care room.

Wireless Communication

Wireless (WL) communication is an extension of an existing wired network environment and uses radio-based systems to transmit data signals through the air without any physical connections. Telemetry is a clinical use of WL communication. Nurses can communicate with other healthcare team members, departments, and offices and with patients through the use of pagers, cellular phones, PDAs, and wireless computers. Nurses can send and receive e-mail, clinical data, and other text messages. The Internet can be accessed on these devices.

WL systems are used by emergency medical personnel to request authorization for the treatments or drugs needed in emergency situations. Laboratories use WL technology to transmit laboratory results to physicians; patients awaiting organ transplants are provided with WL pagers so that they can be notified if a donor is found; and parents of critically ill children carry WL pagers when they are away from a phone. Visiting nurses using a home monitoring system employ WL technology to enter vital signs and other patient-related information. Inpatient nurses can send messages to the admissions department when a patient is being transferred to another unit without having to wait for someone to answer the telephone. Increasingly, whole hospitals utilize WL technology to deploy their information systems to the point of patient care.

New hardware for patient information systems has both advantages and disadvantages. Portable devices, such as PDAs and tablet computers, are less expensive than placing a stationary computer in each patient room. In addition, each caregiver on a shift can be equipped with a device. They allow access to information at the point of care, both for retrieval of information and entry of patient data. Disadvantages of handheld technology stem from their size and portability. They have a small display screen, limiting the amount of data that can be viewed on the screen and the size of the font. They can be put down and forgotten and dropped and broken and are a target for theft. There must also be a convenient and adequate place to store them when they are not in use and to charge their batteries if needed. WL technology may not operate with the speed necessary to advantage busy healthcare workers in fast-paced environments.

Management of the hardware designed to advantage clinical information system software is important. Nursing leaders must make knowledgeable decisions about the type of hardware to use, the education needed to use it effectively, and the proper care and maintenance of the equipment. Important questions to ask include the following: What data and information do we need to gather? When and where should it be gathered? How difficult is the equipment to use? Has the hardware been tested sufficiently to ensure purchase of a dependable product?

COMMUNICATION TECHNOLOGY

Communication technology is an extension of WL technology that enables hands-free communication among mobile hospital workers. Hospital staff members wear a pendant-like badge around their neck and, by simply pressing a button on the badge, can be connected to the person with whom they wish to speak by stating the name or function of the person.

Voice technology may also enhance the use of computer systems in the future. **Speech recognition (SR)** is also known as *computer speech recognition*. The term *voice recognition* may also be used to refer to speech recognition but is less accurate. SR converts spoken words to machine-readable input. SR applications in everyday life include voice dialing (e.g., "Call home"), call routing (e.g., "I would like to make a collect call"), and simple data entry (e.g., stating a credit card or account number). In health care, preparation of structured documents, such as a radiology report, is possible. In all these examples, the computer gathers, processes, interprets, and executes audible signals by comparing the spoken words with a template in the system. If the patterns match, recognition occurs and a command is executed by the computer. This allows untrained personnel or those whose hands are busy to enter data in an SR environment without touching the computer. Voice technology will also allow quadriplegic and other physically challenged individuals to function more efficiently when using the computer. SR systems recognize a large number of words but are still immature. The speaker must use staccato-like speech, pausing between each clearly spoken word; and these systems must be programmed for each user so that the system recognizes the user's voice patterns.

Automating the healthcare delivery process is not an easy task. Patient care processes are often not standardized across settings, and most software vendors cannot customize software for each organization. Some current versions of the electronic patient record have merely automated the existing schema of the chart rather than considering how computers could permit data to be viewed or used differently from manual methods. The complexity of decision making about health information systems software and hardware has given rise to the science of informatics.

INFORMATICS

Informatics is "a science that combines a domain science, computer science, information science, and cognitive science" (Hunter, 2001, p. 180). The term *nursing informatics* was probably first used and defined by Scholes and Barber in 1980 in their address to the International Medical Informatics Association (IMIA) at the conference that year in Tokyo. They defined nursing informatics as "the application of computer technology to all fields of nursing—nursing services, nurse education, and nursing research" (p. 73).

Nursing informatics is now a thriving subspecialty of nursing that combines nursing knowledge and skills with computer expertise. Like any knowledge-intensive profession, nursing is greatly affected by the explosive growth of both scientific advances and technology. Nurse informatics specialists manage and communicate nursing data and information to improve decision making by consumers, patients, nurses, and other healthcare providers. Nurse informatics specialists formed the American Nursing Informatics Association (ANIA) in the early 1990s to provide networking, education, and information resources that enrich and strengthen the roles of nurses in the field of informatics, including the domains of clinical information, education, and administration decision support. In addition, nursing informatics is represented in the American Medical Informatics Association (AMIA) and the IMIA by working groups that promote the advancement of nursing informatics within the larger interdisciplinary context of health informatics.

Many undergraduate and graduate nursing education programs recognize that it is essential to prepare nurses to practice in a technology rich environment (National League of Nursing [NLN], 2008; Warren & Connors, 2007). Noting the federal initiatives pushing the adoption of electronic health records throughout all healthcare institutions by the year 2014, the National League of Nursing stressed that it is imperative that graduates of today's nursing programs know how to use and advantage "informatics tools to ensure safe and quality care" (NLN, 2008, p. 1). Certification as a nurse informatics specialist by the American Nurses Credentialing Center (ANCC) requires specific coursework and specific experience and/or continuing education.

Healthcare informatics, however, is truly interdisciplinary. In its truest form, it focuses on the care of patients, rather than on a specific discipline (Hannah, Ball, & Edwards, 2006). Although specific bodies of knowledge exist for each healthcare profession (e.g., nursing, dentistry, dietetics, pharmacy, medicine), they interface at the patient. Working with integrated clinical information systems demands interdisciplinary collaboration at a high level.

A model for nursing informatics depicted in Figure 11-1 is applicable across healthcare informatics (Graves, Amos, Huether, Lange, & Thompson, 1995). The core of this model is the transformation of data into information and then into knowledge. Data are discrete entities that describe or measure something without interpreting it. Numbers are data; for example, the number *30*, without interpretation, means nothing. Information consists of defined, interpreted, organized, or structured data. The number *30* defined as milliliters, minutes, or hours

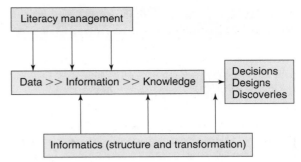

FIGURE 11-1 Nursing informatics conceptual model.

has meaning. Knowledge refers to information that is combined or synthesized so that interrelationships are identified. For example, the number *30*, when included in the statement "All patients who had indwelling bladder catheters for longer than 30 days developed infections," becomes knowledge, something that is known. The transformation of data into knowledge facilitates decision making, new discoveries, and the creation of designs.

In practice, skilled clinicians synthesize data and information quickly, interpreting and comparing new data with previous information about the patient to reach knowledgeable conclusions. Much of the data's potential value is lost, however, if not stored where others can retrieve and use them in a timely manner to synthesize new information and knowledge. Box 11-4 illustrates combining and interpreting data to provide information, which, when synthesized, provides new knowledge.

Data from many patients analyzed and synthesized in scientific studies are combined to provide evidence for best practices in patient care. Either evidence-based practice reassures us that our approach to patient care is correct, or the evidence redirects our thinking. Technology has influenced both the availability and the applicability of evidence for practice.

Knowledge Technology

Knowledge technology consists of systems that generate or process knowledge and provide clinical decision support (CDS). Defined broadly, CDS is a clinical computer system, computer application, or process that helps health professionals make clinical decisions to enhance patient care. The clinical

BOX 11-4 USING THE INFORMATION TRIAD

Several patients in the coronary care unit had fallen at night in the previous 3 weeks. This was very unusual because patients with heart conditions do not usually become disoriented at night. The newly assigned charge nurse became concerned about this and began to look for commonalities among the patients who had fallen. She found that they were all taking the same sleeping medication. She mentioned this at a meeting and found that several other nurses had noticed the same situation. Together, they contacted the pharmacist, who contacted the pharmaceutical representative. He found that the medication dosage had been tested on college students and that the dose was too high for older, less healthy individuals. This is an example of combining data to provide information that, when aggregated and processed, becomes new knowledge.

BOX 11-5 EXPERT DECISION FRAME FOR "GIVE MAXIMUM DOSE OF PAIN MEDICATION"

The Knowledge Base
A. Pain score
B. Invasive procedure scheduled
C. Opiate analgesic ordered
D. Contraindications to the medication
E. History of allergic reaction to opiate analgesics
F. Contraindication to maximum dose of opiate analgesic
G. Time since last dose of opiate analgesic administered
H. Time since surgical procedure

The Inference Engine
Give the maximum dose of pain medication if (A or B) and (C and H <48 hours and G >3 hours) and not (D or E or F)
or:
(C and H <48 hours and G >4 hours) and not (D or E or F)

knowledge embedded in computer applications or work processes can range from simple facts and relationships to best practices for managing patients with specific disease states, new medical knowledge from clinical research, and other types of information. Among the most common forms of CDS are drug-dosing calculators—computer-based programs that calculate appropriate doses of medications after a clinician inputs key data (e.g., patient weight or the level of serum creatinine). These calculators are especially useful in managing the administration of medications with a narrow therapeutic index. Allergy alerts, dose range checking, drug-drug interaction, and duplicate order checking are other common applications of CDS.

Clinical (or diagnostic) decision support systems (CDSSs) are interactive computer programs designed to assist health professionals with decision-making tasks by mimicking the inductive or deductive reasoning of a human expert. The basic components of a CDSS include a knowledge base and an *inferencing mechanism* (usually a set of rules derived from the experts and evidence-based practice). The knowledge base contains the knowledge that an expert nurse would apply to data entered about a patient and information to solve a problem. The inference engine controls the application of the knowledge by providing the logic and rules for its use with data from a specific patient.

Box 11-5 illustrates the use of an expert system for determining the maximum dose of pain medication that can safely be given to a patient after an invasive procedure. The knowledge base contains eight items that are to be considered when giving the maximum dose. The inference engine controls the use of the knowledge base by applying logic that an expert nurse would use in making the decision to give the maximum dose. This decision frame states that if pain is severe (A) or a painful procedure is planned (B), and there is an order for pain medication (C) and the time since surgery is less than 48 hours (H) and the time since the last dose is greater than 3 hours (G), and there are no contraindications to the medication (D) or history of allergy (E) or contraindication to the maximum dose (F), then the "decision" would be to give the dose of pain medication. The rules are those that expert nurses would apply in making the decision to give pain medication.

EXERCISE 11-5

Mr. Jones's heart rate is 54 beats per minute. Tony is about to give Mr. Jones his scheduled atenolol dose. When Tony scans Mr. Jones's armband and the medication bar codes, the computer warns him that atenolol should not be given to a patient with a heart rate less than 60 beats per minute. What should Tony do?

One of the benefits of CDSSs is that they permit the novice nurse to advantage the decision-making expertise and judgment of an expert. Nursing leaders must be aware of the usefulness of decision support systems for nursing, as the development of CDS applicable to nursing practices is just beginning. Clinical experts are needed to develop both the knowledge in the database and the logic used to develop the rules for its application to a particular patient in a particular circumstance. Advanced critical-thinking skills are needed to develop logic and rules. When these are in place, patient care quality can be standardized and improved.

A critical use of information has been in the area of the medication management process. These processes are high-risk and high-volume activities (Malashock, Smith-Shull, & Gould, 2004). New applications provide support for all aspects of the process, thereby improving safety and efficiency (Box 11-6).

EVIDENCE-BASED PRACTICE

Evidence-based practice (EBP) is a systematic approach to clinical decision making to provide the most consistent and best possible care to patients. EBP integrates current research findings that define best practices, clinical expertise, and patient values to optimize patient outcomes as well as their quality of life (Sackett, Straus, Richardson, Rosenberg, & Haynes, 2005). A substantial gap exists between evidence from research findings and practice. Chapter 21 explains the process of translating research into practice.

Realizing the importance of overcoming the obstacles that prevent nursing practices based on evidence, nursing has begun to incorporate EBP in education and practice (Melnyk et al., 2004; Titler et al., 2001). There are a number of models for creating and implementing EBP, all based on the following five key essential elements (Moyer & Elliott, 2004):

1. Ask a clinical question
2. Acquire the evidence
3. Appraise the evidence
4. Apply the evidence
5. Assess the outcomes

Informatics can play an important role in four of these five elements.

Ask a Clinical Question

To acquire evidence for nursing practice, nurses must realize they have an information need. Precisely articulating a clinical question is the first step in the process. For example, nurses might ask, "What is the most reliable method for measuring temperature in an infant younger than 60 days?"

Acquire the Evidence

When clinicians identify a need for information, they must be able to search current literature. Doing a search in a non-electronic format is impossible, given the volume of information available. Clinicians can access electronic evidence summaries via web-based resources such as Clinical Evidence (*www.clinicalevidence.bmj.com/*) and BestBETs (*www.bestbets.org/*). In addition, sites such as the Agency for Healthcare Research and Quality (AHRQ) and the National Guideline Clearinghouse provide searchable databases for published clinical practice guidelines (*www.guideline.gov*). The Cochrane Collaborative is a reliable source of evidence for healthcare practices that seeks to improve decision making in health care through systematic reviews of the literature about patient care interventions (*www.cochrane.org*). Finally, clinicians can electronically access relevant electronic databases (CINAHL, EMBASE, MedLine, OVID, PubMed, and PsycLIT) to retrieve relevant articles and studies to assist them in answering clinical questions. Ideally, the assistance of a clinical librarian can be obtained to fine-tune the clinical question and literature search.

One study about how nurses located and accessed information to answer questions about patient care found that access to a collection of online knowledge-based resources resulted in a significant increase in nurses using the computer-based resources and a decline in seeking information from colleagues, textbooks, or journals (Tannery, Wessel, Epstein, & Gadd, 2007). The value of immediate access to information for patient care is clear.

Appraise the Evidence

Assessing the validity, reliability, and applicability of the literature is time-consuming; however, with practice, assessing the literature becomes easier. Also, this step is important for building the evidence basis for nursing practice. The Centre for Evidence-based

BOX 11-6 INFORMATION TECHNOLOGY: TRENDS IN THE MEDICATION MANAGEMENT PROCESS

Various information technology (IT) devices and software applications are designed to support the medication management process. Each has unique functionality and targets a specific phase of the medication process.

Computerized Provider Order Entry (CPOE)
- Decision support and clinical warnings (e.g., alerts the provider of allergies, pertinent laboratory data, drug-drug and drug-food interactions)
- Automatic dose calculation
- Link to up-to-date drug reference material
- Automatic order notification
- Standardized formulary-compliant order sets
- Legible, accurate, and complete medication orders
- Decreased variations in practice
- Less time clarifying orders
- Fewer verbal orders
- No manual transcription errors

Electronic Medication Administration Record (e-MAR)
- Integration with clinical documentation (in the electronic record)
- Link to up-to-date drug reference material
- Automatic reminders and alarms for approaching or missed medication administration times
- Prompts for associated tasks or additional documentation requirements
- Alert when cumulative dosing exceeds maximum
- Legible record
- Accessible to multiple users
- Improved accuracy of pharmacokinetic monitoring (administration times are reliable)
- Record matches the pharmacy profile
- Generated reports to track medication errors provides visibility to near misses
- Perpetual interface with pharmacy inventory system
- Increase the accuracy of charge capture (at the time of administration vs. when drug is dispensed)

Bar Coding and Radio Frequency Identification (RFID) Scanning
- Medication documentation captured electronically at the time of administration (populates the e-MAR)

- Five rights verified
- Positive patient identification
- Clinician alerted to discrepancies (e.g., wrong drug, wrong dose, wrong time, wrong patient, expired drug)
- Automatic tracking of medication errors and provides visibility to near misses

"Smart" Infusion Pumps (Medication Infusion Delivery System)
- Reduced the need for manual dose/rate calculation
- Institution defined standardized drug library (drugs, concentrations, dosing parameters)
- Software filter prevention of programming errors/programming is within pre-established minimum and maximum limits before the infusion can begin
- Device infusion parameter limits based on patient type or care area
- Interface with the patient's pharmacy profile with capabilities to program the pump electronically
- User alerted to pump setting errors, wrong channel selection, and mechanical failures
- Electronic notification to pharmacy when fluids/medications need to be dispensed
- Interface with the patient's e-MAR (accurate documentation of administration times and volumes infused)
- Memory functions for settings and alarms with a retrievable log
- Electronic recording of reprogramming and limit override activity

Automated Dispensing Unit/Cabinets
- Secure drug storage
- Controlled user access—biometric identification
- Interface with the pharmacy profile—access restricted until order reviewed
- Quick access once medication order reviewed by pharmacist
- Ability to monitor controlled substance waste and utilization patterns
- Perpetual interface with pharmacy inventory

Pharmacy Automation and Robotics
- Increased accuracy and speed of dispensing

From Bell, M.J. (2005). Nursing information of tomorrow. *Healthcare Informatics, 22*(2), 74-78; Larrabee, S., & Brown, M.M. (2003). Recognizing the institutional benefits of bar-code point-of-care technology. *Joint Commission Journal on Quality and Safety, 29*(7), 345-353.

Medicine at Oxford University provides tools that guide the appraisal of randomized controlled trials, systematic literature reviews, and the like. They can be downloaded and printed from the website *(www. cebm.net/critical_appraisal.asp).*

Apply the Evidence

When clinicians identify information that answers a clinical question, a practice change may be required. Practice changes must be addressed with the appropriate governing body (e.g., an interdisciplinary or nurse practice council). The governing body evaluates the information and incorporates needed changes into related policies, procedures, and standards of care. In addition, this group can help communicate and educate nurses about practice changes and help identify process and outcome measurements that should be assessed related to practice changes.

Clinical information systems with appropriate CDS can support the application of evidence-based practice to direct patient care. For example, if a patient is at risk for the development of pressure ulcer over a bony prominence, nurses complete and document a standardized risk assessment and the software suggests the most appropriate interventions to maintain skin integrity.

Assess the Outcomes

Measuring process and outcome changes is a key step in the evidence-based practice model. Information systems play a key role in this process. Measuring daily practice against evidence-based guidelines, standards, or protocols is not a one-time activity. It must be hardwired into a system, whether it is a small primary care office or large hospital. Using technology, real-time reports can detect variation from recommended practice by service, department, or individual practitioner. A regular review must take place to evaluate the findings of these reports. This review will reveal whether there were important reasons to vary, barriers to practice the accepted standard, or new evidence supporting a review of the practice (DePalma, 2002).

Like other healthcare providers, nurses cannot read or retain all the information needed to act effectively for patients. Information technology can provide real-time access to clinical information and integrate evidence-based clinical guidelines in standardized plans for patient care. Easily accessed information about best care practices makes positive patient outcomes more likely than relying on either the nursing interventions learned in basic educational programs or traditional practice experience. Patients' clinical data can be linked to reference literature and drug information, as well as to organizational policies, procedures, patient education materials, and the like.

PATIENT SAFETY

The patient care environment is complex and prone to errors (Ebright, Patterson, Chalko, & Render, 2003). Nurses are the healthcare workers who prevent accidents in patient care and create safety daily (IOM, 2004). In addition to physical challenges, resource challenges, and interruptions characteristic of nursing work, nurses are challenged by inconsistencies and breakdowns in care communication. Communication and information difficulties are among the most common nursing workplace challenges and are frustrating and potentially dangerous for patients.

Information technology is identified as an essential tool for advancing patient safety (Malloch, 2007). Nurses, other health professionals, and patients and families rely increasingly on information technology to communicate, manage information, mitigate error potential, and make informed decisions (Bakken et al., 2004; Marin, 2004). Health information technology has the potential to improve—or obstruct—work performance, communication, and documentation (Ash, Berg, & Coiere, 2004). Because nurses play a key central role in patient care, the extent to which information technology supports or detracts from nurses' work performance can be expected to affect patient outcomes (Kossman & Scheidenhelm, 2008).

Nurses identified that the highest percentage of their top 10 challenges are related to systems and technology put in place to accomplish patient care (Krichbaum et al., 2007). Nurses spend up to 40% of their workday meeting ever-increasing demands from the systems in which they work to provide patient care (Ebright et al., 2003). Nurses rank new, excessive, or changing forms and documentation systems number 2 among the variables contributing most to complexity compression. Only inadequate staffing ranks higher (Krichbaum et al., 2007).

Documentation to meet organizational, accreditation, insurance, state, and federal requirements, as well as provide information needed by other healthcare providers, imposes a heavy demand on nurses' time. Documentation requirements lessen nursing time for direct contact with patients and families. Reduced nursing availability affects patient safety and care quality. Nurses in acute care settings spend, on average, one quarter to one half of their time documenting patient care (Ammenwerth, Mansmann,

Iller, Eichstadter, 2003; Frankel, Cowie, & Daley, 2003; Korst, Eusebio-Angeja, Chamorro, Aydin, & Gregory, 2003; Kossman & Scheidenhelm, 2008). Finishing documentation is one reason nurses do not complete work on time—it is a form of mandatory overtime (Trossman, 2001).

IMPACT OF CLINICAL INFORMATION SYSTEMS

Good decision making requires good information. Clinical information systems that provide access to patient information and provide clinical decision support can reduce errors and inefficiencies (Ball, Weaver, & Abbot, 2003).

Patient information in an electronic clinical information system is organized and legible. Nurses see all of the medications prescribed for a patient in one location; doses are written clearly, and drug names are spelled correctly. The patient problem list shows acute and chronic health conditions and complete allergy information. Abnormal findings are highlighted and can be graphed and compared with interventions. Alerts signal nurses that critical information has been entered in the electronic record. For example, critical test results signal the need for provider notification and intervention. An alert that a patient is at risk for falling signals the need for additional monitoring and interventions to ensure safety. Nursing reminders to perform pressure area care reduce the incidence of this important healthcare-related complication (Frankel, Cowie, & Daley, 2003).

When standards for care are not being followed, clinical information systems can generate alerts, reminders, or suggestions. Rules remind care providers to perform required care. When documentation is not recorded for medication administration, IV tubing change, or wound care, for example, the system generates a reminder based on rules that have been agreed to by providers. Evidence-based practices are integrated in the process of care as providers are guided to select the most appropriate course of action.

Errors are avoided by eliminating the problem of illegible handwriting. Computerized order entry also eliminates the nursing time required for clarification of illegible and incomplete orders. Transcription is no longer required, orders are sent directly to the performing department, and patient care needs are communicated more clearly and quickly to all clinicians. Medication dosing, drug allergy, and drug-drug interaction checking all have significant impact on patient safety (Mekhjian et al., 2002).

Impact on Communication

Integrated information systems allow all members of the interdisciplinary patient care team to see pertinent patient information and plan care based on what is currently happening and what should occur in the future. Everyone knows who is responsible for the patient and who needs to communicate about the patient's care. Clinical information systems provide multiple users with simultaneous, real-time access to patient records. Patient care hand-offs are safer when information is not unavailable or lost in the process. Patient care processes are facilitated, and treatment delays are decreased. The patient's care experience is also improved by decreasing redundant data collection by multiple members of the care team.

Impact on Patient Care Documentation

Nurses spend much time documenting patient care activities. Clinical documentation in an electronic information system improves access to patient information and increases documentation efficiency and organization (Kossman & Scheidenhelm, 2008). In an intensive care setting, automatic downloads of patient vital signs, ventilator settings, and IV intake provide efficiency and timesaving for nurses (Frankel, Cowie, & Daley, 2003). Redundant documentation is eliminated with an integrated clinical information system, and completeness of nursing documentation has increased with some systems (Larrabee et al., 2001).

Impact on Medication Administration Processes

The *United States Pharmacopeia MEDMARX* database includes annual records of medication errors. In 2006, approximately 25% of errors involved some aspect of computer technology as at least one cause of the error. Most errors related to technology involved mislabeled bar codes on medications, mistakes at order entry because of confusing computer screens, or other problems with information management (TJC, 2008). Errors also were related to dispensing devices and human factors, such as failure to scan bar codes or overrides of bar-code warnings.

Computerized provider order entry (CPOE) can be an effective mechanism for improving patient safety. There can be unintended consequences, however, and new kinds of errors can be detected (Ash et al., 2007). Safeguards built into clinical information systems can avert an error, but awareness of the potential for new issues is vital.

Automated medication administration systems that use bar-code technology can ensure that the right patient gets the right medication, in the correct dose, by the appropriate route, and at the specified time. However, it is imperative that this new information technology not impede nurses' care of patients. Faced with urgent or emergent situations with patients, technical difficulties, or poor work re-design, unorthodox and potentially unsafe "work-arounds" are sometimes invented when the medication administration system is not usable and obstructs patient care (Koppel, Wetterneck, Telles, & Karsh, 2008).

Closed-loop electronic prescribing, dispensing, and bar-code patient identification systems reduce prescribing errors and medication adverse events and increase confirmation of patient identity before administration. However, time spent on medication-related tasks increases for physicians, pharmacists, and nurses (Franklin, O'Grady, Donyai, Jacklin, & Barber, 2007).

SAFELY IMPLEMENTING HEALTH INFORMATION TECHNOLOGY

Despite the promise of positive impact from clinical information systems, success is not a guarantee. Remaining alert to its limitations and risks is crucial, because new technology and increasing automation make work less transparent and create opportunities for new types of errors (Reason, 2002). According to McBride (2005):

Information technology is not a panacea, and will not fulfill its promise unless it is harnessed in support of foundational values. That is why every nurse cannot afford to be unconnected to this transformation, but must take an active role in ensuring that IT is used in service to our profession's values. After all, we are knowledge workers. (p. 188)

The Joint Commission warns that as health information technology is adopted, users must be mindful of the safety risks and preventable adverse events that implementation can create (TJC, 2008). The report notes that any form of technology can adversely affect patient care safety and quality if it is designed or implemented improperly. TJC suggests 13 actions, which are presented in Table 11-2.

A clinical information system's success or failure is related to the system's "fit" with the organizational culture, the information needs of its users, and users' work processes and practices (Kaplan, 2001; Kaplan & Harris-Salamone, 2009). Duke University Medical Center informatics experts wrote that they had learned in 1993 that "ongoing planning, adjusting, fitting the technology to the work, and adapting policy formation were more important than the technology itself" (Stead et al., 1993, p. 225). The same is true today!

Relying too heavily on health information technology for communication can reduce teamwork and may negatively affect patient safety and care quality (Ash et al., 2004). Although improved access and better-organized information can eliminate nurses' locating information for other nurses and physicians, information technology will never eliminate the need for personal communication and teamwork.

Successful development and implementation of nursing information technology depend on nurses working in partnership with organizational leadership, information systems vendors, and systems analysts to create tools that truly benefit nurses. When nurses have the systems and tools needed to provide patient care effectively and efficiently, safety and care quality will follow. Direct-care nurses must work with informatics nurses and information system developers and programmers in system development, implementation, and ongoing improvement. Nurses are key partners in every phase of the clinical information life cycle (Benham-Hutchins, 2009). By combining computer and information science with nursing science, the goals of supporting nursing practice and

TABLE 11-2	THE JOINT COMMISSION RECOMMENDATIONS FOR SAFELY IMPLEMENTING HEALTH INFORMATION TECHNOLOGY

	SUGGESTED ACTION
1	Examine work processes and procedures for risks and inefficiencies. Resolve problems identified before technology implementation. Involve representatives of all disciplines—clinical, clerical, and technical—in the examination and resolution of issues.
2	Involve clinicians and staff who will use or be affected by the technology, along with information technology (IT) staff with strong clinical backgrounds, in the planning, selection, design, reassessment, and ongoing quality improvement of technology. Involve pharmacists in planning and implementing any technology that involves medication.
3	Assess your organization's technology needs. Require IT staff to interact with users outside their own facility to learn about real-world capabilities of potential systems from various vendors; conduct field trips; look at integrated systems to minimize the need for interfaces.
4	Continuously monitor for problems during the introduction of new technology and address issues as quickly as possible to avoid workarounds and errors. Consider an emergent issues desk staffed with project experts and champions to help rapidly resolve problems. Use interdisciplinary problem solving to improve system quality and provide vendor feedback.
5	Establish training programs for all clinical and operations staff, designed appropriately for each group and focused on how the technology will benefit staff and patients. Do not allow long delays between training and implementation. Provide frequent refresher courses or updates.
6	Develop and communicate policies delineating staff authorized and responsible for technology implementation, use, oversight, and safety review.
7	Ensure that all order sets and guidelines are developed, tested, and approved by the Pharmacy and Therapeutics Committee (or equivalent) before implementation.
8	Develop a graduated system of safety alerts in the new technology to help clinicians determine urgency and relevancy. Review skipped or rejected alerts. Decide which alerts need to be hard stops in the technology, and provide supporting documentation.
9	Develop systems to mitigate potential computerized provider order entry (CPOE) drug errors or adverse events by requiring department and pharmacy review and sign off. Use the Pharmacy and Therapeutics Committee (or equivalent) for oversight and approval of electronic order sets and clinical decision support (CDS) alerts. Ensure proper nomenclature and printed label design, eliminate dangerous abbreviations and dose designations, and ensure electronic medication administration record (eMAR) acceptance by nurses.
10	Provide environments that protect staff doing data entry from undue distractions when using the technology.
11	Maximize the potential of the technology to maximize safety. Continually reassess and enhance safety effectiveness and error detection. Use error-tracking tools, and evaluate events and near-miss events.
12	Monitor and report errors and near-miss events. Pursue potential system errors or use problems with root cause analysis or other forms of failure-mode analysis. Consider reporting significant issues to external reporting systems.
13	Re-evaluate the applicability of security and confidentiality protocols. Reassess Health Insurance Portability and Accountability Act (HIPAA) compliance periodically to ensure that the addition of technology and the growing responsibilities of IT staff have not introduced new security or compliance risks.

the delivery of high-quality nursing care can be achieved (Delaney, 2007). The Literature Perspective on p. 219 identifies some recommendations related to health information technology (HIT) successes and failures.

For example, imagine that a patient you are caring for complains of light-headedness and nausea. When documenting vital signs, you note that the blood pressure measurement is lower than it was the day before. Graphing the values across several days illustrates a

LITERATURE PERSPECTIVE

Resource: Kaplan, B., & Harris-Salamone, K. D. (2009). Health IT success and failure: Recommendations from the literature and an AMIA workshop. *Journal of the American Medical Informatics Association: JAMIA, 16,* 291-299.

The use of health information technology (HIT) can bring improved healthcare quality and save costs. However, despite best practice research that has identified success factors for HIT projects, many still fail. Success or failure has social, legal, and ethical components.

In 2006, the American Medical Informatics Association (AMIA) sponsored a workshop to examine why too many HIT projects are unsuccessful. Factors influencing success and/or failure include communication, workflow, and quality; the complexity of HIT undertakings; the need to integrate projects, work environments, and regulatory and policy requirements; and the difficulty of getting all the parts and participants in harmony. Workshop participants reviewed more than 70 papers about HIT success and failure and proposed both a research agenda and action items for the association in the "white paper" that reports the outcomes of the workshop.

Implications for Practice
One action item is a call for developing informatics curricula for students and professionals. Were you exposed to information technology during your nursing education? How would you rank your knowledge and skills in computer literacy, information literacy, and the use of information technology? If you think that your educational preparation was lacking, what can you do to enhance your skills with information technology as a practicing nurse?

steady decline in the readings. Reviewing the medication list, you note he is receiving hydralazine (Apresoline). Processing the data that you have collected, you implement "falls precautions," send a communication order to monitor his blood pressure and other symptoms frequently, and notify the physician if the situation has not changed.

EXERCISE 11-6
Think about the data that you gather and document every day: vital signs, intake and output, laboratory and test results, and the patient's responses to care. What data did you automatically combine or reorganize to help you make a decision regarding patient care? How did you use this information to improve your patient's outcome? How and with whom did you communicate the data and information? How did technology combine or organize data?

FUTURE TRENDS AND PROFESSIONAL ISSUES

Biomedical Technology

Developments in biomedical technology are nothing short of astounding. Every year at a major conference on health innovation, the Cleveland Clinic designates the top 10 technologies that will shape health care in the year ahead (Graham, 2008). The list for 2009 comprised the following:

1. Circulating Tumor Cell Technology: A blood test that measures cancer cells that have broken away from an existing tumor and entered the bloodstream can detect recurrent cancer sooner, demonstrate how well treatment is working, and predict the patient's probable outcome.
2. Warm Organ Perfusion Device: When a heart becomes available for transplant, surgeons have just 4 hours before the organ begins to deteriorate. This device re-creates conditions within the body to keep the heart pumping for up to 12 hours.
3. Diaphragm Pacing System: Electrodes connected to nerves on the diaphragm run to and from a control box worn outside the body. When the electrodes are stimulated, the diaphragm contracts, pulling air into the lungs. When not stimulated, the diaphragm relaxes and air is exhaled.
4. Multi-Spectral Imaging Systems: When the system is attached to a standard microscope, researchers can stain tissue samples and examine them with different light wavelengths. This helps understand complicated signaling pathways in cancer cells to develop more targeted therapies.
5. Percutaneous Mitral Valve Regurgitation Repair: Using a tiny, barbed, wishbone-shaped device, the heart valve is repaired noninvasively. A catheter is carefully guided through the femoral vein in the groin, up to the heart's mitral valve. A clip on the tip of a catheter is then clamped on the valve leaflets, which holds them together to prevent regurgitant blood flow.
6. New Strategies for Creating Vaccines for Avian Flu: A new approach that uses a mock version

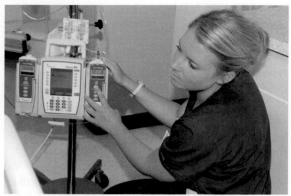

Twenty-first century IV pumps offer safety features, accuracy, advanced pressure monitoring, ease of use, and versatility.

of the avian flu virus called a *virus-like particle (VLP)* may offer a better solution to protect people against infection.

7. LESS and NOTES Applications: LESS (laparo-endoscopic single-site surgery) takes laparoscopic surgery to a new level by reducing the process to a small cut in the belly button. NOTES (natural orifice transluminal endoscopic surgery) permits the surgeon to access the appendix, prostate, kidney, or gallbladder through one of the body's natural cavities, such as the mouth, vagina, or colon.

8. Integration of Diffusion Tensor Imaging: DTI is a new technology that allows neuroscientists to noninvasively probe the long-neglected half of the brain called *white matter.*

9. Doppler-Guided Uterine Artery Occlusion: This is a new, noninvasive treatment for fibroid tumors, which occur in more than 40% of women older than 35 years.

10. Private Sector National Health Information Exchange: This is a comprehensive system of electronic health records that links consumers, general practitioners, specialists, hospitals, pharmacies, nursing homes, and insurance companies.

Information Technology

Health care in the United States is expensive and of variable quality. Recognizing that informatics can play an important role in controlling costs and improving quality, the federal government's economic stimulus plan in 2009 earmarked $20 billion for health information technology. However, the money must be spent wisely, not quickly. One consideration suggested is to use the money to move the health information technology industry toward strong, mandated data standards. Data standards are at the foundation of integrated, interoperable information systems that will permit an emergency department or operating room to transfer data to inpatient hospital units and permit hospitals to send data to a patient's primary care record in the provider's office.

Electronic Patient Care Records

Multiple terms have been used to define electronic patient care records, with overlapping definitions. Both electronic health record (EHR) and electronic medical record (EMR) have gained widespread use, with some health informatics users assigning the term *EHR* to a global concept and *EMR* to a discrete localized record. An EHR refers to an individual patient's medical record in digital format. The EHR is a longitudinal electronic record of patient health information generated across encounters in any care delivery setting. EHR systems coordinate the storage and retrieval of individual records with the aid of computers. The EHR is most often accessed on a computer, often over a network, and may include EMRs from many locations and/or sources. Among the many forms of data often included are patient demographics, health history, progress and procedure notes, health problems, medication and allergy lists (including immunization status), laboratory test results, radiology images and reports, billing records, and advanced directives.

Credit card–like devices called smart cards store a limited number of pages of data on a computer chip. The implementation of computer-based health information systems will lead to computer networks that will store health records across local, state, national, and international boundaries. The smart card serves as a bridge between the clinician terminal and the central repository, making patient information available to the caregiver quickly and cheaply at the point of service because the patients bring it with them. This will help coordinate care; improve quality-of-care decisions; and reduce risk, waste, and duplication of effort. Patients are mobile and consult many practitioners, thereby causing their records to be frag-

BOX 11-7 SMART CARDS

1. Patient demographics/photo identification
2. ICE—In Case of Emergency—contact and other key information
3. Patient medical history: for example, allergies, medications, immunizations, laboratory results
4. Past care encounter summaries, including surgical procedures
5. Patient record locations and electronic address information
6. Ability to upload or download patient information

mented. With the electronic smart card, patients, providers, and notes can be brought together in any combination at any place. Box 11-7 provides examples of the types of data that are recorded on smart cards.

Data Privacy and Security

Data protection, systems' security, and patient privacy are concerns with electronic health records. However, patients' rights to privacy of their data must be maintained whether recorded in a manual or automated system. With computerized data, any person with the proper permission may access the information anywhere in the world and multiple people can do so simultaneously. Data can also be inadvertently sent to the wrong individual or site. Information security and privacy are important concerns as development of electronic health information systems accelerates at the beginning of the twenty-first century.

A firewall protects the information in the central data repository from access by unauthorized users. It is a network security measure that keeps electronic intruders from accessing an organization's data on its private network while allowing members of the organization to reach the Internet. Organizational policies on the use, security, and accuracy of data must be developed and monitored for compliance.

Communication Technology

Telecommunications

Telecommunications and systems technology facilitate clinical oversight of health care via telephone or cable lines, remote monitoring, information links, and the Internet. Telehealth is the use of modern telecommunications and information technologies for the provision of health care to individuals at a distance and the transmission of information to

provide that care. This is accomplished using two-way interactive videoconferencing and high-speed telephone lines, fiberoptic cable, and satellite transmissions. Patients sitting in front of the teleconferencing camera can be diagnosed, treated, monitored, and educated by nurses and physicians. ECGs and radiographs can be viewed and transmitted. Sophisticated electronic stethoscopes and dermascopes allow nurses and physicians to hear heart, lung, and bowel sounds and to look closely at wounds, eyes, ears, and skin. Ready access to expert advice and patient information is available no matter where the patient or information is located. Patients in rural areas and prisons especially benefit from this technology.

Telecommunication also supports distance learning, which has been possible for some years, with enhanced opportunities to engage students in online classrooms. With online or "virtual" classrooms, students from anywhere in the world with computer access can log into a university's online learning system via the Internet. The Internet, which can provide health education and other health information, is a worldwide network of computers that fosters communication, collaboration, resource sharing, and information access. It is a multicultural library that is open 24 hours a day, every day to ordinary computer users.

In addition to formal distance education possibilities, the Internet permits access to nearly limitless information in the form of text, pictures, video, and sound. Web pages contain text and "links" to other documents filled with information. Using the Internet to seek answers to specific questions, promote high-level thinking, and develop problem-solving skills is the objective of WebQuests. WebQuests are described as effective, creative, engaging, student-centered learning activities by nursing faculty. Students develop information and information technology literacy (Russell et al., 2008). Box 11-8 lists websites of interest to nurses.

Although reliable and high-quality information can be found via the Internet, web users need to evaluate the quality. How does one evaluate the credentials of the author of the information or site? Several texts and articles suggest criteria for the evaluation of websites related to health that remain timely today (Goldsborough, 1999; Hollaway, Kripps, Koepke, & Skiba, 2000; Nicoll, 2001). Box 11-9 lists criteria for evaluation of these sites. In addition to recognizing

BOX 11-8 **HEALTH-RELATED WEBSITE UNIFORM RESOURCE LOCATORS (URLS)**

DESCRIPTION	URL
Agency for Healthcare Research and Quality (AHRQ)	www.ahrq.gov
American Heart Association	www.americanheart.org
American Hospital Association (AHA)	www.aha.org
American Nurses Association (ANA)	www.nursingworld.org
American Nurses Credentialing Center (ANCC)	www.nursecredentialing.org
American Organization of Nurse Executives (AONE)	www.aone.org
Centers for Disease Control and Prevention (CDC)	www.cdc.gov
Guide to Evidence-Based Practice	www.cebm.utoronto.ca/
Health on the Net	www.hon.ch/
Healthfinder—U.S. Department of Health & Human Services	www.healthfinder.gov
Institute of Healthcare Improvement (IHI)	www.ihi.org
The Joint Commission (TJC)	www.jointcommission.org
Nursing and healthcare resources	www.intute.ac.uk/nmah/
Resources for nurses and families	http://pegasus.cc.ucf. edu/%7Ewink
World Health Organization	www.who.int/

these criteria when evaluating their own web searches, nurses sharing this information with patients will improve their use of health information websites.

Sending and receiving electronic mail (e-mail) is another increasing use of the Internet within health care. Mail can be sent to individuals in any part of the world through e-mail, or e-mail of particular interest may be obtained by subscribing to a listserv or blog. A *listserv* is a group of people who have similar interests. Subscribers to a listserv become part of the "conversation." All messages sent to the listserv are forwarded to all subscribers, who can then read and respond to them. A blog (a contraction of the term weblog) is a type of website, usually maintained by an individual with regular entries of commentary, descriptions of events, or other material such as graphics or videos. Many blogs provide commentary or news on a particular subject, including healthcare topics. A typical blog combines text, images, and links to other blogs, web pages, and other media related to its topic. The ability for readers to leave comments in an interactive format is an important part of many blogs.

E-mail is becoming a preferred communication method between some healthcare providers and patients. This asynchronous mode of communication allows timely responses to non-emergent healthcare issues at the convenience of both the patient and provider. It prevents "telephone tag" and avoids the interruptions often encountered when paging healthcare providers. E-mail can be a very effective means of delivering health services to people and may be especially effective with patients and families managing chronic illness. For example, current systems permit patients with insulin-dependent diabetes to upload blood sugar measurements into systems shared by their providers and receive e-mail directions for ongoing care. E-mail provides documentation of the patient-provider communication and gives the patient instructions in writing. E-mails can have embedded links to information from a variety of websites the provider recognizes as legitimate sources of sound information. Box 11-10 presents guidelines for the use of e-mail between patients and providers.

Informatics

In 2008, the Health Information Management Systems Society (HIMSS) identified that nearly 60% of American hospitals had implemented some component of an EMR. The American Nurses Association recognized nursing informatics as a specialty nursing practice in 2001. Although more than 8000 nurses are practicing in informatics, many more are needed to achieve widespread development and adoption of effective health information systems (Sensmeier, 2008).

Many opportunities exist to improve the safety, efficiency, and effectiveness of nursing care. The goal of informatics nurses and nursing leaders is to use information technology to ensure that critical information is available to caregivers at the point of care to make health care safer and more effective while improving efficiency. This requires interconnected

BOX 11-9   TEN *C's* FOR EVALUATING INTERNET SOURCES

1. Content
What is the intent of the content?
Are the title and author identified?
Is the content "juried"?
Is the content "popular" or "scholarly," satiric or serious?
What is the date of the document or article?
Is the "edition" current?
Do you have the latest version?

2. Credibility
Is the author identifiable and reliable?
Is the content credible? Authoritative? Should it be?
What is the purpose of the information (i.e., is it serious, satiric, or humorous)?
Is the uniform resource locator (URL) extension .edu, .com, .gov, .org, .net, or .info?

3. Critical Thinking
How can you apply critical-thinking skills, including previous knowledge and experience, to evaluate Internet resources?
Can you identify the author, publisher, edition, etc. as you would with a "traditionally" published resource?
What criteria do you use to evaluate Internet resources?

4. Copyright
Even if the copyright notice does not appear prominently, someone wrote or is responsible for the creation of a document, graphic, sound, or image and the material falls under copyright conventions. "Fair use" applies to short, cited excerpts, usually as an example for commentary or research.
Materials are in the "public domain" if this is explicitly stated. Internet users, as users of print media, must respect copyright.

5. Citation
Internet resources should be cited to identify sources used, both to give credit to the author and to provide the reader with avenues for further research. Standard style manuals (print and online) provide some examples of how to cite Internet documents, although these standards are not uniform.

6. Continuity
Will the Internet site be maintained and updated?
Is it now and will it continue to be free?
Can you rely on this source over time to provide up-to-date information?
Some good .edu sites have moved to .com, with possible cost implications.
Other sites offer partial use for free and charge fees for continued or in-depth use.

7. Censorship
Is your discussion list "moderated"?
What does this mean?
Does your search engine or index look for all words, or are some words excluded?
Is this censorship?
Does your institution, based on its mission, parent organization, or space limitations, apply some restrictions to Internet use?
Consider censorship and privacy issues when using the Internet.

8. Connectivity
If more than one user will need to access a site, consider each user's access and "functionality." How do users connect to the Internet and what kind of connection does the assigned resource require?
Does access to the resource require a graphical user interface?
If it is a popular (busy) resource, will it be accessible in the time frame needed?
Is it accessible by more than one Internet tool?
Do users have access to the same Internet tools and applications?
Are users familiar with the tools and applications?
Is the site "viewable" by all Web browsers?

9. Comparability
Does the Internet resource have an identified comparable print or CD ROM data set or source?
Does the Internet site contain comparable and complete information?
Do you need to compare data or statistics over time?
Can you identify sources for comparable earlier or later data?
Comparability of data may or may not be important, depending on your project.

10. Context
What is the context of your research?
Can you find "anything" on your topic, that is, commentary, opinion, narrative, statistics and your quest will be satisfied?
Are you looking for current or historical information? Definitions? Research studies or articles?
How does the Internet information fit in the overall information context of your subject?
Before you start searching, define the research context and research needs and decide what sources might be best to use to successfully fill information needs without data overload.

The Ten C's were developed 1991-1996 by the University of Wisconsin—Eau Claire; a revision was made June 19, 2003.

BOX 11-10 **PATIENT-PROVIDER E-MAIL COMMUNICATION GUIDELINES**

Patient Responsibilities and Expectations

- Include the patient's name in the body of the e-mail.
- Include the category or type of message in the subject line.
- Review the e-mail to make sure it is clear and that all relevant information is provided before sending to the provider.
- Follow up with the provider as needed to determine whether the intended recipient received the e-mail and when the recipient will respond.
- Take precautions to preserve the confidentiality of the e-mail.
- Inform the provider of e-mail address changes.
- Inform the provider of the types of information the patient does not want to be sent by e-mail.

Provider Responsibilities and Expectations

- Use an encrypted security system.
- Obtain informed consent from the patient before using e-mail communication.
- Establish acceptable types of e-mail messages, and provide clear guidelines regarding emergency subject matter.
- Develop a system for integrating e-mail contact into the patient's record.
- Establish an expected response time for messages.

and integrated healthcare technology across hospitals, healthcare systems, and geographic regions. Standards for data systems that operate efficiently with one another (termed "interoperability") and attention to data security and patient privacy are necessary.

Nurses are working as leaders in several national initiatives to lay the groundwork and guide progress toward the goal of a nationwide health information network. Every nurse can embrace technology to improve nursing practice. Some strategies to accomplish this include (1) involving nurses in every decision about health IT that affects their workflow, (2) investing in training nurses to effectively use technology in their practice, and (3) levering opportunities to use IT to enable quality improvement (Sensmeier, 2008).

Knowledge Technology

Technology has the potential to shorten the many years that currently exist between the development of new knowledge for patient care and the application of that knowledge in real-time practice with patients. Increasingly, patient conditions that are directly influenced by nursing care are part of the Centers for Medicare & Medicaid Services (CMS) pay for performance and The Joint Commission "never events." It is more important than ever to inform nurses of the best knowledge regarding clinical phenomena that are the focus of nursing care: medication management, activity intolerance, immobility, risk for falls and actual falls, risk for skin impairment and pressure ulcer, anxiety, dementia, sleep, prevention of infection, nutrition, incontinence, dehydration, smoking cessation, pain management, patient and family education, and self-care.

Norma Lang, a nursing informatics leader, has described the challenges of bringing the best evidence for practice to bear against nursing care (Lang, 2008). First, there is the challenge of synthesizing the knowledge available in a manner that is useful to clinicians. Then, computerized information systems are needed to provide clinical decision support at the point of care. Finally, the computer system must collect good clinical data to promote ongoing knowledge development for nursing care of patients and families. Several "intelligent" clinical information systems are in development. These systems translate nursing knowledge into reference materials that can be accessed at the point of care. Further, computer applications are in development that assist nurses to take action and execute patient care based on the best evidence for practice (Lang, 2008; Lang et al., 2006; Staggers & Brennan, 2007).

Professional, Ethical Nursing Practice and New Technologies

Technology has and will continue to transform the healthcare environment and the practice of nursing. Nurses are professionally obligated to maintain competency with a vast array of technologic devices and systems. Baseline informatics competency is required for all nurses to function in the twenty-first century.

Because of the increasing ability to preserve human life with biomedical technology, questions about living and dying have become conceptually and ethically complex. Conceptually, it becomes more difficult to define extraordinary treatment and human life because technology has changed our concepts of living and dying. A source of ethical dilemmas is the use of invasive technologic treatment to treat patients with extraordinary means and to prolong life for patients with limited or no decision-making capabilities. Nurses are concerned with individual patient welfare and the effects of technologic intervention on the immediate and long-term quality of life for patients and their families. Patient advocacy remains an important function of the professional nurse.

Safeguarding patients' welfare, privacy, and confidentiality is another obligation of nurses. Security measures are available with computerized information systems, but it is the integrity and ethical principles of system end-users that provide the final safeguard for patient privacy. System users must never share the passwords that allow them access to information in computerized clinical information systems. Each password uniquely identifies a user to the system by name and title, gives approval to carry out certain functions, and provides access to data appropriate to the user. When a nurse signs on to a computer, all data and information that are entered or reviewed can be traced to that password. Every nurse is accountable for all actions taken using his or her password. All nurses must be aware of their responsibilities for the confidentiality and security of the data they gather and for the security of their passwords.

Nurse leaders must promote the existence and use of an ethics committee in their institutions and assign knowledgeable nurses to serve on these committees. Nurse managers must ensure that policies and procedures for collecting and entering data and the use of security measures (e.g., passwords) are established to maintain confidentiality of patient data and information. Nurse managers must also be knowledgeable patient advocates in the use of technology for patient care by referring ethical questions to the organization's ethics committee.

EXERCISE 11-7

Think about the use of the World Wide Web in health care. How do you use it to look up healthcare information? How would you advise a patient to select appropriate sites?

SUMMARY

Biomedical, information, communication, and knowledge technology will form a bond in the future, linking people and information together in a rapidly changing world of health care. With new technology comes the need for a new set of competencies. Nursing participation in designing this exciting future will ensure that the unique contributions of nurses to patient and family health and illness care are clearly and formally represented.

THE SOLUTION

I knew successful implementation of an integrated clinical information system requires active participation of the clinical staff during all phases of the project, including the selection, design, build, and training phases. I made sure each care setting was represented by all types and levels of care providers. Installing a new clinical information system provides an opportunity to transform processes so that the provision of care is more efficient and effective. We used this approach even though it extended the project's completion timeline. The solution was progressive and enthusiastically embraced by users.

One device solution does not meet the needs of a diverse user group working with different software applications. So, we provided a variety of device options at the point of care. Because this approach is more expensive at the initial outlay, we were somewhat reluctant to fund it. However, our project leaders demonstrated how the efficiencies gained in the clinician's daily workflow quickly offset the extra expense.

Information technology is an essential component of a patient safety program. The positive impact of technology is clearly illustrated when applied to the complex medication process. The software enhancements we made provided decision support, patient identification verification, device programming safeguards, accurate automated drug dispensing, alerts, and integrated monitoring systems.

—*Cheri Hunt*

Would this be a suitable approach for you? Why?

THE EVIDENCE

Linder et al. (2009) worked together to improve the documentation and treatment of tobacco use in primary care. These physicians and nurses developed and implemented a three-part enhancement to the electronic health record in use in their setting: (1) an icon that displays each patient's smoking status, (2) tobacco cessation treatment reminders, and (3) a form that facilitates ordering medications and counseling referrals for tobacco users.

The clinical decision support and reminders in the electronic system helped this practice to improve documentation of patient tobacco status from 37% to 54% of patients. Tobacco users were referred more frequently for cessation counseling and more reliably made contact for counseling assistance but were not prescribed more tobacco cessation medication than were patients in the control group. Most important, patients who were tobacco users at the start of the electronic intervention trial were more likely to be recorded as non-users by the end of the study than were their peers in the control group (5.3% vs. 1.9%; $P < .001$).

NEED TO KNOW NOW

- Use the biomedical technology frequently required for patient care in your clinical practice area.
- Access the clinical information systems you will need to find information about the patients assigned your care, and enter data about their status, interventions you provide, the plan of care, and their responses to care.
- Know the standards for information privacy and confidentiality as they are operationalized within your organization.

CHAPTER CHECKLIST

Nurses are the key personnel in the healthcare system to mediate the interaction among science, technology, and the patient because of their unique holistic viewpoint and the "24/7" role of vigilant healthcare providers who preserve the patients' humanity, optimal functioning, and promotion of health. The challenge for the profession is to continue to provide patient-centered care in a technologic society that strives for efficiency and cost-effectiveness. Nurse administrators, managers, and staff must provide leadership in managing information and technology to meet the challenge.

- Informatics is the transformation of data into knowledge. It consists of three core components: data, information, and knowledge.
- Nurses commonly manage three types of information technology: biomedical technology, information technology, and knowledge technology.
- Biomedical technology includes the following:
  - Physiologic monitoring
  - Diagnostic testing
  - Medication administration
  - Therapeutic interventions
- Information technology refers to computers and programs that are used to manage data and information.

- Goals of information management are as follows:
  - Obtain, manage, and use information to improve patient outcomes
  - Improve individual and organizational performance in patient care
  - Improve performance in other organizational processes
- Information systems can be used for the following:
  - Reducing clerical nursing
  - Providing patient census and location
  - Obtaining results from tests and list of medications
  - Accessing nursing policies and procedures
  - Coordinating patient care
  - Monitoring chronic conditions
  - Managing financial billing and statistical reporting
- Placement of computers at the patient's side or using handheld devices has many advantages, including the following:
  - Saves time
  - Improves communication by providing more timely access by others
  - Decreases likelihood of documentation omission

- Adapts to nurse's workflow
- Personalizes patient assessment
- Simplifies care planning
- Knowledge technology involves decision support systems that are used to mimic the informational processing of an expert nurse.
- Evidence-based practice involves both the application of evidence to practice and the building of evidence from practice.
- The electronic health record contains healthcare information for an individual from birth to death, allowing immediate access to comprehensive health information.

- Future trends in biomedical, information, and knowledge technology will occur rapidly and demand that nurses remain involved in their development and implementation.
- Privacy and security issues have become important with increased access to and therefore potential broad misuse of patient care data.
- Ethical decision making in health care becomes more complex with increasing medical technology.

TIPS FOR MANAGING INFORMATION AND TECHNOLOGY

- Create a vision for the future.
- Match your vision to the institution's mission and strategic plan.
- Learn what you need to know to fulfill the vision.
- Join initiatives that are moving in the direction of your vision.

- Be prepared to initiate, implement, and support new technology.
- Use an automated dispensing system.
- Use biometric technology.
- Use bar-coding systems/bar-code technology.
- Never stop learning, or you will always be behind.

REFERENCES

Ammenwerth, E., Mansmann, U., Iller, C., & Eichstadter, R. (2003). Factors affecting and affected by user acceptance of computer-based nursing documentation: Results of a two-year study. *Journal of the American Medical Informatics Association: JAMIA, 10,* 69-84.

Ash, J. S., Berg, M., & Coiere, E. (2004). Some unintended consequences of information technology in health care: The nature of patient care information system-related errors. *Journal of the American Medical Informatics Association: JAMIA, 11,* 104-112.

Ash, J. S., Sittig, D. F., Poon, E. G., Guappone, K., Campbell, E., & Dykstra, R. H. (2007). The extent and importance of unintended consequences related to computerized provider order entry. *Journal of the American Medical Informatics Association: JAMIA, 14*(4), 415-423.

Bakken, S., Cook, S., Curtis, L., Desjardins, K., Hyun, S., Jenkins, M., John, R., Klein, W. T., Paguntalan, J., Roberts, W. D., & Soupios, M. (2004). Promoting patient safety through informatics based nursing education. *International Journal of Medical Informatics, 73,* 581-589.

Ball, M., Weaver, C., & Abbot, P. (2003). Enabling technologies promise to revitalize the role of nursing in an era of patient safety. *International Journal of Medical Informatics, 69,* 29-38.

Benham-Hutchins, M. (2009). Frustrated with HIT? Get involved! *Nursing Management, 40*(1), 17-19.

Bonzheim, K. (2006). *Process and workflow improvements through technology adoption.* Health Information Management Systems Society. Chicago, IL.

Breslow, M. J. (2007). Remote ICU care programs: Current status. *Journal of Critical Care, 22,* 66-76.

Clark, J., & Lang, N. (1992). Nursing's next advance: An International Classification for Nursing Practice. *International Nursing Review, 39*(4), 109-112.

Considine, K., & Botti, V. (2004). Who, when and where? Identification of patients at risk of an in-hospital adverse event: Implications for nursing practice. *International Journal of Nursing Practice, 10,* 21-31.

Delaney, C. (2007). Nursing and informatics for the 21st century. *Creative Nursing, 2,* 4-6.

DePalma, J. (2002). Proposing an evidence-based policy process. *Nursing Administration Quarterly, 26*(4), 55-61.

Drucker, P. (1993). *Post capitalist society.* New York: Harper Business Publishers.

Ebright, P. R., Patterson, E. S., Chalko, B. A., & Render, M. L. (2003). Understanding the complexity of registered nurse work in acute care settings. *Journal of Nursing Administration, 33,* 630-638.

Elfrink, V., Bakken, S., Coenen, A., McNeil, B., & Bickford, C. (2001). Standardized nursing vocabularies: A foundation for quality care. *Seminars in Oncology Nursing, 17*(1), 18-23.

Frankel, D. J., Cowie, M., & Daley, P. (2003). Quality benefits of an intensive care clinical information system. *Critical Care Medicine, 31*, 120-125.

Franklin, B. D., O'Grady, P., Donyai, K., Jacklin, A., & Barber, N. (2007). The impact of a closed-loop electronic prescribing and administration system on prescribing errors, administration errors and staff time: A before-and-after study. *Quality and Safety in Healthcare, 16*, 279-284.

Goldsborough, R. (1999). Information on the net often needs checking. *RN, 62*(5), 22, 24.

Graham, J. (November 13, 2008). 10 medical technologies to watch in 2009. *The Chicago Tribune*, Retrieved March 2, 2010 from http://newsblogs.chicagotribune.com/triage/2008/11/10-medical-tech.html.

Graves, J. R., Amos, L. K., Huether, S., Lange, L. L., & Thompson, C. B. (1995). Description of a graduate program in clinical nursing informatics. *Computers in Nursing, 13*(2), 60-70.

Hannah, K. J., Ball, M. J., & Edwards, K. J. (2006). *Introduction to nursing informatics* (3rd ed.). New York: Springer-Verlag.

HIMSS Analytics, Health Information Management Systems Society. (2008). *EMR Adoption Model*. Retrieved March 2, 2010 from www.himssanalytics.org/hc_providers/emr_adoption.asp.

Hollaway, N., Kripps, B., Koepke, K., & Skiba, D. J. (2000). Evaluating health care information on the Internet. In J. Fitzpatrick & K. S. Montgomery (Eds.), *Internet resources for nurses*. New York: Springer.

Hunter, K. M. (2001). Nursing informatics theory. In V. K. Saba & K. A. McCormick (Eds.), *Essentials of computers for nurses: Informatics for the new millennium* (pp. 179-190). New York: McGraw-Hill.

Institute for Safe Medication Practices (ISMP). (2008). ADC survey shows some improvements, but unnecessary risks still exist. *Safety Briefs, 13*, 1-2.

Institute of Medicine (IOM), Committee on Patient Safety. (2000). *To err is human: Building a safer health care system*. Washington, DC: The National Academies Press.

Institute of Medicine (IOM), Committee on Quality Health Care in America. (July 2001). *Crossing the quality chasm: A new health system for the 21st century*. Washington, DC: National Academy Press.

Institute of Medicine (IOM), Committee on the Work Environment for Nurses and Patient Safety. (2004). *Keeping patients safe: Transforming the work environment of nurses*. Washington, DC: The National Academies Press.

Kaplan, B. (2001). Evaluating informatics applications: Some alternative approaches. *International Journal of Medical Informatics, 64*(1), 39-56.

Kaplan, B., & Harris-Salamone, K. D. (2009). Health IT success and failure: Recommendations from the literature and an AMIA workshop. *Journal of the American Medical Informatics Association: JAMIA, 16*, 291-299.

Koppel, R., Wetterneck, T., Telles, J. L., & Karsh, B. T. (2008). Workarounds to barcode medication administration systems: Their occurrences, causes, and threats to patient safety. *Journal of the American Medical Informatics Association: JAMIA, 15*, 408-423.

Korst, L., Eusebio-Angeja, A., Chamorro, T., Aydin, C., & Gregory, K. (2003). Nursing documentation time during implementation of an electronic medical record. *Journal of Nursing Administration, 33*, 24-30.

Kossman, S. P., & Scheidenhelm, S. L. (2008). Nurses' perceptions of the impact of electronic health records on work and patient outcomes. *CIN: Computers, Informatics, Nursing, 26*, 69-77.

Krichbaum, K., Diemert, C., Jacox, L., Jones, A., Koenig, P., Mueller, C., & Disch, J. (2007). Complexity compression: Nurses under fire. *Nursing Forum, 42*, 86-94.

Lang, N. M. (2008). The promise of simultaneous transformation of practice and research with the use of clinical information systems. *Nursing Outlook, 56*, 232-236.

Lang, N. M., Hook, M. L., Akre, M. E., Kim, T. Y., Berg, K. S., & Lundeen, S. P. (2006). Translating knowledge-based nursing into referential and executable applications in an intelligent clinical information system. In C. Weaver, C. Delaney, P. Webber, & R. Carr (Eds.), *Nursing and informatics for the 21st century* (pp. 291-304). Chicago: Healthcare Information and Management Systems Society (HIMSS).

Larrabee, J. H., Boldreghini, S., Elder-Sorrells, K., Turner, Z. M., Wender, R. G., Hart, J. M., & Lenzi, P. S. (2001). Evaluation of documentation before and after implementation of a nursing information system in an acute care hospital. *Computers in Nursing, 19*, 56-65.

Liewelyn, J., Martin, B., Shekleton, M., & Firlet, S. (1998). Analysis of falls in the acute surgical and cardiovascular surgical patient. *Applied Nursing Research, 1*, 116-121.

Linder, J. A., Rigotti, N. A., Schneider, L. I., Kelley, J. H. K., Brawarsky, P., & Haas, J. S. (2009). An electronic health record based intervention to improve tobacco treatment in primary care. *Archives of Internal Medicine, 169*, 781-787.

Malashock, C., Smith-Shull, S., & Gould, D. A. (2004). Effect of smart infusion pumps on medication errors related to infusion device programming. *Hospital Pharmacy, 39*(5), 460-469.

Malbrain, M. L., Chiumello, D., Pelosi, P., Bihari, D., Innes, R., Ranieri, V. M., Del Turco, M., Wilmer, A., Brienza, N., Malcangi, V., Cohen, J., Japiassu, A., De Keulenaer, B. L., Daelemans, R., Jacquet, L., Laterre, P. F., Frank, G., de Souza, P., Cesana, B., & Gattinoni, L. (2005). Incidence and prognosis of intraabdominal hypertension in a mixed population of critically ill patients: A multiple-center epidemiological study. *Critical Care Medicine, 33*, 315-322.

Malloch, K. (2007). The electronic health record: An essential tool for advancing patient safety. *Nursing Outlook, 55*, 159-161.

Marin, H. (2004). Improving patient safety with technology. *International Journal of Medical Informatics, 73*, 543-546.

Matsuo, A., Shimomura, W., Motas, M., Kamikawa, C., Guy, S., & Kooker, B. (2008). Better patient surveillance. *Nursing Management, 39*, 14-18.

McBride, A. (2005). Nursing and the informatics revolution. *Nursing Outlook, 53*, 183-191.

Mekhjian, H. S., Kumar, R. R., Kuehn, L., Bentley, T. D., Teater, P., Thomas, A., et al. (2002). Immediate benefits realized following implementation of physician order entry at an academic medical center. *Journal of the American Medical Informatics Association. 9*(5), 529-539.

Melnyk, B. M., Fineout-Overholt, E., Fischbeck Feinstein, N., Li, H., Small, L., Wilcox, L., & Kraus, R. (2004). Nurses' perceived knowledge, beliefs, skills, and needs regarding evidence-based practice: Implications for accelerating the paradigm shift. *Worldviews on Evidence-based Nursing, 1*(3), 185-193.

Moyer, V. A., & Elliott, E. J. (Eds.). (2004). *Evidence-based pediatrics and child health* (2nd ed.). London: BMJ Publishing Group.

Myers, M. A., & Reed, K. D. (2008). The virtual ICU (vICU): A new dimension for critical care nursing practice. *Critical Care Nursing Clinics of North America, 20*, 435-439.

National League for Nursing (NLN). (2008). *Position statement: Preparing the next generation of nurses to practice in a technology-rich environment—An informatics agenda.* Retrieved March 2, 2010 from www.nln.org.

Nicoll, L. H. (2001). *Nurses' guide to the Internet* (3rd ed.). Philadelphia: Lippincott.

Ozbolt, J. G., & Saba, V. K. (2008). A brief history of nursing informatics in the United States of America. *Nursing Outlook, 56*, 199-205.

Parker, P. J. (2005). One nurse informatics specialist views the future technology in the crystal ball. *Nursing Administration Quarterly, 29*(2), 123-124.

Reason, J. (2002). Combating omission errors through task analysis and good reminders. *Quality & Safety in Health Care, 11*, 40-44.

Russell, C. K., Burchum, J. R., Likes, W. M., Jacob, S., Graff, J. C., Driscoll, C., Britt, T., Adymy, C., & Cowan, P. (2008). WebQuests: Creating engaging student-centered, constructivist learning activities. *CIN: Computers, Informatics, Nursing, 26*(2), 78-87.

Sackett, D. L., Straus, S. E., Richardson, W. S., Rosenberg, W., & Haynes, R. B. (2005). *Evidence based medicine: How to practice and teach EBM* (3rd ed.). New York: Churchill Livingstone.

Scholes, M., & Barber, B. (1980). Towards nursing informatics. In D. A. D. Lindberg & S. Kaihara (Eds.), *MEDINFO: 1980* (pp. 7-73). Amsterdam, Netherlands: North-Holland.

Sensmeier, J. (2008). Deep impact: Informatics and nursing practice. *Nursing Management IT Solutions Supplement,* September, 2-6.

Simpson, R. (2003). Everything a CNO needs to know about managing information technology. *Nurse Leader, 1*(4), 43-45.

Snyder-Halpern, R., Corcoran-Perry, S., & Narayan, S. (2001). Developing clinical practice environments supporting the knowledge work of nurses. *Computers in Nursing, 19*(1), 17-23.

Staggers, N., & Brennan, P. F. (2007). Translating knowledge into practice: Passing the hot potato! *Journal of the American Medical Informatics Association: JAMIA, 14*, 684-685.

Stead, W. W., Bird, W. P., Califf, R. M., Elchlepp, J. G., Hammond, W. E., & Kinney, T. R. (1993). The IAIMS at Duke University Medical Center: Transition from model testing to implementation. *MD Computing, 10*, 225-230.

Stead, W. W., & Lin, H. S. (Eds.). (2009). *Computational technology for effective health care: Immediate steps and strategic directions.* Washington, DC: National Academies of Science.

Tan, J. (1995). *Health management information systems: Theories, methods, applications.* Gaithersburg, MD: Aspen.

Tannery, N. H., Wessel, C. B., Epstein, B. A., & Gadd, C. S. (2007). Hospital nurses' use of knowledge-based information resources. *Nursing Outlook, 55*, 15-19.

The Joint Commission (TJC). (2008). *Sentinel Event Alert: Safely implementing health information and converging technologies.* Retrieved September 24, 2009, from www.jointcommission. org/SentinelEvents/SentinelEventAlert/sea_42.htm.

The Joint Commission (TJC). (2009). *TJC accreditation manual e-dition.* Retrieved September 24, 2009, from http://e-dition. jcrinc.com/Frame.aspx.

Titler, M. G., Kleiber, C., Steelman, V. J., Rakel, B. A., Budreau, G., Everett, L. Q., Buckwalter, K. C., Tripp-Reimer, T., & Goode, C. J. (2001). The Iowa model of evidence-based practice to promote quality care. *Critical Care Nursing Clinics of North America, 13*(4), 497-509.

Trossman, S. (2001). The documentation dilemma: Nurses poised to address paperwork burden. *The American Nurse, 33*, 1,9,18.

Vidal, M. G., Ruiz Weisser, J., Gonzalez, F., Toro, M. A., Loudet, C., Balasini, C., Canales, H., Reina, R., & Estenssoro, E. (2008). Incidence and clinical effects of intra-abdominal hypertension in critically ill patients. *Critical Care Medicine, 36*, 1823-1831.

Warren, J., & Connors, H. (2007). Health information technology can and will transform nursing education. *Nursing Outlook, 55*, 58-60.

Werley, H. H., & Lang, N. M. (Eds.). (1988). *Identification of the nursing minimum data set.* New York: Springer.

SUGGESTED READINGS

American Nurses Association. (2008). *Nursing informatics: Practice scope and standards of practice.* Silver Spring, MD: Nursesbooks.org.

Englebardt, S. P., & Nelson, R. (2002). *Health care informatics: An interdisciplinary approach.* St. Louis: Mosby.

Hebda, T. L., & Czar, P. (2008). *Handbook of informatics for nurses & healthcare professionals.* Philadelphia: Prentice-Hall.

McGonigle, D. (2008). *Nursing informatics.* Boston: Jones & Bartlett Publishing.

Saba, V., & McCormick, K. A. (2005). *Essentials of nursing informatics.* Hightstown, NJ: McGraw-Hill.

Weaver, C., Delaney, C., Webber, P., & Carr, R. (2006). *Nursing and informatics for the 21st century.* Chicago: Healthcare Information and Management Systems Society (HIMSS).

Managing Costs and Budgets

Trudi B. Stafford

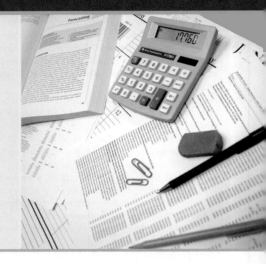

This chapter focuses on methods of financing health care and specific strategies for managing costs and budgets in patient-care settings. Factors that escalate healthcare costs, sources of healthcare financing, reimbursement methods, cost-containment and healthcare reform strategies, and implications for nursing practice are discussed. Various budgets and the budgeting process are explained. In addition to clinical competency and caring practices, understanding the cost issues in healthcare delivery and the ethical implications of financial decisions is essential for nurses to contribute fully to the health and healing of patients and populations.

OBJECTIVES

- Explain several major factors that are escalating the costs of health care.
- Evaluate different reimbursement methods and their incentives to control costs.
- Differentiate costs, charges, and revenue in relation to a specified unit of service, such as a visit, hospital stay, or procedure.
- Value why all healthcare organizations must make a profit.
- Give examples of cost considerations for nurses working in managed care environments.
- Discuss the purpose of and relationships among the operating, cash, and capital budgets.
- Explain the budgeting process.
- Identify variances on monthly expense reports.

TERMS TO KNOW

budget	charges	full-time equivalent (FTE)
budgeting process	contractual allowance	managed care
capital expenditure budget	cost	nonproductive hours
capitation	cost-based reimbursement	operating budget
case mix	cost center	organized delivery system (ODS)
cash budget	fixed costs	payer mix

payers

price

productive hours

productivity

profit

prospective reimbursement

providers

revenue

unit of service

utilization

variable costs

variance

variance analysis

THE CHALLENGE

Marcus Johnson, RN, MSN
Director of Medical-Surgical Services, Central Hospital,
Tempest Health Care System, Detroit, Michigan

Central Hospital (CH) is one of nine acute care hospitals that make up the Tempest Health Care System (THCS). Medical-Surgical Services (MSS) account for 200 of CH's 367 beds. The primary sources of revenue for CH are managed care (42%), Medicare (36%), and self-pay (22%).

Over the past 6 months, the nation has experienced an economic crisis of historic proportion. Locally, three major employers in THCS's market have threatened to file bankruptcy and have laid off thousands of employees.

Revenues for both CH and THCS have declined drastically. Inpatient admissions have decreased, and the payer mix is shifting from managed care to more self-pay. THCS administrators insist that all hospital operations stay budget-neutral. The next fiscally responsible step is to require that variable expenses in hospitals be reduced. Because labor costs are the greatest variable expense in a hospital, such thinking often leads to demands to reduce nursing staff or to substitute lower-paid personnel. As the nurse director of the MSS, my goal is to maintain a high-quality, high-performance work team that adds value for patients. In this situation, what steps can be taken before reducing staff in the MSS? How can I remain budget-neutral during times of economic crisis?

What do you think you would do if you were this nurse?

INTRODUCTION

Healthcare costs in the United States continue to rise at a rate greater than general inflation. In 2009, for example, Americans spent $2.2 trillion for health care—approximately 16.2% of the gross domestic product (GDP). This equals $7026 per person. The health share of the GDP is projected to increase to 19.5% in 2017 (Centers for Medicare & Medicaid Services [CMS], 2008). Yet millions of uninsured and underinsured Americans do not have access to basic healthcare services. With the exception of South Africa, the United States was the only industrialized nation where health care is viewed as a privilege rather than a right.

Despite our huge expenditures, major indicators reveal significant health problems in the United States, as well as large disparities in health status related to gender, race, and socioeconomic status (*Healthy People 2010*, 2001). Our infant mortality rate is among the highest of all industrialized nations, and black infants die at more than twice the rate of white infants. Average life expectancy is lower than that in most developed countries, and men have a life expectancy that is 6 years less than that of women. One in eight women will develop breast cancer during her lifetime, with black and Native American women experiencing a much higher death rate than white women. Violence-related injuries are on the rise, and unintentional injuries, such as motor vehicle accidents, are a leading cause of death. Clearly, we are not receiving a high value return for our healthcare dollar.

The large portion of the GDP that is spent on health care poses problems to the economy in other ways, too. Funds are diverted from needed social programs such as childcare, housing, education, transportation, and the environment. The price of goods and services is increased, and therefore the country's ability to compete in the international marketplace is compromised. The cost of providing health care to automobile manufacturing employees added from $1100 to $1500 to the cost of each of the 4.65 million vehicles General Motors sold in 2004 (Appleby & Carty, 2005). As the amount of the GDP devoted to healthcare expenses rises, the more vulnerable the healthcare industry is to external influences. This creates a major concern for an industry that already expresses concerns about being overregulated.

WHAT ESCALATES HEALTHCARE COSTS?

Total healthcare costs are a function of the prices and the utilization rates of healthcare services (Costs = Price × Utilization) (Table 12-1). *Price* is the rate that healthcare providers set for the services they deliver, such as the hospital rate or physician fee. *Utilization* refers to the quantity or volume of services provided, such as diagnostic tests provided or number of patient visits.

Price inflation and administrative inefficiency are leading contributors to increasing prices for health services. In recent decades, rises in healthcare prices have dramatically outpaced general inflation. Examples of factors that stimulate price inflation are physician incomes that rise faster than average worker earnings and the high prices of prescription drugs, which are often 50% higher than prices in other nations (Bodenheimer & Grumbach, 2009). Administrative inefficiency or waste is primarily a result of the large numbers of clerical personnel whom organizations use to process reimbursement forms from multiple payers. U.S. hospitals spend an average of 20% of their budgets on billing administration alone! This single fact indicates why some hospital administrators advocate for the elimination of multiple payers.

Several interrelated factors contribute to increased utilization of medical services. These include unnecessary care, consumer attitudes, healthcare financing, pharmaceutical usage, and changing population demographics and disease patterns. A substantial amount of unnecessary care does not add health benefits for patients. Inappropriate or ineffective medical procedures are also prevalent and have led to national initiatives to demonstrate efficacy of interventions and to decrease variations in physician practice.

Our attitudes and behaviors as consumers of health care also contribute to rising costs. In general, we prefer to "be fixed" when something goes wrong rather than to practice prevention. When we need "fixing," expensive high-tech services typically are perceived as the best care. Many of us still believe that the physician knows best, so we do not seek much information related to costs and effectiveness of different healthcare options. When we do seek information, it is not readily available or understandable. Also, we are not accustomed to using other, less costly healthcare providers, such as nurse practitioners.

The way health care is financed contributes to rising costs. When health care is reimbursed by third-party payers, consumers are somewhat insulated from personally experiencing the direct effects of high healthcare costs. For example, the huge rise in consumer demand for prescription drugs since 1995 was fueled by low copayments for drugs required by most insurance companies (Heffler et al., 2004). As consumer out-of-pocket expenses for drugs increase, consumer demand should decrease. In most instances, however, consumers do not have many incentives to consider costs when choosing among providers or using services. In addition, the various methods of reimbursement have implications for how providers price and use services.

TABLE 12-1	RELATIONSHIP OF PRICE AND UTILIZATION RATES TO TOTAL HEALTHCARE COSTS			
PRICE ×	**UTILIZATION RATE** =	**TOTAL COST**	**% CHANGE**
$1.00	100	$100.00	0
$1.08*	100	$108.00	+8.0%
$1.08	105†	$113.40	+13.4%
$1.08	110‡	$118.80	+18.8%

*8% increase for inflation.
†5% more procedures done.
‡10% more procedures done.

Evidence of pharmaceutical usage can be seen in advertisements in magazines and on television. No longer do pharmaceutical companies attempt to influence only the prescribers. They go directly to the consumer, who then goes to the prescriber. Because of some typical drug benefit programs, the consumer often is unaware of the total cost of a medication, which may be a "quick fix" (described previously) or a lifestyle enhancement, such as sexual enhancers or skin conditioning.

Changing population demographics also are increasing the volume of health services needed. For example, chronic health problems increase with age and the number of older adults in America is rising. The fastest growing population is the group ages 85 years and older, and Baby Boomers are beginning to move into their senior years. Infectious diseases such as acquired immunodeficiency syndrome (AIDS) and tuberculosis, as well as the growing societal problems of homelessness, drug addiction, and violence, increase demands for health services.

HOW IS HEALTH CARE FINANCED?

On March 23, 2010, historic healthcare reform was signed into law. This phased-in legislation includes some features that take effect quickly and others that are delayed for several years. Pre-existing conditions that often limited an individual's ability to secure health insurance starts with coverage for children. Although the enacted legislation does not cover the entire population, a great majority will be covered. This coverage changes how individuals are insured and thus how they are viewed within the system. Multiple demands for nurses, especially those in advanced practice roles, will continue to emerge over the next several years. As all of these changes unfold, opportunities and challenges exist for the way in which health care will be delivered and paid for, and those changes will alter what nursing does.

Health care is paid for by four sources: government (45%); private insurance companies (35.9%); individuals (15%); and other, primarily philanthropy (4.1%) (Figure 12-1). Three fourths of the government funding is at the federal level. Federal programs include Medicare and health services for members of the military, veterans, American Indians, and federal prisoners. Medicare, the largest federal program, was established in 1965 and pays for care provided to

people 65 years of age and older and some disabled individuals. Medicare Part A is an insurance plan for hospital, hospice, home health, and skilled nursing care that is paid for through Social Security taxes. Nursing home care that is mainly custodial is not covered. Medicare Part B is an optional insurance that covers physician services, medical equipment, and diagnostic tests. Part B is funded through federal taxes and monthly premiums paid by the recipients. Medicare does not cover outpatient medications, eye or hearing examinations, or dental services. The drug benefit plan, effective in 2006, has been viewed as beneficial but very difficult to understand.

Medicaid, a state-level program financed by federal and state funds, pays for services provided to persons who are medically indigent, blind, or disabled and to children with disabilities. The federal government pays between 50% and 83% of total Medicaid costs based on the per capita income of the state. Services funded by Medicaid vary from state to state but must include services provided by hospitals, physicians, laboratories, and radiology departments; prenatal and preventive care; and nursing home and home health-care services.

Private insurance is the second major source of financing for the healthcare system. Most Americans have private health insurance, which usually is provided by employers through group policies. Individuals can purchase health insurance, but typically the rates are very high and provide minimal coverage. Health insurance that is so intertwined with

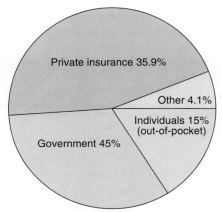

FIGURE 12-1 Sources of financing for health care. These distributions will change as healthcare reform laws take effect.

employment is problematic and contributes to the number of uninsured and underinsured Americans. Many of the uninsured workers are those employed in small businesses that cannot afford to provide group insurance and those who have part-time, seasonal, or service positions.

Individuals also pay directly for health services when they do not have health insurance or when insurance does not cover the service. Costs paid by individuals are called *out-of-pocket expenses* and include deductibles, copayments, and coinsurance. Health insurance benefits often do not cover preventive care, cosmetic surgeries, alternative healthcare therapies, or items such as eyeglasses and nonprescription medications.

REIMBURSEMENT METHODS

Four major payment methods are used for reimbursing healthcare providers: charges, cost-based reimbursement, flat-rate reimbursement, and capitated payments (Zelman, McCue, Millikan, & Glick, 2003). These methods are summarized in Box 12-1. Health-service researchers do not agree on the exact effects of these reimbursement methods on cost and quality. However, considering these effects is important because changes in payment systems have implications for how care is provided in healthcare organizations.

Charges consist of the cost of providing a service plus a markup for profit. Third-party payers often put limitations on what they will pay by establishing usual and customary charges by surveying all providers in a certain area. Usual and customary charges rise over time as providers continually increase their

prices. In cost-based reimbursement, all allowable costs are calculated and used as the basis for payment. Each payer (government or insurance company) determines what the allowable costs are for each procedure, visit, or service. Charges and cost-based reimbursement are retrospective payment methods because the amount of payment is determined after services are delivered. When the reimbursed costs are less than the full charge for the service, a contractual allowance or discount exists. Charges and cost-based reimbursement were the predominant payment method in the 1960s and 1970s but have been largely supplanted by payer fee schedules determined before service delivery.

Flat-rate reimbursement is a method in which the third-party payer decides in advance what will be paid for a service or episode of care. This is a prospective reimbursement method. If the costs of care are greater than the payment, the provider absorbs the loss. If the costs are less than the payment, the provider makes a profit. In 1983, Medicare implemented a prospective payment system (PPS) for hospital care that uses diagnosis-related groups (DRGs) as the basis for payment.

EXERCISE 12-1

What is the contractual allowance when a hospital charges $800 per day to care for a ventilator-dependent patient and an insurance company reimburses the hospital $685 per day? What is the impact on hospital income (revenue) if this is the reimbursement for 2500 patient days?

The DRG system is a classification system that groups patients into categories based on the average number of days of hospitalization for specific medical diagnoses, considering factors such as the patient's age, complications, and other illnesses. Payment includes the expected costs for diagnostic tests, various therapies, surgery, and length of stay (LOS). The cost of nursing services is not explicitly calculated. With a few exceptions, DRGs do not adequately reflect the variability of patient intensity or acuity within the DRG. This is problematic for nursing because the amount of resources (nurses and supplies) used to care for patients is directly related to the patient acuity. Therefore many nurses believe that DRGs are not good predictors of nursing care

BOX 12-1	MAJOR REIMBURSEMENT METHODS
Method	**Inclusions**
Charges	Cost of providing service plus markup
Cost-based (retrospective)	All allowable costs
Flat-rate (prospective)	Rate decided in advance
Capitated	Rate based on designated services over designated time

requirements. Recently, Medicare also began reimbursing home health agencies, nursing homes, and ambulatory care providers through a PPS.

In addition to Medicare, some state Medicaid programs and private insurance companies use a DRG payment system. Although DRGs are not currently used for specialty hospitals (pediatric, psychiatric, and oncology), they are a dominant force in hospital payment. Implementation of a PPS with DRGs resulted in increased patient acuity and decreased LOS in hospitals, along with a greater demand for home care. The need for hospital and community-based nurses also increased.

The resource-based relative value scale (RBRVS) is a flat-rate reimbursement method the federal government uses to pay physicians. Fees in this system are set by estimating the time, cognitive and technical skills, and physical effort required to provide the specific service. Another common flat-rate method is the discounted payments payers negotiate with providers in preferred provider organizations (PPOs).

Capitated payments are based on the provision of specified services to an individual over a set period such as 1 year. Providers are paid a per-person-per-year (or per-month) fee. If the services cost more than the payment, the provider absorbs the loss. Likewise, if the services cost less than the payment, the provider makes a profit. Capitation is the mode of payment characteristic of health maintenance organizations (HMOs) and other managed care systems.

EXERCISE 12-2

Medicare reimburses a hospice $70 for home visits. For one particular group of patients, it costs the hospice an average of $98 per day to provide care. What are the implications for the hospice? What options should the hospice nurse manager and nurses consider?

THE CHANGING HEALTHCARE ECONOMIC ENVIRONMENT

Health care is a major public concern, and rapid changes are occurring in an attempt to reduce costs and improve the health and wellness of the nation. As shown in Box 12-2, strategies shaping the evolving healthcare delivery system include managed care;

BOX 12-2   HEALTHCARE DELIVERY REFORM STRATEGIES

Strategies	Key Features
Managed care	Health plan that includes both service and finance
Organized delivery systems	Networks of organizations; providers and payers
Competition based on price, patient outcomes, and service quality	Basis is cost and quality

---

organized delivery systems (ODSs); and competition based on price, patient outcomes, and service quality. These strategies affect both the pricing and use of health services.

EXERCISE 12-3

For each reimbursement method, think about the incentives for healthcare providers (individuals and organizations) regarding their practice patterns. Are there incentives to change the quantity of services used per patient or the number or types of patients served? Are there incentives to be efficient? List the incentives. How might each method affect overall healthcare costs? (Think in terms of effect on utilization and price.) What do you think the effect on quality of care might be with each payment method?

Managed care is a health plan that brings together the delivery and financing function into one entity, in contrast with a traditional fee-for-service plan, in which insurers pay providers based on costs (Finkler & McHugh, 2007). A major goal of managed care is to decrease unnecessary services, thereby decreasing costs. Managed care also works to ensure timely and appropriate care. HMOs are a type of managed care system in which the primary physician serves as a gatekeeper who determines what services the patient uses. Because HMOs are paid on a capitated basis, it is to the HMO's advantage to practice prevention and use ambulatory care rather than more expensive hospital care. In other forms of managed care, a non-physician case manager arranges and authorizes the services provided. Many insurance companies have used case managers for years. Nurses who work in home health and ambulatory settings often communicate with insurance company case managers to plan the care for specific patients. PPOs

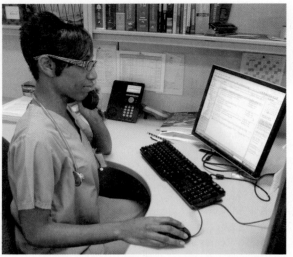

Nurses in ambulatory care settings often work directly with insurance companies to plan patient care.

and point-of-service (POS) plans are other types of managed care plans that give the patient more options than traditional HMOs do for selecting providers and services.

ODSs comprise networks of healthcare organizations, providers, and payers. Typically, this means hospitals, physicians, and insurance companies. The aim of such joint ventures is to develop and market collectively a comprehensive package of healthcare services that will meet most needs of large numbers of consumers. Hospitals, physicians, and payers will share the financial risks of the enterprise. Although hospitals share some risk now with prospective payment, physicians have not generally shared the risk. This risk-sharing is expected to provide incentives to eliminate unnecessary services, use resources more effectively, and improve quality of services.

Competition among healthcare providers increasingly is based on cost and quality outcomes. Decision making regarding price and utilization of services is shifting from physicians and hospitals to payers, who are demanding significant discounts or lower prices. Scientific data that demonstrate positive health outcomes and high-quality services are required. Providers who cannot compete based on price, patient outcomes, and service quality will find it difficult to survive as the system evolves.

WHAT DOES THIS MEAN FOR NURSING PRACTICE?

What does the healthcare economic environment mean for the practicing professional nurse? We must value ourselves as providers and think of our practice within a context of organizational viability and quality of care. To do this, we must add "financial thinking" to our repertoire of nursing skills and we must determine whether the services we provide add value for patients. Services that add value are of high quality, affect health outcomes positively, and minimize costs. The following sections help develop financial thinking skills and ways to consider how nursing practice adds value for patients by minimizing costs.

WHY IS PROFIT NECESSARY?

Private, nongovernmental healthcare organizations may be either for-profit (FP) or not-for-profit (NFP). This designation refers to the tax status of the organization and specifies how the profit can be used. Profit is the excess income left after all expenses have been paid (Revenues − Expenses = Profit). FP organizations pay taxes, and their profits can be distributed to investors and managers. NFP organizations, on the other hand, do not pay taxes and must reinvest all of their profits, commonly called *net income* or *income above expense,* in the organization to better serve the public.

All private healthcare organizations must make a profit to survive. If expenses are greater than revenues, the organization experiences a loss. If revenues equal expenses, the organization breaks even. In both cases, nothing is left over to replace facilities and equipment, expand services, or pay for inflation costs. Some healthcare organizations can survive in the short run without making a profit because they use interest from investments to supplement revenues. The long-term viability of any private healthcare organization, however, depends on consistently making a profit. Box 12-3 presents a simplified example of an income statement from a neighborhood not-for-profit nursing center.

Nurses and nurse managers directly affect an organization's ability to make a profit. Profits can be achieved or improved by decreasing costs or increasing revenues. In tight economic times, many

BOX 12-3   INCOME STATEMENT OF REVENUES AND EXPENSES FROM A NEIGHBORHOOD NURSING CENTER: FYE DECEMBER 31, 2010

Revenues		
Patient revenues	$283,200	
Grant income	60,000	
Other operating revenues	24,000	
TOTAL	$367,200	$367,200
Expenses		
Salary costs	$140,400	
Supplies	64,400	
Other operating expenses (e.g., rent, utilities, administrative services)	79,900	
TOTAL	$284,700	284,700
Excess of revenues over expenses [profit]*		$82,500

FYE, Fiscal year ending.
* Loss would be shown in parentheses ( ) or brackets [ ].

managers think only in terms of cutting costs. Although cost-cutting measures are important, especially to keep prices down so that the organization will be competitive, ways to increase revenues also need to be explored.

EXERCISE 12-4

Obtain a copy of an itemized patient bill from a healthcare organization and review the charges. What was the source and method of payment? How much of these charges were reimbursed? How much was charged for items you regularly use in clinical care?

COST-CONSCIOUS NURSING PRACTICES

Understanding What Is Required to Remain Financially Sound

Understanding what is required for a department or agency to remain financially sound requires that nurses move beyond thinking about costs for individual patients to thinking about income and expenses and numbers of patients needed to make a profit. In a fee-for-service environment, revenue is earned for every service provided. Therefore increasing the volume of services, such as diagnostic tests and patient visits, increases revenues. In a capitated environment in which one fee is paid for all services provided, increasing the overall number of patients served and decreasing the volume of services used is desirable.

With capitation, nurses must strive to accomplish more with each visit to decrease return visits and complications. Many healthcare organizations function in a dual-reimbursement environment—part capitated and part fee-for-service. Nurses need to understand their organization's reimbursement environment and strategy for realizing a profit in its specific circumstances.

Knowing Costs and Reimbursement Practices

As direct caregivers and case managers, nurses are constantly involved in determining the type and quantity of resources used for patients. This includes supplies, personnel, and time. Nurses need to know what costs are generated by their decisions and actions. Nurses also need to know what items cost and how they are paid for in an organization so that they can make cost-effective decisions. For example, nurses need to know per-item costs for supplies so that they can appropriately evaluate lower-cost substitutes.

In ambulatory and home health settings, nurses must be familiar with the various insurance plans that reimburse the organization. Each plan has different contract rules regarding preauthorization, types of services covered, required vendors, and so on. Although nurses must develop and implement their plans of care with full knowledge of these reimbursement practices, the payer does not totally drive the care. Nurses still advocate for patients in important ways while also working within the cost and contractual constraints. Moreover, when nurses understand the reimbursement practices, they can help patients maximize the resources available to them.

In hospitals, the cost of nursing care usually is not calculated or billed separately to patients; instead, it is part of the general per-diem charge. One major problem with this method is the assumption that all patients consume the same amount of nursing care. Another problem with bundling the charges for nursing care with the room rate is that nursing as a clinical service is not perceived by management as generating revenue for the hospital. Rather, nursing is perceived predominantly as an expense to the organization. Although this perception may not matter in a capitated setting in which all provider services are considered a cost, accurate nursing care cost data are needed to negotiate managed care contracts. In addition, patients do not see direct charges and so have no way to understand the monetary value of the services they receive.

EXERCISE 12-5

How was nursing care charged on the bill you obtained? What are the implications for nursing in being perceived as an expense rather than being associated with the revenue stream? Why will this perception be less important in a capitated environment?

Capturing All Charges in a Timely Fashion

Nurses also help contain costs by ensuring that all possible charges are captured. Several large hospitals report more than $1 million a year lost from supplies that were not charged. In hospitals, nurses must know which supplies are charged to patients and which ones are charged to the unit. In addition, the procedures and equipment used need to be accurately documented. In ambulatory and community settings, nurses often need to keep abreast of the codes that are used to bill services. These codes change yearly, and sometimes items are bundled together under one charge and sometimes they are broken down into different charges. Turning in charges in a timely manner is also important because delayed billing negatively affects cash flow by extending the time before an organization is paid for services provided. This is particularly significant in smaller organizations.

In home health, hospice, and long-term care organizations, billing is closely integrated with the clinical information system. For example, to ensure reimbursement, the physician's plan of care and documentation that the patient meets the criteria for admission must be noted on the clinical record. Typically, nurses are responsible for documenting this information.

EXERCISE 12-6

You used three intravenous (IV) catheters to do a particularly difficult venipuncture. Do you charge the patient for all three catheters? What if you accidentally contaminated one by touching the sheet? How is the catheter paid for if not charged to the patient? Who benefits and who loses when patients are not charged for supplies?

Using Time Efficiently

The adage that time is money is fitting in health care and refers to both the nurse's time and the patient's time. When nurses are organized and efficient in their care delivery and in scheduling and coordinating patients' care, the organization will save money. With capitation, doing as much as possible during each episode of care is particularly important to decrease repeat visits and unnecessary service utilization. Because LOS is the most important predictor of hospital costs (Finkler, Kovner, & Jones, 2007), patients who stay extra days cost the hospital a considerable amount. Decreasing LOS also makes room for other patients, thereby potentially increasing patient volume and hospital revenues. Nurses can become more efficient and effective by evaluating their major work processes and eliminating areas of redundancy and rework. Automated clinical information systems that support integrated practice at the point of care will also increase efficiency and improve patient outcomes.

EXERCISE 12-7

The Visiting Nurse Association (VNA) cannot file for reimbursement until all documentation of each visit has been completed. Typically, the paperwork is submitted a week after the visit. When the number of home visits increases rapidly, the paperwork often is not turned in for 2 weeks or more. What are the implications of this routine practice for the agency? Why would the VNA be very vulnerable financially during periods of heavy workload? What are some options for the nurse manager to consider to expedite the paperwork?

Discussing the Cost of Care with Patients

Talking with patients about the cost of care is important, although it may be uncomfortable. Discovering during a clinic visit that a patient cannot afford a specific medication or intervention is preferable to finding out several days later in a follow-up call that the patient has not taken the medication. Such information compels the clinical management team to explore optional treatment plans or to find resources to cover the costs. Talking with patients about costs is important in other ways, too. It involves the patients in the decision-making process and increases the likelihood that treatment plans will be followed. Patients also can make informed choices and better use the resources available to them if they have appropriate information about costs.

EXERCISE 12-8

A new patient visits the clinic and is given prescriptions for three medications that will cost about $120 per month. You check her chart and discover that she has Medicare (but not Part D) and no supplemental insurance. How can you determine whether she has the resources to buy this medicine each month and if she is willing to buy it? If she cannot afford the medications, what are some options?

Meeting Patient Rather Than Provider Needs

Developing an awareness of how feelings about patients' needs influence decisions can help nurses better manage costs. A nurse administrator in a home health agency recently related an account of a nurse who continued to visit a patient for weeks after the patient's health problems had resolved. When questioned, the nurse said she was uncomfortable terminating the visits because the patient continued to tell her he needed her help. Later, the patient revealed that he had not needed nursing care for some time, although he had continued telling the nurse he did because he thought she wanted to keep visiting him. This illustrates how nurses need to verify whose needs are being met with nursing care.

Evaluating Cost-Effectiveness of New Technologies

The advent of new technologies is presenting dilemmas in managing costs. In the past, if a new piece of equipment was easier to use or benefited the patient in any way, nurses were apt to want to use it for everyone, no matter how much more it cost. Now they are forced to make decisions regarding which patients really need the new equipment and which ones will have good outcomes with the current equipment. Essentially, nurses are analyzing the cost-effectiveness of the new equipment with regard to different types of patients to allocate limited resources. This is a new and sometimes difficult way to think about patient care and at times may not feel like a caring way to make decisions regarding patient care. However, such decisions conserve resources without jeopardizing patients' health and thus create the possibility of providing additional healthcare services.

EXERCISE 12-9

Last year, a new positive-pressure, needleless system for administering IV antibiotics was introduced. Because the system was so easy to use and convenient for patients, the nurses in the home infusion company where you worked ordered it for everyone. Typically, patients get their IV antibiotics four times each day. The minibags and tubing for the regular procedure cost the agency $22 a day. The new system costs $24 per medication administration, or $96 a day. The agency receives the same per-diem (daily) reimbursement for each patient. Discuss the financial implications for the agency if this practice is continued. Generate some optional courses of action for the nurses to consider. How should these options be evaluated? What secondary costs, such as the cost of treating fewer needle-stick injuries, should be included?

Predicting and Using Nursing Resources Efficiently

Because healthcare organizations are service institutions, the largest part of their operating budget typically is for personnel. For hospitals, in particular, nurses are the largest group of employees and often account for most of the personnel budget. Staffing is the major area nurse managers can affect with respect to managing costs, and supply management is the second area. To understand why this is so, it is helpful to understand the concepts of fixed and variable costs.

The total fixed costs in a unit are those costs that do not change as the volume of patients changes. In other words, with either a high or a low patient census, expenses related to rent, loan payments, administrative salaries, and salaries of the minimum number of staff to keep a unit open must be paid. Variable costs are costs that vary in direct proportion to patient volume or acuity. Examples include nursing personnel, supplies, and medications. Break-even analysis is a tool that uses fixed and variable costs for determining the volume of patients needed to just break even (Revenue = Expenses) or to realize a profit or loss.

In hospitals and community health agencies, patient classification systems are used to help managers predict nursing care requirements (see Chapter 14). These systems differentiate patients according to acuity of illness, functional status, and resource needs. Some nurses do not like these systems because they believe the essence of nursing is not captured. However, we need to remember that these are tools to help managers predict resource needs. Describing all nursing activities and judgments is not necessary for a tool to be a good predictor. Misguided efforts to sabotage classification systems with the hope for better staffing work primarily to prevent the development of tools to better manage practice. Used appropriately, patient classification systems can help evaluate changing practice patterns and patient acuity levels as well as provide information for budgeting processes.

EXERCISE 12-10
Given the definitions for fixed and variable costs, why do you think nurse managers have the greatest influence over costs through management of staffing and supplies?

Managing staffing and decreasing LOS can achieve the most immediate reductions in costs. Hospitals strive to lower costs so that they will attract new contracts and be attractive as partners in provider networks. Therefore staffing methods and patient care delivery models are being closely scrutinized. Work redesign, a process for changing the way to think about and structure the work of patient care, is the predominant strategy for developing systems that better utilize high-cost professionals and improve service quality. Increased staff retention, patient safety, and positive patient outcomes result from effective work redesign processes.

Using Research to Evaluate Standard Nursing Practices

Nurses use research to restructure their work to ensure they add value for patients. Koelling, Johnson, Cody, and Aaronson (2005) studied the effect of patient education by a nurse educator on the clinical outcomes of patients with heart failure. In this randomized, controlled trial, one group of patients received standard discharge information and the other group of patients received standard discharge information and 1 hour of one-on-one education from a nurse educator. All subjects were followed by telephone after discharge to collect data concerning post-hospitalization clinical events, symptoms, and self-care practices. Patients who received the additional 1-hour teaching session with the nurse

---

📖 LITERATURE PERSPECTIVE

Resource: Virkstis, K. L., Westheim, J., Boston-Fleischhauer, C., Matsui, P. N., & Jaggi, T. (2009). Safeguarding quality: Building the business case to prevent nursing-sensitive hospital-acquired conditions. *The Journal of Nursing Administration, 39*(7/8), 350-355.

In October 2008, The Centers for Medicare & Medicaid Services (CMS) initiated a program that would negatively affect reimbursement for 11 hospital-acquired patient conditions that were judged reasonably preventable. CMS took the stand that it would decrease reimbursement if these conditions were not documented to be present on admission to the hospital. Four of the 11 conditions (catheter-associated urinary tract infections, falls and trauma, vascular catheter–associated infections, and stages III and IV pressure ulcers) have been identified as nursing-sensitive indicators. This article presents a review of the literature related to two of these nursing-sensitive indicators—patient falls and pressure ulcers. They found that the average cost burden for a hospital-acquired pressure ulcer ranged anywhere from $3,529 per case to $52,931 per case. The average cost burden for a patient fall in the hospital averaged $15,418. The article includes tools that nursing leadership can use to estimate potential cost avoidance savings that can be recognized in their individual facilities for falls and pressure ulcers. Through their analysis, these authors found that the strongest business case for nursing leadership is to concentrate their efforts on cost savings through prevention of these two hospital-acquired conditions.

Implications for Practice
The findings from this study show that significant cost savings are associated with the prevention of two nursing-sensitive, hospital-acquired conditions—specifically, falls and pressure ulcers.

educator showed improved clinical outcomes, increased adherence to self-care management, and reduced costs of care because of a reduction in re-hospitalizations. The costs of care, including the costs associated with the additional education session, resulted in a savings of $2823 per patient in the education group as compared with the control group. The findings from this economic evaluation support the implementation of nursing education programs for patients with chronic heart failure as evidenced by improved patient outcomes and reduced costs. Box 12-4 summarizes some cost-conscious strategies for nursing practice. Further, the Literature Perspective on p. 240 describes the need for a business case related to outcomes.

BUDGETS

The basic financial document in most healthcare organizations is the budget—a detailed financial plan for carrying out the activities an organization wants to accomplish for a certain period. An organizational budget is a formal plan that is stated in terms of dollars and includes proposed income and expenditures. The budgeting process is an ongoing activity in which plans are made and revenues and expenses are managed to meet or exceed the goals of the plan. The management functions of planning and control are tied together through the budgeting process.

A budget requires managers to plan ahead and to establish explicit program goals and expectations. Changes in medical practices, reimbursement methods, competition, technology, demographics, and regulatory factors must be forecast to anticipate

their effects on the organization. Planning encourages evaluation of different options and assists in more cost-effective use of resources.

EXERCISE 12-11

A community nursing organization performs an average of 36 intermittent catheterizations each day. A prepackaged catheterization kit that costs the organization $17 is used. The four items in the kit, when purchased individually, cost the organization a total of $5. What factors should be considered in evaluating the cost-effectiveness of the two sources of supplies?

TYPES OF BUDGETS

Several types of interrelated budgets are used by well-managed organizations. Major budgets that are discussed in this chapter include the operating budget, the capital budget, and the cash budget. The way these budgets complement and support one another is depicted in Figure 12-2. Many organizations also use program, product line, or special purpose budgets. Long-range budgets are used to help managers plan for the future. Often, these are referred to as *strategic plans* (Finkler & McHugh, 2007).

Operating Budget

The operating budget is the financial plan for the day-to-day activities of the organization. The expected

---

BOX 12-4	STRATEGIES FOR COST-CONSCIOUS NURSING PRACTICE

1. Understanding what is required to remain financially sound
2. Knowing costs and reimbursement practices
3. Capturing all possible charges in a timely fashion
4. Using time efficiently
5. Discussing the costs of care with patients
6. Meeting patient, rather than provider, needs
7. Evaluating cost-effectiveness of new technologies
8. Predicting and using nursing resources efficiently
9. Using research to evaluate standard nursing practices

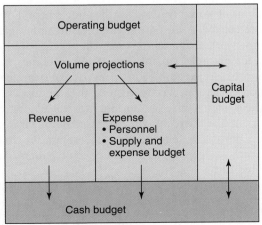

FIGURE 12-2 Interrelationships of the operating, capital, and cash budgets.

TABLE 12-2	WORKLOAD CALCULATION (TOTAL REQUIRED PATIENT CARE HOURS)				
PATIENT ACUITY LEVEL*	HOURS OF CARE PER PATIENT DAY (HPPD)†	×	PATIENT DAYS‡	=	WORKLOAD§
1	3.0		900		2,700
2	5.2		3,100		16,120
3	8.8		4,000		35,200
4	13.0		1,600		20,800
5	19.0		400		7,600
Total			10,000		82,420

* *1*, Low; *5*, high.
†HPPD is the number of hours of care on average for a given acuity level.
‡1 patient per 1 day = 1 patient day.
§Total number of hours of care needed based on acuity levels and numbers of patient days.

revenues and expenses generated from daily operations, given a specified volume of patients, are stated. Preparing and monitoring the operating budget, particularly the expense portion, is often the most time-consuming financial function of nurse managers.

The expense part of the operating budget consists of a personnel budget and a supply and expense budget for each cost center. A cost center is an organizational unit for which costs can be identified and managed. The personnel budget is the largest part of the operating budget for most nursing units. (See The Evidence section on p. 248.)

Before the personnel budget can be established, the volume of work predicted for the budget period must be calculated. A unit of service measure appropriate to the work of the unit is used. Units of service may be, for example, patient days, clinic or home visits, hours of service, admissions, deliveries, or treatments. Another factor needed to calculate the workload is the patient acuity mix. The formula for calculating the workload or the required patient care hours for inpatient units is as follows: Workload volume = Hours of care per patient day × Number of patient days (Table 12-2).

In some organizations, the workload is established by the financial office and given to the nurse manager. In other organizations, nurse managers forecast the volume. In both situations, nurse managers should inform administration about any factors that might affect the accuracy of the forecast, such as changes in physician practice patterns, new treatment modalities, or changes in inpatient versus outpatient treatment practices.

The next step in preparing the personnel budget is to determine how many staff members will be needed to provide the care. (This topic is discussed in more detail in Chapter 14.) Because some people work full-time and others work part-time, full-time equivalents (FTEs) are used in this step rather than positions. Generally, one FTE can be equated to working 40 hours per week, 52 weeks per year, for a total of 2080 hours of work paid per year. One half of an FTE (0.5 FTE) equates to 20 hours per week. The number of hours per FTE may vary within an organization in relation to staffing plans, so it is important to check.

The 2080 hours paid to an FTE in a year consist of both productive hours and nonproductive hours. Productive hours are paid time that is worked. Nonproductive hours are paid time that is not worked, such as vacation, holiday, orientation, education, and sick time. Before the number of FTEs needed for the workload can be calculated, the number of productive hours per FTE is determined by subtracting the total number of nonproductive hours per FTE from total paid hours. Alternatively, payroll reports can be reviewed to determine the percentage of paid hours that are productive for each FTE. Finally, the total

BOX 12-5   PRODUCTIVE HOURS CALCULATION

Method 1:   **Add all nonproductive hours/FTE and subtract from paid hours/FTE**

Example:	Vacation	15 days
	Holiday	7 days
	Average sick time	4 days
	TOTAL	26 days

26 × 8* hours = 208 nonproductive hours/FTE
2080 − 208 = 1872 productive hours/FTE

Method 2:   **Multiply paid hours/FTE by percentage of productive hours/FTE**

Example: Productive hours = 90%/FTE
(1872 productive hours of total 2080 = 90%)
2080 × 0.90 = 1872 productive hours/FTE

Total FTE Calculation

Required Patient Care Hours	÷	Productive Hours Per FTE	=	Total FTEs Needed
82,420	÷	1872		= 44 FTEs

FTE, Full-time equivalent.
*Based on an 8-hour shift pattern.

number of FTEs needed to provide the care is calculated by dividing the total patient care hours required by the number of productive hours per FTE (Box 12-5).

The total number of FTEs calculated by this method represents the number needed to provide care each day of the year. It does not reflect the number of positions or the number of people working each day. In fact, the number of positions may be much higher, particularly if many part-time nurses are employed. On any given day, some nurses may be scheduled for their regular day off or vacation and others may be off because of illness. Also, some positions that do not involve direct patient care, such as nurse managers or unit secretaries, may not be replaced during nonproductive time. Only one FTE is budgeted for any position that is not covered with other staff when the employee is off.

> **EXERCISE 12-12**
> Change the number of patients at each acuity level listed in Table 12-2, but keep the total number of patients the same. Recalculate the required total workload. Discuss how changes in patient acuity affect nursing resource requirements.

The next step is to prepare a daily staffing plan and to establish positions (see Chapter 14). Once the positions are established, the labor costs that comprise the personnel budget can be calculated. Factors that must be addressed include straight-time hours, overtime hours, differentials and premium pay, raises, and benefits (Finkler & McHugh, 2007). Differentials and premiums are extra pay for working specific times, such as evening or night shifts and holidays. Benefits usually include health and life insurance, Social Security payments, and retirement plans. Benefits often cost an additional 20% to 25% of a full-time employee's salary.

> **EXERCISE 12-13**
> If the percentage of productive hours per FTE is 80%, how many worked or productive hours are there per FTE? If total patient care hours are 82,420, how many FTEs will be needed?

The supply and expense budget is often called the *other-than-personnel services (OTPS) expense budget.* This budget includes a variety of items used in daily unit activities, such as medical and office supplies, minor equipment, and books and journals; it also includes orientation, training, and travel. Although different methods are used to calculate the supply and expense budget, the previous year's expenses usually are used as a baseline. This baseline is adjusted for projected patient volume and specific circumstances known to affect expenses, such as predictable personnel turnover, which increases orientation and training expenses. A percentage factor is also added to adjust for inflation.

The final component of the operating budget is the revenue budget. The revenue budget projects the income that the organization will receive for providing patient care. Historically, nurses have not been directly involved with developing the revenue budget, although this is beginning to change. In most hospitals, the revenue budget is established by the financial office and given to nurse managers. The anticipated revenues are calculated according to the price per patient day. Data about the volume and types of patients and reimbursement sources (i.e., the case mix and the payer mix) are necessary to project revenues in any healthcare organization. Even when nurse managers do not participate in developing the revenue budget, learning about the organization's revenue base is essential for good decision making.

Capital Expenditure Budget

The capital expenditure budget reflects expenses related to the purchase of major capital items such as equipment and physical plant. A capital expenditure must have a useful life of more than 1 year and must exceed a cost level specified by the organization. The minimum cost requirement for capital items in healthcare organizations is usually from $300 to $1000, although some organizations have a much higher level. Anything below that minimum is considered a routine operating cost.

Capital expenses are kept separate from the operating budget because their high cost would make the costs of providing patient care appear too high during the year of purchase. To account for capital expenses, the costs of capital items are depreciated. This means that each year, over the useful life of the equipment, a portion of its cost is allocated to the operating budget as an expense. Therefore capital expenditures are subtracted from revenues and, in turn, affect profits.

Organizations usually set aside a fixed amount of money for capital expenditures each year. Complete well-documented justifications are needed because the competition for limited resources is stiff. Justifications should include projected amount of use;

services duplicated or replaced; safety considerations; need for space, personnel, or building renovation; effect on operational revenues and expenses; and contribution to the strategic plan.

Cash Budget

The cash budget is the operating plan for monthly cash receipts and disbursements. Organizational survival depends on paying bills on time. Organizations can be making a profit and still run out of cash. In fact, a profitable trend, such as a rapidly growing census, can induce a cash shortage because of increased expenses in the short run. Major capital expenditures can also cause a temporary cash crisis and so must be staggered in a strategic way. Because cash is the lifeblood of any organization, the cash budget is as important as the operating and capital budgets (Finkler & McHugh, 2007).

The financial officer prepares the cash budget in large organizations. Understanding the cash budget helps nurse managers discern (1) when constraints on spending are necessary, even when the expenditures are budgeted and (2) the importance of carefully predicting when budgeted items will be needed.

THE BUDGETING PROCESS

The steps in the budgeting process are similar in most healthcare organizations, although the budgeting period, budget timetable, and level of manager and employee participation vary. Budgeting is done annually and in relation to the organization's fiscal year. A fiscal year exists for financial purposes and can begin at any point on the calendar. In the title of some financial reports, a phrase similar to "FYE June 30, 2010" appears and means that this report is for the fiscal year ending on the date stated.

Major steps in the budgeting process include gathering information and planning, developing unit budgets, developing the cash budget, negotiating and revising, and using feedback to control budget results and improve future plans (Finkler & McHugh, 2007). A timetable with specific dates for implementing the budgeting process is developed by each organization. The timetable may be anywhere from 3 to 9 months. The widespread use of computers for budgeting is reducing the time span for budgeting in many organizations. Box 12-6 outlines the budgeting process.

Modified from Finkler, S. A., Kovner, C. T., & Jones, C. (2007). *Financial management for nurse managers and executives* (3rd ed.). St. Louis: Saunders.

The information-gathering and planning phase provides nurse managers with data essential for developing their individual budgets. This step begins with an environmental assessment that helps the organization understand its position in relation to the entire community. The assessment includes, for example, the changing healthcare needs of the population, influential economic factors such as inflation and unemployment, differences in reimbursement patterns, and patient satisfaction.

Next, the organization's long-term goals and objectives are reassessed in light of the organization's mission and the environmental analysis. This helps all managers situate the budgeting process for their individual units in relation to the whole organization. At this point, programs are prioritized so that resources can be allocated to programs that best help the organization achieve its long-term goals.

Specific, measurable objectives are then established, and the budgets must meet these objectives. The financial objectives might include limiting expenditure increases or making reductions in personnel costs by designated percentages. Nurse managers also set operational objectives for their units that are in concert with the rest of the organization. This is where units or departments interpret what effect the changes in operational activities will have on them.

For instance, how will using case managers and care maps for selected patients affect a particular unit? Establishing the unit-level objectives is also a good place for involving staff nurses in setting the future direction of the unit.

Along with the specific organization and unit-level operating objectives, managers need the organization-wide assumptions that underpin the budgeting process. Explicit assumptions regarding salary increases, inflation factors, and volume projections for the next fiscal year are essential. With this information in hand, nurse managers can develop the operating and capital budgets for their units. These are usually developed in tandem because each affects the other. For instance, purchasing a new monitoring system will have implications for the supplies used, staffing, and staff training.

The cash budget is developed after unit and department operating and capital budgets. Then the negotiation and revision process begins in earnest. This is a complex process because changes in one budget usually require changes in others. Learning to defend and negotiate budgets is an important skill for nurse managers. Nurse managers who successfully negotiate budgets know how costs are allocated and are comfortable speaking about what resources are contained in each budget category. They also can clearly and specifically depict what the effect of not having that resource will be on patient, nurse, or organizational outcomes.

EXERCISE 12-14

If you can interview a nurse manager, ask to review the budgeting process. Ask specifically about the budget timetable, operating objectives, and organizational assumptions. What was the level of involvement for nurse managers and nurses in each step of budget preparation? Is there a budget manual?

The final and ongoing phase of the budgeting process relates to the control function of management. Feedback is obtained regularly so that organizational activities can be adjusted to maintain efficient operations. Variance analysis is the major control process used. A variance is the difference between the projected budget and the actual performance for a particular account. For expenses, a favorable, or positive, variance means that the budgeted amount was greater than the actual amount spent. An unfavorable, or negative, variance means that the budgeted amount was less than the actual amount spent. Positive and negative variances cannot be interpreted as good or bad without further investigation. For example, if fewer supplies were used than were budgeted, this would appear as a positive variance and the unit would save money. This would be good news if it means that supplies were used more efficiently and patient outcomes remained the same or improved. A problem might be suggested, however, if using fewer or less-expensive supplies led to poorer patient outcomes. Or it might mean that exactly the right amount of supplies was used but that the patient census was less than budgeted. To help managers interpret and use variance information better, some institutions use flexible budgets that automatically account for census variances.

EXERCISE 12-15

Examine Table 12-3 and identify major budget variances for the current month. Are they favorable or unfavorable? What additional information would help you explain the variances? What are some possible causes for each variance? Are the causes you identified controllable by the nurse manager? Why or why not? Is a favorable variance on expenses always desirable? Why or why not?

MANAGING THE UNIT-LEVEL BUDGET

How is a unit-based budget managed? At a minimum, nurse managers are responsible for meeting the fiscal goals related to the personnel and the supply and expense part of the operations budget. Typically, monthly reports of operations (see Table 12-3) are sent to nurse managers, who then investigate and

TABLE 12-3   STATEMENT OF OPERATIONS SHOWING PROFIT AND LOSS FROM A NEIGHBORHOOD NURSING CENTER: MARCH 31, 2010

| CURRENT MONTH | | | | YEAR-TO-DATE | | |
BUDGET	ACTUAL	VARIANCE	REVENUES	BUDGET	ACTUAL	VARIANCE
Patient Revenues						
21,500	22,050	550	Insurance payment	64,500	66,150	1,650
1,500	1,550	50	Donations	4,500	4,750	250
23,000	23,600	600	Net Patient Revenues	69,000	70,900	1,900
Non-Patient Revenues						
5,000	5,000	0	Grant income (#138-FG)	15,000	15,000	0
500	500	0	Rent income	1,500	1,500	0
5,500	5,500	0	Net Non-patient Revenues	16,500	16,500	0
28,500	29,100	600	Net Revenues	85,500	87,400	1,900
Expenses						
			Personnel			
7,750	8,500	(750)	Managerial/professional	23,250	24,400	(1,150)
2,000	1,800	200	Clerical/technical	6,000	5,800	200
9,750	10,300	(550)	Net salaries and wages	29,250	30,200	(950)
1,200	1,400	(200)	Benefits	3,600	4,000	(400)
10,950	11,700	(750)	Net Personnel	32,850	34,200	(1,350)
			Non-personnel			
2,500	2,500	0	Office operating expenses	7,500	7,500	0
2,000	2,100	(100)	Supplies and materials	3,000	3,050	(50)
300	450	(150)	Travel expenses	900	450	450
4,800	5,050	(250)	Net Non-personnel	11,400	11,000	400
15,750	16,750	(1,000)	Net Expenses	44,250	45,200	(950)
Revenues Over/Under Expenses						
3,750	3,350	(400)	Net Income	11,250	11,800	550

explain the underlying cause of variances greater than 5%. Many factors can cause budget variances, including patient census, patient acuity, vacation and benefit time, illness, orientation, staff meetings, workshops, employee mix, salaries, and staffing levels. To accurately interpret budget variances, nurse managers need reliable data about patient census, acuity, and LOS; payroll reports; and unit productivity reports.

Nurse managers can control *some* of the factors that cause variances, but not all. After the causes are determined and if they are controllable by the nurse manager, steps are taken to prevent the variance from occurring in the future. However, even uncontrollable variances that increase expenses might require actions of nurse managers. For example, if supply costs rise drastically because a new technology is being used, the nurse manager might have to look for other areas where the budget can be cut. Information learned from analyzing variances also is used in future budget preparations and management activities. The Research Perspective below shows an example of why analysis of the literature and its translation into practice needs to be studied in light of cost impact.

 RESEARCH PERSPECTIVE

Resource: Brooks, J. M., Titler, M. G., Ardery, G., & Herr, K. (2009). Effect of evidence-based acute pain management practices on inpatient costs. *Health Services Research, 44*(1), 245-263.

This randomized study was undertaken to estimate hospital cost changes associated with implementation of "translating research into practice" (TRIP) acute pain management practices and to estimate the direct effect that these practices has on inpatient cost. The program was designed to increase the use of evidence-based pain management practices for patients hospitalized with hip fractures. The average cost of implementing the TRIP intervention within a hospital was $17,714, which included increased cost of nursing services, special operating rooms, and therapy services. The cost savings per inpatient stay was over $1500. This study concluded that hospitals treating more than 12 patients with hip fractures can lower overall cost by implementing the TRIP intervention.

Implications for Practice
The findings from this economic evaluation support the implementation of evidence-based practices for pain management for patients with hip fractures that will more than pay for itself in hospitals that treat more than 12 patients with hip fractures.

In addition, nurse managers monitor the productivity of their units. Productivity is the ratio of outputs to inputs; that is, productivity equals output/ input. In nursing, outputs are nursing services and are measured by hours of care, number of home visits, and so forth. The inputs are the resources used to provide the services such as personnel hours and supplies. Only decreasing the inputs or increasing the outputs can increase productivity. Hospitals often use hours per patient day (HPPD) as one measure of productivity. For example, if the standard of care in a critical care unit is 12 HPPD, then 360 hours of care are required for 30 patients for 1 day. When 320 hours of care are provided, the productivity rating is 113% (360/320 = 1.13), meaning productivity was increased or needed care was not delivered. One must consider the quality component into any productivity model related to care. In home health, the number of visits per day per registered nurse is one measure of productivity. If the standard is 5 visits per day but the weekly average was 4.8 visits per day, then productivity was decreased. Variances in productivity are not inherently favorable or unfavorable and thus require investigation and explanation before judgments can be made about them. For example, an explanation of the variance (4.8 visits per day) might include the fact that one visit took twice the amount of time normally spent on a home visit because of patient needs, thus preventing the nurse from making the standard 5 visits per day. The extra time spent on one patient was productive time but not adequately accounted for by this measure of productivity (visits per day).

Although they do not have a direct accountability for the budget, staff nurses play an important role in meeting budget expectations. Many nurse managers find that routinely sharing the budget and budget-monitoring activities with the staff fosters an appreciation of the relationship between cost and the mission to deliver high-quality patient care. Providing staff with access to cost and utilization data allows them to identify patterns and participate in selecting appropriate, cost-effective practice options that work for the staff and patients. Managers and staff who work in partnership to understand that cost versus care is a dilemma to manage rather than a problem to solve will develop innovative, cost-conscious nursing practices that produce good outcomes for patients, nurses, and the organization.

THE SOLUTION

I began by investigating the reasons for our decreased admissions and shift in payer mix. I discovered that one of our highest admitting physicians is now admitting his patients to a competitor hospital. I met with him to determine why his admission pattern had changed. Most of his patients are employed in local industry, and their health care provider is Reform Health Insurance (RHI). THCS recently dropped our contract with RHI. His patients are requesting hospitalization at our competitor to stay in-network with their health insurance plan.

In an effort to reduce labor costs without compromising quality patient care, I focused on staffing appropriately to census and patient acuity. During times of low census, staff are now flexed and floated to other MSS units with greater staffing needs. In return, during times of high census, nurses from other units are flexed and floated to our unit.

Our Staff Nurse Council developed an initiative to reduce overtime. The reason for most of our overtime is charting at the end of shift. The overtime reduction initiative emphasizes improved teamwork and concurrent charting to reduce end-of-shift charting.

THCS secured a new contract with RHI, which resulted in an increase in census. Flexing and floating staff continues to be challenging. Nurses prefer to work on their "home" unit but appreciate that their hours are not cut if they float to another MSS unit. The staff-driven initiative regarding overtime has been our biggest success. In an effort to ensure that no nurse has overtime at the end of their shift, the nurses are collaborating, communicating, and supporting each other throughout the shift to facilitate concurrent charting. This effort has improved our financial performance and our employee engagement through a stronger sense of teamwork. Because of the combined efforts of nursing leadership, collaboration with physicians, and innovative initiatives by the frontline staff, we have had no staff reductions, and our financial performance is better than budget.

—Marcus Johnson

Would this be a suitable approach for you? Why?

THE EVIDENCE

Anderson and Shelton (2006) share the experiences of two merging hospitals and their use of the same nursing department scheduling system. One hospital used the system for staff scheduling, whereas the other hospital used it for workload measure and management decision making. Staff and leadership personnel were taught the entire content of the system, because information from this system would influence decision making at all levels within the organization. Consistent use of the product produced data that could be drilled down by cost center on FTEs overall, per patient day, overtime, and professional time. This collection of data proved to be invaluable for managers at all levels for both scheduling and overall labor management. Recently, an additional tool included in the system has been instituted to automate shift selections for staff. This feature allows managers to post openings in shifts 6 weeks in advance. Through the computerized system, nurses can easily pick up these additional open shifts. Employee satisfaction has improved as nurses gained more control over their schedules. Full use of the department scheduling system has been linked to improved nurse recruitment and retention. The nurse vacancy rate dropped from 14% to 3%, and nurse turnover dropped to 4% to 5%.

NEED TO KNOW NOW

- Determine the most commonly used equipment and how much it costs so that you know that aspect of care.
- Know the costs and charges (if applicable) of the 20 most frequently used supplies on your unit.
- Know how to retrieve literature related to best practice in staffing according to patient acuity and patient census.
- Know how to retrieve literature related to cost savings in nursing practice.

CHAPTER CHECKLIST

Financial thinking skills are the cornerstone of cost-conscious nursing practice and are essential for all nurses. Nurses must also determine whether the services they provide add value for patients. Services that add value are of high quality, positively affect health outcomes, and minimize costs.

Understanding what constitutes profit and why organizations must make a profit to survive is basic to financial thinking. Knowing what is included in operating, capital, and cash budgets; how they interrelate; and how they are developed, monitored, and controlled is also important. Considering the ethical implications of financial decisions and collectively managing the cost-care dilemma are imperative for cost-conscious nursing practice.

- U.S. health indicators suggest that, as a nation, we are not getting a high value return on our healthcare dollar.
- Total healthcare costs are a function of price and utilization of services.
- The government and insurance companies are the major payers for healthcare services. Individuals are the third major payer.
- Health care has moved toward managed care, organized delivery systems, and competition based on cost and quality outcomes.
- All private healthcare organizations must make a profit to survive.
- Nurses and nurse managers directly influence an organization's ability to make a profit.
- Cost-conscious nursing practices include the following:
  - Understanding what is required to remain financially sound
  - Knowing costs and reimbursement practices
  - Capturing all possible charges in a timely fashion
  - Using time efficiently
  - Discussing the costs of care with patients
  - Meeting patient, rather than provider, needs
  - Evaluating cost-effectiveness of new technologies
  - Predicting accurately and using nursing resources efficiently
  - Using research to evaluate standard nursing practices
- Nurse managers have the most influence on costs in relation to managing personnel and supplies.
- Variance analysis is the major control process in relation to budgeting.

TIPS FOR MANAGING COSTS AND BUDGETS

- Know the major changes in the organization and how they might affect the organization's budget.
- Analyze the supplies you use in providing care and what is commonly missing as one way to make recommendations about supply needs.
- Evaluate what each of your patients would find most helpful during the time you will be caring for them.
- Decide which of your actions create costs for the patient or the organization.
- Be aware of how changes in patient acuity and patient census affect staffing requirements and the unit budget.
- Know how charges are generated and how the documentation systems relate to billing.
- Examine the upsides and downsides of the cost-care polarity thoughtfully.

REFERENCES

Anderson, D. J., & Shelton, W. (2006). Clarify your financial picture with staff management tools. *Nursing Management*, 37(7), 49-51.

Appleby, J., & Carty, S. S. (June 22, 2005). Ailing GM looks to scale back health benefits. *USA Today*. Retrieved October 9, 2009, from www.usatoday.com/money/autos/2005-06-22-gm-healthcare-usat_x.htm.

Bodenheimer, T., & Grumbach, K. (2009). *Understanding health policy: A clinical approach* (5th ed.). New York: McGraw-Hill.

Brooks, J. M., Titler, M. G., Ardery, G., & Herr, K. (2009). Effect of evidence-based acute pain management practices on inpatient costs. *Health Services Research*, 44(1), 245-263.

Centers for Medicare & Medicaid Services (CMS). (2008). *National health expenditure fact sheet.* Retrieved October 9, 2009, from www.cms.hhs.gov/NationalHealthExpendData/25_NHE_Fact_Sheet.asp#TopOfPage, 2008.

Finkler, S. A., Kovner, C. T., & Jones, C. (2007). *Financial management for nurse managers and executives* (3rd ed.). St. Louis: Saunders.

Finkler, S. A., & McHugh, M. (2007). *Budgeting concepts for nurse managers* (4th ed.). St. Louis: Saunders.

Healthy People 2010. (2001). Retrieved October 9, 2009, from www.healthypeople.gov.

Heffler, S., Smith, S., Keehan, S., Clemens, M. K., Zezza, M., & Truffer, C. (2004). Health spending projections through 2013. *Health Affairs, (Suppl. Web exclusives), W4,* 79-93.

Koelling, T. M., Johnson, M. L., Cody, R. J., & Aaronson, K. D. (2005). Discharge education improves clinical outcomes in patients with chronic heart failure. *Circulation, 111,* 179-185.

Virkstis, K. L, Westheim, J., Boston-Fleischhauer, C., Matsui, P. N., & Jaggi, T. (2009). Safeguarding quality: Building the business case to prevent nursing-sensitive hospital-acquired conditions. *The Journal of Nursing Administration, 39*(7/8), 350-355.

Zelman, W., McCue, M. J., Millikan, A. R., & Glick, N. D. (2003). *Financial management of health care organizations: An introduction to fundamental tools, concepts, & applications* (2nd ed.). Malden, MA: Blackwell.

SUGGESTED READINGS

Aiken, L. H. (2008). Economics of nursing. *Policy, Politics, & Nursing Practice, 9*(2), 73-79.

Blegen, M. A., Vaughn, T., & Vojir, C. P. (2007). Nurse staffing levels: Impact of organizational characteristics and registered nurse supply. *Health Services Research, 43*(1, Part 1), 154-173.

Chang, C., Price, S., & Pfoutz, S. (2001). *Economics and nursing: Critical professional issues.* Philadelphia: F.A. Davis.

Clarke, S. P. (2007). Nurse staffing in acute care settings: Research perspectives and practice implications. *Joint Commission Journal on Quality and Patient Safety, 33*(Suppl. 11), 30-44.

Feldstein, P. J. (2004). *Health care economics* (6th ed.). Clifton Park, NY: Thomson Delmar Learning.

Finkler, S. A., Ward, D. M., & Baker, J. J. (2007). *Essentials of cost accounting for health care organizations* (3rd ed.). Sudbury, MA: Jones & Bartlett.

Ghosh, B., & Cruz, G. (2005). Nurse requirement planning: A computer-based model. *Journal of Nursing Management, 13,* 363-371.

Huber, D. (2010). *Leadership & nursing care management* (4th ed.). St. Louis: Saunders.

Johnson, B. (1996). *Polarity management: Identifying and managing unsolvable problems.* Amherst, MA: HRD Press.

Junttila, K., Meretoja, R., Seppala, A., Tolppanen, E., Ala-Nikkola, T., & Silvennoinen, L. (2007). Data warehouse approach to nursing management. *Journal of Nursing Management, 15,* 155-161.

Needleman, J. (2008). Is what's good for the patient good for the Hospital? Aligning incentives and the business case for nursing. *Policy, Politics, & Nursing Practice, 9*(2), 80-87.

Newbold, D. (2008). The production economics of nursing: A discussion paper. *International Journal of Nursing Studies, 45,* 120-128.

Shi, L., & Singh, D. (2007). *Delivering health care in America: A systems approach* (4th ed.). Boston, MA: Jones & Bartlett.

Sultz, H., & Young, K. (2005). *Health care USA: Understanding its organization* (5th ed.). Boston, MA: Jones & Bartlett.

Ward, W. (1988). *An introduction to health care financial management.* Owings Mills, MD: National Health Publishing.

Welton, J. M., Unruh, L., & Halloran, E. J. (2006). Nurse staffing: Nursing intensity, staff mix, and direct nursing care costs across Massachusetts hospitals. *Journal of Nursing Administration, 36*(9), 416-425.

Wesorick, B., Shiparski, L., Troseth, M., & Wyngarden, K. (1997). *Partnership council field book: Strategies and tools for co-creating a healthy work place.* Grand Rapids, MI: Practice Field Publishing.

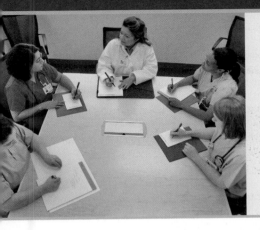

Care Delivery Strategies

Susan Sportsman

This chapter introduces nursing care delivery models used in healthcare agencies to organize care. The historical development and structure of the case method; functional nursing; team nursing; primary nursing, including hybrid forms of this approach; and nursing case management are presented. The discussion summarizes the benefits and disadvantages of each model with an explanation of the nurse manager's and staff nurse's role. In addition, strategies that influence care delivery, such as disease management, differentiated practice, and "transforming care at the bedside," are discussed

OBJECTIVES

- Differentiate the characteristics of nursing care delivery models used in health care.
- Determine the role of the nurse manager and the staff nurse in each model.
- Describe the implementation of a disease-management program.
- Summarize the differentiated nursing practice model and related methods to determine competencies of nurses who deliver care.
- Consider the impact of "transforming care at the bedside" (TCAB) on the delivery of care in a specific nursing unit.

TERMS TO KNOW

advanced generalist
associate nurse
case-management model
case manager
case method
charge nurse
clinical nurse leader
critical path or pathway
differentiated nursing practice
disease management

expected outcomes
functional model of nursing
Magnet Recognition Program®
nursing care delivery model
nursing case management
outcome criteria
partnership model
patient-focused care
patient outcomes
primary nurse

primary nursing
staff mix
Synergy Model
team nursing
total patient care
Transforming Care at the
    Bedside (TCAB)
unlicensed assistive (or nursing)
    personnel
variance

THE CHALLENGE

Jacqueline Ward, RN, BSN
Assistant Director of Nursing, Texas Children's Hospital, Houston, Texas

The charge nurses on a newly designed 36-bed hematology-oncology unit were having increased difficulty in making patient assignments because of the layout and design of the 36,000-square-foot unit. In addition, throughout the shift, the nursing staff members were having difficulty remaining engaged with the activities on the unit because of the distance between bedside stations. Also, the layout of the unit made it difficult for a nurse to ask for help when needed.

After occupying the unit for several months and trying diverse methods to enhance teamwork and communication among the staff, it was apparent that a more formal process was needed to resolve these problems. The assistant director of nursing was assigned to coordinate the resolution of the problem.

What do you think you would do if you were this nurse?

INTRODUCTION

A **nursing care delivery model** is the method used to provide care to patients. Because nursing care is viewed by some as a cost rather than a source of revenue, it is logical for institutions to evaluate their method of providing patient care for the purpose of saving money while still providing quality care. In this chapter, various models of nursing care delivery are discussed, including case method (total patient care); functional nursing; team nursing; primary nursing including hybrid forms; and nursing case management. In addition, the influence of disease-management programs, differentiated nursing practice, and "Transforming Care at the Bedside" is introduced.

Each nursing care delivery model has advantages and disadvantages, and none is ideal. Some methods are conducive to large institutions, whereas other systems may work better in smaller community settings. Managers in any organization must examine the organizational goals, the unit objectives, patient population, staff availability, and the budget when selecting a care delivery model. This historical overview of the common care models is designed to convey the complexity of how care is delivered. This perspective is important because each of these approaches is still used within the broad range of healthcare organizations. In addition, these models often serve as the foundation for new innovative care delivery models.

CASE METHOD (TOTAL PATIENT CARE)

The **case method,** or **total patient care** method, of nursing care delivery is the oldest method of providing care to a patient. This model should not be confused with nursing case management, which is introduced later in the chapter.

The premise of the case method is that one nurse provides total care for one patient during the entire work period. This method was used in the era of Florence Nightingale when patients received total care in the home. Today, total patient care is used in critical care settings where one nurse provides total care to one or two critically ill patients. Nurse educators often select this method of care when students are caring for patients. Variations of the case method exist, and it is possible to identify similarities after reviewing other methods of patient care delivery described later in this chapter.

Model Analysis

During an 8- or 12-hour shift, the patient receives consistent care from one nurse. The nurse, patient, and family usually trust one another and can work together toward specific goals. Usually, the care is patient-centered, comprehensive, continuous, and holistic. But the nurse may choose to deliver this care with a task orientation that negates the holistic perspective (Tiedeman & Lookinland, 2004). Because the nurse is with the patient during most of the shift, even subtle changes in the patient's status are easily noticed (Figure 13-1).

In today's costly healthcare economy, total patient care provided by a registered nurse (RN) is very expensive. Is it realistic to use the highly skilled and extremely knowledgeable professional nurse to provide all the care required in a unit that may have 20 to 30 patients? Who oversees the care coordination in a 24-hour period (Tiedeman & Lookinland, 2004)?

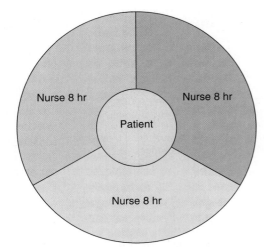

FIGURE 13-1 Case method of patient care for an 8-hour shift.

In times of nursing shortages, there may not be enough resources or nurses to use this model.

Nurse Manager's Role

When using the case method of delivery, the manager must consider the expense of the system. He or she must weigh the expense of an RN versus the expense of licensed practical (vocational) nurses (LPNs/LVNs) and unlicensed assistive (or nursing) personnel in the context of the outcomes required. Unlicensed assistive personnel (UAPs), as the name connotes, are not licensed as healthcare providers. In nursing, they are technicians, nurse aides, and certified nursing assistants. When the patient requires 24-hour care; the nurse manager must decide whether the patient should have RN care or RN-supervised care provided by LPNs/LVNs or unlicensed assistive personnel.

Staff RN's Role

In the case method, the staff RN provides holistic care to a group of patients during a defined work time. The physical, emotional, and technical aspects of care are the responsibility of the assigned RN. This model is especially useful in the care of complex patients who need active symptom management provided by an RN, such as the care of the patient in a hospice setting or an intensive care unit. This care delivery model requires the nurse who is assigned to total patient care to complete the complex functions of care, such as

assessment and teaching the patient and family, as well as the less complex functional aspects of care, such as personal hygiene. Some nurses find satisfaction with this model of care because no aspect of nursing care is delegated to another, thus eliminating the need for supervision of others (Tiedeman & Lookinland, 2004).

> **EXERCISE 13-1**
> You have recently accepted a position at a home health agency that provides 24-hour care to qualified patients. You are assigned a patient who has care provided by an RN during the day, an LPN/LVN in the evening, and a nursing assistant at night. You are the day RN. You are concerned that the patient is not progressing well, and you suspect that the evening and night shift personnel are not reporting changes in the patient's status. What specific assessments should you make to validate your concerns? How would you justify any change in staffing? What recommendations would you make to the nurse manager, and why?

FUNCTIONAL NURSING

The functional model of nursing care delivery became popular during World War II when there was a severe shortage of nurses in the United States. Many nurses joined the armed forces to care for the soldiers. To provide care to patients at home, hospitals began to increase the number of LPNs/LVNs and unlicensed assistive personnel.

The functional model of nursing is a method of providing patient care by which each licensed and unlicensed staff member performs specific tasks for a large group of patients. These tasks are in part determined by the scope of practice defined for each type of caregiver. For example, the RN must be responsible for all assessments, although the LPN/LVN and UAPs may collect data that can be used in the assessment. Regarding treatments, an RN may administer all intravenous (IV) medications and do admissions, one LPN/LVN may provide treatments, another LPN/LVN may give all oral medications, one assistant may do all hygiene tasks, and another assistant may take all vital signs (Figure 13-2). This division of aspects of care is similar to the assembly line system used by manufacturing industries. Just as an auto worker becomes an expert in attaching fenders to a new vehicle, the staff nurse becomes expert in the tasks expected in functional nursing. A charge nurse

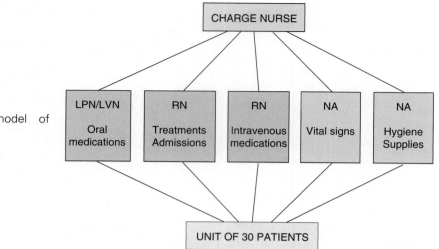

FIGURE 13-2 Functional model of nursing care delivery.

coordinates care and assignments and may ultimately be the only person familiar with all the needs of any individual patient.

Model Analysis

There are several advantages to this model of patient care delivery. First, each person becomes efficient at specific tasks, and much work can be done in a short time. Another advantage is that unskilled workers can be trained to perform one or two specific tasks very well. The organization benefits financially from this model because care can be delivered to a large number of patients by mixing staff with a fixed number of RNs and a larger number of UAPs.

Although financial savings may be the impetus for organizations to choose the functional system of delivering care, the disadvantages may outweigh the savings (Figure 13-3). A major disadvantage is the fragmentation of care. The physical and technical aspects of care may be met, but the psychological and spiritual needs may be overlooked. Patients become confused with so many different care providers per shift. These different staff members may be so busy with their assigned tasks that they may not have time to communicate with each other about the patient's progress. Because no one care provider sees patient care from beginning to end, the patient's response to care is difficult to assess. Critical changes in patient status may go unnoticed. Fragmented care and ineffective communication can lead to patient and family dissatisfaction and frustration. Exercise 13-2 provides an opportunity to imagine how a patient would react to the functional method and also to imagine how the nurse may feel.

EXERCISE 13-2

Imagine your mother is a patient at a hospital that uses the functional model of patient care delivery. She just had her knee replaced, and when you ask the nursing assistant for something for pain, she says, "I'll tell the medication nurse." The medication nurse comes to the room and says that your mother's medication is to be administered intravenously and the IV nurse will need to administer it. The IV nurse is busy starting an IV on another patient and cannot give your mother the medication for at least 10 minutes. This whole communication process has taken 40 minutes, and your mother is still in pain. Discuss your perception of the effectiveness of the functional method of patient care in this situation. How effective do you think communication among staff is when a patient has a problem? What could be done to improve this situation?

Nurse Manager's Role

In the functional model of nursing, the nurse manager must be sensitive to the quality of patient care delivered and the institution's budgetary constraints. Because staff members are responsible only for their specific task, the role of achieving patient outcomes becomes the nurse manager's responsibility.

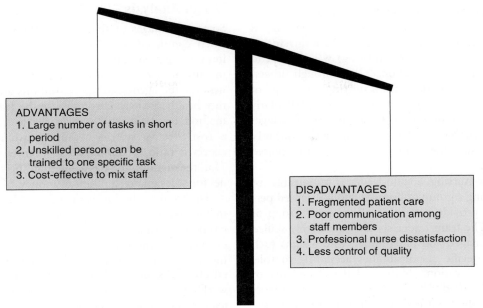

FIGURE 13-3 Advantages and disadvantages of functional nursing.

Staff members can view this system as autocratic and may become discontented with the lack of opportunity for input. By using effective management and leadership skills, the nurse manager can improve the staff's perception of their lack of independence. The manager can rotate assignments among staff within legal and organizational contexts to alleviate boredom with repetition. Staff meetings should be conducted frequently. This encourages staff to express concerns and empowers them with the ability to communicate about patient care and unit functions.

Staff RN's Role

The staff RN becomes skilled at the tasks that are usually assigned by the charge nurse. Clearly defined policies and procedures are used to complete the physical aspects of care in an efficient and economical manner. However, the functional model of nursing may leave the professional nurse feeling frustrated because of the task-oriented role. Nurses are educated to care for the patient holistically, and providing only a fragment of care to a patient may result in unmet personal and professional expectations of nurses.

> **EXERCISE 13-3**
> After 6 months of working on a unit that accommodates patients who have had general surgery, you realize that you are bored and frustrated with the functional model of delivering care. You have been administering all the IV medications and pain medications for your assigned patients. You have minimal opportunity to interact with the patients and learn about them, and you cannot be innovative in your care. Discuss strategies you could use to resolve this dissatisfaction with the functional model of nursing care delivery.

The functional method of delivering care works well in emergency and disaster situations. Each care provider knows the expectations of the assigned role and completes the tasks quickly and efficiently. Subacute care agencies, extended-care facilities, and ambulatory clinics often use the functional model to deliver care quictly.

TEAM NURSING

After World War II, the nursing shortage continued. Many female nurses who were in the military came home to marry and have children instead of returning to the workforce. Because the functional model received criticism, a new system of team nursing (a modification of functional nursing) was devised to improve patient satisfaction. "Care through others" became the hallmark of team nursing. This type of nursing care delivery remains in use, particularly when reduced reimbursement and nursing shortages have resulted in organizations changing the staff mix and increasing the ratio of unlicensed to licensed personnel.

In team nursing, a team leader is responsible for coordinating a group of licensed and unlicensed personnel to provide patient care to a small group of patients. The team leader should be a highly skilled leader, manager, and practitioner, who assigns each member specific responsibilities according to role, licensure, education, ability, and the complexity of the care required. The members of the team report directly to the team leader, who then reports to the charge nurse or unit manager (Figure 13-4). There are several teams per unit, and patient assignments are made by each team leader.

Model Analysis

Some advantages of the team method, particularly when compared with the functional approach, are improved patient satisfaction, organizational decision making occurring at lower levels, and cost-effectiveness for the agency. Many institutions and community health agencies currently use the team nursing method. Inpatient facilities may view team nursing as a cost-effective system because it works with an expected ratio of unlicensed to licensed personnel. Thus the organization has greater numbers of personnel for a designated amount of money.

The team method of patient care delivery has one major disadvantage, which arises if the team leader has poor leadership skills. The team leader must have excellent communication skills, delegation and conflict management abilities, strong clinical skills, and effective decision-making abilities to provide a working "team" environment for the members. The team leader must be sensitive to the needs of the patient and, at the same time, attentive to the needs of the staff providing the direct care (Moore, 2004). When the team leader is not prepared for this role, the team method becomes a miniature version of the functional method and the potential for fragmentation of care is high.

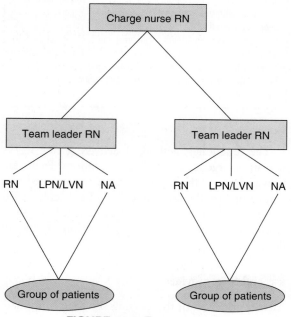

FIGURE 13-4 Team nursing.

EXERCISE 13-4

Think of a time when you worked with a group of four to six people to achieve a specific goal or accomplish a task (perhaps in school you were grouped together to complete a project). How did your group achieve the goal? Was one person the organizer or leader? How was the leader selected? Who assigned each member a component, or did you each determine what skills you possessed that would most benefit the group? Did you experience any conflict while working on this project? How did the concepts of group dynamics and leadership skills affect how your group achieved its goal? What similarities do you see between the team nursing system of providing patient care and your group involvement to achieve a goal?

Nurse Manager's Role

The nurse manager, charge nurse, and team leaders must have management skills to effectively implement the team nursing method of patient care delivery. In addition, the nurse manager must determine which RNs are skilled and interested in becoming a charge nurse or team leader. Because the basic education of baccalaureate-prepared RNs emphasizes critical-thinking and leadership concepts, they are likely candidates for such roles. The nurse manager should also provide an adequate staff mix and orient team members to the team nursing system by providing continuing education about leadership, management techniques, delegation, and team interaction (see Chapters 1, 3, 4, 18, and 26). By addressing these factors, the manager is aiding the teams to function optimally.

The charge nurse functions as a liaison between the team leaders and other healthcare providers, because nurse managers are often responsible for more than one unit and/or have other managerial responsibilities that take them away from the unit. The charge nurse provides support for the teams on a shift-by-shift basis. Appropriate support requires the charge nurse to encourage each team to solve its problems independently.

The team leader plans the care, delegates the work, and follows up with members to evaluate the quality of care for the patients assigned to their team. In the ideal circumstance, the team leader updates the nursing care plans and facilitates patient care conferences. Time constraints during the shift may prevent scheduling daily patient care conferences or prevent some team members attending those that are held.

The team leader must also face the challenge of changing team membership on a daily basis. Diverse work schedules and nursing staff shortages may result in daily changes in the staff mix of a team and a daily assignment change for team members. The team leader assigns the professional, technical, and ancillary personnel to the type of patient care they are prepared to deliver. Therefore the team leader must be knowledgeable about the legal and organizational limits of each role.

Staff RN's Role

Team nursing uses the strengths of each caregiver. The staff nurses, as members of the team, develop expertise in care delivery. Some members become known for their expertise in the psychomotor aspects of care. If one nurse is skilled at starting IVs, she will start all IVs for her team of patients. If a nurse is especially skillful in motivating postoperative patients to use the incentive pyrometer and ambulate, he or she should be assigned to the surgical patients. Under the guidance and supervision of the team leader, the collective efforts of the team become greater than the functions of the individual caregivers.

PRIMARY NURSING

A cultural revolution occurred in the United States during the 1960s. The revolution emphasized individual rights and independence from existing societal restrictions. This revolution also influenced the nursing profession, because nurses were becoming dissatisfied with their lack of autonomy. In addition, the hierarchical nature of communication in team nursing caused further frustration. Institutions were also aware of the declining quality of patient care. The search for autonomy and quality care led to the primary nursing system of patient care delivery as a method to increase RN accountability for patient outcomes.

Primary nursing, an adaptation of the case method, was developed by Marie Manthey as a method for organizing patient care delivery in which one RN functions autonomously as the patient's primary nurse throughout the hospital stay (Manthey, Ciske, Robertson, & Harris, 1970).

Primary nursing brought the nurse back to direct patient care. The primary nurse is accountable for the patients' care 24 hours a day from admission through discharge. Conceptually, primary nursing care provides the patient and the family with coordinated, comprehensive, continuous care (Tiedeman & Lookinland, 2004). Care is organized, using the nursing process. The primary nurse collaborates, communicates, and coordinates all aspects of patient care with other nurses as well as other disciplines (Tiedeman & Lookinland, 2004). Advocacy and assertiveness are desirable leadership attributes for this care delivery model.

The primary nurse, preferably at least baccalaureate-prepared, is held accountable for meeting outcome criteria and communicating with all other healthcare providers about the patient (Figure 13-5). For example, a patient is admitted to a medical unit with pulmonary edema. His primary nurse admits him and then provides a written plan of care. When his primary nurse is not working, an associate nurse implements the plan. The associate nurse is an RN

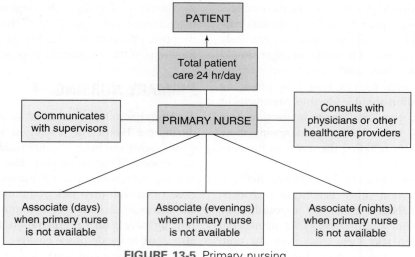

FIGURE 13-5 Primary nursing.

who has been delegated to provide care to the patient according to the primary nurse's specification. If the patient develops additional complications, the associate nurse notifies the primary nurse, who has 24-hour accountability and responsibility. The associate nurse provides input to the patient's plan of care, and the primary nurse makes the appropriate alterations.

Model Analysis

Tiedeman and Lookinland (2004) cited numerous works that speak to the quality of care and patient satisfaction with primary care. Some studies cited in their work speak to increased quality of care and patient satisfaction, whereas others find no difference in these parameters when compared with team nursing. RNs practicing primary nursing must possess a broad knowledge base and have highly developed nursing skills. In this system of care delivery, professionalism is promoted. Nurses experience job satisfaction because they can use their education to provide holistic and autonomous care for the patient. This high level of accountability for patient outcomes encourages RNs to further their knowledge and refine skills to provide optimal patient care. If the primary nurse is not motivated or feels unqualified to provide holistic care, job satisfaction may decrease.

In primary nursing, patients and families are typically satisfied with the care they receive, because they establish a relationship with the primary nurse and identify the caregiver as "their nurse." Because the patient's primary nurse communicates the plan of care, the patient can move away from the sick role and begin to participate in his or her own recovery. By considering the sociocultural, psychological, and physical needs of the patient and family, the primary nurse can plan the most appropriate care with and for the patient and family.

A professional advantage to the primary nursing method is a decrease in the number of unlicensed personnel. The ideal primary nursing system requires an all-RN staff. The RN can provide total care to the patient, from bed baths to patient education, even both at the same time! Unlicensed personnel are not qualified to provide this level of inclusive care (Figure 13-6).

A disadvantage of the primary nursing method is that the RN may not have the experience or educational background to provide total care. The agency needs to educate staff for an adequate transition from the previous role to the primary role. In addition, one has to ask whether the RN is ready and willing and capable of handling the 24-hour responsibility for patient care. In addition, the nurse practice acts must be evaluated to determine whether primary nurses can be held accountable when they are not physically present.

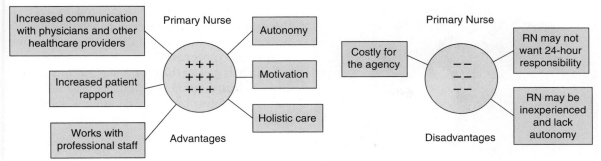

FIGURE 13-6 Advantages and disadvantages of primary nursing.

EXERCISE 13-5

Mr. Faulkner is admitted to the medical unit with exacerbated congestive heart failure. Mike Ross, RN, BSN, is Mr. Faulkner's primary nurse and will provide total care to Mr. Faulkner. Mike notes that this is Mr. Faulkner's third admission in 6 months for congestive heart failure–related symptoms. This is the first admission for which Mr. Faulkner has had a primary nurse. What do you think will be different about this admission with Mike providing primary nursing to Mr. Faulkner? Do you think there will be any difference in continuity of care? How involved do you think Mr. Faulkner will be with his own care in the primary nursing system?

In times of nursing shortage, primary nursing may not be the model of choice. This model will not be effective if a unit has a large number of part-time RNs who are not available to assume the primary nurse role (24-hour responsibility). In addition, with the arrival of managed care in the 1990s, patients' hospital stays were shorter than in the 1970s, when primary nursing became popular. Expedited stays make it challenging for primary nurses to adequately provide the depth of care required by primary nursing. If the patient is admitted on Monday and discharged on Wednesday, the primary nurse has a difficult time meeting all patient needs before discharge if he or she is not working on Tuesday. The primary nurse must rely heavily on feedback from associates, which defeats the purpose of primary nursing. In addition, the reduction in reimbursement to hospitals and other organizations associated with managed care caused administrators to consider ways to reduce the cost of care delivery. Because labor costs are the largest expense in care delivery and the nursing staff makes up the largest portion of the labor costs, attention was given to reducing these costs with changes in the model of care delivery.

EXERCISE 13-6

Imagine you are a primary nurse at an inpatient psychiatric facility. The patients you are assigned to are usually suicidal. How would you feel about the added responsibility for patients even when you were not at work? Is it realistic to expect the nurse to assume the role of the primary nurse with 24-hour responsibility? How would this responsibility affect your personal life? How would you make decisions about the patients and your home life?

Nurse Manager's Role

The primary nursing system can be modified to meet patient, nursing, and budgetary demands while maintaining the positive components that spawned its conception. The nurse manager needs to determine the desire of staff to become primary nurses and then educate them accordingly. The associate nurses and all other healthcare providers need clearly defined roles. They also need to be aware of the primary nurse's role and the importance of communicating concerns directly to that nurse.

The nurse manager who implements this care delivery model experiences some benefits. Primary nursing provides the nurse manager an opportunity to demonstrate leadership capabilities, clinical competencies, and teaching abilities to serve as a role model for professional practice. In addition, the roles of budget controller and unit quality manager remain. The traditional roles of delegation and decision

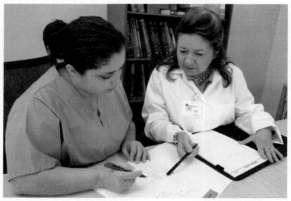

The nurse manager functions as a role model, advocate, coach, and consultant.

making must be relinquished to the autonomous primary nurse. The nurse manager functions as a role model, advocate, coach, and consultant.

Staff RN's Role

The primary nurse uses many facets of the professional role—caregiver, advocate, decision maker, teacher, collaborator, and manager. Because primary nurses cannot be present 24 hours a day, they must depend on associate nurses to provide care when they are not available. The associate nurse provides care using the plan of care developed by the primary nurse. Changes to the plan of care can be made by the associate nurse in collaboration with the primary nurse. This model provides consistency among nurses and shifts. To function effectively in this setting, staff nurses will need experience and opportunities to be mentored in this role.

Because it usually is not financially possible for an agency to employ only RNs, true primary nursing rarely exists. Some institutions have modified the primary nursing concept and implemented a partnership model to incorporate their current staff mix.

Primary Nursing Hybrid: Partnership Model

In the partnership model (or *co-primary nursing model*) of providing patient care, an RN is paired with a technical assistant. The partner works with the RN consistently. When the partner is unlicensed, the RN allows the assistant to perform basic nursing functions consistent with the state delegation rules. This

frees the RN to provide "semi-primary care" to assigned patients. A partnership between an RN and an LPN/LVN allows the LPN/LVN to take more responsibility, because the scope of practice for an LPN/LVN is greater than that of a UAP. In some settings, the partnership is legitimized with an official contract to formalize the relationship. Rehabilitative care settings often use the partnership model to deliver care.

EXERCISE 13-7
You are a primary nurse in a surgical intensive care unit of a small hospital. The unit you work on uses an RN–LPN/LVN partnership to decrease the number of RNs required per shift. You and your partner are assigned four surgical patients. Mr. Jones had a lobectomy 5 hours ago and is on a ventilator; Mrs. Martinez had a quadruple cardiac bypass 14 hours ago; Mr. Wong had a nephrectomy 2 days ago and is receiving continuous peritoneal dialysis; and Mr. Smith has a fractured pelvis and is comatose from a motor vehicle accident 24 hours ago. How would you distribute the staff to provide primary care to these four patients? Do you think it is possible to provide primary care in this situation? What responsibilities would you assume as the primary nurse, and what could you share with the LPN/LVN?

Primary Nursing Hybrid: Patient-Focused Care

Another view of primary care is the care delivered in a patient-focused care unit. Developed in the late 1980s, the patient-focused care model integrates principles from business and industry. The goals for this model of care included (1) improving patient satisfaction and other patient outcomes, (2) improving worker job satisfaction, and (3) increasing efficiencies and decreasing costs (Seago, 1999). This model features decentralized, streamlined, and localized care (Graham, 2003). The multidisciplinary team formulates the plan of care after the primary nurse and the physician have assessed the patient.

Patient-focused care units require a change in the physical environment where care is delivered. Services required by patients are decentralized. Satellite laboratories, radiology facilities, pharmacies, and supply rooms are geographically proximate to the patient rooms (Seago, 1999).

Original models of a patient-focused care unit included an RN paired with a cross-trained

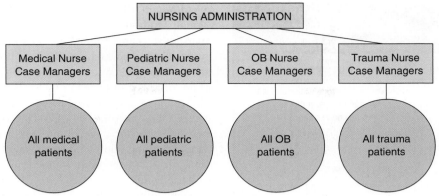

FIGURE 13-7 Nursing case management model in which all patients are assigned to a nurse case manager. *OB,* Obstetric.

technician who provided patient-side care, including respiratory therapy, phlebotomy, and electrocardiographs. Modifications in this nurse-managed model include team members who provide direct care activities such as recording vital signs, drawing blood, and bathing patients.

In a patient-focused care unit, the role and scope of the nurse manager expand. No longer is the individual just a manager of nurses. Now the nurse manager assumes the accountability and responsibility to manage nurses and staff from other, traditionally centralized departments. Because the care is focused on the needs of the patient and not the needs of the department, the role of the manager becomes more sophisticated. The nurse manager orchestrates all the care activities required by the patient and family during the hospitalization. Implementing this philosophy and model of care requires new learning about one's beliefs, attitudes, and practices toward care (Graham, 2003).

NURSING CASE MANAGEMENT

Another nursing care delivery model that requires a complex set of expectations is the process of nursing case management. Case management is the process of coordinating health care by planning, facilitating, and evaluating interventions across levels of care to achieve measurable cost and quality outcomes. It was first seen in the early 1900 by social workers and public health nurses working in the public sector to identify and obtain resources for the needy. In the 1960s, insurers began to use nursing case management (NCM) as a strategy to manage the needs of complex patients who require coordination over the course of treatment. Acute care hospitals used nurses in this role under the term of *utilization management,* particularly when federal regulations required this service for all Medicare and Medicaid patients (Zander, 2002).

In the mid-1980s, when acute care hospitals began to be reimbursed based upon a certain diagnosis, nursing case management became a popular and effective method to manage shortened lengths of stay for patients and to prevent expensive hospital readmissions. Tufts New England Medical Center Hospital in Boston and Carondelet St. Mary's Hospital in Tucson, Arizona, were leaders in the trend to implement a collaborative system that focuses on comprehensive assessment and intervention and holistic care planning with appropriate referrals to meet the healthcare needs of the patient and the family (Figure 13-7) (Zander, 2002). The nursing case-management process may be "within the walls" of the hospital or "beyond the walls." The success of nursing case-management models has been demonstrated in all healthcare settings, including acute, subacute, and ambulatory settings and long-term care facilities, as well as health insurance companies and the community. Table 13-1 identifies some of the service settings using this care delivery model.

The case-management model of patient care delivery maintains quality care while streamlining costs and seeks the active involvement of the patient, the

TABLE 13-1   NURSING CASE-MANAGEMENT SERVICE AREAS

CATEGORY	SERVICE SETTING
Acute	Orthopedics, cardiovascular, critical care, high-risk perinatal, oncology, emergency department
Subacute	Skilled nursing centers, rehabilitation units
Ambulatory	Physicians' offices, clinics
Long-term care	Nursing homes, group homes, assisted-living facilities
Insurance companies	Health maintenance organizations (HMOs), preferred provider organizations (PPOs), Workers' Compensation, Medicaid, Medicare
Community	Nurse-managed centers, home health agencies, urgent care centers, schools, rural settings

Adapted from information presented in Cohen & Cesta (2004); Curtis, Lien, Grove, & Morris (2002); Huber (2010).

family, and diverse healthcare professionals. Healthcare organizations have tailored the case-management system to meet their specific needs. The elements of the case-management model are the case manager and the critical pathway.

Case Manager

Nurses, social workers, and other disciplines may work as case managers, bringing with them their discipline-specific skills and knowledge. Regardless of preparation, the Center for Case Management has identified the following seven core content areas in which a case manager should be proficient (Zander, 2002):

1. Identification of at-risk populations
2. Assessment of clinical system components
3. Development of strategies to manage at-risk populations
4. Leadership for change
5. Market assessment and strategic planning
6. Human resource management
7. Program evaluation through outcomes management

Although there is inconsistency among professional standards about the education for nurse case managers, many prefer master's-prepared clinical nurse specialists who have advanced preparation with the specific populations being served. However, this is no longer emphasized in the core competences for clinical nurse specialists. The case manager is patient-focused and outcome-oriented. The goal is to provide cost-effective care through integration of clinical services in combination with financial services. In addition, the NCM serves as an advocate for the patient and the family.

Depending on the facility, there may be several case managers to coordinate care for all patients or a case manager may be assigned to a specific high-risk population (see Figure 13-7 on the previous page). The case manager may be responsible for coordinating care for up to 20 patients. It is essential that the case manager has frequent interaction with the patient and the healthcare provider to achieve and evaluate expected outcomes.

CLINICAL PATHWAYS

The tool that case managers use to achieve patient outcomes is a clinical pathway. Also referred to as a *multidisciplinary care pathway, integrated care pathway, critical path,* or *collaborative care pathway,* these patient-focused documents describe the clinical standards, necessary interventions, and expected outcomes for the patient at each stage throughout the treatment process or hospital stay. Clinical pathways are not appropriate for all patients and cannot replace professional clinical judgment; however, they do facilitate coordinated, efficient, and evidence-based care (D'Entremont, 2009).

Clinical pathways are grids that outline the critical or key events expected to happen each day of a patient's hospitalization (Cohen & Cesta, 2004). If a patient's progress deviates from the normal path, a variance is indicated. A variance is anything that occurs to alter the patient's progress through the normal critical path. Analysis of variance is essential for effective utilization of a path. Circumstances that can cause a variance include operational, provider, patient, or clinical elements (Cohen & Cesta, 2004). Operational causes include broken equipment or interdepartmental delays. Changes in the practice pattern of the healthcare provider can affect the pathway and cause a variance. Complications in the patient's condition, such as a hemorrhage into the joint after total knee replacement, may increase total hospital days. A complication can inhibit the ability of the patient to meet the clinical indicator, and a patient's or family's refusal of a specific component of care can create a variance.

Variances can be positive or negative. A negative variance is an undesired outcome, whereas a positive variance is an outcome that is achieved before it is expected (Cohen & Cesta, 2004). A patient undergoing a second hip replacement who attended preoperative classes and engaged in activities to "ready himself" for the surgery may actually leave the hospital sooner than predicted in a clinical path. The NCM on the orthopedic unit and the insurance company's case manager would view this as a positive variance, as typically would the patient.

Model Analysis

Nursing case management is a process for providing comprehensive care for those with complex health problems. Case management provides a well-coordinated care experience that can improve the care outcome, decrease the length of stay, and use multiple disciplines and services efficiently. Families and patients receive care across a continuum of settings, often from diverse institutions. NCMs can often break down invisible institutional barriers for the patient. Nurses receive a sense of satisfaction knowing that the patient and family received coordinated, quality care in a cost-effective manner across the spectrum of the illness or injury.

However, major obstacles exist in the implementation of case-management services. Financial barriers, lack of administrative support, human resource inequities, turf battles, and the lack of information support systems have been identified as obstacles in the implementation of case-management services (Zander, 2002). Case management is not a revenue-generating activity but, rather, a "revenue-protecting" activity. It minimizes costs for those case types with the potential of high resource consumption. Consequently, case management may be seen as an expense if the organization is being paid on a fee-for-service basis.

The development of collaborative models of healthcare management incorporating nurses, social workers, and case managers has demonstrated significant cost savings. Some institutions have developed departments of healthcare case management. In this setting, the NCM works with the "medically complex," the social worker with the "socially complex," and utilization management for utilization review. This team of case managers, each with identified core functions, also has specialty functions based on the specific scope of responsibility (Cohen & Cesta, 2004).

Nurse Manager's Role

The nurse manager has increased demands when leading the case-management system. Quality improvement is constantly assessed to ensure that the clinical pathway is diagnosis-related group (DRG)–appropriate and that case managers are adequately managing their caseloads. Reimbursement for the care delivered is tied to effective planning and care delivery within the case-management process. Patient satisfaction is also pertinent to evaluate for quality. If patients are not satisfied with the system, the census may decline.

Communication among all systems must be coordinated. Because the NCM works with all departments, the nurse manager may need to facilitate interdepartmental communication. Educating the staff of other departments about the NCM's role and responsibilities will increase the effectiveness of the case-management process.

Staff RN's Role

The staff nurse working with a patient who has a case manager as the coordinator of care provides patient care according to the case manager's specifications and must know the extent of the case manager's role. Effective communication to facilitate care is the responsibility of both the case manager and the staff RN.

CARE STRATEGIES THAT INFLUENCE CARE DELIVERY

Disease Management

Disease management has been in existence for many decades. However, in the late 1990s, disease management became a model of care that coordinates healthcare interventions and communication for those individuals whose self-care needs are significant (Gorski, 2003). Those with chronic conditions who are high consumers of healthcare dollars are the recipients of disease-managed care. Disease-management programs for patients dealing with chronic illness build on the relationship with the healthcare team to prevent exacerbations and complications using evidence-based guidelines and patient empowerment techniques to improve the overall health and well-being of the patient and family. The focus of this model of care is the concept of wellness—living well with a chronic disease. Determining the barriers to self-care is an essential element of successful disease-management programs.

Disease-management programs consist of assessment to identify a specific population, comprehensive patient and family self-management education, use of evidence-based practice guidelines, medical management based on treatment algorithms, and focused visits with the healthcare team in an ambulatory setting to assist with adherence to the treatment protocol (Cohen & Cesta, 2004; Gorski, 2003). NCMs often decide whether a patient meets the specific criteria for a disease-managed program. Patients with complex healthcare needs and multiple diagnoses will continue to need extensive nursing case management and will not be eligible for a specific disease-management program (Goldstein, 1998).

other strategies

DIFFERENTIATED NURSING PRACTICE

One of the factors that makes development and implementation of any nursing care delivery model difficult is the variation in competence based on education and experience. Over the past 50 years, as multiple entry points in nursing (LPN/LVN, associate degree in nursing [ADN], diploma, bachelor of science in nursing [BSN], and advanced generalist [MSN]) have grown and more is known about the length of time required for a nurse to move from being a novice to competent nurse (Benner, 2001), efforts have been made to document and validate differentiated practice.

Background of Differentiated Practice

Differentiated nursing practice models are models of clinical nursing practice that are defined or dif-

ferentiated by level of education, expected clinical skills or competencies, job descriptions, pay scales, and participation in decision making (AACN, AONE & NOADN, 1995): The "Model for Differentiated Nursing Practice" (AACN, AONE, & NOADN, 1995) notes that the associate degree nurse (ADN) role functions primarily at the bedside in an institutional setting and in less-complex patient care situations. The time frame for care provided by the ADN is defined within a shift or limited period of time, based on activities that provide comfort, physiologic stabilization, or assistance to a peaceful death. The guiding principles of the ADNs' work are found in nursing standards, protocols, and pathways. In this model, the ADN nurses are called *associate nurses* (AACN, AONE, and NOADN, 1995).

The BSN role is conceptualized as operating across time from preadmission to post-discharge. The guiding principles of this role are found in the unusual and often unpredictable response of the patient that goes beyond needs addressed in the standards or pathways. Collaborating with other disciplines and agencies, the BSN intervenes to design and facilitate a comprehensive, well-prepared discharge based on the unique needs of the patient and family (AACN, AONE, and NOADN, 1995; AACN, 2009).

The advanced practice registered nurse (APRN) role is based on master's of science in nursing (MSN) or doctorate of nursing practice (DNP) competencies. The APRN perspective is supported by in-depth education in physiology, physical assessment, pharmacology, and a broad healthcare systems perspective. The MSN/DNP creates and defines protocols and pathways and assists with development of standards on emerging new healthcare phenomena. The MSN/DNP role is not bound by setting but, instead, provides a continuum of care across all settings, working with the patient and family throughout wellness or illness or until death (AACN, AONE, & NOADN, 1995).

The varied educational backgrounds and philosophies of the nurses' implementing a model of practice have a significant impact on the success of the delivery system and the satisfaction of the nurse and the patients. This variation is further complicated by the experience of the nurse in the practice arena. Benner (2001), based on the Dreyfus model of skill acquisition, identified five stages of clinical competence for nurses: novice, advanced beginner, competent, proficient, and expert. She suggests that competence is typified by a nurse who has been on the job in the same or similar situations 2 to 3 years. This would suggest that nurses who are either new graduates or in a new area of clinical practice may require more assistance than those with more experience. A group of nurses who are all at the novice or advanced beginner stage would be less likely than their more experienced counterparts to implement any type of delivery model effectively.

In an effort to clarify the competence level of new graduates, some states, such as Texas, have identified the specific variations in competence among the various educational levels. These competencies can be used by educational programs for curriculum development and evaluation and by employers to determine the specific roles and responsibilities of these graduates. In 1993, the Board of Nurse Examiners and the Board of Vocational Nurse Examiners in Texas adopted the "Essential Competencies of Texas Graduates of Education Programs of Nursing." These competencies identified the knowledge, judgment, skills, and professional values expected of graduates of LVN, diploma/ADN, and BSN programs, varying in complexity, depth, and breadth of the various types of nursing programs. In 2002, these competencies, including competency statements related to provider of care, coordinator of care, and member of the profession, were revised and educational programs were accountable for demonstrating inclusion of these competencies into their curriculum (Poster et al., 2005). These competencies are being updated to address the changing roles of nurses and to enhance their use for service as well as education.

Differentiated Practice in the Clinical Setting

Refinements in differentiated practice have been in place in various clinical settings. Sioux Valley Hospital in Sioux Falls, South Dakota, one of the first hospitals to use differentiated practice, has used this practice model in combination with a case-management model. Associate, primary, and advanced practice nurses were the cornerstone of the model. The associate nurse in the Sioux Valley Model was responsible for the assigned patient during a shift (Foss & Koerner, 1997). Critical paths guided the care

delivered. The primary nurse coordinated care from admission to discharge for those with complex psychosocial, educational, or discharge planning needs (Foss & Koerner, 1997). Clinical nurse specialists and nurse practitioners were responsible for care throughout the illness episode. They interacted and collaborated with multiple disciplines to coordinate ongoing care across all healthcare settings (Foss & Koerner, 1997).

As the complexity of healthcare increases and the pressures of managed care exert their influence, areas such as communication and critical thinking are paramount. Differentiated practice in nursing can respond to these changing healthcare systems, payment strategies, and rising acuities and complex healthcare needs seen in patients and their families.

Incentives for implementing differentiated practice found in the literature include the following (Bellack & Loquist, 1999):

1. The ability to identify the differences in preparation of nurses by level of education
2. The ability to use different levels of nurses to meet the total needs of the patient
3. Improved clinical outcomes that are cost-effective
4. Enhanced prestige of nursing through the identification of different levels of nursing to the public, the payers, and healthcare administration
5. Effective utilization of nursing resources to meet the diverse needs of managed care
6. Career satisfaction with equitable compensation

However, despite a variety of efforts to differentiate the roles and competencies of nurses with various educational and experience backgrounds, the demands of the workplace, the chronic shortage of nurses, and exploding technology have made it difficult to differentiate nursing practice in many clinical settings.

Clinical Nurse Leader

In response to lack of differentiated practice in many worksites and the increased emphasis on patient safety, the American Association of Colleges of Nursing (AACN) developed the clinical nurse leader role in the early 2000s. The clinical nurse leader, which is a protected title for those who successfully complete the clinical nurse leader (CNL) certification examination, is an advanced generalist clinician with education at the master's degree, in contrast to advanced practice registered nurses, whose designation includes clinical nurse specialists, nurse practitioners, nurse midwives, and nurse anesthetists. The CNL oversees the lateral integration of care for a distinct group of patients and may actively provide direct patient care in complex situations. The CNL uses evidence-based practice to ensure that patients benefit from the latest innovations in care delivery. The CNL collects and evaluates patient outcomes, assesses cohort risk, and has the decision-making authority to change care plans when necessary. This nurse functions as part of the inter-professional team by communicating, planning, and implementing care directly with other healthcare professionals including physicians, pharmacists, social workers, clinical nurse specialists, and nurse practitioners. The CNL is a leader in the healthcare delivery system in all settings in which health care is delivered, and implementation of the role may vary across settings (AACN, 2008). Box 13-1 outlines the fundamental aspects of the CNL role, as defined by the AACN white paper on the role of the clinical nurse leader (AACN, 2007).

The Synergy Model

Similar to the work of the AACN in developing the CNL, the American Association of Critical-Care Nurses adopted the Synergy Model as the framework for nursing practice as well as for the certification examination for the critical care nurse and the clinical nurse specialist. Some healthcare organizations have adopted this model as their model of care. However, the Synergy Model identifies patient characteristics as "drivers" of the necessary competencies for nurses. When there is a match between the competencies of the nurse and the characteristics of the patient, the best patient outcomes and safe passage through a hospital stay will be achieved (Brewer, 2006).

The Synergy Model describes the following eight patient characteristics: resiliency, vulnerability, stability, complexity, resource availability, participation in care, participation in decision making, and predictability. The eight nurse competencies are clinical judgment, advocacy and moral agency, caring practices, facilitation of learning, collaboration, systems thinking, response to diversity, and clinical require-

---

BOX 13-1   FUNDAMENTAL ASPECTS OF THE CLINICAL NURSE LEADER (CNL)

- Leadership in the care of the sick in and across all environments
- Design and provision of health-promotion and risk-reduction services for diverse populations
- Provision of evidence-based practice
- Population-appropriate health care to individuals, clinical groups/units, and communities
- Clinical decision making
- Design and implementation of plans of care
- Risk anticipation
- Participation in identification and collection of care outcomes
- Accountability for the evaluation and improvement of point-of-care outcomes
- Mass customization of care
- Client and community advocacy
- Education and information management
- Delegation and oversight of care delivery and outcomes
- Team management and collaboration with other health professional team members
- Development and leverage of human, environmental, and material resources
- Management and use of client-care and information technology
- Lateral integration for specified groups of patients

From AACN. (2007). *White paper on the role of the clinical nurse leader.* Website: www.aacn.nche.edu/Publications/WhitePapers/ClinicalNurseLeader.htm.

---

ment (Brewer, 2006). Each of the competencies is essential in providing holistic care to the patient. Depending on the acuity of the patient, some competencies emerge as priorities whereas others are used to a lesser extent (Hardin & Hussey, 2003). When there is synergy between the patient characteristics and the competency of the nurse, patient care is optimized (Rohde & Moloney-Harmon, 2001). The American Association of Critical-Care Nurses website (*www.aacn.org*) provides information about the Synergy Model and its application in numerous and diverse care settings.

Magnet Recognition Program®

In 1983, the American Academy of Nursing's (AAN) task force on nursing practice in hospitals conducted a study of 163 hospitals to identify and describe variables that created an environment that attracted and retained well-qualified nurses who promoted quality care. Forty-one of these institutions were described as "magnet" hospitals because of their ability to attract and retain professional nurses. In 1990, the American Nurses Credentialing Center (ANCC), building on the concepts of the 1983 "magnet" hospital study, developed a program that recognized excellence in the nurses' work environment. Prominent in the designation process is the hospital's documentation of the presence of the "Forces of Magnetism."

The **Magnet Recognition Program**® is designed for hospitals to achieve recognition of excellent nursing care through a self-nominating, self-appraisal process to achieve. The rigorous self-appraisal process is lengthy. The petitioning organization must assess its ability to meet the program standards and typically works for 2 years or more in the development of the application (Havens & Johnston, 2004). The hospital makes application for Magnet™ status, submits documentation to demonstrate its compliance with the Magnet™ standards, and hosts a site visit by Magnet™ appraisers. When the application process is successful, Magnet™ status is awarded for 4 years. In 2004, *U.S. News and World Report* added Magnet™ status to the criteria used in its judging of "best hospitals" (Trossman, 2004). For additional information on Magnet™ credentialing, see *www.nursecredentialing. org/magnet/index.html*.

TRANSFORMING CARE AT THE BEDSIDE

The variety of care delivery models and the complexity of patient needs, organizational structures, and technologic advances require individual action to improve practice patterns in specific units. In 2003, the Robert Wood Johnson Foundation and the Institute of Healthcare Improvement joined to create, test, and implement changes to dramatically improve care on medical/surgical units and improve staff satisfaction. The transforming-care-at-the-bedside (TCAB) initiative was implemented to redesign the work environment of nurses. A group of healthcare experts developed a guiding framework to redesign the work of nurses in medical/surgical units (Viney, Batcheller, Houston, & Belcik, 2006).

| BOX 13-2 | TRANSFORMING CARE AT THE BEDSIDE (TCAB) PREMISES |

- Patient-centered work redesign can create value-added care processes and result in better clinical outcomes and reduced costs.
- Effective care teams can have a positive impact on patient outcomes.
- Management practices and organizational culture have a significant impact on the work environment.
- Matching staff's knowledge and capabilities with work responsibilities enhances job satisfaction.
- Eliminating inefficiencies through work redesign enhances staff satisfaction and morale.

From Viney, M., Batcheller, J., Houston, S., & Belcik, K. (2006). Transforming care at the bedside: Designing new complex systems in an age of complexity. *Journal of Nursing Care Quality, 21*(2), 143-150.

| BOX 13-3 | TRANSFORMING CARE AT THE BEDSIDE (TCAB) OBJECTIVE/DESIGN THEMES |

- Reliability: The care for moderately sick patients who are hospitalized is safe, reliable, effective, and equitable.
- Vitality: Effective care teams continually strive for excellence within a joyful and supportive environment that nurtures professional formation and career development.
- Patient-centeredness: Patient-centered care on medical/surgical units honors the whole person and family, respects individual values and choices, and ensures continuity of care.
- Increased value: All care processes are free of waste and promote continuous flow.

Adapted from Viney, M., Batcheller, J., Houston, S., & Belcik, K. (2006). Transforming care at the bedside: Designing new complex systems in an age of complexity. *Journal of Nursing Care Quality, 21*(2), 143-150.

The TCAB initiative is based on a set of premises (Box 13-2), which then serve as the underpinnings of four key design themes. These include reliability, vitality and teamwork, patient-centered care, and value-added care processes (Box 13-3). According to Viney et al. (2006), both the themes and the premises serve as a framework for teams charged with changing care processes.

The TCAB initiative was initially implemented at three pilot hospitals and subsequently moved to other hospitals across the country. Small groups in each hospital came together, first, to learn about the TCAB process and to ask themselves "what do we know" about their work environment related to a particular design theme. The group then was encouraged to tell stories about their work environment consistent with this theme. After the story-telling opportunity, the group participated in a brainstorming session to develop as many innovations as possible that would contribute to the themes they had chosen. Innovations requiring minimal time and resources were then prioritized and selected for a rapid cycle trial.

Critical to practice changes, rapid cycle change is a process that encourages testing creative change on a small scale while determining potential impact. The process involves four stages—plan, do, study, and act (PDSA). During the *plan phase,* the team had to define the objectives and predict how the identified change would contribute to a design, how the change would occur, and what data collection methods were needed. During the *do phase,* the team had to focus on whether the changed occurred as expected and, if not, what interfered with the plan. In the *study phase,* the team had to determine if the innovation worked as predicted and what knowledge was gained. The *act phase* required the team to plan the next actions.

The team and staff participating in the study rated the innovation in terms of adoption, adaptation, or discontinuation. The innovations were implemented for a short period (from a day to several weeks) at least twice during the prototype testing phase and the pilot testing phase. If the outcomes of testing the innovation are positive, the new design can be easily spread to other participating sites.

CONCLUSIONS

Each patient care delivery model has identified strengths and weaknesses. There is no perfect method for delivering nursing care to groups of patients and their families. Based on the variety of settings and sizes of organizations, no one model addresses all needs. In addition, in times of local or national emergencies, the typical model of care may be replaced with one designed to best fit the emergency. (See Table 13-2 for examples of structure and process in organization that might influence the delivery of care used.) Lencioni (2006) emphasizes that organizational departments and disciplines can no longer afford to operate in solitude and must effectively collaborate to maximize positive outcomes.

TABLE 13-2 STANDARDIZED SET OF ORGANIZATIONAL CRITERIA		
ORGANIZATIONAL STRUCTURES	**ORGANIZATIONAL PROCESSES**	**PATIENT CARE DESCRIPTORS**
Governance	Care planning	Case mix severity
Teaching status	Patient assessment/ monitoring	Intensity of service/skills
Aggregated units	Documentation	Length of stay
Technology level	Policies/procedures	Diagnosis-related groups (DRGs)
Case mix	Patient education	
Operating budget	Supplies	
Nursing hours/day	Implementation of physicians' orders	
Skill mix	Patient/family communication	
Nurse : Patient ratio	Symptom management	
Use of temporary staff	Staff communication	
Nursing education/experience	Medication administration	
Support for professional development	Standards of care	
Continuing education	Unit activities	
Expert resources		
Support personnel		
Physical layout		

Adapted from Deutschendorf, A. (2003). From past paradigms to future frontiers: Unique care delivery models to facilitate nursing work and quality outcomes. *Journal of Nurse Administration, 33*(1), 51-58.

RESEARCH PERSPECTIVE

Resource: Kimball, B., Joynt, J., Cherner, D., & O'Neil, E. (2007). The quest for new innovative care delivery models. *Journal of Nursing Administration, 37*(9), 392-398.

Kimball, Joynt, Cherner, and O'Neil describe the impact of the Institute of Medicine's 2001 report, *Crossing the Quality Chasm: a New Health System for the 21st Century,* on healthcare delivery, particularly related to patient safety and quality improvement. The article describes the 2005 research inquiry of a Boston, Massachusetts, healthcare provider and a human resource consulting firm to determine what new innovative care delivery models were being tested across the United States that have the potential to change or reinvent healthcare delivery. Each of the models identified were evaluated according to (1) what promise they held, (2) the roles nurses play, (3) their impact on quality of care, (4) the extent to which they are cost-effective, and (5) their adaptability to different regions or markets. The criteria the delivery models were required to meet included the following:

- Service primarily adult patients
- Rely on nurses to play a primary role in care delivery
- Include an acute care hospital component
- Integrate technology, support systems, and new roles
- Improve quality, efficiency, and cost

The five innovative approaches identified as particularly effective were the following:

- The 12-bed hospital at Baptist Hospital of Miami
- The Primary Care Team Model at the Seton Family of Hospitals in Austin, Texas
- The Collaborative Patient Care Management Model at High Point Regional Health System in North Carolina
- The Transitional Care Model at the University of Pennsylvania
- The Hospital at Home developed at Johns Hopkins Bayview Medical Center in Baltimore, Maryland

The researchers identified the common elements in the new care delivery models, which included elevated RN roles, sharpened focus on the patient, smoothing patient transitions and hand-offs, leveraging technology to enable care model redesign, and driven by results. In addition, these new care delivery models also included early and regular involvement of caregivers in the design and implementation of new models.

Implications for Practice
Innovative care delivery models are being developed as healthcare organizations are responding to changes in reimbursement, technology, and characteristics of patients served. This study suggests that the common elements in the models evaluated to be effective should be considered when organizations make changes in their care delivery models.

 LITERATURE PERSPECTIVE

Resource: Burritt, J., Wallace, P., Steckel, C., & Hunter, A. (2007). Achieving quality and fiscal outcomes in patient care: The clinical mentor care delivery model. *Journal of Nursing Administration, 37*(12), 558-563.

Burritt, Wallace, Steckel, and Hunter describe the implementation and evaluation of the clinical mentor care delivery model, in which seasoned nurses demonstrating proficient and expert nursing practice (clinical mentors) are relieved of direct patient care responsibilities to assume clinical mentor roles. This model is based upon Benner's framework regarding development of clinical competence, Tanner's work on clinical judgment, and mentoring and reflective thinking. Clinical mentors are assigned to each shift and are accountable for safe, quality care to all patients. They assess, monitor, and evaluate care provided by the primary nurse and other team members to ensure that it is appropriate and efficacious. The mentors engage staff members in the process of reflective thinking to facilitate practice development. This process of learning involves focused "real-time" discussions to connect patient care experience to existing abstract, conceptual knowledge. The clinical mentors also use role modeling in complex, challenging patient care situations to promote learning.

This model of care was implemented in a 372-bed acute care facility in Southern California and evaluated in the context of the

hospital's quality management program, using Donabedian's framework of structure, process, and outcomes. According to the Donabedian model, leveraging of the proficient and expert practice of the clinical mentors across all patients is suggested as a key mediating factor in linking structure, process, and patient-outcome variables. Pre-existing metrics included fall rates, nosocomial pressure ulcers, failure to rescue, length of stay, and complications rate. Nurse satisfaction was measured using Lake's modification of the Nursing Work Index–Revised and the Practice Environment Scale of the Nursing Work Index. Data were collected on adult patients hospitalized at the facility as part of the hospital's quality program 6 months before and after the introduction of the clinical mentor role. The results suggest that the clinical mentor care delivery model can have a significant impact on nurse-sensitive outcomes of care and organizational efficiency through reduced length of stay.

Implications for Practice
Although the evaluation reported in this article was done in only one hospital over a discrete period of time, the results suggests that providing structured mentoring in a clinical environment has positive implications for patient outcomes. Additional research to validate these findings is warranted.

This chapter describes the traditional patient care delivery models that have been used over the past half century. The complexity of the current healthcare system, the shortage of health professionals, and the pressures to ensure patient safety and cost-effective care have led many organizations to explore alternative models to deliver patient care. New models of care are being tested, as demonstrated by the Research Perspective on p. 269 and the Literature Perspective on p. 269.

THE SOLUTION

As an assistant director of nursing, I am responsible for ensuring the delivery of excellent patient care to patients admitted to our hematology-oncology unit. The nurses on the unit were committed to this approach but were faced with communication challenges. Collaborating with other members of the leadership team, receiving feedback from the staff nurses, and seeking out best practices from my peers in the healthcare community produced a solution. We initiated a sit-down report for all nurses called the "huddle" and established a "nurse buddy" system.

The "huddle" is conducted at the beginning of the shift after each nurse has obtained report from the nurse on the previous shift and has had the opportunity to review each patient's plan of care. The nurses are paged and notified that the "huddle" will occur. The "huddle" is facilitated by the charge nurse, who surveys each nurse on his or her workload and the projected times he or she would need assistance with patient care.

The "nurse buddy" system was initiated to provide the patient-side nurse with an immediate resource—someone other than the charge nurse. These two nurses provide each other with assistance on an "as-needed" basis. The "buddy" is assigned at the time all patient assignments are made and is in close proximity.

The feedback is very positive. The charge nurse has a clearer picture of the status of the patients, families, and staff. Because the staff nurses are more engaged, they state that they are involved with the unit's operational needs for the day. Patient care is planned collaboratively so that each nurse is available to the "buddy" at times of need. Overall, teamwork and communication have been enhanced.

—*Jacqueline Ward*

Would this be a suitable approach for you? Why?

THE EVIDENCE

Wolf and Greenhouse (2007) recognize the need for healthcare system change and the importance of a well-developed care delivery model in addressing these changes. They suggest that it is not necessary to "start from scratch" in developing a model; many valuable lessons, learned from experience and scientific evidence, can be incorporated into new models. The authors suggest three factors beyond the experience of the past that should be considered in developing a new model. First, major healthcare trends, such as changes in patients, providers, information technology, and reimbursement, as well as medical advances, must be considered. Second, identifying what patients want and need is important. Some of the patient needs identified by the authors are those traditionally expected, such as a competent provider to meet their physical, emotional, and spiritual needs. However, an identified need that has not always been expected was "someone to help sort through available information for a solution effective for them." Third, Wolf and Greenhouse suggest that developers must make structural (who will do what?), process (how will it get done?), and outcome (what difference will it make?) decisions to ensure that the new model is in strategic alignment with the organization, sustainable over time, and can be replicated. The article provides specific questions that can be helpful in making these structural, process, and outcome decisions.

NEED TO KNOW NOW

- Consider the usual model of care delivery when selecting a position for employment.
- Anticipate that a national or local emergency could alter normal care delivery.
- Determine if there are experienced nurses who provide clinical leadership in specific settings.

CHAPTER CHECKLIST

The roles of the nurse manager and staff nurse vary with each nursing care delivery model. Regardless of the model, the nurse manager must have strong leadership and management skills for the model to be effective. Numerous issues must be considered when a care delivery model is implemented. Without a competent manager, none of the discussed models would be effective.

- A care delivery model is the method nurses use to provide care to patients.
- There are five models of patient care delivery, each with its advantages and disadvantages:
  - The case method focuses on total patient care for a specific time period.
    - The nurse manager must consider the expense of this system and identify all staff members' level of education and communication skills.
  - The functional model of nursing emphasizes task-oriented care for a large group of patients.
    - The nurse manager is responsible for achieving patient outcomes, whereas staff members are responsible only for their specific tasks.
    - The functional model is most often used in subacute care facilities.
  - In the team method, a small team provides care to a small group of patients.
    - The nurse manager in this model needs strong management, critical thinking, and leadership skills.
    - The modular method is a modification of team nursing that focuses on the geographic location of patient rooms and assignments of staff members.
  - In the primary nursing method, a primary nurse provides total patient care and directs patient care from admission to discharge.
    - The nurse manager functions as role model, advocate, coach, consultant, budget controller, and unit quality manager.
    - The partnership model, or co–primary nursing model, pairs an RN with a technical assistant.

- The patient-focused care unit employs a primary nurse and multi-skilled team members.
- The nursing case-management system is outcome-based and is facilitated by a case manager, who directs unit-based care using a critical path.
  - The nurse manager in this care delivery system faces increased demands to move the patient through the system as quickly as possible.
  - Managed care is a way of organizing patient care delivery with cost savings as the main goal.
- The nurse manager and charge nurse are responsible for directing patient care regardless of the delivery system. Key leadership and management concepts for directing patient care include the following:
  - Accountability
  - Delegation
  - Critical thinking
  - Communication
  - Promotion of autonomy
  - Collaboration
- Disease-management programs assist those with chronic illness to manage their self-care to achieve their optimal health.
- The nurse case manager plays a vital role in the management of care.
- The concept of differentiated practice emphasizes two levels of nursing practice: technical and professional.
- Each level has specific roles and responsibilities that depend on the nurse's educational preparation, experience, and clinical expertise.
- All the nursing roles complement each other.
- Emerging models of professional nursing practice continue to evolve.

▎TIPS FOR SELECTING A CARE DELIVERY MODEL*

- Look at the organization and the population being served when selecting a care delivery model.
- Consider the organizational structure and processes when selecting the care delivery model.
- There are advantages and disadvantages to any model; there is no ideal approach.

- Know that every model has specific expectations for both managers and staff.
- Determine if there are experienced nurses who provide clinical leadership in specific settings.

*These tips would be useful also for new graduate nurses evaluating employment opportunities.

REFERENCES

AACN. (2007). *White paper on the role of the clinical nurse leader.* American Association of Colleges of Nursing. Retrieved October 2009, from www.aacn.nche.edu/Publications/WhitePapers/ClinicalNurseLeader.htm.

AACN. (2008). *CNL frequently asked questions.* Retrieved October 2009, from www.aacn.nche.edu/CNL/faq.htm.

AACN. (2009). *DNP fact sheet.* Retrieved October 2009, from www.aacn.nche.edu/DNP/index.htm.

AACN, AONE, & NOADN. (1995). *A model for differentiated nursing practice.* American Association of Colleges of Nursing. Retrieved October 2009, from www.aacn.nche.edu/publications/model.htm.

American Association of Critical-Care Nurses. (2009). Retrieved October 2009, from www.aacn.org.

Bellack, J. P., & Loquist, R. S. (1999). Employer responses to differentiated nursing education. *Journal of Nursing Administration, 29*(9), 4-8, 32.

Benner, P. (2001). *From novice to expert: Excellence and power in clinical nursing practice.* Upper Saddle River, New Jersey: Prentice Hall.

Brewer, B. (2006). Is patient acuity a proxy for patient characteristics of the AACN Synergy Model for patient care? *Nursing Administration Quarterly, 30*(40), 351-357.

Burritt, J., Wallace, P., Steckel, C., & Hunter, A. (2007). Achieving quality and fiscal outcomes in patient care: The clinical mentor care delivery model. *Journal of Nursing Administration, 37*(12), 558-563.

Cohen, E., & Cesta, T. (2004). *Nursing case management: From essentials to advanced practice applications* (4th ed.). St. Louis: Mosby.

Curtis, K., Lien, D., Chan, A., Grove, P., & Morris, R. (2002). The impact of trauma case management on patient outcomes. *Journal of Trauma, 53*(3), 477-482.

D'Entremont, B. (2009). Clinical pathways: The Ottawa Hospital experience. *Canadian Nurse, 105*(5), 8-9.

Foss, N., & Koerner, J. (1997). The advanced practice nurses roles in differentiated practice: Martha's story. *AACN: Advanced Critical Care, 8*(2), 262-270.

Goldstein, R. (1998). The disease management approach to cost containment. *Nursing Case Management, 3*(3), 99-103.

Gorski, L. (2003). A disease management program for heart failure: Collaboration between a home care agency and a care management organization (electronic version). *Lippincott's Case Management, 8*(6), 265-273.

Graham, I. (2003). Leading the development of nursing within a nursing development unit: The perspectives of leadership by the team leader and professor of nursing (electronic version). *International Journal of Nursing Practice, 9*(4), 213-222.

Hardin, S., & Hussey, L. (2003). AACN Synergy Model for patient care: Case study of a CHF patient (electronic version). *Critical Care Nurse, 23*(1), 73-76.

Havens, D. S., & Johnston, M. A. (2004). Achieving Magnet hospital recognition: Chief nurse executives and Magnet coordinators tell their stories (electronic version). *Journal of Nursing Administration, 34*(12), 579-588.

Huber, D. (2010). *Leadership and nursing case management* (4th ed.). St. Louis: Saunders.

Kimball, B., Joynt, J., Cherner, D., & O'Neil, E. (2007). The quest for new innovative care delivery models. *Journal of Nursing Administration, 37*(9), 392-398.

Lencioni, P. (2006). *Silos, politics, and turf wars: A leadership fable about destroying the barriers that turn colleagues into competitors.* San Francisco: Jossey-Bass.

Manthey, M., Ciske, K., Robertson, P., & Harris, I. (1970). Primary nursing: A return to the concept of "my nurse" and "my patient." *Nursing Forum, 9*, 65-83.

Moore, N. (2004). Notes from the floor (electronic version). *Nursing Administration Quarterly, 28*(4), 258-264.

Poster, E., Adams, P., Clay, C., Garcia, B., Hallman, A., Jackson, B., Klotz, L., Lumpkins, R., Ried, H., Sanford, P., Slaton, K., & Yuill, N. (2005). The Texas Model of Differentiated Entry-Level Competencies of Graduates of Nursing Programs. *Nursing Education Perspectives, 26*(1), 18-23.

Rohde, D., & Moloney-Harmon, P. A. (2001). Pediatric critical care nursing: Annie's story. *Critical Care Nurse, 21*(5). Retrieved July 3, 2005, from www.aacn.org/WD/Certifications/content/synprac12.pcms?pid=1&&menu=.

Seago, J. (1999). Evaluation of a hospital work redesign: Patient-focused care. *Journal of Nursing Administration, 29*(11), 31-38.

Tiedeman, M., & Lookinland, S. (2004). Traditional models of care delivery: What have we learned (electronic version)? *Journal of Nursing Administration, 34*(6), 291-297.

Trossman, S. (2004). A magnetic force: ANCC program gains recognition in ensuring excellence in nursing services (electronic version). *American Journal of Nursing, 104*(12), 68-69.

Viney, M., Batcheller, J., Houston, S., & Belcik, K. (2006). Transforming care at the bedside: Designing new care systems in an age of complexity. *Journal of Nursing Care Quality, 21*(2), 143-150.

Wolf, G., & Greenhouse, P. (2007). Blueprint for design: Creating models that direct change. *Journal of Nursing Administration, 37*(9), 381-387.

Zander, K. (2002). Nursing case management in the 21st century: Intervening where margin meets mission. *Nursing Administration Quarterly, 26*(5), 58-67.

INTERNET RESOURCES

American Association of Colleges of Nursing. *White paper on the role of the clinical nurse leader.* Website: www.aacn.nche.edu/Publications/WhitePapers/ClinicalNurseLeader.htm.

American Case Management Association. Website: www.acmaweb.org.

American Nurses Credentialing Center. *History of the Magnet program.* Website: www.nursecredentialing.org/Magnet/ProgramOverview/HistoryoftheMagnetProgram.aspx.

Case Management Society of America. Website: http://cmsa.org.

Clinical Practice Guidelines Online. Agency for Healthcare Research and Quality (AHRQ). Website: www.ahrq.gov/clinic/cpgonline.htm.

RWJ Foundation launches Transforming Care at the Bedside Virtual Resource Center. Website: www.rwjf.org/pr/product.jsp?id=31512.

Transforming Care at the Bedside. Institute for Healthcare Improvement. Website: www.ihi.org/ihi/search/searchresults.aspx?searchterm=Transforming+Care+at+the+Bedside&searchtype=basic.

Transforming Care at the Bedside (TCAB)-Tool Kit. Robert Wood Johnson Foundation. Website: www.rwjf.org/pr/product.jsp?id=30051&c=EMC-CA137.

SUGGESTED READINGS

Brown, J., Smith, C., Stewart, M., Trim, K., Freeman, T., Beckhoff, C., & Kasperski, M. (2009). Level of acceptance of different models of maternity care. *Canadian Nurse, 105*(1), 19-23.

Burritt, J., Wallace, P., Steckel, C., & Hunter, A. (2007). Achieving quality and fiscal outcomes in patient care: The clinical mentor care delivery model. *Journal of Nursing Administration, 37*(12), 558-563.

Duffy, J., Baldwin, J., & Mastorovich, M. (2007). Using the Quality-Care Model to organize patient care delivery. *Journal of Nursing Administration, 37*(12), 546-551.

Heath, J., Johanson, W., & Blake, N. (2004). Healthy work environments: A validation of the literature. *Journal of Nursing Administration, 34*(11), 524-530.

Kimball, B., Joynt, J., Cherner, D., & O'Neil, E. (2007). The quest for new innovative care delivery models. *Journal of Nursing Administration, 37*(9), 392-398.

Lookinland, S., Tiedeman, M., & Crosson, A. (2005). Nontraditional models of care delivery: Have they solved the problem? *Journal of Nursing Administration, 35*(2), 74-80.

Tachibana, C., & Nelson-Peterson, D. (2007). Implementing the clinical nurse leader role using the Virginia Mason Production system. *Journal of Nurse Administration, 37*(11), 477-479.

Wiggins, M. (2008). The Partnership Care Delivery Model: An examination of the core concept and the need for a new model of care. *Journal of Nursing Management, 16,* 629-638.

14

Staffing and Scheduling

Susan Sportsman

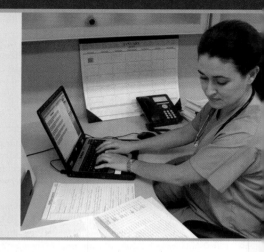

This chapter explores research regarding the relationship between nurse staffing and various nurse and patient outcomes. It discusses the interrelationship between the personnel budget and the staffing plan. Measures for evaluating unit productivity and the impact of various staffing and scheduling strategies on overall nursing satisfaction and continuity of patient care are discussed. These key points are critical to nurse managers' ability to deliver safe and effective care in their areas of responsibility while maintaining a high degree of employee satisfaction on the unit. Understanding the impact of nurse-sensitive indicators on patient outcomes helps nurse managers control the unit's labor expenses. Their ability to use this information and communicate about staffing to employees is critical to effectively managing productive services and being a valuable member of the leadership team.

OBJECTIVES

- Evaluate the impact of patient and hospital factors, nurse characteristics, nurse staffing, and other organizational factors that influence nurse and patient outcomes.
- Integrate current research into principles to effectively manage nurse staffing.
- Analyze activity reports to determine the effectiveness of a unit's productivity.
- Examine personal scheduling needs in relation to patients' requirements for continuity of care and positive outcomes, as well as the nurse manager's need to create a schedule that is balanced and fair for all team members.
- Relate floating, mandatory overtime, and the use of supplemental agency staff to nurse satisfaction and patient care outcomes.

TERMS TO KNOW

average daily census (ADC)
average length of stay (ALOS)
cost center
direct care hours
factor evaluation system
fixed FTEs
forecast
full-time equivalents (FTEs)
indirect care hours
labor cost per unit of service

mandatory overtime
nonproductive time
nurse outcomes
nurse-sensitive data
nursing productivity
overtime
patient outcomes
percentage of occupancy
productive time
prototype evaluation system

scheduling
staffing
staffing plan
staffing regulations
units of service
variable FTEs
variance report
workload

THE CHALLENGE

Mary Ellen Bonczek, BSN, RN, MPA, NEA-BC
Senior Vice President and Chief Nurse Executive, New
* Hanover Regional Medical Center, Wilmington, North*
* Carolina*

The inpatient general surgical units of a large regional medical center total 54 beds, and the surgical trauma intensive care unit (STICU) has 16 beds. The organization was faced with severe capacity constraints as it prepared to begin a master site facility plan that would result in an additional 120 beds over the next 3 years. There was a particular void in service, because there was no step-down unit for surgical patients. The coronary care unit (CCU), medical intensive care unit (MICU), and cardiovascular intensive care unit (CVICU) all have step-down units to which they can transfer patients and free up beds for truly critical patients. Beds that were already filled with general surgery patients were targeted to be the step-down unit for the STICU.

The challenge to develop the surgical step-down unit included the identification of the appropriate number of step-down beds needed by considering the volume of patients in STICU that could be transferred to the surgical step-down unit. Admission and discharge criteria for this step-down unit needed to be developed and approved by the medical staff. New equipment needs also had to be identified. The staff competencies necessary to provide appropriate care to these patients had to be considered and education plans developed. In addition, a staffing plan had to be outlined. Communication to the nursing staff was critical—some feared that they would lose their jobs because the critical care staff would assume their positions.

What do you think you would do if you were this nurse?

INTRODUCTION

Healthcare costs are escalating at a furious pace, and revenues continue to decelerate. Healthcare organizations have recognized that controlling labor costs is critical for overall cost reduction. Because nursing salaries constitute some of the major drivers of labor costs in a healthcare organization, nurse leaders are increasingly challenged to tightly manage both staffing and scheduling within their assigned cost centers. Staffing, which involves planning for hiring and deploying qualified human resources to meet the needs of a group of patients, is a primary responsibility of the nurse manager. It is also a major way in which a nurse in that role can influence quality of care. Scheduling, on the other hand, is a function of implementing the staffing plan by assigning unit personnel to work specific hours and days of the week.

Nurse managers must make skilled staffing and scheduling decisions to ensure that safe and cost-effective care is provided by the appropriate level of caregiver. No matter what the practice setting—acute care, home care, or long-term care—there is an increased focus on manager accountability for establishing and monitoring effective and efficient staffing systems.

THE STAFFING PROCESS

AHRQ Nurse Staffing Model

Because of the emphasis on patient safety and ensuring positive patient outcomes in health care, research to define the "best practices" of staffing has been a high priority in the past 15 years. Consistently over that period, the research suggests that increasing the numbers of registered nurses results in many positive benefits to patients, such as a reduction in hospital-related mortality and failure to rescue, both nurses-sensitive outcomes (Kane, Shamliyan, Mueller, Duval, & Wilt, 2007). None of these studies demonstrated a causal relationship. Further, hospitals with an overall commitment to high-quality care through sufficient staffing also invested in other actions that improve quality (Kane et al., 2007).

The results of the meta-analysis by Kane et al. (2007) is published in an Agency for Healthcare Research and Quality (AHRQ) report "Nursing Staffing and Quality of Patient Care" (*www.ahrq.*

gov/clinic/tp/nursesttp.htm). Based on the relevant research, the authors developed a conceptual framework (Figure 14-1) illustrating the complex relationships between nurse staffing and the quality of patient care. The framework considers the impact of patient and hospital factors, nurse staffing, nurse characteristics, nurse outcomes, medical care, and organizational factors on patient outcomes. Hyun, Bakken, Douglas, and Stone (2008) suggest that although data available to decide how to effectively allocate scarce nursing resources in practice are still limited, existing principles, frameworks, and guidelines provide a foundation for evidence-based nurse staffing. So, despite the complex relationships apparent in the AHRQ framework, it can be useful not only for further research but also for nurse managers to develop "best practices" for staffing.

Patient Factors

The acuity or severity of patients' conditions, influenced by their age, primary diagnosis, co-morbidity

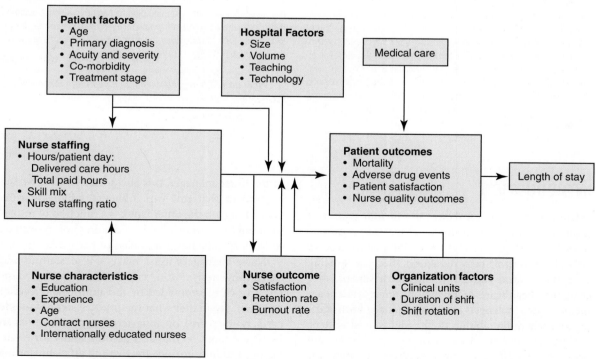

FIGURE 14-1 Conceptual framework of nurse staffing and patient outcomes.

and treatment stage, is a key component in determining the staffing required for safe care. However, the dynamic nature of patient care often makes it difficult to quantify the care needs of patients at any given time.

Patient classification systems have been developed in an effort to give nurse managers the tools and language to describe the acuity of patients on their unit. "Sicker" patients receive higher classification scores, indicating that more nursing resources are required to provide patient care. Nurse managers use the classification data to adjust the unit's staffing plan for a given time or to quantify acuity trends over longer periods as they forecast their staffing needs during the budget process.

Patient Classification Types

Two basic types of patient classification systems exist: prototype and factor. A prototype evaluation system is considered both subjective and descriptive. It classifies patients into broad categories and uses these categories to predict patient care needs. The relative intensity measures (RIMs) system is a prototype system. This system classifies patient care needs based on their diagnosis-related group (DRG). The data are then fed to a decision support system that integrates clinical and financial information.

A factor evaluation system is considered more objective than a prototype evaluation system. It gives each task, thought process, and patient care activity a time or rating. These associations are then summed to determine the hours of direct care required, or they are weighted for each patient. Each intervention is given a name and a definition and is further specified to incorporate a list of all associated interventional activities. The list of interventions is comprehensive and applicable to inpatient, outpatient, home care, and long-term care patients.

Typically, organizations use a combination of systems. Some patient types with a single healthcare focus, such as maternal deliveries or outpatient surgical patients, would be appropriately classified with a prototype system. Patients with more complex care needs and a less predictable disease course, such as those with pneumonia or stroke, are more appropriately evaluated with a factor system.

Numerous potential problems exist with patient classification systems. The issue most often raised by administrators relates to the questionable reliability and validity of the data collected through a self-reporting mechanism. Another concern with patient classification data relates to the inability of the organization to meet the prescribed staffing levels outlined by the patient classification system. Administrators worry that they risk potential liability if they do not follow the staffing recommendations of the patient classification system. If the classification data indicate that six caregivers are needed for the upcoming shift but the organization can provide only five caregivers, what are the potential consequences for the organization if an untoward event occurs?

Concern over the accuracy of biased data and the inability to meet predicted staffing levels outlined by the patient classification systems has caused many healthcare organizations to abandon patient classification as a mechanism for determining appropriate staffing levels. Staff morale is at risk when acuity models indicate one level is necessary and the organization cannot increase staffing to meet those needs. Likewise, staff morale is at risk without acuity models when it is clear to staff that patient needs exceed care capacity. A truer approach is to measure and monitor patient outcomes and participate in national databases that monitor staffing effectiveness. For example, the National Database of Nursing Quality Indicators® (NDNQI®) provides a benchmarking report comparing "like" participating organizations and units around the country.

National Database of Nursing Quality Indicators®

The NDNQI® (*www.nursingworld.org/Main MenuCategories/ThePracticeofProfessionalNursing/ PatientSafetyQuality.aspx*) is the only national nursing database that provides quarterly and annual reporting of structure, process, and outcome indicators to evaluate nursing care at the unit level. This large, longitudinal database is built upon the 1994 American Nurses Association (ANA) Patient Safety and Quality Initiative. This initiative involved a series of pilot studies across the United States to identify nurse-sensitive indicators to use in evaluating patient care quality. These nurse-sensitive indicators include both structures of care and care processes, which in turn influence care outcomes. Nurse-sensitive indicators are distinct and specific to nursing and different from medical indicators of care quality (Montalvo, 2009).

Data for the NDNQI® database are collected for eight types of units: critical care, step-down, medical, surgical, combined medical-surgical, rehabilitation, pediatric, and psychiatric. RN survey data are collected for all hospital unit types including outpatient and interventional units (Dunton, Gajewski, Klaus, & Pierson, 2007). Hospitals may join the NDNQI® project, submitting data regarding nurse-sensitive indicators. Hospitals can benchmark (or compare) their own data against other similar hospitals and participate in the ongoing research on nurse-sensitive data. Table 14-1 outlines the nurse-sensitive indicators included in the NDNQI® project.

A component of the NDNQI® database is the hours per patient day (HPPD) required to provide the necessary care for patients on the unit. This figure may include the HPPD of total nursing care provided or the HPPD of RN care provided. The NDNQI®

TABLE 14-1   NURSE-SENSITIVE INDICATORS INCLUDED IN THE NDNQI® PROJECT

INDICATOR	SUB-INDICATORS	MEASURE(S)
1. Nursing Hours per Patient Day*†	a. Registered Nurses (RNs) b. Licensed Practical/Vocational Nurses (LPNs/LVNs) c. Unlicensed Assistive Personnel (UAP)	Structure
2. Patient Falls*†		Process & Outcome
3. Patient Falls with Injury*†	a. Injury Level	Process & Outcome
4. Pediatric Pain Assessment, Intervention, Reassessment (AIR) Cycle		Process
5. Pediatric Peripheral Intravenous Infiltration Rate		Outcome
6. Pressure Ulcer Prevalence*	a. Community Acquired b. Hospital Acquired c. Unit Acquired	Process & Outcome
7. Psychiatric Physical/Sexual Assault Rate		Outcome
8. Restraint Prevalence†		Outcome
9. RN Education/Certification		Structure
10. RN Satisfaction Survey Options*‡	a. Job Satisfaction Scales b. Job Satisfaction Scales—Short Form c. Practice Environment Scale (PES)†	Process & Outcome
11. Skill Mix: Percent of total nursing hours supplied by Agency Staff*†	a. RNs b. LPNs/LVNs c. UAP	Structure
12. Voluntary Nurse Turnover†		Structure
13. Nurse Vacancy Rate		Structure

14. Healthcare-Associated Infection
  a. Urinary catheter–associated urinary tract infection (UTI)†
  b. Central line catheter–associated bloodstream infection (CABSI)*†
  c. Ventilator-associated pneumonia (VAP)†
		Outcome

From Montalvo, I. (September 2007). The National Database of Nursing Quality Indicators™ (NDNQI®). *OJIN: The Online Journal of Issues in Nursing,* *12*(3), 2.
*Original American Nurses Association (ANA) nursing-sensitive indicator.
†National Quality Forum (NQF)–endorsed nursing-sensitive indicator "NQF-15."
‡The RN survey is annual, whereas the other indicators are quarterly.

project reports a number of findings related to the HPPD required by patients. For example, Dunton, et al. (2007) suggest that:

- Lower falls rates were related to higher total nursing hours (including RN, licensed practical nurse/licensed vocational nurse [LPN/LVN] and unlicensed nursing assistants) per patient day and a higher percentage of nursing hours supplied by RNs.
- For every increase of 1 hour in total nursing HPPD, fall rates were 1.9% lower.
- For every increase of 1 percentage point in the nursing hours supplied by RNs, the fall rate was 0.7% lower (Dunton et al., 2007).

Nurse managers may also use clinical or human resource indicators other than those identified by NDNQI® to evaluate the effectiveness of the staffing and quality of patient care. Box 14-1 identifies some of these indicators.

Nurse Staffing

Over the past 10 years, as the evidence regarding nurse-sensitive indicators has grown, there has been significant controversy regarding the level of nurse staff required for various groups of patients, primarily

---

BOX 14-1   OTHER INDICATORS OF STAFFING EFFECTIVENESS

Clinical or Service Indicators
- Family complaints
- Patient complaints
- Adverse drug events
- Injuries to patients
- Postoperative infections
- Upper gastrointestinal bleeding
- Shock/cardiac arrest
- Length of stay

Human Resource Indicators
- Overtime
- Staff vacancy rate
- Staff turnover rate
- Understaffing as compared with the hospital's staffing plan
- Nursing care hours per patient day
- Staff injuries on the job
- On-call or per diem use
- Sick time

---

in acute care hospitals. In 2008, the ANA polled more than 10,000 nurses nationally to determine their perceptions of the impact of staffing levels on their work environment. Of the nurse respondents, 73% did not believe the staffing on their unit or shift was sufficient and 59.8% said they knew of someone who left direct care because of concerns about safe staffing. Of the 51.9% of respondents who were considering leaving their current position, 46% cited inadequate staffing as the reason. Almost 52% of the respondents said that they thought the quality of nursing care on their unit had declined in the past year, and 48.2% would not feel confident having someone close to them receiving care in the facility where they work (American Nurses Association [ANA], 2008).

The recognition that the number of nurses providing care to patients is associated with better patient outcomes in acute care leads to a discussion regarding the best model to ensure sufficient staffing. Two major approaches have been put forward. The first requires a specific number of patients cared for by one nurse per shift (mandated nurse-patient ratios). Legislation to mandate specific nurse-patient ratios was implemented in California in 1999 (Keepnews, 2007).

The second approach requires the development of a staffing plan, which holds hospitals accountable for projecting the nursing needs on each unit for a period of time, typically for 6 months or a year. Hospitals are also responsible for monitoring the extent to which actual staffing matches the staffing plans, making revisions as necessary. These plans often require that direct care nurses are part of the nurse staffing committee to ensure that safe nurse-to-patient ratios are based on patient needs and other related criteria. The first legislation mandating such a committee was passed by the Texas state legislature in 2002. As of October 2008, seven states had some sort of legislation requiring a nursing staffing plan in acute care hospitals (Haebler, 2008).

Those who support a specified nurse-patient ratio based on the type of unit (e.g., ICU, medical-surgical) believe this approach will require hospitals to either find sufficient numbers of nurses to meet the ratio or shut down units. Those who prefer the nurse staffing plan approach believe that use of a staffing plan is built on nursing judgment that will allow staffing to be flexible, depending on patient acuity, nurse experience, configuration of the unit, and other factors. The

ANA has developed a website *(http://safestaffing-saveslives.org/)* devoted specifically to staffing. This website, *Safe Staffing Saves Lives*, includes the principles of safe staffing developed by ANA that apply to all clinical care settings (Box 14-2). Review the website for more information.

24-Hour Staffing

Most of the research regarding safe staffing has been done in acute care hospitals or long-term care facili-

---

BOX 14-2   ANA PRINCIPLES FOR NURSE STAFFING

Principles

The nine principles identified by the expert panel for nurse staffing and adopted by the ANA Board of Directors on November 24, 1998, are listed below. A discussion of each of the three categories is available through ANA.

I. Patient Care Unit Related

a. Appropriate staffing levels for a patient care unit reflect analysis of individual and aggregate patient needs.

b. There is a critical need to either retire or seriously question the usefulness of the concept of nursing hours per patient day (HPPD).

c. Unit functions necessary to support delivery of quality patient care must also be considered in determining staffing levels.

II. Staff Related

a. The specific needs of various patient populations should determine the appropriate clinical competencies required of the nurse practicing in that area.

b. Registered nurses must have nursing management support and representation at both the operational level and the executive level.

c. Clinical support from experienced RNs should be readily available to those RNs with less proficiency.

III. Institution/Organization Related

a. Organizational policy should reflect an organizational climate that values registered nurses and other employees as strategic assets and exhibit a true commitment to filling budgeted positions in a timely manner.

b. All institutions should have documented competencies for nursing staff, including agency or supplemental and traveling RNs, for those activities that they have been authorized to perform.

c. Organizational policies should recognize the myriad needs of both patients and nursing staff.

---

ties. As a result, these findings must be applied to other healthcare settings with some caution. In addition, there has been little research regarding the differences in staffing in any clinical environment during off-peak hours (nights and weekends). Despite the fact that hospital activity is at its peak from 7 AM to 7 PM weekdays, when maximum resources are available in the nurse's work environment, this time represents only 36% of the time that nurses work in acute care or long-term care. During the remaining 64% of the time, nurses work in off-peak environments with (1) scaled-back ancillary personnel, (2) fewer (often less-experienced) staff, (3) minimal supervision, and (4) strained communication with on-call healthcare providers (Hamilton, Eschiti, Hernandez, & Neill, 2007).

The problems identified by Hamilton et al. (2007) are corroborated in other studies. Researchers have associated weekends and nights with increased mortality in hospitals for more than 25 diagnoses/patient groups. For example, Becker (2007) found acute myocardial infarction more likely to result in death among Medicaid patients admitted on weekends and Goldfarb and Rowan (2000) reported mortality after night discharge from ICU to a general unit to be 2.5 times greater compared with discharge during the day. Peberdy et al. (2008) found lower survival rates from inpatient cardiology units at nights and on weekends, even after adjusting for potentially confounding factors. Although the reasons for the differences in risk in off-peak hours are under investigation, nurse managers must be cognizant of these differences and staff during off-peak times in a prudent manner to minimize patient risk.

External Factors Influencing Staffing

An important source for guidance in projecting staffing requirements is the licensing regulations of the state, typically through the department of health, which often reflect legislation discussed earlier. Staffing regulations or recommendations can relate to the minimum number of professional nurses required on a unit at a given time or to the amount of minimum staffing in an extended-care facility or prison.

However, it is important to note that licensing standards and staffing regulations by state departments of health are not the only regulatory bodies that affect staffing plans. There are a number of national organizations with missions related to continuous improvement in the safety and quality of health care provided to the public. The Joint Commission (TJC) is an example of this type of organization. TJC works to support performance improvement in healthcare organizations through establishing standards and survey accreditation processes. To comply with the 2008 TJC patient care standards related to staffing, for example, an institution must provide an adequate number and mix of staff consistent with the hospital's staffing plan to meet the care, treatment, and service needs of the patients. TJC is not prescriptive as to what constitutes "adequate" staffing. However, in response to increasing public concerns about patient care safety and quality, TJC correlates an organization's clinical outcome data with its staffing patterns to determine the effectiveness of the overall staffing plan.

During the TJC accreditation process, the surveyor reviews the staffing plans developed by the nurse manager for any obvious staffing deficiencies—for example, a shift or series of shifts in which the unit staffing plan is not met. The surveyor also interviews staff nurses outside of the presence of nurse managers to inquire about staff perceptions of the units' staffing adequacy. Surveyors may review the staffing effectiveness data for that unit as it compares with any variations from the staffing plan to identify quality-of-care concerns. Nurse managers are well advised to prepare a balanced staffing plan that supports a unit's unique patient care needs and the scrutiny of TJC survey process. They also should post this staffing plan and compliance reports for staff to see on a routine basis. In some states, this posting is required.

Additional regulatory agencies that provide accreditation services similar to those provided by TJC include the American Osteopathic Association (AOA), the Center for Accreditation of Rehabilitation Facilities (CARF), the Accreditation Association for Ambulatory Health Care (AAAHC), the Det Norske Veritas (DNV), the National Committee for Quality Assurance in Behavioral Health, and the Community Health Accreditation Program. Other groups are emerging.

Consumer expectations may also play a role in the development and implementation of the staffing plans. Exceeding the expectations of consumers for care and services is a major strategy for maintaining and improving the long-term viability of any healthcare organization. Recognizing that the patient expects to receive high-quality nursing care that is delivered promptly and efficiently by nurses who are satisfied with their workload has a significant influence on the development of a staffing plan.

Organizational policies and clear expectations communicated to staff are essential to manage high and low volume as well as changes in acuity. Proposed personnel budgets and staffing plans that cannot flex up or down when patient acuity or volumes change put the nurse manager in a position in which patient safety may not be maintained and financial obligations cannot be met. In addition, there must be mechanisms in place and internally publicized that allow staff to ask for additional help as needed. Patient, staff, and physician satisfaction; service and care improvement; and patient safety improvement are all outcomes of a solid staffing plan. Nurse managers are obligated to consider these variables when preparing the personnel budget.

Nurse Characteristics

Kane et al. (2007) define nurse characteristics as the age, experience, and education of the nurse who is providing care. In addition, the use of supplemental (agency/contract) nurses and internationally educated nurses is a variable that influences nurse staffing. Although not specifically identified in the AHRQ conceptual framework, other factors such as the use of float pools and overtime also may affect patient outcomes.

Ridley (2008), in reviewing literature from 1986 to 2006 regarding the relationship between patient safety and nurse education level, found that when studies discriminate between registered nurses and other types of nursing personnel (LPN/LVNs or unlicensed assistive personnel), there is evidence that an increased number of RNs and a larger percentage of RNs relative to other nursing personnel decrease adverse patient outcomes sensitive to nursing care. In 2003, Aiken, Clarke, Cheung, Sloane, and Silber examined whether the proportion of hospital RNs educated at the baccalaureate level or higher was associated with risk-adjusted 30-day mortality and failure to rescue; interest in this idea has persisted. Further research is necessary to validate this claim (Ridley, 2008). However, Dunton et al. (2007) found that for every increase of a year in average RN experience, the fall rate was 1% lower and the number of hospital-acquired pressure ulcers was reduced by 0.7%.

Overtime

Kane et al. (2007) reviewed seven descriptive studies that used survey methodology to find that nurses are working long hours. Because more nurses are choosing to work 12-hour shifts, the risk of working more than 12 hours is high, given that nurses often cannot finish their work by the end of their scheduled shift. There is beginning evidence that working more than 12 hours and rotating shifts can lead to errors that compromise patient safety. This suggests that requiring nurses to work rotating shifts should be avoided and that nurses should be educated about the effect of fatigue on the quality of their practice (Kane et al., 2007).

Requiring staff to stay on duty after their shift ends to fill staffing vacancies is called mandatory overtime. Professional nursing organizations and state boards of nursing across the country are discussing the issue of mandatory overtime. It has become a major negotiating point for nurses in unionized settings, and some state nursing associations that use workplace advocacy strategies to improve the work environment in their states have developed legislation that prohibits mandatory overtime. The ANA and other nursing organizations oppose mandatory overtime, because it is seen as a risk to both patients and nurses.

In contrast, *requesting* staff to stay on duty after their shift ends to fill staffing vacancies is called overtime. This differs from mandatory overtime because there are no employment consequences to the staff response to the request. In addition, in a given week, nurses may work in more than one employment setting as a means of increasing their income. Although this practice is an individual decision, tired and overworked nurses are more likely to have compromised decision-making abilities and technical skills because of fatigue.

Research has been done related to the impact of fatigue on patient safety from nurses working overtime. Berney and Needleman (2003), as evaluated by Kane et al. (2007), examined the association between overtime hours and patient outcome and found that every additional 10% of overtime hours

was associated with a 1.3% increase in hospital-related mortality.

> **EXERCISE 14-1**
>
> Review a healthcare organization's policies on overtime. Is mandatory overtime covered in the policy? Are the consequences for failing to work mandatory overtime when requested to do so by a supervisor outlined in the policy?
>
> How would you respond to a nurse manager who required you to stay on the job after your shift was over? Develop a list of questions you might ask on a job interview relating to use of overtime in the organization.
>
> What does the state board of nursing in your state allow regarding mandatory overtime? As a nurse manager, how would you respond to a staffing shortage without mandatory overtime as an option? Develop a list of strategies for eliminating mandatory overtime, if such exists.

Float Pools and Agency Staff

Many nurses choose to work for staffing agencies. They may be hired by the nursing unit as an independent contractor for a shift, a week, or longer. There are advantages to the nurse to work for an agency, such as higher hourly rates of pay, diversity in work assignments, exposure to a variety of work teams, and the ability to travel.

Organizations may use supplemental (contract or agency) staff to fill temporary staff vacancies. Despite the response to an unexpected vacancy, nurse managers must consider the potential negative aspects of depending on supplemental staff to meet the unit's staffing plan. Patients should be unable to distinguish agency staff from unit staff. However, the ability to provide that level of orientation to agency or contract staff is often difficult.

The evidence regarding the impact of the use of contract nurses on patient outcome is mixed. Cho (2002), as cited in Kane et al. (2007), showed no association between hours worked by a contract nurse and the rates of urinary tract infection, pneumonia, pressure ulcers, surgical wound infections, and bloodstream infections. In contrast, Kane et al. (2007) reviewed research by Cho (2002) and Donaldson, et al. (2005), which found that an increase in rates of patient falls corresponded to use of additional contract hours.

Another strategy that may be used to deal with unanticipated staff vacancies involves "floating" nurses from one clinical unit to another to fill the vacancy. In studies included in the 2007 research, two studies indicated the use of "float" nurses was associated with an increased risk of nosocomial infections and rate of bloodstream infections (Kane et al., 2007); however, further research is necessary to validate this finding. In practice, the use of float nurses may be effective if the nurses are deployed from a centralized flexible staffing pool and they have the competencies to work on the unit to which they are assigned. Nurses willing to work as float nurses are generally experienced nurses who maintain a broad range of clinical competencies. They often receive added compensation for their willingness to be flexible and to float to a variety of units on short notice.

When an organization does not have the flexibility of a staffing pool, the organization may expect nurses to float across clinical units to fill vacancies. To ensure patient safety and nurse satisfaction, the organization must develop a policy regarding the reassignment of the staff to clinically similar units. If staff nurses are asked to be reassigned to an area outside of their sphere of clinical competence, they should be asked to support only basic care needs and not assume a complete and independent assignment. This practice should be used only on an emergency basis or with the nurse's agreement, because being required to float is often a "dissatisfier" for nurses.

Hospital Factors

According to the AHRQ conceptual model, hospital factors include the size of the hospital, the volume of patients seen, whether the hospital is a teaching hospital, and the extent to which technology is used in the hospital. Kane et al. (2007) reviewed a study by Seago, Spetz, and Mitchell (2004) that found that for-profit hospitals and systems had fewer RN productive hours for medical-surgical nursing. A number of studies have found that the type of unit affected hospital RN staffing. Intensive care, pediatric, and maternity units had significantly higher RN staffing than medical/surgical or gynecologic units. Controlling for size, rural hospitals also had higher RN staffing (Kane et al., 2007). Studies exploring the relationship between increased RN-to-patient ratio found that the effect of increasing the number of RNs to patients was greater in surgical patients and in ICUs. The evidence

of the effect of increased RN-to-patient ratios in medical units is less consistent and needs further investigation (Kane et al., 2007). The nurse surveillance capacity of a hospital (those factors that strengthen or weaken the nurses' ability to observe patients for signs of difficulty) also affects the quality of care given. Nurse surveillance capacity is composed of nurse staffing, education, expertise, and experience, as well as nurse practice environment characteristics. Kutney-Lee, Lake, and Aiken (2009) found that greater nurse surveillance capacity was significantly associated with better quality of care and fewer adverse events. (See the Literature Perspective below.)

Regardless of the characteristics of the hospital, managers must be concerned with the financial health of the institution. As a result, hospital financial officers are often reluctant to increase the number of RN staff because of fear of escalating costs. However, Dall, Chen, Seifert, Maddox, and Hogan (2009) found that for each additional patient care RN employed at 7.8 HPPD, over $60,0000 annually will be saved from reduced medical cost and improved national productivity (accounting for 72% of labor costs). This is only a partial estimate of the economic value of nursing because it omits the intangible benefits of reduced pain and suffering by patients and family members,

LITERATURE PERSPECTIVE

Resource: Kutney-Lee, A., Lake, E. T., & Aiken, L. H. (2009). Development of the hospital nurse surveillance capacity profile. *Research in Nursing* & *Health, 32*(2), 217-228.

Surveillance by nurses is a key component of improved patient care. This article defines, operationalizes, measures, and evaluates **nurse surveillance capacity,** which includes organizational features that enhance or weaken nurse surveillance. Nurse surveillance capacity is composed of nurse staffing, education, expertise, and experience, as well as nurse practice environment characteristics. This study found that greater nurse surveillance capacity was significantly associated with better quality of care and fewer adverse events.

Implications for Practice
Evaluating the nurse surveillance capacity in a particular nursing work environment may assist the nurse manager to improve nurse surveillance and patient outcomes on his or her unit.

the reduced risk of rehospitalization, benefits to the hospital such as improved reputation and reduced malpractice claims, and other indirect costs. Unfortunately, from the hospital administrators' perspective, healthcare facilities realize only a portion of the economic value of professional nursing, because under current reimbursement systems, the incentive is for hospitals to staff at levels below where the benefit to society equals the cost to employ an additional nurse (Kane et al., 2007).

Nurse Outcomes

Nurse outcomes include staff vacancy rate, nurse satisfaction, staff turnover rate, retention rate, and nurse burnout rate. Kane et al. (2007) noted that while patient outcomes are the ultimate concern, nurse outcomes can interact with nurse staffing to affect patient outcomes. In addition, patient outcomes will, in turn, affect length of stay (LOS), and greater complication rates may increase the length of stay for patients.

A number of studies evaluated by Kane et al. (2007) focused on the impact of nurse satisfaction on patient outcomes. In a survey of 8760 nurses, Sochalski (2004), as described by Kane et al. (2007), examined the relative risk of adverse events among Medicare patients in relation to perceived quality of care. Nurses responded to the survey question, "In general, how would you describe the quality of nursing care delivered to patients in your unit on your last shift?" A reduction by 16% in the relative risk of patient falls and medication errors corresponded to a 30% increase in nurses satisfied with the care provided. However, Kane et al. (2007) also reviewed a number of studies that did not detect a significant improvement in patient satisfaction in relation to nurse satisfaction.

Kane et al. (2007) reported on the impact of nurse autonomy and nurse turnover in relation to patient outcomes. For example, they cite a study by Seago, Spetz, and Mitchell (2004) that found that a 2% increase in nurse autonomy accompanied a 0.5% reduction in pressure ulcer rates.

Organizational Factors That Affect Staffing Plans

Organizational factors described in the AHRQ conceptual framework include issues such as types of clinical units and the duration of the shift nurses work, as well as the extent to which shifts are rotated. These factors are typically addressed in the structure and philosophy of the nursing service department, organizational staffing policies, organizational supports, and services offered.

Structure and Philosophy of the Nursing Services Department

A nursing philosophy statement outlines the vision, values, and beliefs about the practice of nursing and the provision of patient care within the organization. The philosophy statement is used to guide the practice of nursing in the various nursing units on a daily basis. Nurse managers must propose a staffing plan and a personnel budget that allow consistency between the written philosophy statement and the observable practice of nursing on their units. It is demoralizing for nurses to feel that they cannot comply with their nursing philosophy statement or professional values because of problems associated with consistently inadequate staffing.

The philosophy statement also guides the establishment of the overall structure of the nursing service department and the staffing models that are used within the organization. The staffing model adopted by the organization plays a major role in determining the mix of professional and assistive staff needed to provide patient care.

Organizational Staffing Policies

Nurse managers are guided in their development of unit personnel budgets by the organization's staffing policies. For example, the organization develops a policy that identifies the rate at which an employee earns overtime and other benefit time. Therefore nurse managers will be in compliance with these laws if they adhere to their organizational staffing policies.

Organizational Support Systems

A critical variable that affects the development of the nursing personnel budget is the presence, or absence, of organizational systems that support the nurse in providing care. If the organization has recognized the need to keep the professional nurse at the bedside, support systems to allow that to happen will be evident. Examples of support systems that enhance the nurse's ability to remain on the unit and provide direct care to patients include transporter services, clerical support services, and hospitality services.

However, professional nurses often work in organizations that require them to function in the role of a multipurpose worker, particularly in acute or long-term care. Because nurses in these settings are generally scheduled to work 24 hours a day, 7 days a week, they may be required to provide services for other professionals who provide more limited hours of care to patients. It is wise for nurse managers to identify what costs are being incurred in the unit as a result of the absence of adequate organizational support systems and to develop strategies to put those systems into place or justify the budget accordingly. Important to this consideration is the study by Upenieks, Akhavan, and Kotlerman (2008), which found that a number of activities that were not actual direct care activities performed at the patient's bedside were considered value-added activities, because they represented a direct benefit to the patient. (See the Research Perspective below.)

 RESEARCH PERSPECTIVE

Resource: Upenieks, V., Akhavan, J., & Kotlerman, J. (2008). Value-added care: A paradigm shift in patient care delivery. *Nursing Economic$ 6*(5), 294-300.

The purpose of the study was to (1) gain an understanding of how much time frontline RNs spent in value-added care and (2) determine whether increasing the combined level of RNs and unlicensed assistive personnel (UAP) increased the amount of time spent in value-added care compared with time spent in necessary tasks and waste. The study found that a number of activities that were not actual direct-care activities performed at the patient's bedside, including collaborating with team members, reviewing charts, preparing medications, teaching activities, and communicating with family members, were considered value-added activities, since they represented a direct benefit to the patient.

Implications for Practice
This study validated the work done by Robert Wood Johnson's Foundation's initiative, *Transforming Care at the Bedside*, designed to increase the amount of time nurses spend in value-added activities and to reduce time spent in non–value-added activities to improve workflow efficiency, encourage care processes free of waste, and promote continuous flow of patient activities through the appropriate use of nurses and UAPs.

Services Offered

When developing a staffing budget, nurse managers must consider the services offered on the unit, as well as organizational plans to provide new or expanded clinical services. For example, a manager of an inpatient surgical unit must consider the potential effect of offering a new surgical procedure to the community. What projections have been made for this market? What is the expected length of stay for patients undergoing this new procedure? What are the national standards for care for this type of patient? A nurse manager will use this information to project added staff to manage these changes in service.

Conversely, nurse managers must also be aware of any organizational plans to delete an existing service that their unit supports. For example, if a nurse manager in a home care setting knows that reimbursement for a certain procedure in the home has declined to the point that this service must be discontinued, allowances for fewer required staffing resources in the coming year must be made.

FORECASTING UNIT STAFFING REQUIREMENTS

Recognizing factors, including related research, that influence staffing can inform decisions regarding development of the staffing plan. However, other issues must be considered when determining an appropriate staffing level for a specific unit. The staffing plan for a unit is initiated in concert with the development of the personnel budget. The person(s) responsible for projecting staffing needs of the unit should consider a number of factors when forecasting the unit's workload for the upcoming year, including the following:

1. Projected units of services (UOS)
2. Historical staffing requirements
3. Effectiveness of the current staffing plan
4. Trends in acuity on the unit
5. Anticipated skill mix or other personnel changes
6. Experience and education of staff
7. New physicians, programs, services, or technology anticipated to affect staffing
8. Patient outcomes
9. Need for educational updates driven by changes in patient care guidelines

Various mathematical formulations are used to create personnel budgets and staffing patterns. However, these formulas were developed when the average length of stay and reimbursement patterns were much different than they are today. The current difficulties related to staffing in health care suggest that current methods used to predict personnel budgets and staffing patterns have become increasingly complex and ineffective. Fitzpatrick & Brooks (2010) suggest the use of optimization models that rely on computer and logistic sciences to identify the best solution to particular staffing problems (Fitzpatrick & Brooks, 2010). (See the Literature Perspective below.)

Units of Service

Units of service (UOS) are productivity targets, such as nursing hours per patient day (HPPD) or hours per visit for emergency departments. The UOS multiplied by the volume for a clinical area determines the number of staff needed in a given time period. The formula can be adjusted for total paid staff or just for those required for the delivery of direct patient care.

To develop an adequate personnel budget, the amount of work performed by a nursing unit, or cost center, is referred to as its workload. Workload is measured in terms of the units of service defined by the cost center. Nurse managers must understand the nature of the work in their area of responsibility to define the units of service that will be used as their workload statistic and to forecast, or project, the volume of work that will be performed by their cost center during the upcoming year.

Calculation of Full-Time Equivalents

Nurse managers use the unit's forecasted workload to calculate the number of full-time equivalents (FTEs) that will be needed to construct the unit's overall staffing plan. It is important to remember that there is a distinction between an employee in a position and an FTE. Chapter 12 describes FTEs and how they are calculated. To achieve a balanced staffing plan, nurse managers must determine the correct combination of full-time and part-time positions that will be needed.

Nurse managers must also consider the effect of productive and nonproductive hours when projecting the FTE needs of the unit. Productive time is the paid hours that are actually worked on the unit. Productive hours can be further defined as direct or indirect. Direct care hours are used to pay for the care of patients. Indirect care hours are used to pay for other required unit activities, such as staff meetings or continuing education attendance.

Nonproductive time (see Chapter 12) includes those hours of benefit time that are paid to an employee for vacation, holiday, personal, or sick time in some organizations or for an employee attending orientation or continuing education activities. In most practice settings, nurses must be replaced when they are off duty and accessing their paid benefit time off. Managers must be aware of the average benefit hours required for their unit, or they will understate their FTE needs. This requires nurse managers to consider carefully how to allocate their budgeted FTEs

 LITERATURE PERSPECTIVE

Resource: Fitzpatrick, T., & Brooks, B. (2010). The nurse leader as logistician: Optimizing human capital. *JONA 40*(2), 69-74.

Ten-day hospital length of stays, cost-based reimbursements, and unlegislated staffing ratios were common when the mathematical formulas currently used to create personnel budgets and staffing patterns were developed. However, healthcare delivery has become much more dynamic and complex in the twenty-first century and the old formulas, based on averages, are no longer adequate. Because these formulas use a single number, usually an average, to represent uncertain outcomes, the "flaw of averages" tends to promote zero-sum solutions. For example, if the solutions meet financial goals, staff satisfaction are sacrificed. Conversely, if staff satisfaction is achieved, financial targets are not met.

The authors suggest that optimization models, using the power of computer science and logistics science, can simulate solutions for complex staffing problems. These solutions consider myriad constraints and variables and arrange them is such a way to produce the optimal answer solution. For example, the real-world problems are defined as a set of mathematical equations, addressing *objectives* (minimize cost, maximize preferences, and perfect coverage), *variables* (skill and staff mix, demand fluctuation, and cost differentials) and *constraints* (staff availability, union rules) to determine the best solution.

Implications for Practice
Although these modeling tools and techniques have not yet been widely used in health care, they are available. The authors suggest that executive teams should include experts with these modeling and analytical skills. In addition, nurse executives also may want to gain these skills.

into full-time and part-time positions to meet the staffing requirements for the unit when a portion of the staff is taking paid time off. In addition, looking at the number of employees being paid for any specific day may not reflect the number actually providing care. So, the nurse manager's role must include competencies in finances, information technology, and automation of staffing and scheduling programs.

EXERCISE 14-2

Select a hospital-based department and determine the hours of operation. Assess the master scheduling plan and determine how many RNs are needed to ensure that each shift has one RN present. Assuming that a 36-hour work week (three 12-hour shifts) will equal one FTE, convert the required number of registered nurse positions to FTEs. Complete the exercise assuming a 40-hour work week (five 8-hour shifts) and compare the FTE variance.

Distribution of Full-Time Equivalents

Nurse managers must consider a number of variables when they begin the process of distributing FTEs into the unit staffing plan. The staffing plan, which is based on the unit's approved personnel budget AND the projected staffing needs to ensure patient safety, as previously discussed, serves as a guide for creating the unit's schedules for the upcoming year. Variables that must be considered by managers when creating master staffing plans include the following:

1. The hours of operation of the unit
2. The basic shift length for the unit
3. Known activity patterns for the unit at various times of day
4. Maximum work stretch for each employee
5. Shift rotation requirements
6. Weekend requirements
7. Personal and professional requirements and requests for time off (e.g., school schedule, meetings for professional development, and support for models of shared governance)

Each of these variables interrelates with the others, so few "absolutes" are possible. For example, initially one might think that a 24/7 unit might require more staff than a 7 AM to 6 PM area. If the 24/7 unit, however, is providing basic care all day and few activi-

ties at night (e.g., a long-term care facility), fewer staff might be needed than for the 7 AM to 6 PM area if that were, for example, a day surgery unit.

The master staffing plan must consider the distribution of fixed FTEs in the plan. Fixed FTEs are held by those employees who will be scheduled to work, no matter what the volume of activity. These employees generally hold an exempt or salaried position, meaning their compensation does not depend on the unit's workload. Examples of employees who typically hold a fixed FTE include the nurse manager, the clinical nurse specialist, and the education staff.

The manager then distributes the variable FTEs into the staffing plan. Variable FTEs are held by those employees who are scheduled to work based on the workload of the unit. These employees are considered non-exempt or hourly wage employees, meaning their compensation depends on the actual number of hours worked in a given pay period. Examples of employees who typically hold a variable FTE position include staff nurses, clerical staff, and other ancillary support staff assigned to the unit.

SCHEDULING

Scheduling is a function of implementing the staffing plan by assigning unit personnel to work specific hours and specific days of the week. The nurse manager is often challenged to take the FTEs that are allotted through the personnel budget, distribute them appropriately, and create a master schedule for the unit that also meets each employee's personal and professional needs. Although completely satisfying each individual staff member is not always possible, a schedule can usually be created that is both fair and balanced from the employee's perspective while still meeting the patient care needs. Creating a flexible schedule with a variety of scheduling options that leads to work schedule stability for each employee is one mechanism likely to retain staff, which is within the control of nurse managers.

Constructing the Schedule

Mechanisms are typically in place within an organization for staff to use in requesting days off and to know when the final schedule will be posted. In addition, most organizations have written policies and procedures that must be followed by nurse managers to ensure compliance with state and federal labor laws relative to scheduling. These policies also aid managers in making scheduling decisions that will be perceived as fair and equitable by all employees.

Schedules are usually constructed for a predetermined block of time based on organizational policy—for example, weekly, biweekly, or monthly. The unit schedule may be prepared in a decentralized fashion by nurse managers or by unit staff through a self-scheduling method. In some organizations, centralized staffing coordinators may oversee all of the schedules prepared for the patient care units. Each method of schedule preparation has pros and cons.

Decentralized Scheduling—Nurse Manager

One decentralized method for preparing the schedule involves nurse managers developing the schedule in isolation from all other units. In this model, the nurse managers approve all schedule changes and actually spend time on a regular basis drafting the staff schedule, considering only the staffing needs of the unit. In other decentralized models, managers do the preliminary work on schedules and then submit them to a centralized staffing office for review and for the addition of any needed supplemental staff. The advantage of this decentralized model is that the accountability for submitting a schedule in alignment with the established staffing plan rests with managers. These individuals are ultimately the ones responsible for maintaining unit productivity in line with the personnel budget, so the incentive to manage the schedule tightly is strong. The negative aspect of this decentralized method relates to the inability of any individual nurse manager to know the "big picture" related to staffing across multiple patient care units. Requests for time off are approved in isolation from all other units, and there is a real potential with this model that each manager will make a decision at the unit level that will be felt in aggregate as a "staffing shortage" across multiple units.

Staff Self-Scheduling

A self-scheduling process has the potential to promote staff autonomy and to increase staff accountability. In addition, team communication, problem-solving, and negotiating skills can be enhanced through the self-scheduling process. Successful self-scheduling is achieved when each individual's personal schedule is balanced with the unit's patient care needs.

Self-scheduling has become more complicated in the wake of care delivery changes and the decentralization of many activities to the individual patient care units. The professional nursing staff cannot work in isolation of other care members when creating a schedule. Assessing the readiness of support staff to participate in this type of initiative is critical as resource utilization and cost containment continue to be major focal points of concern.

Self-scheduling or flexible scheduling needs to be properly managed. Although personal needs of the staff are important to meet, the patient care needs on the unit are the paramount focus for building a schedule. Unit standards for a staffing plan are established, and then a negotiated schedule that results in meeting the needs of staff and patients is the expected and ultimate outcome.

Centralized Scheduling

One benefit to centralized scheduling is that the staffing coordinator is usually aware of the abilities, qualifications, and availability of supplemental personnel who may be needed to complete the schedule. In many organizations, the centralized staffing coordinator is also aware of each unit's personnel budget and any constraints it may impose on the schedule. On the other hand, a disadvantage to centralized staffing is the limited knowledge of the coordinator relative to changing patient acuity needs or other patient-related activities on the unit. Developing a mechanism for the centralized staffing coordinator to share unit-specific knowledge with the respective nurse manager can resolve this disadvantage satisfactorily.

Many organizations have invested in computer software designed to create optimal schedules based on the approved staffing plans for individual units. The centralized staffing coordinator maintains the integrity of the computerized databank for each unit; enters schedule variances daily; generates planning sheets, drafts, and final schedules; and runs any specialized productivity reports requested by nurse managers. Nurse managers review the initial schedule created by the computer, make necessary modifications, and approve the final schedule.

Variables That Affect Staffing Schedules

Nurse managers must consider many variables to create a fair and balanced schedule. Examples of

- Hours of operation
- Shift rotations
- Weekend rotations
- Approved benefit time for the schedule period—for example, vacations and holidays
- Approved leaves of absence/short-term disability
- Approved seminar, orientation, and continuing education time
- Scheduled meetings for the schedule period
- Current filled positions and current staffing vacancies
- Number of part-time employees

- Volume statistic: number of units of service for the reporting period
- Capacity statistic: number of beds or blocks of time available for providing services
- Percentage of occupancy: number of occupied beds for the reporting period
- Average daily census (ADC): average number of patients cared for per day for the reporting period
- Average length of stay (ALOS): average number of days that a patient remained in an occupied bed

Formulas for Calculating Volume Statistics
Assume that a 20-bed medical-surgical unit *(capacity statistic)* accrued 566 patient days in June *(volume statistic)*. Ninety-eight of these patients were discharged during the month.

Average Daily Census (ADC) on this unit is 18.9:
Formula: patient days for a given time period divided by the number of days in the time period
a. 30 days in June
b. 566 patient days/30 days = ADC of 18.9

Percentage of Occupancy for June is 95%:
Formula: daily patient census (rounded) divided by the number of beds in the unit
19 patients in a 20-bed unit =
19 patients/20 beds = 95% occupancy

Average Length of Stay for June is 5.8
Formula: number of patient days divided by the number of discharges
566 patient days/98 patient discharges = 5.8 (rounded)

variables nurse managers can anticipate and must consider as they prepare the unit's schedule are found in Box 14-3. Other unanticipated variables can complicate the best-prepared schedule. When faced with call-ins for illness, funeral leaves, jury duty, or an emergent need for a leave of absence (LOA), nurse managers must attempt to fill a shift vacancy on short notice. Requesting staff to add hours over their planned commitment, floating staff from another unit or securing someone from a staffing pool, contracting with agency nursing staff, and seeking overtime are examples of strategies that nurse managers may be compelled to use to ensure safe staffing of their units. However, as discussed, many potential negative consequences are associated with using these strategies.

EXERCISE 14-3
Assume you are going on a job interview. Considering your personal preferred work schedule, what scheduling practices would be most satisfying to you and might lead you to accept employment with the organization? What scheduling practices might cause you to look elsewhere for a job? Develop a list of questions to ask your potential employer regarding scheduling practices in his or her organization.

EVALUATING UNIT STAFFING AND PRODUCTIVITY

Nurse managers are increasingly pressed to justify their staffing decisions to their staff, senior management, and accrediting agency. The unit activity/production report, which provides a variety of measures of unit workload, can be helpful in such justification. In addition, a review of the extent to which the actual staffing over a specific time period matches the staffing plan, particularly coupled with various outcomes over the same period, gives a picture of the productivity and effectiveness of the unit. Although the format of these reports may vary, the kinds of information typically available to nurse managers in an activity report are included in Box 14-4.

In the inpatient setting, the average daily census (ADC) is one measure considered by nurse managers to project the potential workload of the unit. The ADC is a simple measure of the average number of patients being cared for in the available beds on the unit trended over a specific period. The formula for calculating the ADC is found in Box 14-4. If a unit's ADC is trending upward, the nurse manager should propose additional personnel to manage this increase

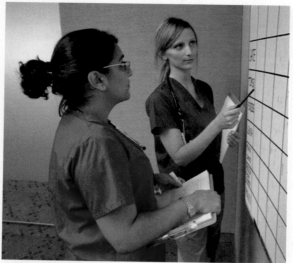

Calculating the percentage of occupancy is essential when developing a unit's staffing plan.

in patient volume. If the ADC is trending downward, the nurse manager should propose the need for fewer resources to manage this downward census trend. In the acute care setting, a unit's ADC can be extremely volatile based on the patterns of admissions, transfers, and discharges on the unit. In a long-term care setting, however, the unit's ADC may be very stable over prolonged periods. Nurse managers may note census trends based on a particular shift, the day of the week, or the season of the year. The addition of new physicians, the creation of new programs or services, and many other variables may also affect a unit's average daily census. Admissions and discharge increases staffing demands. Nurse managers must maintain a strong grasp on these measures of workload to prepare an adequate staffing plan for their unit.

Another way of assessing a unit's activity level is to calculate the percentage of occupancy. The unit's occupancy rate can be calculated for a specific shift, on a daily basis, or as a monthly or annual statistic. The formula for calculating the percentage of occupancy is also found in Box 14-4. Nurse managers use the percentage of occupancy to develop the unit's staffing plan. Optimal occupancy rates may vary by practice setting. In a long-term care facility, the organization would desire 100% occupancy rates.

However, in an acute care facility, 85% occupancy rates would ensure the best potential for patient throughput.

Another measure of unit activity that may be considered by nurse managers is the average length of stay (ALOS), or the average number of days each patient stays in an occupied bed. As reimbursement dollars have decreased, so have lengths of stay. However, the cost of treating the patient has not decreased as dramatically because patient acuity is greater; essentially, hospitals need to provide more care in less time for fewer dollars with the same, if not better, outcomes. For this reason, as a unit's ALOS trends downward, the need for staffing resources may not change substantially or it may actually climb. The formula for calculating the average length of stay is also found in Box 14-4.

The measures just mentioned provide the nurse manager with an understanding of the number of patients who have been admitted to the unit over a period of time. The nurse is then charged with matching the needs of these patients with the appropriate number of staff members. Managers have positions and subsequent budgeted nursing salary dollars in the personnel budget based on the estimated units of service that will be provided in the unit. If managers can provide more care to more patients while spending the same or fewer salary dollars, they have increased their unit productivity. Conversely, if the same or more salary dollars are spent to provide less care to fewer patients, managers have decreased their unit productivity.

Nursing productivity is a formula-driven calculation. Unit of service (UOS) multiplied by the volume (patient days or emergency department visits) equals hours available to create direct productive staffing plans. Those hours multiplied by a nonproductive factor (e.g., 1.12) to account for paid time off equals the total hours available for the staffing plan. It is essential to set a ratio of patients to RN. This is then applied to the total hours available, and the support structure (nursing assistants or unit clerks) then can be built accordingly. Patient type, scope of service, and acuity and/or classification of the patient are all factors correlated with patient outcomes that drive staffing decisions. Meeting these productivity standards is important to ensure the financial well-being of the organization. However, if the safety needs of the patients are put at risk to achieve this productivity level, the consequences are harmful to patients, staff, and the organization as a whole.

Calculating nursing productivity is challenging for nurse managers because it is difficult to quantify the efficiency and effectiveness of individual nurses providing care to patients. Individual nurses can vary greatly in their critical-thinking abilities, their skill levels, and their ability to make timely and accurate decisions that affect patient outcomes.

Variance Between Projected and Actual Staff

Organizations can use labor cost or a straight FTE model for comparison of actual with projected staff. Labor cost per unit of service is a simple measure that compares budgeted salary costs per budgeted volume of service (productivity target) with actual salary costs per actual volume of service (productivity performance). This measure requires managers to staff according to their staffing plan because the plan reflects the approved personnel budget. Box 14-5 shows an analysis of labor costs per units of service.

Typically, nurse managers must evaluate and explain changes in productivity resulting in a difference between the projected staffing plan and the actual schedule, using a variance report. If managers compare the two numbers and the actual productivity performance number is higher than the target, they have spent more money for care than they budgeted. A number of variables may cause the labor costs to be higher than anticipated, such as increased overtime, paying bonus pay for regular staff, using costly agency resources, or a higher-than-anticipated amount of indirect education or orientation time.

If managers compare the two numbers and the actual productivity performance number is lower than the target, they have spent less money for care than they budgeted. Managers must also explain this high degree of productivity. One variable that may cause the labor costs to be lower than anticipated is an increased nonprofessional skill mix or consistently understaffing their unit.

It cannot be said that having a productivity performance number that is either higher or lower than that planned represents effective management. Assuming that staffing plans were an accurate reflection of the conditions on the specific units, if managers compare

the actual productivity performance with their productivity target and the two numbers match, the managers have probably managed effectively. However, given the dynamic nature of patient care, an ongoing evaluation of the conditions on the unit as well as the extent to which proposed staffing levels are reached or exceeded should be monitored on an ongoing basis. Variance reports provide an opportunity for such evaluation.

BOX 14-5   ANALYSIS OF LABOR COSTS PER UNIT OF SERVICE

1. A manager of a cardiac telemetry unit proposes the following in the personnel budget. These are the unit's productivity targets.
   Total patient days: 5840
   - ADC = 16
   - Staffing plan for ADC of 16:
     - Day shift: 3 RNs and 3 UAP (50% RN skill mix)
     - Evening shift: 3 RNs and 3 UAP (50% RN skill mix)
     - Night shift: 3 RNs and 1 UAP (75% RN skill mix)
   - Direct care labor costs are also projected by the manager based on the average RN and UAP salaries for this unit
   - Target = $139.32 per patient, or $2229.12 per day
2. The manager actually staffs as follows:
   - ADC = 16
   - Actual staffing for ADC of 16:
     - Day shift: 4 RNs and 2 UAP (66% RN skill mix)
     - Evening shift: 4 RNs and 2 UAP (66% RN skill mix)
     - Night shift: 3 RNs (100% RN skill mix)
   - Direct labor costs for this day = $145.44 per patient, or $2327.04 per day
3. The manager has incurred a variance:
   - Exceed target by $6.12 per patient, or $97.92 for the day

ADC, Average daily census; *RN,* registered nurse; *UAP,* unlicensed assistive personnel.

EXERCISE 14-4

Assume you are working in the charge nurse role. One of the staff assigned to work with you becomes ill and must go home suddenly, leaving his designated patient assignment to be assumed by someone else. As a charge nurse, what factors would you consider as you determine how to reassign this work to other nurses? If you were a co-worker on the shift, instead of the charge nurse, what effective follower behaviors might you demonstrate to support the charge nurse in this situation? Can you identify behaviors of co-workers that would complicate the staffing situation further?

Impact of Leadership on Productivity

Nurse managers must possess staffing and scheduling skills to prepare a staffing plan that balances organizational directives with unit needs for care and services. They must spend time each month evaluating their unit's productivity performance. Yet it is also important that nurse managers improve unit productivity by spending more of their work time coaching and mentoring staff and providing them with clear information and direction related to meeting unit productivity goals. Nurse managers are the chief retention officers and need to perform their duties accordingly.

SUMMARY

Staffing and scheduling are some of the greatest challenges for a nurse manager. When these functions are performed well, the resulting satisfaction of the unit staff contributes to positive patient outcomes. When they are not performed well, low morale and discontent result. The manager has various data available to help in planning the staffing patterns for the unit. Success, however, depends on the unit staff and the manager working collaboratively to meet the needs for care.

THE SOLUTION

A staff meeting was called to discuss the impact of the transition of a number of beds for surgical trauma ICU (STICU) step-down patients on the inpatient general surgery unit. Information was given to all staff regarding the potential size of the step-down unit and the methods for staffing this unit. Staff members were assured that no jobs would be lost and that appropriate training would be provided to current staff to ensure their competence.

Six beds were determined to be the initial number of step-down beds to be incorporated into the surgical inpatient unit. Staff members were involved in the design of the space from the perspective of identifying which rooms were to be used and what in-room supplies and equipment would be necessary. Continuous pulse oximetry and bedside computers were among the top equipment needs identified.

A staffing plan was established for the step-down unit, and staff members on the general surgery unit were first to be offered the positions. The unit's staffing plan was filled with staff members from the general surgical unit, as well as a related unit. Educational plans were developed and the STICU nursing staff members were open and welcoming when the new step-down staff rotated and

partnered with the STICU staff in the critical care environment. The new step-down staff completed didactic education, and the same STICU nurses provided backup for them when the unit opened.

Continuous discussions were held with the medical staff involved through a champion who was identified within the department of general surgery. Talking points were distributed to the medical staff and the other hospital staff to keep everyone current with the progress. Interdisciplinary teams were developed around the care models and are now engaged in daily patient care conferences to monitor progress of patients.

The unit has been open for 6 months and is a success. There are no vacant positions, critical care beds are more available, medical staff are pleased with the care delivered, patient satisfaction for this unit is very good, and the staff feel accomplished and proud of their contribution to the overall capacity challenge!
—*Mary Ellen Bonczek*

Would this be a suitable approach for you? Why?

THE EVIDENCE

Kane et al. (2007), in a meta-analysis of 94 observational studies done between 1990 and 2006, found consistent evidence that suggests an increase in the number of registered nurses (RNs) relative to the number of patients on a unit was associated with a reduction in hospital-related mortality, failure to rescue, and other nurse-sensitive outcomes. The increased number of nurses also influenced a reduced length of stay after adjustment for patient characteristics is considered. However, none of these studies demonstrated a causal relationship. Kane et al. (2007) noted that hospitals with an overall commitment to high-quality care through sufficient staffing may also invest in other actions that improve quality.

NEED TO KNOW NOW

- Know what your state nurse practice act and related rules say about staffing requirements.
- Know how staffing is determined for the unit where you work or are considering working.

- Know to ask for help if your assignment is limiting your ability to provide safe patient care.

CHAPTER CHECKLIST

This chapter addresses the managerial functions of staffing and scheduling and asserts that skills in both functions are needed by the nurse manager to maintain unit productivity and patient and staff satisfaction.

- The nurse manager must consider the impact of patient and hospital factors, nurse staffing, nurse characteristics, and organizational factors on nurse and patient outcomes.
- The nurse manager must also consider the following internal variables when preparing the budget and the unit staffing plan:
  - Organizational staffing policies
  - Structure and philosophy of the nursing services department
  - Organizational support services
  - Changes in services and programs
  - Projected units of service
- When forecasting the personnel needs for the unit, the nurse manager must consider the following:
  - The staffing model of the unit
  - The skill mix of the nursing staff
- The number of positions and FTEs needed to meet the anticipated units of service
- The amount of nonproductive paid-benefit time allotted to each staff member
- Patient outcomes
- Availability of resources
- When constructing the unit schedule, the nurse manager must consider the following:
  - Unit hours of operation
  - Shift or weekend rotations required in the unit
  - Approved paid time off for vacations, holidays, and other benefit hours
  - Staffing vacancies
  - Availability of automation
  - Organizational policies on overtime and use of agency personnel
- When evaluating unit productivity, the nurse manager should consider the following:
  - Acuity trends identified through patient classification systems and/or staff input
  - Labor cost per unit of service
  - Periodic unit activity reports

TIPS FOR STAFFING AND SCHEDULING

- Know state laws and voluntary accreditation (professional society and institutional) standards for staffing.
- Integrate ongoing research regarding the impact of various factors on patient outcomes into staffing plans.
- Identify current demands for staff and anticipate externally imposed changes such as services offered and availability of RNs and LPNs/LVNs.

- Value the various responses to short staffing from the manager, staff, and patient perspectives.
- Recognize the complexity of staffing issues and how they relate to staff satisfaction, community perception, budget, and accreditation standards.

REFERENCES

Aiken, L. H., Clarke, S. P., Cheung, R. B., Sloane, D. M., & Silber, J. H. (2003). Educational levels of hospital nurses and surgical patient mortality. *JAMA: the Journal of the American Medical Association, 290*(12), 1617-1623.

American Nurses Association (ANA). (2008). *Principles for nurse staffing*. Washington, DC: Author. Retrieved September 28, 2009, from http://safestaffingsaveslives.org/.

Becker, D. J. (2007). Do hospitals provide lower quality care on weekends? *Health Services Research*, 42(4), 1589-1612.

Berney, B. L., & Needleman, J. (2003). *Use, trends, and impacts of nurse overtime in New York hospitals 1995-2000* (PhD dissertation), Boston University.

Cho-S-H. (2002). *Nurse staffing and adverse patient outcomes* (PhD dissertation), University of Michigan.

Dall, T., Chen, Y., Seifert, R., Maddox, P., & Hogan, P. (2009). The economic value of professional nursing. *Medical Care*, 47(1), 97-104.

Donaldson, N., Bolton, L. B., Aydin, C., Brown, D., Elashoff, J. D., & Sandhu, M. (2005). Impact of California's licensed nurse-patient ratios on unit-level nurse staffing and patient outcomes. *Policy, Politics & Nursing Practice*, 6(3), 198-210.

Dunton, N., Gajewski, B., Klaus, S., & Pierson, B. (2007). The relationship of nursing workforce characteristics to patient outcomes. *Online Journal of Issues in Nursing*, 12(3).

Fitzpatrick, T., & Brooks, B. (2010). The nurse leader as logistician: Optimizing human capital. *JONA*, 40(2), 69-74.

Goldfarb, C., & Rowan, K. (2000). Consequences of discharge from intensive care at night. *Lancet*, 355(9210), 1138-1142.

Haebler, J. (2008). Safe staffing legislation: Win-win for Ohio and others. *Nevada RNformation*, August, September, October 15.

Hamilton, P., Eschiti, V. S., Hernandez, K., & Neill, D. (2007). Differences between weekend and weekday nurse work environments and patient outcomes: A focus group approach to model testing. *Journal of Perinatal Neonatal Nursing*, 21(4), 331-341.

Hyun, S., Bakken, S., Douglas, K., & Stone, P. (2008). Evidence-based staffing: Potential roles for informatics. *Nursing Economic*, 26(3), 151-173.

Kane, R. L., Shamliyan, T., Mueller, C., Duval, S., & Wilt, T. (March 2007). *Nursing staffing and quality of patient care:*

Evidence report/technology assessment No. 151. (Prepared by the Minnesota Evidence-based Practice Center under Contract No. 290-02-0009.) AHRQ Publication No. 07-E0005. Rockville, MD: Agency for Healthcare Research and Quality.

Keepnews, D. (2007) Evaluating nurse staffing regulations. *Policy, Politics, and Nursing Practice*, 8(4), 235-236.

Kutney-Lee, A., Lake, E. T., & Aiken, L. H. (2009). Development of the hospital nurse surveillance capacity profile. *Research in Nursing & Health*, 32(2), 217-228.

Montalvo, I. (2009). The national database of nursing quality indicators® (NDNQI®). *OJIN: The Online Journal of Issues in Nursing*, 12(3), Manuscript 3. Retrieved September 28, 2009, from www.nursingworld.org/MainMenuCategories/ANAMarketplace/ANAPeriodicals/OJIN/TableofContents/Volume122007/No3Sept07/NursingQualityIndicators.aspx.

Peberdy, M. A., Ornato, J. P., Larkin, G. L., Braithwaite, R. S., Kashner, T. M., Carey, S. M., Meaney, P. A., Cen, L., Nadkarni, V. M., Praestgaard, A. H., & Berg, R. A. (2008). Survival from in-hospital cardiac arrest during nights and weekends. *JAMA: the Journal of the American Medical Association*, 299(7), 785-792.

Ridley, R. T. (2008). The relationship between nurse education level and patient safety: An integrative review. *Journal of Nursing Education*, 47(4), 149-156.

Seago, J., Spetz, J., & Mitchell, S. (2004). Nurse staffing and hospital ownership in California. *Journal of Nursing Administration*, 34(5), 228-231.

Sochalski, J. (2004). The relationship between nurse staffing and the quality of nursing care in hospitals. *Medical Care*, 42(Suppl. 2), 1167-1173.

Upenieks, V., Akhavan, J., & Kotlerman, J. (2008). Value-added care: A paradigm shift in patient care delivery. *Nursing Economic$*, 6(5), 294-300.

SUGGESTED READINGS

Boswell, C., Gatson, Z., Baker, D., Vaughn, G., Lyons, B., Chapman, P., & Cannon, S. (2008). Application of evidence-base practice through a float project. *Nursing Forum*, 43(3), 126-132.

Clarke, S. (2007). Registered nurse staffing and patient outcomes in acute care: Looking back, pushing forward. *Medical Care*, 45(12), 1126-1128.

Garrett, C. (2008). The effect of nurse staffing patterns on medical errors and nurse burnouts. *AORN Journal*, 87(6), 1191-1204.

Hofler, L. (2008). Nursing education and transition to the work environment: A synthesis of national reports. *Journal of Nursing Education*, 47(1), 5-12.

Mamaril, M., Sullivan, E., Clifford, T., Newhouse, R., & Windle, P. (2007). Safe staffing for the post anesthesia care unit: Weighing the evidence and identifying the gaps. *Journal of PeriAnesthesia Nursing*, 22(6), 393-399.

Mittmann, N., Seung, S., Pusterzu, L., Isogai, S., & Michaels, D. (2008). Nursing workload associated with hospital patient care. *Managed Health Outcomes*, 16(1), 53-56.

Newbold, D. (2006). The production economics of nursing: A discussion paper. *International Journal of Nursing Studies*, 45, 120-128.

Pappas, S. (2008). The cost of nurse-sensitive adverse events. *Journal of Nursing Administration*, 38(5), 230-236.

Thomas-Hawkins, C., Flynn, L., & Clarke, S. (2008). Relationships between registered nurse staffing, processes of nursing care, and nurse-reported patient outcomes in chronic hemodialysis units. *Nephrology Nursing Journal*, 35(2), 123-145.

Van den Heede, K., Clarke, S., Sermeus, W., Vleugels, A., & Aikens, L. (2007). International experts' perspectives on the state of the nurse staffing and patient outcomes literature. *Journal of Nursing Scholarship*, 39(4), 290-297.

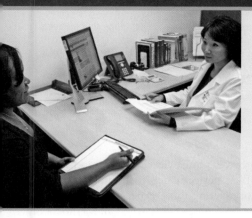

Selecting, Developing, and Evaluating Staff

Diane M. Twedell

Two of the most important functions of a manager are interviewing and hiring employees for an organization. It is essential that individual employees understand role expectations.

Role theory is a useful organizing framework for the manager and the employee to follow throughout all aspects of role performance. Effective communication of roles and role expectations among all members can facilitate improvements in performance, worker satisfaction, and most important, quality of care delivered. The role of the manager as a coach who empowers employees to grow as followers and develop their leadership skills in a learning environment is explored.

OBJECTIVES

- Relate concepts of role theory to position descriptions.
- Distinguish key points for the interview of a potential employee.
- Delineate the various performance appraisal processes.
- Examine specific guidelines for performance feedback.

TERMS TO KNOW

coaching
empowerment
halo effect

performance appraisal
position description
role ambiguity

role conflict
role theory

THE CHALLENGE

Janee Klipfel, RN, BSN, CURN
Lake City, Minnesota

I faced many challenges when assuming the role of nurse manager for a large and dynamic surgical patient care unit. It was a major time of unit transition because the previous nurse manager had been in the position for 26 years. A large number of positions on the unit were open. I created a spreadsheet of the staff members who were currently on the unit and their years of experience. It became clear to me that we were functioning at the most basic levels. What we needed most was more staff!

What do you think you would do if you were this nurse?

INTRODUCTION

Healthcare delivery systems are businesses that are economically driven. Whether the setting is inpatient or outpatient, the emphasis is on providing the highest quality of care at an affordable price. The nurse manager is a key individual whose leadership can directly influence many environmental functions. Today's nurse manager needs strong leadership skills to navigate changes, with a focus on the patient and safe, reliable care (Steanncyk, Handcock, & Meadows, 2013). Other functions begin with the selection of the right person for the right position and having the manager function in the role of coach. As a coach, the nurse manager can assist and encourage employees to perform at their highest levels in an empowered and self-directed manner. The nurse manager also clarifies the organization's mission and expectations.

The role of follower cannot be overrated! A strong patient care unit has both effective leadership and team members who understand their role in meeting the goals for quality patient care. Professional healthcare providers must clearly understand what is expected of their performance, including the ramifications of not meeting those expectations. This performance can be achieved only when all members of the organization have clearly defined roles and overall objectives. Ambiguous roles are more detrimental to role performance and employee work satisfaction than is conflict within the role.

ROLE CONCEPTS AND THE POSITION DESCRIPTION

The acquisition of a role requires an individual to assume the personal as well as the formal expectations of a specified role or position. Many individuals function within multiple roles. As discussed in the Theory Box below, role theory provides an appreciable framework for the development and evaluation of staff. Today's professional nurse is often a parent, spouse, and community volunteer and maintains full-time employment outside the home. Many skills are necessary for each role. In addition, the role-taker

THEORY BOX

Role Theory

THEORY/CONTRIBUTOR	KEY IDEAS	APPLICATION TO PRACTICE
Role Theory and Role Dynamics in Organizations Kahn, Wolfe, Quinn, Snoek, & Rosenthal (1964) developed this theory.	Roles within organizations affect an individual's interactions with others. Acquisition of these roles is time-dependent and varies based on individual experiences and value systems. For effective communication to take place, role expectations for performance must be understood by all individuals involved.	The role of the professional nurse is complex. Role acquisition, role clarity, and role performance are enhanced by the use of clear position descriptions and evaluation standards.

(i.e., the individual actually performing the role) has specified performance objectives within the social context in which the role is enacted. The social context includes the physical and social environment.

Role ambiguity in the workplace creates an environment for misunderstanding and hinders effective communication. In this situation, individuals do not have a clear understanding of what is expected of their performance or how they will be evaluated. In contrast, role conflict is easier to recognize. Employees know what is expected of them, but they are either unwilling or unable to meet the requirements.

Employees must have clear role expectations and perceive that their contributions are valued. Empowerment and control for certain aspects of the environment have been linked to increased personal health, job satisfaction, and individual performance. They are then more likely to be committed to the organization and to provide a higher level of patient care. These principles are applicable to both managers and staff members. A consistent focus on developing staff creates a learning environment directed toward excellence.

Acquisition of the role is time-dependent; individuals apply their life experiences to each role and interpret the role within their own value system. As roles become more complex, the individual may take longer to assimilate the components of each particular role. Nursing graduates enter the profession with various levels of educational and life experiences. The nurse manager plays an integral role in assisting these individuals in the development and acquisition of the complex role of the professional nurse. It is important to remember that role development evolves over time and considers individual needs. Role acquisition is something that nurses can encounter numerous times during their career. The RN who completes additional academic education and becomes an advanced practice registered nurse takes on a new role. The staff RN who moves to a new or different specialty acquires a new role. Coaching is a technique that the manager can use to facilitate individual development; this technique is discussed within the context of performance appraisal.

The position description provides written guidelines detailing the roles and responsibilities of a specific position within the organizational context. The position description reflects functions and obligations of a specific work position. It is a contract for the individual that describes responsibilities of the work assignment, as well as to whom the individual reports.

EXERCISE 15-1

Obtain a position description for a registered nurse from a community nursing service and a hospital. Compare them. Analyze the general categories (e.g., communication, responsibilities) and the specific behaviors. What competencies do you already have? How will you develop other competencies? What are common competencies for registered nurses?

The position description should reflect current practice guidelines for individuals and may have competency-based requirements. As paradigms of nursing delivery systems shift to the home and community, professional nurses must have a clear understanding of the performance that is expected. The nurse is also responsible for clearly understanding the position descriptions of the paraprofessionals to whom care is delegated. Clear and concise position descriptions for all employees are extremely important because they provide the basis for roles within the organization. Example statements from a position description for a staff nurse in a medical/surgical patient care unit appear in Box 15-1.

SELECTING STAFF

The selection of staff would seem to be a relatively simple process. The manager wants the most qualified

---

BOX 15-1 EXCERPTS FROM A POSITION DESCRIPTION FOR AN RN STAFF NURSE

- Accountable for the coordination of nursing care, including direct patient care, patient/family education, and discharge planning
- Maintains basic cardiac life support (BCLS) competency
- Is required to accurately assess and prioritize patient-care needs and delegate care appropriately to licensed practical nurses (LPNs) and patient care assistants (PCAs)
- Works collaboratively with multidisciplinary team members

individual for the position. Choosing the right individual is the challenge! Brooke (2008, p. 50) notes that the cost of recruiting and orienting a new nurse "drives home the necessity of carefully selecting nurses who'll work well within your hospital's culture." Health care is centered on caring for people, and nurses with appropriate people skills are essential for producing satisfied patients and families. For example, if an applicant values that the needs of the patient come first and this value is also articulated via the organization, he or she has similar values related to the work of the organization. The applicant and the manager must agree on what defines quality care and the manner in which it should be delivered. The manager must also decide whether members of the existing staff are to be included in the screening and interview process for new employees. The following guidelines are suggestions for the manager and staff, as well as for the prospective employee.

The manager's focus before and during the interview is to be prepared and have well-thought-out questions. The environment should be comfortable and provide privacy without interruptions. The interview questions can be related to the applicant's experience or be directed to evaluate values and critical-thinking skills. This may be accomplished by asking the applicant to describe his or her reactions to challenging situations previously experienced. Dye (2007, p. 116) notes that highly effective interviewers focus heavily on asking what are known as behavioral questions: "These are questions that seek demonstrated examples of behavior from the candidates' past experiences and concentrate on job related functions and accomplishments." A question related to teamwork in an interview could be, *Tell me about a time when you were working in a group and there were problems with other individuals who were not pulling their weight. What did you do to maintain a team environment?*

Technical skills, such as specific certificates, are also important for the work environment and, therefore, also must be discussed or validated. The applicant may be given a case study to read and discuss with the interviewer. The case study could describe a situation for the unit in which the applicant is being interviewed; the content of the case study may require the applicant to prioritize the care of one patient or a group of patients. Questions from the applicant should be answered honestly. Jackson and Thurgate (2011, 247), stated, "The most important thing to remember is that the interview is a two-way process: the applicant is there to find out information about the organization, job, or course as much as the interviewer is there to find out about the applicant." A tour of the unit and a review of the position description are helpful to give the applicant information about the expectations of the role. Staff members also may be included in the interview and can provide information to the applicant as appropriate. At the conclusion of the interview, it is important for the nurse manager to clarify concrete issues. According to McConnell (2008, p. 53), "All applicants interviewed for a position deserve informational closure after the fact. An indication of follow-up should be more than a don't call us, we'll call you." Applicants should know the time line of when they can expect to hear about their interview result, who will contact them, and how they will be contacted. Thank applicants for the interview, and end interviews on a positive note.

The applicant also has responsibilities in preparation for the employment interview. It is important to be on time and appropriately dressed. Conservative dress is always acceptable. A uniform is not necessary and usually not even preferable. First impressions may be lasting impressions. Previous review of the organization's goals and mission statement, as well as a review of the position description for which the interview is being conducted, is also appropriate. The applicant should be prepared to answer each question honestly and thoughtfully. It is as important to the prospective employee to make the right decisions as it is to the employer. The manager and the applicant must have a clear understanding of the values and organizational goals for nursing care to ensure that the applicant is well-suited for the role. The applicant should focus on the topic and avoid irrelevant conversations. He or she must prepare for any questions that might be discussed. In addition to describing previous situations and how they were handled, the applicant may be asked to describe personal strengths and weaknesses. At the end of the interview, the applicant should thank the manager for his or her time and verify when the selection will be made and how it will be communicated. It is also appropriate to send the manager a brief note of appreciation for the interview. More information appears in Chapter 29.

DEVELOPING STAFF

Once the interview and offer are completed and an applicant has accepted the position, strategies are used to help the individual acclimate to the new organization and/or role. Some larger organizations use residency programs for new graduates. These may last as long as 1 year and are designed to help new graduates transition from the role of student to that of professional nurse. Other strategies that exist in every organization, and may last for very brief times or as long as several weeks, focus on orientation to the role and the organization. Orientation to the organization usually is a structured program that is generally applicable to all new employees. It may include outlining the mission, benefits, safety programs, and other specific topics. Orientation to the work area usually depends on the specialty area involved, the skills that need to be verified, and the environment itself. Every individual brings various experiences and skills to a new position. A nurse manager will assist new employees by advising them about educational programs and experiences that will aid in their entry to the organization. It is imperative that the orientation period be used efficiently for both the employee and the organization. Retention of new nursing personnel begins on the day of their hire. Robert Wood Johnson Foundation (2006, p. 8) noted "that the cost of replacing just one medical surgical nurse is $92,442." This dollar figure includes human resource expenses, temporary replacement costs, lost productivity, training, and terminal payouts. Although the amount might be cited differently, the cost of replacement is high.

Orientation can accomplish a variety of things. It is a time for new employees to learn the work environment and the staff. Many institutions provide preceptors, who are considered to be expert clinicians and resources. Moore (2008, p. E-14) emphasized that "preceptorships are key to help staff integrate new skills and knowledge into practice, thereby helping nursing departments achieve their healthcare mission and goals." Preceptors teach newly hired nurses in the clinical setting. In some settings, the Kolb (1985) "Learning-Style Inventory" (LSI) may be administered to new employees and the information then shared with the preceptors and the new employees. When preceptors understand the learning styles of new employees, a better focus for implementation of the orientation goals is provided. After learning styles have been identified, new employees work with preceptors who understand specifically how to address the individualized learning needs of new employees in a manner that enhances learning.

Continued development of the staff is a unique role for the nurse manager. It is a challenge to merge a group of individuals with varying levels of expertise and experience. If the focus is centered on professional socialization and development, a common thread will "weave" itself throughout all employees. That common thread may be a particular philosophy of care delivery, further development of critical-thinking skills for a specific specialty, or political activities in which members are involved. Some units encourage a monthly journal club or a brief presentation by employees to summarize information learned from a conference. One nursing unit could send a staff member to monthly open meetings of the state board of nursing. This staff member then could summarize the report of the meeting for the rest of the staff to keep them informed of the legal aspects of professional nursing.

Empowerment strategies are useful for individual professional development, as well as for overall staff development. Empowerment is a process that acknowledges the values and judgment of individuals and trusts that their decisions will be the correct ones. In The Challenge and The Solution sections in this chapter, employee self-development and professional empowerment were the results of intervention.

For individuals to feel empowered, the environment must be open and they must feel safe to explore and develop their own potential. The organizational environment must encourage individuals to employ the freedom of making decisions while retaining accountability for the consequences of those decisions. Management must release control to followers so that the followers might work more effectively, both individually and as a team. Specific environmental challenges and situations can influence employee attitudes, feelings of empowerment, and performance within roles. These challenges can affect commitment to the organization and individual work satisfaction. Positive feedback or coaching, achievement recognition, and support for new ideas may enhance employees' feelings of empowerment and their ability to perform effectively. According to McDonald and colleagues (2010), today's nurses expect to be able to participate in the governance of the organization, especially when their practice is involved.

One strategy for staff empowerment is providing timely feedback for performance contributions, not simply during the annual performance appraisal. Supporting the implementation of innovative ideas and providing opportunities for mentoring relationships are also valuable approaches for the manager and staff. Many organizations use shared governance as a guide for accountability. A premise of shared governance is that power, control, and decision making can empower staff and enhance individual and group accountability.

PERFORMANCE APPRAISALS

Feedback to employees regarding their performance is one of the strongest rewards an organization can provide. Performance appraisals are individual evaluations of work performance. Ideally, evaluations are conducted on an ongoing basis, not just at the conclusion of a predetermined period. Evaluations, however, are usually done annually and also may be required after a scheduled orientation period for new employees. Chandra (2006), p. 24 identifies the following:

> Administrators may conduct performance appraisals to monitor performance quality and quantity, evaluate job standards and expectations, provide a basis for personnel decisions (e.g., promotions, transfers, releases, staffing needs), and provide other information that may signal potential problems or successes of daily operations. (p. 34)

The process of providing feedback, for either an above-average or a below-average performance, is best received at a time closest to the incidents being evaluated. The actual appraisal is sometimes viewed as a negative experience. Many nurse managers perceive the appraisal as a time-consuming process of endless paperwork. Instead, nurse managers should embrace the appraisal process as a key time for assisting with staff development. Chandra (2006, p. 37) notes that "the actual interactive conference between the employee and the evaluator should be a productive session." Appraisals should be designed so that they can be supported in court if the need arises.

Court decisions can be made based on the evidence, or lack of evidence, presented in the evaluation instrument. Consider, for example, the individual who has been fired for reasons of poor work performance. The employee must be provided written notice that performance is unsatisfactory, and that notice must specify what the employee must accomplish for satisfactory performance. This simple condition can make the difference for either the employee or the employer to justify the fairness for termination. Performance appraisals can be either formal or informal. Performance appraisals may also include personal and peer evaluations, as well as managerial components.

An informal appraisal might be as simple as immediately praising the individual for performance recognized. A compliment from a family member or patient might be conveyed. Some units have a specific bulletin board for thank-you notes from patients and their families. Sometimes a simple "Thank you for all your hard work today!" can be extended from the manager to the staff. In addition, staff members have a responsibility to show the manager their appreciation and give positive and negative feedback.

The formal performance appraisal involves written documentation according to specific organization guidelines. Whether the evaluation is informal or formal, it does not preclude interim evaluations. The primary reason for an interim evaluation is so that praise or corrections are made as close to an episode as possible.

Brief anecdotal notes entered into the employee's file on a regular basis are important. These anecdotal notes, when accumulated over time, provide a more accurate cumulative appraisal. The anecdotal note describes an occurrence, either favorable or unfavorable, in a brief and concise manner. The purpose is to assist the manager with information throughout an entire rating period.

These notes, combined with variance reporting, are another means of documenting employee performance and provide a more conclusive appraisal that reflects the entire rating period. Variance reporting identifies specific occurrences, based on benchmarks or specific standards. As an example, "The employee will have CPR certification by January 1." If the employee does not meet this deadline, a variance is recorded along with the specific circumstances or discipline planned.

Example of an Anecdotal Note: Nurse "Johnson"

2/14/09: Patient (Joyce Allen) and family described the wonderful care that she received from Ms. Johnson during this hospitalization. All members of the family noted that when Ms. Johnson was in the room, "We felt like we were the most important people in the world." She made the patient feel "special and not just like another number." Compliment relayed to employee on 2/15/09. (Note in employee's anecdotal record with a signature and date by nurse manager.)

> **EXERCISE 15-2**
> Select a partner. Observe some clinical or classroom behavior and prepare an anecdotal note. Ask your partner for feedback about the content.

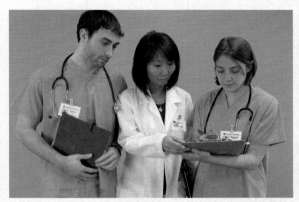

Coaching can promote team building and optimal performance of the employees.

Additional methods may be incorporated into the performance appraisal in the form of competency assessment tools. Windsor, Douglas, and Harvey (2012, p. 213) explain, "The competency movement is about creating a more flexible and mobile labour force to increase productivity, and it does so by redefining work as a set of transferable or 'soft' generic skills that are transportable and is the possession of the individual." Integration of relevant competency assessment data into the evaluation process further enhances the individual employee's sense of empowerment, as well as accountability for the evaluation process.

Coaching

The overall evaluative process can be enhanced if the manager employs the technique of coaching. Coaching is a process that involves the development of individuals within an organization. This coaching process is a personal approach in which the manager and the employee interact on a frequent and regular basis with the ultimate outcome that the employee performs at an optimal level. Coaching can be individual or may involve a team approach; when implemented in a planned and organized manner, it can promote team building and optimal performance of the employees. Coaching is a learned behavior for the nurse manager and takes time and effort to be developed. The rewards for both the employee and the nurse manager are significant; communication is enhanced, and the performance appraisal process is an active one between the employee and the manager.

The formal performance appraisal usually involves some type of predetermined evaluation tool or instrument. The tool may be a simple one or may involve the integration of a variety of measuring methods. The instruments should reflect the philosophy of the organization and be as objective and specific as possible regarding the employee's performance. Numerous instruments and a variety of simple to complex scoring methods for each exist. The new employee must have a clear understanding of timing and the content of the appraisal tool at the onset of employment. The example in Box 15-2 illustrates a type of peer-appraisal method in which a staff nurse could evaluate another staff nurse within the area-specific context of assessment documentation.

> **EXERCISE 15-3**
> Think back to your last performance appraisal, either in the clinical situation as a professional nurse or in the role of nursing student. Did you feel you were fairly and adequately evaluated? Were the comments reflective of your current practice and made by someone who had directly observed the care that you provided? What was the environment like for the interview? Were you comfortable with the evaluator? Was feedback given, both positive and negative? How did you feel at the conclusion of the interview? Taking the time to think about the answers to these questions might provide you insight and direction before your next performance appraisal interview.

The scoring procedures for evaluations can be as simple as *satisfactory/unsatisfactory*. A more complex scoring system that includes a numerical rating scheme (using a range of 1 to 4, with *1* meaning "rarely meets standards," to *4* meaning "always exceeds standards") also appears in Box 15-2. The results from the peer-review process are then summarized and incorporated into the manager's formal performance appraisal.

PERFORMANCE APPRAISAL TOOLS

The type of appraisal tool used is not as important as how it is used, and, as the Research Perspective at right shows, there is little consistency across organizations in what they use. A formal written tool may have specific guidelines or a more open-ended format. General topics may be addressed in an anecdotal or "incident" type of format. The tool or evaluation form should facilitate accurate appraisal of the individual's performance and provide an opportunity to identify personal goals of the individual and goals of the organization. The Literature Perspective at right illustrates one example of aligning individuals with the organization through the appraisal process.

There are primarily two categories of performance appraisal tools: structured and flexible. Box 15-3 summarizes examples of structured and flexible tools.

RESEARCH PERSPECTIVE

Resource: Hamilton, K. E., Coates, V., Kelly, B., Boore, J., Cundell, J. H., Gracey, J., McFetridge, B., McGonigle, M., & Sinclair, M. (2007). Performance assessment in healthcare providers: A critical review of evidence and current practice. *Journal of Nursing Management, 15,* 773-791.

This article focuses on the evaluation methods of performance assessment through an international literature review and a survey of current practice. A comprehensive literature review was completed, and performance appraisal processes and tools from across Ireland were submitted. Results indicated that a diverse range of assessments were identified. Each method had advantages and disadvantages. The conclusion noted that no single method of performance appraisal is appropriate for assessing clinical performance. Multiple strategies are needed to capture employee performance accurately.

Implications for Practice
If organizations link performance appraisal tools to their mission, finding a wide variety of assessments is logical. Knowing the advantages and disadvantages of each is important.

LITERATURE PERSPECTIVE

Resource: Topjian, D. F., Buck, T. F., & Kozlowski, R. (2009). Employee performance for the good of all. *Nursing Management, 40*(4), 24-29.

This article focuses on the development of objective performance metrics for a variety of nursing personnel in a health system that aligns with overall strategic initiatives and organizational goals. A task force was formed to (1) develop a model of evaluation that was understandable and easily used by staff nurses and managers; (2) align staff with achievement of success at both unit and individual levels; (3) provide clear criteria to distinguish *meeting* from *exceeding* expectations; and (4) develop a tool that would avoid bias.

The article provides concrete examples of how a peer or manager could evaluate a nurse's performance. A specific number of criteria must be successfully met to hit the threshold of *exceeds expectations*. The methodology used could be very helpful in assisting nurses and managers to assess performance.

Implications for Practice
Using examples of other tools can help organizations develop their own tools. Having a specific number of criteria to achieve clarifies for everyone what the expected behaviors are.

BOX 15-2	PEER PERFORMANCE APPRAISAL, STAFF NURSE

Area of Responsibility
Assessment/Diagnosis: Provides continuous holistic assessment to include physical, psychosocial, spiritual, and educational needs. Directs outcome criteria so that discharge plans are timely and optimal quality care is delivered.

a. Completes database (history/physical assessment) within 12 hours of admission (Score 4)

b. Illustrates documentation reflective of continuous assessment per unit guidelines (e.g., neurovascular assessment of extremity after cardiac catheterization) (Score 3)

c. Initiates plan of care according to critical path guidelines within 12 hours of admission (Score 4)

d. Provides for safe environment (Score 4)

Structured Performance Appraisal Tools
Graphic Rating Scales

Graphic rating scales are another example of a structured approach to evaluation. They comprise a numbering system that indicates high and low values for evaluating performance. The rating scale is popular because it is easy to construct and easy to use. Problems with this type of scale are that it lacks specificity and may promote a halo effect. Chandra (2006) defines the halo effect as follows:

> … a common example of a personality bias in which the rating is based on a characteristic of the individual that actually has nothing to do with the work trait being considered. Managers may give higher ratings to individuals they like (a positive halo effect) and lower ratings to individuals they do not like (a negative halo effect). (p. 36)

It is important for information about employee performance to be gathered over the entire evaluation period. Chandra (2006) notes that evaluations should not be a reflection of isolated incidents. It is human nature to remember incidents that are recent or sensational because those that deviate from the norm make a greater impression. However, these are usually a poor basis for overall evaluations.

Anecdotal notes compiled consistently over the entire rating period are a much more equitable method for providing an accurate summary of the employee's performance. Some managers use small notes with adhesive backs to place inside an employee's informal file to document behaviors quickly as situations warrant. A sheet of paper for notes placed in the front of each file would also serve the same purpose. The manager might also keep secured electronic data files for the same purpose. Security of the files, electronic or paper, is important to maintain confidentiality.

Rating Scales

Rating scales are relatively easy to construct and easy to complete (Table 15-1). On the downside, they usually consist of generalizations, not specific behaviors, and the rating is relatively subjective in nature. Some managers never give a "5," with the rationale that no employee always exceeds expectations.

Flexible Performance Appraisal Tools

The evaluation focus can also be conducted with a collaborative approach. How can the manager assist the individual to develop professionally?

Behaviorally Anchored Rating Scales

Behaviorally anchored rating scales (BARS) can be implemented as a collaborative or flexible approach. The focus is on behavior and should include employees in the development. BARS combine ratings with critical incidents (specific examples that have occurred) or criterion references (examples usually based on standards of practice or competency-based standards). The criteria used for this scale are specific

---

BOX 15-3 EXAMPLES OF STRUCTURED AND FLEXIBLE PERFORMANCE APPRAISAL TOOLS

Structured (Traditional Method)
- Graphic rating scale
- Rating scales

Flexible (Collaborative Method)
- Behaviorally anchored rating scales (BARS)
- Management by objectives (MBO)
- Peer review

TABLE 15-1 EXAMPLE OF A RATING SCALE

CRITERIA	ALMOST NEVER				ALWAYS EXCEEDS
1. Completes nursing care in a professional and competent manner	1	2	3	4	5
2. Is reliable; comes to work on time	1	2	3	4	5
3. Provides patient teaching as appropriate	1	2	3	4	5

to the specialty of nursing delivered and preestablished outcomes. This scale is also considered more advantageous in terms of litigation. BARS describe the employee's performance both quantitatively and qualitatively. Staff who are involved in the development of these instruments are more likely to understand the importance of evaluation for each criterion selected and to have an understanding of their performance expectations. This is another example of clarification of roles and role expectations within the organization. The primary drawback of this scale is that it is expensive to develop and time-consuming to implement; it must be designed for each specific position description or standard of practice. However, it provides the manager with concrete information regarding an employee's performance, with minimal subjective interference. Box 15-4 provides an example of how established nursing standards of practice, or protocols for practice, can be incorporated into the appraisal process using peer review. The data might also be used in an outcome review process as a component of a continuous quality-improvement program. The final result would be summarized by the manager and incorporated into the employee's performance appraisal.

Management by Objectives

One method that has been used for many years is management by objectives (MBO), which was popularized by Peter Drucker (1954). Performance goals are established jointly between the manager and the employee for the upcoming evaluation period. Progress regarding the accomplishment of these goals is documented throughout the rating period. An MBO approach requires that the employee establishes clear and measurable objectives at the beginning of each rating period. Then, during the performance appraisal evaluation, both the employee and the manager address these objectives individually and in writing. In effect, the employee has created a "performance contract," as well as defined goals for future professional performance. Box 15-5 illustrates goals and accomplishments.

Peer Review

Peer review is also a flexible or contemporary strategy. If the guidelines are developed collaboratively, peer review may also be considered a developmental method of evaluation; that is, employees are involved in the development and implementation process. Nurses tend to function in their normal patterns in the presence of peers, and this can be a very solid rating method. However, it is important to obtain objective ratings based on performance, not subjective ratings based on personal friendships. This method should not be used if the manager is attempting to institute team-building strategies or if the unit is unstable and employees do not like each other. The employees must trust and respect each other to participate willingly in the peer-appraisal process. George and Haag-Heitman (2011, p. 255) state, "Nursing peer review is a critical component to addressing the variations and inadequacies in the quality of nursing care."

BOX 15-4	EXAMPLE OF A BEHAVIORALLY ANCHORED RATING SCALE

Emergency room (ER) staff nurse responsibilities for patient admitted with chest pain: (ER records evaluated per protocol; minimum 10/rating period). Met/Unmet

1. Vital signs recorded within 5 min of admission _____
2. Cardiac monitor, IV, lab tests, and ECG done within 15 min _____
3. If sublingual nitroglycerin given, vital signs recorded every 5 min for 30 min _____
   a. Chest pain changes evaluated per protocol _____
   b. Post–chest pain 12-lead ECG documented _____

BOX 15-5	LEARNING GOALS AND ACCOMPLISHMENTS

Learning Goals
1. Prepare for and take advanced cardiac life support (ACLS) certification examination
2. Participate in shared governance committee as unit representative

Accomplishments (12 Months Later—Summary)
1. Successfully passed ACLS certification
2. Participated in monthly meetings; chaired task force for development and implementation of new delivery system; presented in-service class to staff on several units

Summary of Appraisal Instruments

Which instrument/method of appraisal is best? The missions and goals of the organization determine the tools used. A combination of several tools is probably superior to any one method. The primary success of any performance appraisal lies in the skills and communication abilities of the manager. It is also the manager's responsibility to educate employees about the process and tools for performance appraisals. Role ambiguity and uncertainty of standards of practice and methods for evaluation are significant contributors to decreased work satisfaction. The best-designed instrument will fail if the manager is ineffective and cannot communicate with the employee. Finally, some linkage of the outcomes of the appraisal process to salary and benefits conveys a reinforcement of the process of appraising and its importance for individual professional development.

EXERCISE 15-4

Obtain a performance appraisal tool from the local healthcare organization from which you obtained a position description. Based on the descriptions provided, how would you characterize it? Is it structured or flexible? Is it quantitatively based, qualitatively based, or both? How does the tool reflect the position description?

Appraisal Interview Environment

The appraisal instrument is not the only factor in the evaluation process. The interview should be conducted professionally and in a positive manner. It is an ideal time for communication between the employee and the manager. Chandra (2006, p. 37) states to "make certain that the employee knows about the appraisal conference well in advance so that he or she can plan for it." There should be no interruptions, if possible. This time is important for clarification of employee and organizational goals. Evaluation of employee performance should be objective and unemotional. The evaluation instruments should be clearly completed, and time should be allowed for discussion. Goals may be established. The manager and the employee should sign the appraisal forms, and each should be provided a copy. The effectiveness of the entire appraisal method relies on the manner in which the manager uses the tools and the feedback that the employee receives. Effective communication between the manager and employees can prevent potential performance problems on a unit. Specific behaviors by the manager enhance the actual appraisal process (Box 15-6).

BOX 15-6	**KEY BEHAVIORS FOR THE PERFORMANCE APPRAISAL SESSION**

- Provide a quiet, controlled environment, without interruptions.
- Maintain a relaxed but professional atmosphere.
- Put the employee at ease; the overall objective is for the best job to be done.
- Review specific examples for both positive and negative behavior (keep an anecdotal file for each employee).
- Allow the employee to express opinions, orally and in writing.
- Write future plans and goals, training needs, and such (a "performance contract" for the future).
- Set follow-up date as necessary to monitor improvements, if cited.
- Show the employee confidence in his or her performance.
- Be sincere and constructive in both praise and criticism.

THE SOLUTION

Energy was focused on basic daily operations. Nurses were hired and oriented. The nursing education specialist and clinical nurse specialist developed critical-thinking scenarios to be administered to new staff by more experienced staff. Physician colleagues were instrumental in providing educational sessions that were relevant to the diverse surgical population and included experiences in our Multidisciplinary Simulation Center. A 6-month formal progress review and a 9-month informal meeting were implemented to continue to follow the large volume of new nurses after orientation in their first year. About 1 year later, unit-level surveys revealed that the staff's number-one goal was to get to know each other. This was a sign of obvious growth to me. Planning commenced immediately for hospitality and social functions. Trust developed through interaction over time. Personal development and esteem needs surfaced and were nurtured. These included certification, shared decision making, degree planning, poster presentations, and celebrations

THE SOLUTION—cont'd

of achievement awards and service anniversaries. We have significantly reduced turnover rates and have maintained these reduced rates into a second year. Patient satisfaction ratings of overall quality met or exceeded peer benchmarks as measured by our research vendor, and staff satisfaction ratings increased by 35 percentage points. Our unit vision statement was just created. The key to leadership success—I believe that it lies in listening to your team, knowing where its members are, and meeting them as often as possible a little above that.

—*Janee Klipfel*

Would this be a suitable approach for you? Why or why not?

THE EVIDENCE

The first year of a nurse's career can be a very difficult time for retention in the acute care setting. Recruiting, orienting, and providing ongoing education to a newly hired nurse are costly processes. Thus it is important to use best practices to retain in the acute care environment. Funderbunk (2008) reviews the benefits of mentoring and how to establish a mentoring program and provides information about mentoring of leadership and goals of a program. A comprehensive view of how to establish a mentoring program and what supports are necessary is detailed.

NEED TO KNOW NOW

- Look for a fit of the position and the organization.
- Review position descriptions and performance appraisal.
- Know what developmental activities are available.

CHAPTER CHECKLIST

The manager plays a key role in the selection and development of staff. As a role model, the manager is also key in the establishment of the type of work environment that exists. Managers must be supportive and develop their staff to their highest potential. They must have accurate position descriptions and tools for evaluation of employee performance. These are integral to role development and professional socialization. Managers must also use various communication methods to empower their employees. Coaching and implementation of empowerment strategies positively contribute to overall staff performance as well.

- The interviewer should do the following:
  - Prescreen the applicants.
  - Prepare questions in advance.
  - Control the environment.
  - Provide role clarification.
  - Be a good listener.
  - Answer questions honestly.
  - Provide closure.
  - Inform the applicant when he or she will be notified.
- The applicant should do the following:
  - Be on time and dressed appropriately.
  - Review the organization's mission and goals.
  - Prepare questions in advance.
  - Answer questions honestly and completely.
  - Note appreciation for the interview.
- Development of the staff includes the following:
  - Organized and efficient orientation/residency
  - Plans for education, team building, and professional socialization
  - Active coaching
  - Implementation of empowerment strategies
- Development of accurate position descriptions and tools for evaluation of employees is integral to role development and professional socialization.

Nurse managers should use various communication methods, including coaching techniques.

- Role theory describes how individuals perceive their position in an organization.
- Distinction and clarity among the various positions are imperative if partnerships in quality patient care are to exist.
- The position description serves several purposes:
  - Provides written guidelines that describe roles and responsibilities
  - Reflects the position's overall function and obligations
  - Serves as a contract between manager and employee

- Reflects current practice guidelines for the position
- Performance appraisals are a method of providing feedback to the employee in relation to individual performance.
  - Types of structured (traditional) performance appraisals include the following:
    - Graphic rating scales
    - Rating scale
  - Types of flexible (collaborative) performance appraisals include the following:
    - Behaviorally anchored rating scales (BARS)
    - Management by objective (MBO)
    - Peer review

TIPS FOR CONDUCTING AN INTERVIEW

- Prescreen the applicant, and schedule a time for the interview.
- Prepare questions in advance. Be concise but thorough.
- Control the environment for noise and interruptions.

- Explain and clarify the role for which the applicant is interviewing.
- Be a good listener.
- Answer questions honestly.
- Inform the applicant when he or she will be informed of the decision.

REFERENCES

Brooke, P. (2008). Hiring and firing: Know the consequences. *Nursing Management, 39*(9), 50-52.

Chandra, A. (2006). Employee evaluation strategies for healthcare organizations: A general guide. *Hospital Topics, 84*(2), 34-38.

Drucker, P. F. (1954). *The practice of management* (1st ed.). New York: Harper.

Dye, C. F. (2007). Hiring: Get it right the first time. *Healthcare Financial Management, 61*(3), 116-118.

Funderbunk, A. (2008). Mentoring: the retention factor in the acute care setting. *Journal for Nurses in Staff Development, 24*(3), E1-E5.

George, V. & Haag-Heitman, B. (2011). Nursing peer review: the manager's role. *Journal of Nursing Management, 19*, 254-259.

Hamilton, K. E., Coates, V., Kelly, B., Boore, J., Cundell, J. H., Gracey, J., McFetridge, B., McGonigle, M., & Sinclair, M. (2007). Performance assessment in healthcare providers: A critical review of evidence and current practice. *Journal of Nursing Management, 15*, 773-791.

Jackson, C. & Thurgate, C. (2011). Applications and interviews: preparing for success. *British Medical Journal of Healthcare Assistants, 5*(5), 246-249.

Kahn, R. L., Wolfe, D. M., Quinn, R. P., Snoek, J. D., & Rosenthal, R. A. (1964). *Occupational stress: Studies in role conflict and ambiguity*. New York: Wiley.

Kolb, D. A. (1985). *Learning-Style Inventory*. Boston: McBer.

McConnell, C. R. (2008). Conducting the employee selection interview: How to do it effectively while avoiding legal obstacles. *JONA's Healthcare Law, Ethics and Regulation, 10*(2), 48-56.

McDonald, S. F., Tullai-McGuinness, S., Madigan, E. A., & Shively, M. (2010). Relationship between staff nurse involvement in organizational structures and perception of empowerment. *Critical Care Nursing Quarterly, 33*(2), 148-162.

Moore, M. L. (2008). Preceptorships: Hidden Benefits to the Organization. *Journal for Nurses in Staff Development, 24*(1), E9-E15.

Robert Wood Johnson Foundation (RWJF). (2006). Wisdom at work: *The importance of the older and experienced nurse in the workplace*. Retrieved October 2, 2009, from www.rwjf.org.

Steanncyk, A., Handcock, B., & Meadows, M. T. (2013). The nurse manager: change agent or change coach? *Nursing Administration Quarterly, 37*(1), 13-17.

Topjian, D. F., Buck, T. F., & Kozlowski, R. (2009). Employee performance for the good of all. *Nursing Management, 40*(4), 24-29.

SUGGESTED READINGS

Harrison, T., Stewart, S., Ball, K., & Meyer-Bratt, M. (2007). Clinical focus program: Enhancing the transition of senior nursing students to independent practice. *Journal of Nursing Administration, 37*(6), 311-317.

Keahey, S. (2008). Against the odds: Orienting and retaining rural nurses. *Journal for Nurses in Staff Development, 24*(2), E15-E20.

Westendorf, J. (2007). The nursing shortage: Recruitment and retention of current and future nurses. *Plastic Surgical Nursing, 27*(2), 93-97.

Windsor, C., Douglas, C., & Harvey, T. (2012). Nursing and competencies—a natural fit: the politics of skill/competency formation in nursing. *Nursing Inquiry, 19*(3), 213-222.

PART 3

Changing the Status Quo

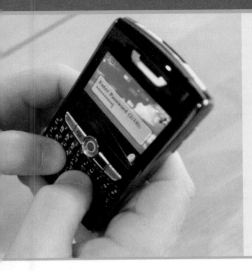

Strategic Planning, Goal-Setting, and Marketing

Mary Ellen Clyne

This chapter discusses the actualization of several organizational elements of planning for the future, with a focus on the strategic planning process, goal-setting, management by objectives, and marketing. Specific examples of planning and marketing strategies as used in healthcare organizations are presented when appropriate.

OBJECTIVES

- Articulate the value and importance of conducting an environmental assessment.
- Explore the planning process.
- Review the purpose of a mission statement, a philosophy, and established goals and objectives.
- Apply goal-setting and strategic planning.
- Explain the process of strategic planning in establishing a product line in an acute care setting.
- Determine the value of marketing plans in health care.

TERMS TO KNOW

marketing
strategic planning

THE CHALLENGE

Nancy Holecek, MPA, RN
Senior Vice President of Patient Care Services, Saint Barnabas
Health Care System, West Orange, New Jersey

In an effort to ensure patient safety, nurse managers were concerned with the interruptions facing the staff nurses administering medications. Specifically, the staff nurses were interrupted from medication administration to answer phone calls and random questions, redirect visitors, request medications, and verify stat orders

for other patients. The nurse managers and the staff nurses wanted to bring their vision of ensuring patient safety to the process of medication administration. Bringing the vision to reality was a challenge.

What do you think you would do if you were this nurse?

Given the turbulent times we face in health care, as well as the aging population in our society, now, more then ever, healthcare organizations are under enormous pressure to reduce expenses and contain costs. Major reforms are required, and the healthcare system has responded by restructuring the following imperatives:

- Empowering patients
- Ensuring care across the continuum that is both coordinated and comprehensive
- Securing appropriate utilization of resources, advanced technology, and work force
- Focusing on health promotion and prevention

Nurses are instrumental in the development of planning and executing new strategies for the future and thus in influencing the direction of health care. As technology advances, it is paramount for nurses to be at the forefront of this paradigm shift. This paradigm shift will require nurses to embrace, apply, and evaluate the use of such new technology. By demonstrating our ability to adopt and use new technology, we will be able to provide nursing with the expertise and earn the credibility to serve as advisors, directors, and influencers of technology. Thus, by our active participation and expertise, we can ensure that technology will be used to meet nursing's information needs, to advance nursing practice, and to ensure nursing's continued viability. In the twenty-first century, technology will connect care across the delivery system (Atkins & Cullen, 2013).

The operational definition of *proactive* is simply "aggressive planning." It provides direction for one's efforts and toward which others must then react. Thus greater control is possible so that one's vision becomes a probability, not just a possibility. The importance of proactive, thoughtful, deliberate planning in the face of uncertainties cannot be overestimated. *Proactive* means that everyone in the organization manages his or her work and professional life and how he or she relates to the organization's goals and missions.

STRATEGIC PLANNING

Strategic planning is a process by which the guiding members of the organization envision their future and develop the necessary and appropriate procedures and operations to actualize that future. Focus is designed to encompass the organization's emphasis on mission statements, strategic action plans, changes in policies and procedures, environmental factors affecting the organization, and the development and execution of new services.

The strategic planning process shown in Figure 16-1 consists of the following series of steps:

- Search the internal, external, and organizational environment to determine those forces or changes that may affect the work of the organization or that may be crucial to its survival.
- Analyze the organization's strengths, weaknesses, opportunities, threats (SWOT analysis) and its potential for dealing with change.
- Develop and evaluate the various strategies available to the organization to meet these opportunities and threats.
- Revise organizational mission, philosophy, goals, and objectives based on the above.
- Select the best strategic option that balances the organization's potential with the challenges of changing conditions, taking into account the values of its management and its social responsibilities.

Cutouts?

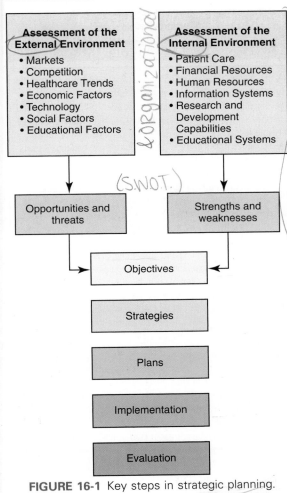

Assessment of the External Environment	Assessment of the Internal Environment
• Markets • Competition • Healthcare Trends • Economic Factors • Technology • Social Factors • Educational Factors	• Patient Care • Financial Resources • Human Resources • Information Systems • Research and Development Capabilities • Educational Systems

(Organizational)

(S.W.O.T.)

Opportunities and threats	Strengths and weaknesses

Objectives

Strategies

Plans

Implementation

Evaluation

FIGURE 16-1 Key steps in strategic planning.

outline only!

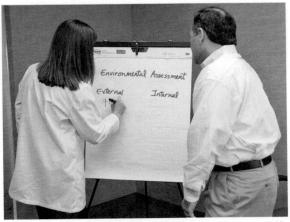

Environmental Assessment
External   Internal

A strong and dynamic strategic plan results in efficient and effective use of resources.

life, and provides direction and improvement for operational activities of the organization. Furthermore, a strong and dynamic strategic plan, if used, results in efficient and effective use of resources and reflects the organizational culture and customer focus. Numerous reasons exist for nurse leaders to plan in a proactive, systematic manner and include the following: (1) knowledge regarding philosophy, goals, and external and internal operations of the organization is necessary; and (2) an understanding of the planning process is paramount.

Phases of the Strategic Planning Process

The strategic planning process is proactive, vision-directed, action-oriented, creative, innovative, and oriented toward positive change. Strategic planning precedes strategic management and the development of a system such as a balanced scorecard that supports accountability using performance metrics (Higginbotham & Church, 2012). In addition to evidence-based accountability, the ever-changing healthcare marketplace demands agility and alignment of mission, values, and resources (Higginbotham & Church, 2012).

A strong and dynamic strategic plan results in the efficient and effective use of resources. The term *strategic planning process* is the development of a plan of action covering 3 to 5 years. The initial phase is the most difficult.

- Prepare the strategy.
- Execute and evaluate the strategy.

IF

Reasons for Planning

In today's healthcare environment, which is marked by extreme turbulence and complexity, strategic planning for healthcare organizations must be more than an outline of a business plan. Therefore, to survive the ongoing change and restructuring of the healthcare system, the strategic plan becomes the fundamental tool for creating and sustaining the organizational vision for the future. This process leads to achievement of goals and objectives, gives meaning to work

strategic planning

efficient & effective use of resources

Visionary leaders ensure that those around them understand the direction in which the organization is going (Kohles, Bligh, & Carsten, 2012). These visionaries search for a new path through a vigorous dialog with various constituents, both internally and externally, because great visions will not actualize from solitary analysis. Using a follower-centric approach to implement a shared vision promotes adoption of organizational goals (Kohles, Bligh, & Carsten, 2012). Although strategic planning is often achieved at the executive level of an organization, staff and managers provide a valuable perspective. Also, if a vision is accepted, understood, and adopted by followers, employee commitment, satisfaction, and positive performance increase (Kohles, Bligh, & Carsten, 2012).

Phase 1: Assessment of the External and Internal Environment

External Environmental Assessment. Assessment of the external environment is the initial phase in the strategic-planning process. The economic, demographic, technologic, social-cultural, educational, and political-legal factors are assessed in terms of their impact on opportunities and threats within the environment. Healthcare leaders can assess the effect of competitors on their environment, thus plan and monitor their own operations, and develop other creative and visionary programs as they work within the framework of their institutional mission and goals. Coyne and Horn (2009) suggested that leaders of an organization must anticipate how their competitors might respond to the strategic plan. Once that is known, the response can be incorporated into the plan. An example appears in Box 16-1.

EXERCISE 16-1

What is your opinion about the demographic situation in the city in which you live and work? What is the cultural makeup of the area? What is the gap between the real needs and services provided to patients in your organization?

Internal Environmental Assessment. The internal assessment of the environment relates to the institution of health care and includes a review of the effectiveness of the structure, size, programs, financial resources, human resources, information systems,

---

BOX 16-1   AN EXAMPLE OF ENVIRONMENTAL ASSESSMENT

A community-based acute care hospital is undertaking a study to examine accessibility, availability, quality, and effectiveness of developing an Orthopedic Center of Excellence. One of the initial steps is to conduct an environmental scan. The factors considered are the following:

- Economic forces and the escalating rates of healthcare costs
- The numbers and types of health professionals, including board-certified orthopedic physicians who are specializing in innovative joint replacement, operating room (OR) orthopedic nurses and OR orthopedic surgical technicians (certified), orthopedic staff nurses (certified), case managers, social workers, physical and occupational therapists, and pain management specialists
- Cost of orthopedic implants and reimbursement
- The social, political, and regulatory forces, including strategic priorities of the government in health promotion and disease prevention
- The diagnostic services available, including magnetic resonance imaging (MRI) and nuclear diagnostic imaging
- Community Outreach and educational opportunities

Patient Trends

- Demographic and population trends (population, employment, socioeconomic indicators, education, ethnicity, and lifestyle issues, with particular emphasis on minority groups)
- Trends in health care (increased emphasis on wellness programs and enhanced technologies)
- Prospective users' input about current and future services

---

and research and development capabilities of the organization. In addition, education and training of staff and public demands are reviewed. The management team involves all levels of staff in this process and focuses on the purpose of the organization; the mission and goals; the capabilities, skills, and relationships of various professional and related staff; and the weaknesses and strengths of staff in such areas as leadership, planning, coordination, research, and staff development.

Organizational Environmental Assessment. The organizational environment assessment relates to the hospital administration, service departments, and medical staff. The process is considered an informal evaluation of relationships that define the organizational boundaries to assess for structure and loyalties that may affect the achievement of work.

Also, the organizational climate must be assessed because it can shape the strategic direction of the organization.

Phase 2: Review of Mission Statement, Philosophy, Goals, and Objectives

Mission Statement. A mission statement reflects the purpose and direction of the healthcare organization or a department within it. A statement of philosophy provides direction for the organization and/or department within it. The content usually specifies organizational beliefs regarding the rights of individuals, beliefs regarding health and nursing, expectations of practitioners, and commitment of the organization to professionalism, education, evaluation, and research. The importance of the mission statement cannot be overstated, yet it is questionable how many individuals in an organization, when questioned directly, can articulate their mission statement or the philosophy.

Covey (1990) identified that the mission statement is vital to the success of an organization and believes that everyone should participate in the development of the mission statement: "The involvement process is as important as the written product and is the key to its use" (p. 139). "An organizational mission statement, one that truly reflects the deep shared vision and values of everyone within that organization, creates a unity and tremendous commitment" (p. 143).

EXERCISE 16-2

Select a healthcare organization with which you have been affiliated. How effective is the organizational structure (i.e., is the organization operating effectively and efficiently)? What overall human resources are present (e.g., table of organization, various titles, and numbers of people)? What information systems are used? Critique these questions as they apply to the nursing component only.

An example of a mission statement for a newly developed joint replacement program might be to provide quality, to be integrated, and to use the patient-focused healthcare model.

Goal-Setting. Goal-setting is the process of developing, negotiating, and formalizing the targets or objectives of an organization. If goals are not appro-

priate to the organization, frustration and poor performance could result (Bungay, 2011).

Using the example from Box 16-1, the joint replacement program might have five goals:

1. Provide comprehensive patient/family education across the continuum of care.
2. Develop protocols for standardized patient care programs in terms of activities of daily living, physical and occupational therapy, recreational exercise, and pain management.
3. Incorporate a multidisciplinary approach to patient care through the use of physicians, nurse practitioners, nurses, case managers, social workers, physical and occupational therapists, dietitians, home care personnel, and clergy.
4. Enhance community support programs for arthritic patients.
5. Ensure that the website is current, with information and services available to patients.

EXERCISE 16-3

Obtain and review a healthcare organization's mission statement. Based on what it says and means to you, create a goal statement that fits.

Practical insights from these studies that are critical to nurse administrators are that specific goals are more likely to lead to higher performance than are vague or very general goals, such as "try to do your best." Feedback, or knowledge of results, is more likely to motivate individuals toward higher performance levels and commitment to goal achievements. For example, as organizations have become more focused on their data related to care, they have been able to focus on specific goals and behaviors that result in better care.

Four key steps in implementing a goal-setting program are as follows:

1. Set goals that are specific, and adhere to a deadline.
2. Promote goal commitment by providing instructions and support to employees and managers.
3. Support the achievement of goals with appropriate feedback as soon as possible.
4. Monitor performance at appropriate intervals.

Objectives. The ability to write clear and concise objectives is an important aspect of nursing leadership. Effective objectives are known as *S.M.A.R.T. objectives* and include the following:

Specific The objective statement is properly constructed and describes exactly what is to be accomplished.

- It begins with the word *to,* followed by an action verb.
- It specifies a single result to be achieved.
- It specifies a target date for its attainment.

Measurable The objectives are measurable.

- They provide the level of accomplishment of the end result.
- They leave no question as to what is expected.

Agreed On The objectives are agreed on by all parties.

- There is mutual agreement by all parties who will be responsible for execution and monitoring.

Realistic The objectives must be created within the realm of possibility and a challenge.

- The objectives should not be unrealistic or unattainable.
- They must be written in the span of control for the specific team working toward the goals.
- The team has to be accountable for follow-through.

Time Bound The objectives should establish a time frame for which the activity or improvement must be achieved.

- Timelines and deadlines are adhered to.
- The time line must be well-defined by avoiding statements such as "in the future."

Phase 3: Identification of Strategies

The third phase of the strategic planning process involves identifying major issues, establishing goals, and developing strategies to meet the goals. The term *strategy* can be defined as an organized and innovative plan that assists an organization to achieve its objectives. All departmental managers are involved in this process and are responsible for preparing a detailed plan of action, which may include the following: development of short-term and long-term objectives, formulation of annual department objectives, allocation of resources, and preparation of the budget.

EXERCISE 16-4

You are a staff nurse at an acute care community hospital. The Chair of the Professional Practice Committee has assigned you to work on a planning committee. The purpose of the committee is to devise long-term and short-term departmental goals for nursing.

The population of the town is 55,000, and the population is aging. The senior population probably will increase over the next 5 years. Many in the community are seeking assistance for arthritis complications such as building better bones and exercise programs, physical therapy opportunities, and community education.

The hospital has both an inpatient and an outpatient rehabilitation program with a specialized orthopedic unit; the unit is staffed with nurses who are nationally certified in orthopedics and with world-renowned, board-certified orthopedic surgeons.

Considering the concepts of this strategic planning situation, in what direction should this nursing department consider moving during the next 5 years? How will you determine between long-term and short-term plans? What additional information will your committee need to plan realistically for the next 5 months and the next 5 years?

Table 16-1 identifies an action plan for creating, implementing, and evaluating an orthopedic center of excellence based on the environmental assessment in Box 16-1 on p. 314.

Phase 4: Implementation

The fourth phase of strategic planning is that the specific plan for action is executed in order of priority. This entails open communication with staff (this is paramount) regarding the priorities for the next year and subsequent periods; development of revised policies and procedures regarding the changes; and the creation of area and individual objectives related to the plan. The specific plan needs to be focused on marketing, programs, operations, budget, and human resource.

Phase 5: Evaluation

On a consistent basis, at regular intervals, the strategic plan is reviewed at all levels to determine whether the execution of goals, objectives, and activities is on target. As stated, a sense of flexibility regarding the objectives is important to consider, and objectives may change as a result of legislation, budget changes, and change in structure or other environmental

TABLE 16-1 STRATEGIC PLAN OF ACTION FOR THE DEVELOPMENT, IMPLEMENTATION, AND EVALUATION OF AN ORTHOPEDIC CENTER OF EXCELLENCE

OBJECTIVE	ACTIVITIES	RESPONSIBLE COUNCIL	TIME FRAME
1. To develop an Orthopedic Center of Excellence	1.1 To conduct a needs assessment • Primary and secondary service area • Demographic review • Out migration	Director of nursing Orthopedic product line manager Strategic planning and marketing director	January 2012
	1.2 To conduct a literature review related to each of these topics: • Orthopedic product lines • Innovative orthopedic joint replacement procedures • Programs related to the orthopedics evidenced-based practices for joint replacement	Orthopedic product line manager Operating room (OR) director Vice president of medical affairs Director of rehabilitative services Nurse practitioner Staff nurse	January 2012
	1.3 To form an advisory committee comprising community representatives to oversee the development and implementation of the center	Patient satisfaction director Physician champion Vice president of patient care services Orthopedic staff across the continuum of care Director of rehabilitation services Vice president of medical affairs	February 2012
	1.4 To develop the organizational structure, mission statement, philosophy, and objectives, and revise accordingly	All parties	March 2012
	1.5 To develop policy and procedure manuals for staff in all areas	Orthopedic staff across the continuum of care Medical staff Standards staff Nurse practitioners Director of education Staff nurses	Ongoing
	1.6 To determine the business structure of the organization (i.e., legalities regarding partnerships, corporations, and proprietorship)	Nurse practitioners Medical staff Vice president of medical affairs Orthopedic product line manager Vice president of patient care services Assistant vice president of patient care services Office of General Counsel	Ongoing
	1.7 To develop a budget	Assistant vice president of patient care services Orthopedic product line manager/nurse manager	March 2012 Ongoing

Continued

TABLE 16-1	STRATEGIC PLAN OF ACTION FOR THE DEVELOPMENT, IMPLEMENTATION, AND EVALUATION OF AN ORTHOPEDIC CENTER OF EXCELLENCE—cont'd		
OBJECTIVE	**ACTIVITIES**	**RESPONSIBLE COUNCIL**	**TIME FRAME**
	1.8 To develop a business site for the organization: • All renovations • Equipment • Supplies	Consultants and orthopedic product line manager	April 2012
	1.9 To develop a marketing program (newspapers, telephone, signs, and direct mailings)	Nurse practitioners Orthopedic product line manager Director of strategic planning and marketing Medical staff Staff nurses	February 2012 Ongoing
2. To implement and evaluate the effectiveness and efficiency of these programs	2.1 To develop patient questionnaires related to satisfaction regarding care provided	Nurse practitioners Orthopedic product line managers Director of patient satisfaction Orthopedic frontline staff across the continuum Staff nurses	April 2012
	2.2 To develop cost-effective analysis studies to evaluate each of the programs being provided	Orthopedic product line manager	Ongoing
	2.3 To collect and collate data related to utilization of services by orthopedic patients	Nurse practitioners Staff across the continuum of care Pharmacists Medical staff Orthopedic product line manager Quality director	Ongoing

factors. Therefore, alternative activities may need to be adapted to the situation. For example, one agency was informed that the budget had to be decreased by $250,000 over the next 3 months. The staff became involved in the development of creative methods for ensuring that the necessary changes occurred. Savings were realized with restructuring, reducing expense, and, when appropriate, converting intravenous (IV) to oral (PO) medication administration.

MARKETING

Marketing is about identifying and meeting both human and social needs (Kotler & Keller, 2009). Bryce and Dyer (2007) suggested that marketing enables the organization to assess the needs of the customers in order to develop and execute services to meet those needs by establishing a niche, or specially focused, market. The benefits of marketing include increased customer satisfaction; the potential to become the hospital of choice for both patients and employees; improved resource attraction; and improved operational efficiency. The underlying assumption is that marketing helps manage the exchange of goods and services in a more efficient manner. Marketing has rarely been an integral aspect of nursing. The Literature Perspective on p. 319 identifies why nursing services can be a dimension of a healthcare system's marketing.

LITERATURE PERSPECTIVE

Resource: Montoya & Kimball. (2012). Nursing services: an imperative to healthcare marketing. *Journal of Nursing Education and Practice, 2*(4), 187-193.

Nursing is the largest service sector in health care and as such often constitutes the face of the organization to the patients in that facility. Good nursing care can be one of the strongest marketing positions a healthcare system adopts. This is especially true as both patient- and family-centered care are organized and executed in a healthcare system. This paper illustrates the many ways nurses can be an asset of a marketing program.

Implications for Practice
Nurses have the opportunity to advertise and promote a positive marketing image for a healthcare organization.

RESEARCH PERSPECTIVE

Resource: Clyne, M., Dilligard, R., Langish, R., Ruddy, K., & Vega, D. (2009). *Knowledge, attitudes, beliefs and practices regarding breast cancer screening in female health care workers in an acute care hospital in Northern New Jersey.* Unpublished researched—Sigma Theta Tau Poster Session, Seton Hall University, South Orange, NJ.

A convenience sample of female healthcare workers (n = 411) in an acute care hospital setting was used for this study to examine the knowledge, attitudes, beliefs, and practices regarding breast cancer screening. For this descriptive study, a 12-item, 5-point Likert questionnaire was distributed to all female healthcare workers as a paycheck attachment in October (Breast Cancer Awareness Month).

Half of the respondents had a family history of cancer, 80% performed a self-examination of the breast, 79% indicated their physician encouraged them to have a mammogram, and 95% had insurance. Perceptions about receiving a recommendation for a mammogram tended to be positive, and mammogram was believed to be more effective than examination by self or the physician.

Implications for Practice
This study has specific implications for designing marketing strategies, including the authors' recommendations regarding developing educational programs in the acute care hospitals regarding the importance of screening, prevention, and early detection of breast cancer. Furthermore, nurses need to advocate for the availability of searchable databases so patients can find important information.

Nursing also impacts the marketing of ideas and information that are essential for patient health. The Research Perspective at the right assesses the knowledge, attitudes, beliefs, and practices regarding breast cancer screening of selected healthcare workers.

Strategic Marketing Planning Process

The strategic marketing planning process is similar in nature to the strategic planning process and the nursing process. Figure 16-2 offers a comparative chart outlining the steps in the process.

The steps of the strategic marketing planning are as follows:

- Analyze the organization-wide mission, objectives, goals, and culture to which the marketing strategy must contribute.
- Assess organizational strengths, weaknesses, opportunities, and threats (SWOT analysis) presented by the external environment.
- Analyze the future environment the marketer is likely to face with respect to the public served; competition; and the social-cultural, political, technologic, and economic environment.
- Determine the marketing mission, objectives, and specific goals for the relevant planning period.
- Formulate the core marketing strategy to achieve the specified goals.

- Implement the necessary organizational structure and the systems within the marketing function to ensure proper follow-through of the designed strategy.
- Establish detailed programs and tactics to carry out the core strategy for the planning period, including a timetable of activities and the assignment of specific responsibilities.
- Establish benchmarks to measure interim and final achievements of the program.
- Execute the planned program.
- Monitor performance, and adjust the core strategy, tactical details, or both as needed.

Although healthcare organizations have marketing departments, nurses are involved in the process because of their direct involvement with the users of service—the patients.

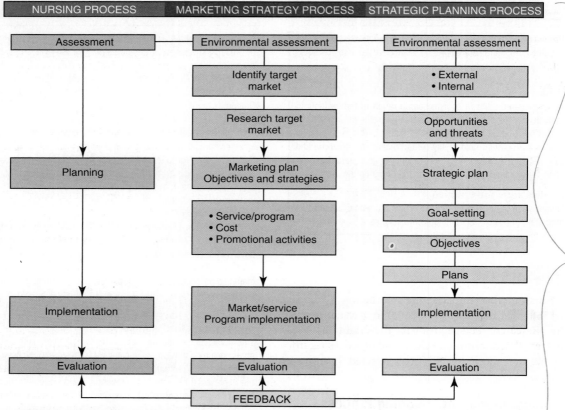

FIGURE 16-2 Marketing framework as compared to using the nursing process and strategic planning.

Assessment

Determining Organization-Level Missions, Objectives, and Goals

A marketing plan is developed by the executive leaders of the organization and advisory board to do the following:

1. Determine the organization-level long-term culture, mission, objectives, and goals.
2. Assess the organization's potential future external environment.
3. Assess the organization's current and potential strengths, weaknesses, opportunities, and threats.

Analyzing Organizational Strengths and Weaknesses

In the marketing process, an environmental assessment is conducted to identify and research the target market. An example of this is conducting a needs assessment of the services currently provided by an organization to develop new services or promotional activities to meet the needs of the population being served.

Focus groups may consist of interviews with key staff; review of documents; observation of staff; visits to competitors; and overview of advertisements, brochures, and other documents as deemed appropriate. Nurses often have great insight about needs because patients convey their desires and lack of services during care delivery.

Analyzing External Threats and Opportunities

The three components of the external environment are (1) the public environment, which consists of groups and organizations that affect the organization (e.g., public, media, regulatory agencies); (2) the competitive environment, which consists of other organizations that vie for the attention and loyalty of customers; and (3) the macro-environment, which consists of demographic, economic, technologic, political, and social forces to which the organization must adapt.

Setting Marketing Mission, Objectives, and Goals

The marketing mission, objectives, and goals must align with the organizational mission, objectives, and goals. The marketing focus is geared to changing market conditions, much as a financial advisor evaluates changing investment market conditions. The market, comprising both external and internal markets, influences the way an organization moves toward its vision.

Planning

The environmental assessment is followed by the development of a marketing plan. This plan outlines the service or program to be provided, includes a detailed budget-cost analysis, and describes the promotional activities designed to promote the program. "Predicting the future" is difficult in turbulent times. To anticipate problems and plan for the future, forecasting involves considering multiple factors that could occur. The process requires several components:

- Assessing the current and potential future situation
- Identifying the strengths, weaknesses, opportunities, and threats
- Defining the driving forces in the environment
- Developing optional scenarios
- Identifying the preferred action
- Developing a plan of action
- Executing the plan of action
- Evaluating and monitoring the plan

Forecasts should be estimates of how accurately a situation can provide optional futures and learning experiences and be considered for their influence in convincing managers of the need for change, be cost-effective, and be used for their ritualistic purpose. Rather than using the "shooting at a target" metaphor, it may be more appropriate to think of forecasters as art teachers, helping line (and clinical) managers

paint updated pictures of their future. For example, in forecasting the number of patients who will need orthopedic services in a community, a manager needs to consider an environmental scan comprising the aging population and morbidity and mortality related to inactivity underlying orthopedic problems.

Implementation and Execution

The implementation, or execution, phase includes the establishment of the program and promotional activities designed to communicate benefits of the service or program to patients. Forms of promotion may include media releases, brochures, pamphlets, newsletters, and "word-of-mouth" advertising. Pamphlets and brochures are promotional materials that inform individuals about the benefits of a healthcare agency's programs and services.

Evaluation and Monitoring

The evaluation may incorporate customer satisfaction surveys, interviews with customers, and further research studies designed to assess reasons that customers are using or not using a service, program, or product. Feedback is an essential component of the marketing process.

Box 16-2 represents steps in the strategic marketing planning process in relation to the delivery of breast cancer screening services to female healthcare workers in an acute care community hospital in a suburban area of Belleville, New Jersey.

Nurses can play an active role and be given responsibilities relating to planning, goal-setting, and marketing. Each of us has some sense of what is important today and sustainable for tomorrow in the context of our cultural perspective. Most of us sense the difference between fads and trends and how each affects us personally and professionally. Nursing leaders are accountable for setting goals, including their followers in those activities, and aligning tasks with the mission and goals of the organization. As nursing leaders represent the profession, organization, or community, they are marketing each of those elements. Nurse leaders can positively contribute to formal marketing strategies through various activities such as focus groups or evaluating responses to marketing materials. However, the focus should be on how nurse leaders' actions contribute to future quality.

BOX 16-2 MISSION STATEMENT, GOALS, AND OBJECTIVES OF A NORTHERN NEW JERSEY BREAST CANCER SCREENING PROGRAM

Mission Statement

To reduce the leading cause of cancer deaths in women by delivering a comprehensive, organized, and evaluated breast cancer screening program for female healthcare workers in an acute care setting in Belleville, New Jersey. The Breast Cancer Screening Program is committed to deliver a program that is sensitive to women's needs, builds on health-promoting behaviors, and fosters partnerships with interest groups in the healthcare community.

Overall Goals

To integrate health promotion strategies and medical practice to reduce mortality from breast cancer by having 100% of eligible female healthcare workers participate in annual mammography screening and conduct self–breast examinations.

Objectives

- To detect breast cancer earlier than would occur if organized screening were not available
- To develop and implement a hospital mobilization plan for the program
- To develop and implement a social marketing plan, including a health education component for the program
- To articulate protocols and standards for healthcare professionals associated with the program
- To establish protocols for the interaction of the target population with the program
- To develop and implement training and technical assistance for those associated with the delivery of the program
- To develop a partnership with healthcare professionals that will facilitate program delivery
- To establish a regional breast screening service so that all women in the target population have equal access to breast screening
- To document the follow-up of all women in whom an abnormality has been detected
- To provide screening that is sensitive and acceptable to the target population
- To evaluate the program on a continual basis, including needs assessment and measurement of process, economic, and outcome variables

THE SOLUTION

Trying to find common ground to achieve the vision of patient safety at the time of medication administration for the nursing staff and the nursing management team was of utmost importance. Given the fact that we had developed a system-wide Professional Practice Council and Nursing Research Council, I thought this might be a great starting place for the staff to develop a creative way to bring their vision to actuality. These councils also exist at each affiliate of the Saint Barnabas Health Care System. Therefore the evidenced-based practices could be reviewed and standardized at the local level and then brought up to the system councils. This is truly an empowered group with decision-making capacity for nursing in the system.

1. The literature was reviewed and disseminated among the members of the Professional Practice Council at the system level and at each affiliate level. Dialog ensued, and staff were very interested in the research findings.
2. There was an opportunity for one affiliate to participate in a national study regarding this topic. The staff nurses at the affiliate site were enthusiastic about such an opportunity. They gladly participated because the results would undoubtedly have a profound impact on enhancing patient safety during medication administration for the system.
3. The findings and implications of the study were reviewed and discussed with the Professional Practice Councils. Final decision making about how we were going to embrace this newly found evidenced-based practice and decision making was conducted by the council members.

4. I wanted this to be a win-win moment for the staff and made sure they had all the appropriate resources available to them in making changes to our policies and procedures. I ensured that all potential barriers were removed for success in making their vision come true.
5. The staff felt a strong sense of ownership to this vision and were instrumental in the success of the changes. In addition, the vice presidents of the system were all in full support of the Professional Practice Councils' recommendations and vision.

The utilization of these Professional Practice Councils truly provided the staff nurses with a new perspective that they can in fact make a difference in the delivery of care at the bedside and be recognized for the value of their expertise to resolve patient safety issues. This is an empowered group of professionals who had the opportunity to see their vision turn into a reality based on nursing research and best practices. The Professional Practice Council members take great pride in their accomplishments and are wonderful role models and mentors to others. Their commitment to excellence in patient care does not go unnoticed.

—*Nancy Holecek*

Would this be a suitable approach for you? Why or why not?

THE EVIDENCE

Drenkard (2012) proposes that development of a nursing strategic plan leads to effective goal accomplishment, an essential for obtaining and maintaining Magnet™ status.

The strategic planning process includes assessing the current status of nursing services, researching the ideal state of nursing care delivery and evidence-based practice, and conducting a gap analysis between the ideal and the real (Drenkard, 2012). From this process a shared vision for nursing can be developed that will optimize nursing services in a healthcare organization.

Drenkard (2012) notes that an action plan for the accomplishment of that shared vision includes establishing measurable goals, developing specific tactics to accomplish those goals, and creating accountability systems. A key consideration for this activity is the inclusion of major stakeholders, such as members of the finance and human resource departments, in the planning process that nursing undertakes.

NEED TO KNOW NOW

- Consider how the vision and mission statement of the organization would affect your practice.

- Know the strengths, weaknesses, opportunities, and threats facing your healthcare organization.
- Listen for ideas about needs from your patients.

CHAPTER CHECKLIST

The operational effectiveness of any organization depends on its strategic planning. Nurse leaders/managers must be knowledgeable of the critical elements to facilitate the process. Setting goals and defining marketing strategies for product line development are part of the role of professional nurses to achieve effective organizational results in creating a niche market in healthcare services.

- The strategic planning process leads to attainment of goals and objectives and provides meaning to work life and direction for the organizational activities.
- Strategic planning is similar in nature to the nursing process and involves the following:
  - Assessment of the environment (internal, external, and operational)
  - Appraisal of the organization's strengths and weaknesses

  - Identification of the major opportunities and threats
  - Development of strategies to meet these opportunities
  - Implementation and evaluation of the strategies
- Marketing strategies play a vital role in healthcare settings as competition increases to provide services and programs to consumers. The steps in the strategic marketing planning process are as follows:
  - Assessment
  - Planning
  - Implementation
  - Evaluation
- Nurses can play a pivotal role in the development of visionary programs and services that meet the needs of the customers.

TIPS FOR PLANNING, GOAL-SETTING, AND MARKETING

- Be clear about the organization's mission and vision, ensure they meet the needs of those you serve, and stay true to them.
- Read and listen to wide sources of data to determine what is happening and what trends could affect you and your organization, and be flexible if changes are eminent.

- Be clear about your role in the organization and its success. Actively participate in the process.
- Think about what messages others need to hear about you and the services you provide.

REFERENCES

Atkins, D. & Cullen, T. (2013). The future of health information technology: implications for research. *Medical Care, 51*(3), Supp 1.

Bryce, D., & Dyer, J. (2007). Strategies to crack well-guarded markets. *Harvard Business Review, 85*(5), 84-92.

Bungay, S. (2011). How to make the most of your company's strategy. *Harvard Business Review, 89*(1/2), 133-140.

Clyne, M., Dilligard, R., Langish, R., Ruddy, K., & Vega, D. (2009). *Knowledge, attitudes, beliefs and practices regarding breast cancer screening in female health care workers in an acute care hospital in Northern New Jersey.* Unpublished researched—Sigma Theta Tau Poster Session, Seton Hall University, South Orange, NJ.

Covey, S. (1990). *The seven habits of highly effective people.* Toronto: Simon & Schuster.

Coyne, K., & Horn, J. (2009). Predicting your competitor's reaction. *Harvard Business Review, 87*(4), 90-97.

Drenkard, K. (2012). Strategy as solution: developing a nursing strategic plan. *Journal of Nursing Administration, 42*(5), 242-243.

Higginbotham, E. J. & Church, K. C. (2012). Strategic planning as a tool for achieving alignment in academic health centers. *Transactions of the American Clinical and Climatological Association, 123,* 292-303.

Kohles, J. C., Bligh, M. C. & Carsten, M. K. (2012). A follower-centric approach to the vision integration process. *The Leadership Quarterly, 23,* 476-487.

Kotler, P., & Keller, K. (2009). *Marketing management.* Upper Saddle River, NJ: Prentice Hall.

Montoya, I. D., & Kimball, O. M. (2012). Nursing services: An imperative to health care marketing. *Journal of Nursing Education and Practice, 2*(4), 187-193.

SUGGESTED READINGS

Elliott, R. W. (2012). Strategic planning: is it really necessary? *Nephrology Nursing Journal, 39*(1), 11.

Harmon, R. B., Fontaine, D., Plews-Ogan, M., & Williams, A. (2012). Achieving transformational change: Using appreciative inquiry for strategic planning in a school of nursing. *Journal of Professional Nursing, 28*(2), 119-124.

Jasper, M. & Crossan, F. (2012). What is strategic management? *Journal of Nursing Management, 20*(7), 838-846.

Jeffs, L., Merkley, J., Richardson, S., Eli, J., & McAllister, M. (2011). Using a nursing balanced scorecard approach to measure and optimize nursing performance. *Nursing Leadership, 24*(1), 47-58.

Perryman, M. M. & Rivers, P. A. (2011). Strategic groups in healthcare: a literature review. *Health Services Management Research, 24*(3), 151-159.

Shirey, M. R. (2013). Lewin's theory of planned change as a strategic resource. *Journal of Nursing Administration, 43*(2), 69-72.

Shirey, M. R. (2012). Cultivating strategic thinking skills. *Journal of Nursing Administration, 42*(6), 311-314.

Shoemaker, L. K. & Fischer, B. (2011). Creating a nursing strategic planning framework based on evidence. *Nursing Clinics of North America, 46*(1), 11-25.

White, J. (2012). Reflections on strategic nurse leadership. *Journal of Nursing Management, 20*(7), 835-837.

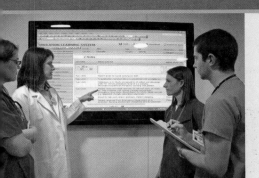

Leading Change

Mary Ann T. Donohue

This chapter describes the general nature of change in healthcare organizations. The theories and models, processes, responses, principles, and strategies typically involved in creating and leading change are presented. The manager's primary role is that of change facilitator. This role includes functions that anticipate, create, and manage the dynamic forces of change for desired outcomes and goal achievement. Choosing how to react to imposed change is a frequent responsibility and leading proactively offers multiple opportunities to better enhance outcomes. Therefore the effective change agent ensures staff empowerment to achieve change outcomes. The term change agent *is used in this chapter to describe the nurse leader who is responsible and accountable for achieving a defined set of management-oriented outcomes through the orchestrated efforts of any defined group.* Change *refers to an alteration in the work environment that is new or different from what existed previously.* Change management *refers to the overall processes and strategies used to moderate and manage the preparation for, effect of, responses to, and outcomes of conditions that are new and different from those that existed previously.*

OBJECTIVES

- Analyze the general characteristics of change in open-system organizations.
- Relate the models of planned change to the process of low-level change.
- Evaluate nonlinear theories for managing high-level change.
- Evaluate the use of select functions, principles, and strategies for initiating and managing change.
- Formulate desirable qualities of effective change agents.

TERMS TO KNOW

barriers	chaos theory	low-complexity change
change agents	cybernetic theory	negative feedback
change management	facilitators	nonlinear change
change outcome	high-complexity change	planned change
change process	informal change agent	strategies
change situations	learning organization	

Sharon McEvoy, RN
Nurse Manager, Clara Maass Medical Center, Belleville, New
*   Jersey*

As a nurse manager on a large medical/surgical unit, I often noticed that our nursing assistants did a lot of running around in and out of patients' rooms. They often answered call bells for the same things, over and over, all day long. In addition, I saw that the professional nursing staff could not always locate the nursing assistants because they were so spread out over the geographic layout of the unit. Around the same time, patient satisfaction and staff satisfaction had either reached a plateau or remained low. I heard a presenta-

tion about hourly rounding and then found some articles explaining how the practice had been introduced in many hospitals across the country. I brought the articles to my staff and introduced the concept to them. The challenge, I told them, is to anticipate patients' needs rather than respond to them as we all had been doing for years. How could I make hourly rounding work on our unit without resistance? Would our patient and staff satisfaction increase? How would the staff adjust to the change?

What do you think you would do if you were this nurse?

INTRODUCTION

Change is a natural social process of individuals, groups, organizations, and society. The forces of change may have their origins external, internal, or both to healthcare organizations. We do know that change is constant, inevitable, pervasive, and unpredictable and varies in rate and intensity, which unavoidably influences individuals, technology, and systems at all levels of every organization. Even if we did not want to change, the rapidity and the volume of changes affecting the healthcare environment dictate that we must embrace a new imperative: the future. If we do not, we risk inevitable frustration and dissatisfaction and, perhaps, expend more energy obstructing growth than promoting opportunities for success.

Because most healthcare organizations operate as open systems, they are especially receptive to a wide variety of influences. The impact of organization-wide change depends on the organization's particular stage of development, degree of flexibility, and history of response to change. The role of change agents is to lead change efforts. Their activities are rooted in thinking that is systems-based and theory-based, quite tolerant of ambiguity, and ever mindful of the bigger picture. Therefore the management of change in organizations requires moving easily back and forth from an emphasis on long-range planning and established goals to a greater focus on managing competing, dynamic forces in change situations. The successful manager of change constantly moves the group toward a set of predetermined, achievable outcomes. Balancing change in the long and short views

is always a key challenge in any given situation, and the capacity to manage change is one of the marks of a true leader.

CONTEXT OF THE CHANGE ENVIRONMENT

Change is a challenging process and leaders must know how to navigate it (Salmela, Eriksson & Fagerstrom, 2011). In an increasingly uncertain world, managers and leaders in our profession are challenged to be skilled in using change theory, serving as change agents, and supporting staff during times of change. According to the American Organization of Nurse Executives (AONE) (2005), managers and leaders need to do the following:

- Use change theory to plan for the implementation of organizational change
- Serve as change agent, assisting others in understanding the importance, necessity, and processes of change
- Support staff during times of difficult transitions
- Recognize one's own reaction to change, and strive to remain open to new ideas and approaches
- Adapt leadership style to situational needs

Nursing entities are open systems that must be responsive to external and internal stimuli and that must be capable of dynamic change essential for survival (Meyer & O'Brien-Pallas, 2010). Using planned linear change was useful when cycles in society and health care were somewhat stable (low-complexity change). The highly complex, accelerated, and unpredictable change situations of today still require planning, but on a constantly changing basis.

Nurses are key players in healthcare delivery. They are partners with multiple care providers and pivotal players in open-systems organizations. In their classic work, Begun and White (1995) said that it was important for nursing to consider its dominant logic as a source of structural inertia. Using chaos theory components, they suggested that nursing in certain organizations is too "stuck" and thus too unresponsive and unable to adapt to the influences of rapid change. Today, nursing organizations that achieve designation by the American Nurses Credentialing Center (ANCC) with Magnet™ status are typically ones that are flexible, adaptive, and innovative. They can lead change by putting into place programs that capitalize on rapid change and thus improve patient safety and nurses' work environment and achieve quality outcomes. One way the nurse leader can alter the dominant logic is shown in Box 17-1. Using this methodology, the manager becomes adept at address-ing an emergent approach to change that takes place over a long period rather than sporadic and episodic reactions to change (Shanley, 2007). Scenario planning (i.e., raising multiple "what if" questions with many possible alternative answers) is an example of the needed flexibility and creativity urgently needed in nursing today.

There are two approaches commonly referred to in the literature on change: linear and nonlinear. Planned change models, or linear approaches, can guide directional, incremental, low-level, less-complex changes. Examples are reorganizing the storage of unit supplies and publishing staff development courses for nurses. Changes that represent higher-level thinking, on the other hand, are characteristically more fluid and complex because of the number of interactions and the activities of multiple players and their influences across the organization. Usually, nonlinear change approaches are found in complexity/chaos and learning organization theories. They offer helpful approaches for understanding dynamic, open-system healthcare organizations and for guiding change agents in managing accelerated, increasingly uncertain change environments (Dattee & Barlow, 2010). Change agents in planned changes focus on specific goals and the incremental steps needed to attain those goals. Change agents in nonlinear, complex changes serve as monitors of the environment, negotiators of influences on a change, and precise forecasters of possible scenarios and their anticipated outcomes.

BOX 17-1	GUIDELINES FOR ALTERING THE DOMINANT LOGIC

Decrease	Increase
• Long-term forecasting	• Short-term forecasting
• Preplanned strategies	• Emergent strategies
• Emphasis on past successes	• Search for new opportunities
• One future vision	• Multiple scenarios
• Rigid, permanent structures	• Self-organizing, temporary structures
• Structural isolation in the workplace	• Structural interdependence in the workplace
• Stability of leadership	• Leadership turnover
• Standardization	• Innovation, experimentation, diversity
• Insulation from other professions and marketplace	• Cooperation and competition
• Marketplace "passivity"	• Marketplace "aggression"
• Expectation of job security	• Self-learning

From Begun, J.W., & White, K.R. (1995). Altering nursing's dominant logic: Guidelines from complex adaptive systems theory. *Complexity and Chaos in Nursing*, 2(1), 10. Used with permission of Angela E. Vicenzi, Editor, *Chaos and Complexity in Nursing*.

PLANNED CHANGE USING LINEAR APPROACHES

Most planned change models—linear models—advocate that change can occur in a sequential and directional fashion when guided by effective change agents. The early planned change models, such as those of Lewin (1947); Lippitt, Watson, and Westley (1958); and Havelock (1973), explain the nature of change processes and offer systematic problem-solving methods designed to achieve change. The use of planned change can be useful for low-level change in more stable environments. Flexibility in implementing the plan and moderating the situational factors, as is advocated by nonlinear approaches, can then be introduced to improve the overall outcomes. However, to make change happen, the group has to progress through it. The group cannot let only a few make the changes. Sticking with and advancing the change is daily work that requires the undivided focus of all team members.

Lewin (1947) suggested that an analysis of change situations, which he called *force field analysis,* includes early and ongoing assessment of barriers and facilitators. Barriers in change situations are factors that can hinder the change process; facilitators are factors that can expedite the process. These elements may originate with people, technology, structure, or values. For change to be effective, the force of facilitators must exceed the force of barriers; thus the work of change agents is to reduce the barriers in the situation and support or enhance the facilitators. Figure 17-1 illustrates an example of how to diagram forces so that a visual portrays the strengths and barriers of any change. In this case, the strengths outweigh the barriers.

Lewin (1947) describes change as having three stages:

- Unfreezing
- Experiencing the change
- Refreezing

Unfreezing refers to the awareness of an opportunity, need, or problem for which some action is necessary; it also requires subsequent mental readiness to approach the issue. This phase may occur naturally as a progressive development, or it may result from a deliberate activity as a first step in planning a change.

For example, when the current way of communicating shift-to-shift reports is ineffective, as evidenced by a lack of hand-off communication, the staff becomes aware of the problem and the need for change to occur. As in The Challenge section on p. 326, changes in how patients' needs were anticipated on an hourly basis, with formal scripting processes introduced to the staff on one unit, brought about unfreezing.

EXERCISE 17-1

Identify the facilitators and barriers in the following situation. Rate the potential strength of each in hindering or expediting attainment of the change. Use "+5" for the highest positive strength toward change occurring and "−5" for the greatest negative strength against the change:

The inpatient psychiatric unit is about to convert 12 of its 20 voluntary beds into short-term care facility (STCF) beds for patients who are involuntarily committed. These beds would co-exist with the voluntary beds that are already on the unit. The involuntary beds were transferred from the license of a nearby facility. The talent and the expertise of the former facility were highly desirable to help with the transition to a unit with a higher acuity with sicker patients; therefore 12 of the former facility's nursing staff members were hired. So far, staff's reaction to the merger has been mixed. Individuals from the former facility, while welcomed enthusiastically by the staff from the present unit, were less than enthusiastic. Added to the change was the news that the former facility has filed for bankruptcy, leaving the former employees without their retirement pensions and other benefits.

Experiencing the change or solution leads to incorporation of what is new or different into work and interpersonal processes (Lewin, 1947). Deciding to begin to use the change or being unexpectedly thrust into the change can result in potential integration of the new way of thinking or doing.

Refreezing occurs when the participants in the change situation accept and use the new attitude or behavior (Lewin, 1947). Acceptance is assumed once most staff members integrate the change into their work processes. Surveys, structured or unstructured observations, or other data-collection methods can be conducted at various points after the implementation of a specific change to measure the effectiveness of the new approach. Analysis of these data can help evaluate the degree of implementation and identify additional alterations needed to ensure an effective change outcome.

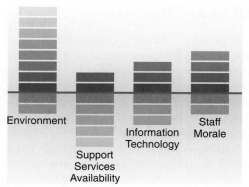

FIGURE 17-1 Examples of forces of change: facilitators and barriers.

Although Havelock's (1973) six-stage model for planning change had particular application to educational entities (see the Theory Box below), it shows similarities in the elements of the directional phases recommended by other planned-change models. Two adjuncts to Havelock's model advocate development of the effective change agent and use of his model as a rational problem-solving process. The rational problem-solving process is "how change agents can organize their work so that successful innovation will take place" (p. 3).

Lippitt, Watson, and Westley's (1958) model suggests seven sequential phases to use to plan change (see the Theory Box below). Inherent in this model is the change agent's appraisal of the "change and resistance forces which are present in the client system

---

THEORY BOX

Theories for Planned Change

KEY CONTRIBUTORS	KEY IDEA	APPLICATION TO PRACTICE
Six Phases of Planned Change* Havelock (1973) is credited with this planned change model.	Change can be planned, implemented, and evaluated in six sequential stages. The model is advocated for the development of effective change agents and used as a rational problem-solving process. The six stages are as follows: 1. Building a relationship 2. Diagnosing the problem 3. Acquiring relevant resources 4. Choosing the solution 5. Gaining acceptance 6. Stabilizing the innovation and generating self-renewal	Useful for low-level, low-complexity change.
Seven Phases of Planned Change† Lippitt, Watson, and Westley (1958) are credited with this planned change model.	Change can be planned, implemented, and evaluated in seven sequential phases. Ongoing sensitivity to forces in the change process is essential. The seven phases are as follows: 1. The client system becomes aware of the need for change. 2. The relationship is developed between the client system and change agent. 3. The change problem is defined. 4. The change goals are set, and options for achievement are explored. 5. The plan for change is implemented. 6. The change is accepted and stabilized. 7. The change entities redefine their relationships.	Useful for low-level, low-complexity change.
Innovation-Decision Process‡ Rogers (2003) is credited with formulating this process.	Change for an individual occurs over five phases when choosing to accept or reject an innovation/idea. Decisions to not accept the new idea may occur at any of the five stages. The change agent can promote acceptance by providing information about benefits and disadvantages and encouragement. The five stages are as follows: 1. Knowledge 2. Persuasion 3. Decision 4. Implementation 5. Confirmation	Useful for individual change.

* Adapted from Havelock, R.G. (1973). *The change agent's guide to innovation in education.* Englewood Cliffs, NJ: Educational Technology Publications.
† Adapted from Lippitt, R., Watson, J., & Westley, B. (1958). *The dynamics of planned change.* New York: Harcourt Brace.
‡ Adapted from Rogers, E.M. (1995). *Diffusion of innovations* (4th ed.). New York: The Free Press.

at the beginning of the change process as well as others which may be revealed as the process advances. Being continuously sensitive to the constellation of change forces and resistance forces is one of the most creative parts of the change agent's job" (p. 92).

More recently, the innovation-decision process (Rogers, 2003) has been used to explain the decision to accept or reject a new idea for use in practice (see the Theory Box on p. 329). According to Rogers' work, the individual's decision-making actions pass through five sequential stages. The decision to not accept the new idea may occur at any stage. However, the change agent can facilitate movement by others through these stages by encouraging the use of the idea and providing information about its benefits and disadvantages.

NONLINEAR CHANGE: CHAOS AND LEARNING ORGANIZATION THEORIES

Chaos Theory

Organizations can no longer rely on rules, policies, and hierarchies to enforce change and achieve outcomes in rigid and inflexible ways. According to chaos theory, the rapidly changing nature of human and world factors underscores how an emphasis on rules and policies is shortsighted, wastes time, and fails to accomplish goals in the long run. Organizations are open systems operating in complex, fast-changing environments. The term *open* by itself suggests that such systems (organizations/services) are affected by and simultaneously affect their environment. These systems are similar to semipermeable membranes, allowing some exchanges between the internal and external environments. Non–human-induced responses are characterized by random-appearing yet self-organizing patterns. Constant adaptation and the mere anticipation of change force organizations to remain relevant in their environment. The cycle of change dictates that, typically, organizations experience periods of stability interrupted by periods of intense transformation, thus demonstrating "spurts" of change rather than continuously steady, incremental change. Although not immediately predictable in the long run, small changes in the internal or external environment can certainly result in significant consequences to organizational work processes and outcomes. Chaos theory

further explains that the conditions present in a particular organizational change will not occur again in the same form (Vicenzi, White, & Begun, 1997). Figure 17-2 illustrates the contrasting patterns.

Organizations have always been self-organizing systems with the potential for self-renewal. Magnet™ organizations, as a key example, illustrate how organizations dedicated to excellence capitalize on a vision of quality to create shared values and beliefs. Furthermore, the focus on interrelationships (chief nursing officer [CNO] to and from staff, nurses with physicians, and employees with patients) creates fertile landscapes for potential change. Their emphasis on evidenced-based outcomes practice models, in addition to innovations in nursing research scholarship, has been exemplary, for example. Such intellectual advancement supports the value of continuous learning as a matter of organizational philosophy and further promotes adaptation to constant, accelerated change.

Learning Organization Theory

Learning organization theory emerged to describe organizations that place emphasis on flexibility and responsiveness (Senge, 1990). Specifically, complex organizations that are responsive to internal and external influences are trying to survive in an unpredictable healthcare environment. They can best respond and adapt when members of the organization

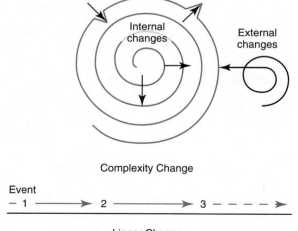

FIGURE 17-2 Contrasting patterns of linear and complexity theories.

complete their work with others using a learning approach. Enactment of Senge's five disciplines is essential to achieving learning organization status. *Disciplines* refers to the grouping that comprises critical and interrelated elements; this grouping can function effectively only when all elements are present, linked, and interacting. For example, an automobile with a working engine and other essential operational features but no tires could not be driven as designed. Without the knowledge of the interrelatedness of the automobile's operational features, one might not be able to take the right action to use this form of transportation.

Senge's (1990) five disciplines of learning organizations are the following:

1. Systems thinking
2. Personal mastery
3. Mental models
4. Shared vision
5. Team learning

Dialog (two-way discussion) promotes the individual, group, and organizational learning process. *Systems thinking* refers to the need for the organization to view the world as a set of multiple visible and invisible parts that interact constantly. When the organization values and facilitates development of the deeper aspirations of its members in addition to professional proficiency, it successfully matches organizational learning and personal growth or *personal mastery*. Each individual and each organization base their activities on a set of assumptions, beliefs, and mental pictures about the way the world should work. When these invisible *mental models* are uncovered and consciously evaluated, it is possible to begin to determine, in a "learningful" (Senge, 1990, p. 9) way, their influence on work accomplishment. Building *shared vision* occurs when leaders involve all members in moving personal visions of the future into a consolidated yet ongoing vision common to members and leaders. *Team learning* refers to the need for a cohesive group to learn together to benefit from the abilities of each member, thereby enhancing the overall outcomes of the team's efforts. Organizations value employees who can learn continuously, interact and communicate effectively as team members, and seek to meet their potential as team members.

An example of the application of chaos and learning organization theories is a community hospital that has been sensitive to and has adapted to external and internal environmental influences, such as the need to make changes in reimbursement and accreditation policies. The process of adaptation involves times of fluctuation interrupted with times of stability. The implications of managed care mandated by major insurance players may not be predictable, but they have significant consequences for the financial survival of the community hospital. New reimbursement strategies have forced community hospitals and other area hospitals to interact to seek consolidation for all to survive. Accelerated change of such magnitude has created change that, at times, appears chaotic. However, the result is that all hospitals are transformed and we can observe that some degree of order exists in the middle of perceived general chaos. It is likely that these exact conditions will not occur again for these hospitals. Yet, hospital administrators and other personnel have shown resilience and assumed a "learning" philosophy to seek overall organizational adaptation and, when able to do so, have thrived. The more telling reality is that many more community hospitals have closed or faced bankruptcy.

MAJOR CHANGE MANAGEMENT FUNCTIONS

Change agents selectively use change management functions and activities to assist in the creation and management of change to reach specific outcomes. They may or may not be used sequentially; they may be applied simultaneously, based on the nature of the change process. Flexibility and appropriateness of use are essential. The five functions are as follows:

1. Planning (includes assessment)
2. Organizing
3. Implementing
4. Evaluating
5. Seeking feedback

Feedback functions in conjunction with the first four management functions as a way to assess the ongoing status of the change process and movement toward desired change outcomes.

Planning is simply the activity of looking ahead to decide how to achieve some result, goal, or outcome. For any plan to be effective, both those who will implement the plan and those who will be affected by the changes must participate in the change-planning process from the beginning. Planning ideally occurs before implementation. Part of the initial and ongoing planning activity includes assessing the "who, what, when, where, how, and why" of the situation needing change and the factors desired to achieve the change. It is important to carefully assess factors in the change situation that will predictably support or interfere with the progress of a change (Lewin, 1947). This information clarifies the conditions and direction of the advancing plan. Putting general plans for change in writing can establish a visual method to communicate ideas, decisions, and responsibilities to others.

Organizing entails making decisions about reaching outcomes in terms of time, personnel, materials, communication, or other activities and resources. For reasons of efficiency, it is important to weigh the costs and benefits of options to reach several possible change outcomes. Organizing builds clarity into the plan by formalizing the desired sequence and means of accomplishing the change.

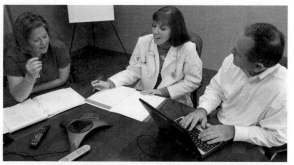

Converting to an electronic health record has to be an inclusive process to be successful.

Implementing ideally occurs after a plan is established. However, unexpected change may sometimes require immediate action. Plans made quickly after the change can facilitate handling the effects of the change. Successful implementation, or putting the plan into action, depends on the appropriateness of the change and the involvement of those who are part of the change. An important aspect of change is that change in one part of a system can affect the function in other, related systems.

Evaluating entails continually judging the degree to which the change process is moving acceptably toward desired outcomes or goals and whether or when outcomes are met. Monitoring, or ongoing data collection, assists the change agent to recognize and correct process problems early. Judging whether an outcome has been fully or partially met occurs in the final stage of the change process.

Effective change agents *seek feedback* by continuously gathering accurate, comprehensive, timely information about the progress of the change process through a variety of sources. Classic references (Ashby, 1957; Cadwallader, 1959) describe that cybernetic theory purports that access to what the theory calls negative feedback establishes communication networks that act as monitors of specific types of information. Analysis of this negative feedback, or information indicating a correction must occur within the system, informs the change agent where problems exist: whether the course of the accelerated change process has veered away from its progress toward desired outcomes or some action is needed to facilitate continued progress toward a particular goal. Although some typical organizational feedback

---

EXERCISE 17-2

From the perspective of a manager applying these functions to a change process, consider the manager's and clinical educator's responsibility to orient two nurses to staff a new infusion center for a small community hospital, and identify the appropriate functions.

Both nurses were long-term employees; one was from the medical/surgical float pool, and the other was the bed coordinator whose position was eliminated because of budget reductions. Ideally, the manager, the clinical educator, and the assistant vice president with oversight for this area will map out in writing (1) the goals of the program, (2) the activities for meeting orientation goals, and (3) a schedule for accomplishing them. The nurse manager and the clinical educator agree to "check in" with each other daily, as well as to meet weekly for a more formal review of the team's progress. Part of this plan includes the option to alter the plan based on unexpected changes. The two nurses will begin the position in 4 weeks and put the prearranged outline of activities into action. The nurse manager's responsibility will be to guide and support the education of the nurses. Unexpected occurrences, such as the nurse manager extending her medical leave of absence by a few days, will create the need to modify the goal, activities, or time frame of the orientation plan (dynamic quality of process). New information (feedback) guides the overall process.

mechanisms include computerized data findings, town hall–style meeting discussions, and informal or formal observations such as in "round-the-clock" CNO meetings or scheduled staff meetings, negative feedback sources are found specifically in the reports of exceptions, such as risk management incident reports, variances in budget expenditures, or new clinical policies. Multiple sources of feedback produce information to build a picture of success for the change process.

Another way to view the approach to change is described by Hirschhorn (2002). He suggests that there are three aspects to effecting a change and that each aspect is equally important to the success of a change. Described as *campaigns,* these three aspects are political, marketing, and military. Table 17-1 illustrates the key concepts of each of the campaigns and provides an example of each. The key, however, is that these are three interrelated efforts that must be addressed for change to be effective.

Furthermore, it is critical to use emotional intelligence rather than knowledge intelligence. This means that a change agent has to have the knowledge of both the nature of the change and the nature of the people with whom he or she is working to effect the

change. Lakoff (2004) suggests that we think in frames and that if the knowledge we are given does not fit our frame about a topic or event, we dismiss the information. It is a challenge when working with another to help that other person adjust the frames. Consider what it is like when working with a group of people with multiple frames and helping them exchange a well-entrenched frame for something new. The critical issues are to help people change their behavior and to realize that communication more likely involves people's emotions and feelings rather than their intellect. Therefore, to bring about change, a leader of change must be equally skilled at knowing the various elements of the change and how to affect them and at knowing how to "read" people and their relationships with the change at hand.

RESPONSES TO CHANGE

Change, whether proactively initiated at the point of change or imposed from external sources, affects people, technology, and systems. Change can be mandated by higher administration, or it can originate within any department or unit or at the level of care delivery. Often, those in high-level administration

TABLE 17-1	EXAMPLES OF THE THREE CAMPAIGNS FOR CHANGE	
TYPE OF CHANGE	**DESCRIPTION**	**EXAMPLE**
Political	Coalition-building to create more influence Changes in structures	Working with pharmacy to effect a change in the delivery of medications to patients Creating new communication approaches to enhance patient-safety outcomes
Marketing	Listening to what is important to team members Working with key groups such as physicians who typically admit patients to a given unit Creating a theme	Explaining to patients' families why certain approaches are taken Determining what motivates others to change Creating huddles to map out the plan for the day Using messages to convey a full set of values around a change (e.g., nothing about me without me ... a theme for patient safety)
Military	Engaging with resistance by providing attention, testing beachheads, and creating a war room	Paying attention (asking questions about, seeking reports about) to the change outcomes Determining the tough choices that need to be made and going after them strategically Creating a space for resources and meetings about the change that symbolizes to others that the change is moving ahead

Adapted from Hirschhorn, L. (2002). Campaigning for change. *Harvard Business Review, 80*(7), 98-104.

create a change for managerial staff to integrate new habits into their work areas. Therefore it follows that the responses that arise across the organization will depend on how change is perceived. Effective change agents anticipate possible responses and apply strategies to deal with them for the best possible change outcomes.

Organizational culture and staff readiness influence responses to change. Knowing values and beliefs of work groups (staff and their managers and administrators—all part of organizational culture) is critical to identifying responses to change. Readiness can be viewed as individuals' current attitudes or willingness, as well as their nursing abilities. Assessment of organizational culture and the readiness of staff and others to engage in making or participating in a change, whether minor or extensive, sets the stage for the selection and use of strategies. For example, in Exercise 17-2, the willingness of the two nurses to learn new skills and the combined talents of the nursing, clinical education, and administrative managerial staff to work together successfully helped achieve the very different nursing and organizational skills required by the new infusion center. Answering the self-assessment questions in Table 17-2 can help determine how receptive one is to change and innovation.

EXERCISE 17-3
Answer the self-assessment questions in Table 17-2.

Human Side of Change

The *human side* of managing change refers to staff responses to change that either facilitate or interfere with change processes. Responses to all or part of the change process by individuals and groups may vary from full acceptance and willing participation to outright rejection or even rebellion. Some nurses may manifest their dissatisfactions visibly; others may quietly undermine the change. There are individuals, in all of our professional careers, who may consistently reject any new thinking or ways of doing things, just to disagree.

The initial responses to change may be, but are not always, reluctance and resistance. Reluctance and resistance are common when the change threatens personal security. For example, changes in the structure of an organization can result in changes of

---

TABLE 17-2   SELF-ASSESSMENT: HOW RECEPTIVE ARE YOU TO CHANGE AND INNOVATION?

Read the following items. Circle the answer that most closely matches your attitude toward creating and accepting new or different ways.

	Yes	Depends	No
1. I enjoy learning about new ideas and approaches.	Yes	Depends	No
2. Once I learn about a new idea or approach, I begin to try it right away.	Yes	Depends	No
3. I like to discuss different ways of accomplishing a goal or end result.	Yes	Depends	No
4. I continually seek better ways to improve what I do.	Yes	Depends	No
5. I commonly recognize improved ways of doing things.	Yes	Depends	No
6. I talk over my ideas for change with my peers.	Yes	Depends	No
7. I communicate my ideas for change with my manager.	Yes	Depends	No
8. I discuss my ideas for change with my family.	Yes	Depends	No
9. I volunteer to be at meetings when changes are being discussed.	Yes	Depends	No
10. I encourage others to try new ideas and approaches.	Yes	Depends	No

If you answered "yes" to 8 to 10 of the items, you are probably receptive to creating and experiencing new and different ways of doing things. If you answered "depends" to 5 to 10 of the items, you are probably receptive to change conditionally based on the fit of the change with your preferred ways of doing things. If you answered "no" to 4 to 10 of the items, you are probably not receptive, at least initially, to new ways of doing things. If you answered "yes," "no," and "depends" an approximately equal number of times, you are probably mixed in your receptivity to change based on individual situations.

position for personnel. Eliminating a critical care nurse position and referring that nurse to the only open position, perhaps that of home health nurse, can certainly result in the nurse feeling angry, displaced, and even temporarily incompetent and isolated.

The change agent's recognition of the ideal and common patterns of individuals' behavioral responses to change can facilitate an effective change (Rogers, 1995). These responses and brief descriptions are as follows:

- *Innovators* thrive on change, which may be disruptive to the unit stability.
- *Early adopters* are respected by their peers and thus are sought out for advice and information about innovations/changes.
- *Early majority* prefer doing what has been done in the past but eventually will accept new ideas.
- *Late majority* are openly negative and agree to the change only after most others have accepted the change.
- *Laggards* prefer keeping traditions and openly express their resistance to new ideas.
- *Rejectors* oppose change actively, even use sabotage, which can interfere with the overall success of a change process.

The change agent's challenge is to deal with these behavioral patterns of individuals by providing opportunities to channel their responses into those supportive of the change process. Helping innovators "test" new ideas might be accomplished in a contained manner so that they are not disruptive yet they feel supported. In this very important sense, the work of the Institute for Healthcare Improvement (IHI) has benefited organizations that use this approach. The focus of IHI is to accelerate rapid small tests of change, often at the point of care *(www.ihi.org/ihi)*. Unit-based decision making to change processes and policies revolves around the staff members working on the unit and depends highly on their ongoing adaptation to evolving realities. For example, a staff nurse champion of change may report to her unit colleagues that she is frustrated with many interruptions while preparing and administering medications, leading to an increased likelihood for error. Discussing the problem may lead to the trial of a solution to the interruptions, such as wearing a prominently colored vest that says, "Do not disturb: Medication administration in process." We do know that the more rapidly change can be incorporated, the more effective the organization is at remaining relevant. Connecting early adopters, such as the unit-based champions, to new ideas and to innovators, such as national peers of an IHI web-based learning community, keeps them at the cutting edge. When these two groups are supported, an early majority can occur. The challenge of working with the laggards is to make them feel comfortable enough to transition to new practices. Thus the equal challenge is to help them feel sufficiently uncomfortable that remaining where they are is no longer the place of comfort. Finally, the goal of working with the rejectors, in effect the low performers, is to minimize their effects and to encourage them to find work that is more satisfying. The change agent's challenges are to be sensitive to employees' stages of loss and to promote transition by responding with appropriate interventions.

Systems and Technological Side of Change

The *systems and technological side of managing change* refers to responses that influence the efficiency and effectiveness of work processes and outcomes. The change agent's challenge is to monitor, recognize, and apply appropriate strategies to minimize responses that are destructive and maximize those that support the dynamics of an ongoing change.

Organizational systems and technology can both influence and be influenced by change. System responses to change may emerge as signs of more or less efficiency or effectiveness. Changes in the type of staff or technology used to deliver care may lead to initial responses of confusion, followed by a period of adaptation by the staff and other systems. The quality of care and the morale of staff may change. Productivity and safety outcomes may be different. Reparation of the breakdowns in the affected work processes can restore efficient and effective functioning. Managing uncertainty is critical.

STRATEGIES

The change agent uses various strategies to facilitate both planned and nonlinear change processes (Figure 17-3). Strategies are approaches designed to achieve a particular purpose based on anticipation and consideration of myriad human, technologic, and system

Situation	Education	Support	Facilitation	Communication	Participation	Negotiation	Manipulation	Cooptation	Coercion	Learning	Visioning	Relationships	Information
Staff is not sure of the next best step in the change process	√	√	√	√						√	√	√	√
Two staff members reluctantly try change	√	√	√	√	√	√				√		√	√
Staff has heard rumors about new program	√			√						√	√		√
Several staff members propose a different method		√	√		√					√	√	√	√
One nurse consistently lags behind in accepting a change	√		√		√					√	√	√	√
A group of staff expresses loss of previous roles		√	√	√						√		√	√
Three staff members challenge the need for a change	√		√	√	√	√				√	√		√
Staff member avoids change in task force membership				√		√		√		√		√	√
Four staff members have become change agents with manager	√	√	√	√	√					√	√	√	√
A group of staff verbalizes satisfaction with status quo	√			√	√	√	√	√		√	√	√	√
One nurse disrupts the change process with other ideas	√			√	√	√	√	√		√	√	√	√
Two nurses try to get others to oppose change	√			√		√	√	√	√				

FIGURE 17-3 Matching strategies to situations.

responses. The intent of the change agent and those supporting the change includes the following (Devereaux et al., 2006):

- Consider the demographic variables, such as age and years of experience
- Establish and promote constant feedback communication loops
- Support training that is convenient and just in time
- Involve the early adopters from the beginning
- Include change implementation in annual performance appraisals
- Create project priorities so staff is not unduly pressured or overwhelmed
- Promote prioritization and accountability throughout the entire process

Strategies such as those identified by Lehman (2008) include the following:

- Identifying what process will be replaced, affected, or created
- Creating a description of the current state of the process being changed or affected
- Determining how this change is aligned with the organization's key mission statements
- Evaluating the deriving and restraining forces
- Identifying stakeholders potentially affected by this change

As supported by chaos and learning organization theories, the change agent also uses vision development, relationship building, information management strategies, and people skills to achieve change.

Communication and *education* refer to interchanges among the change agent, the change participants, and others for the purpose of integrating the elements of the change process. Staff meetings, focus groups, town hall meetings, and other informal discussion groups inform staff and clarify change activities. One effective strategy is the Leadership Rounding Tool developed by the Studer Group. The following are examples of actions the leaders are encouraged to practice weekly (Studer, 2009):

- Establish and maintain a human rapport with their staff (*How are your children? What was your vacation like last week?*).
- Ask what is working well for the staff as they perform their daily functions (*Can you tell me something that is working well for you today?*).
- Ask what is not working well (*Can you tell me something that is a barrier for you today?*).
- Ask if there is someone whom they would like to especially recognize as a contributor to outstanding patient care.
- Answer any tough questions (*Is there anything you've been thinking about asking me that you'd like to know?*).

Active and empathetic listening is always essential. However, staff members need much more than listeners—they need energetic, accountable "do-ers." Feeding information back to the staff creates trust and a belief that leaders are there to help them meet patients' needs. An effective strategy is "walking a mile in my shoes," when a leader periodically shadows a staff member for a defined period (e.g., 4 to 12 hours) to experience firsthand what it is like to work on any particular unit. Coaching, confirming, and coordinating with a unit's informal leaders, can facilitate

change in a positive environment and lead to better outcomes such as staff satisfaction and decreased turnover (Salmela, Eriksson & Fagerstrom, 2011).

Empowerment of staff through *participation* and *involvement* promotes ownership of both the process and the decisions made during the process. It is important to incorporate staff at all levels at the beginning or as early as possible and then throughout the change process.

Facilitation and *support* strategies typically are used to reassure and assist those in the change situation who do not accept a change because of anxiety and fear. When personal security is threatened or when loss and grief are experienced, people tend to want to continue doing what they have always done. A staff member with financial problems may believe that a new benefit plan or implementation of a no-mandatory-overtime policy will result in less take-home pay. The change agent can reassure that person by providing the actual calculation to show that the fear is unfounded if, in fact, that is true. On the other hand, it would be important to deal directly and answer the tough questions and admit when fears have a foundation in reality.

Individuals or groups in a change situation may have the power or resources to adversely affect the success of a particular change. *Negotiation* and *agreement* strategies can revise the terms of the change to accommodate the involved parties and embrace diversity.

Cooptation usually entails manipulated involvement through an appointed or assigned role. An example of this strategy is appointing a highly resistant individual to a change task force that necessitates that the individual be more involved in the change process. *Manipulation* appeals to the motivational needs of others and influences them to participate in change when they might not do so on their own initiative. Expecting staff to be cooperative by participating in a pilot project of the proposed change on a 3-month basis can identify barriers and reduce them whenever possible.

Coercion involves the use of power to force others to make a change, particularly when time is critical to implementation. An example of coercion would be offering to retain a staff member's position during staff reductions if that individual accepts certain conditions.

The ongoing creation of goals and visions (*visioning*) by all the change participants or change teams shows overt responsiveness to the dynamic nature of change (Senge, 1990). This required dialog continually redefines the future, whether for the organization or for a project. To facilitate change nurse leaders must lead relationships, lead the culture, and lead processes with the patient at the center (Salmela, Eriksson & Fagerstrom, 2011). Change agents build work environments that support the time needed to create a shared vision and accept varied beliefs of staff (Senge, 1990).

Information management by the change agent focuses on delivery of the right information to the right place at the right time. Information may produce decisions that are relevant and flexible!

Managing *relationships* involves how individual capabilities and potential can facilitate creative solutions to projected organizational outcomes and is essential to change management. Formal position titles become irrelevant. Matching a staff member who has the needed abilities and attitudes with the demands of an appropriate project, for example, can lead to more creative outcomes. Peers can become coaches and teachers to help develop others' competencies.

The strategies discussed are useful when used appropriately. It is important to recognize cognitive responses or concerns, for example, that can be met with education, information, or other forms of communication. Participation, facilitation, and support can be choices to address the emotional components of accepting change, such as fear, anxiety, or grief. When the issue is sustained lack of motivation or unwillingness to cooperate, the more effective strategies may be manipulation, cooptation, or coercion. Effective change agents develop work environments that support continuous individual and group learning. Because of the dynamic nature of accelerated change environments, effective change agents stay focused on the dynamics of change by consistently managing information, relationships, and vision.

Diffusion theory (Rogers, 2003) describes how the innovation is communicated and spreads over time throughout the members of a specific culture or group. It is different or special from other types of communication, because it is restricted to information about a new idea. It may be planned, as with the introduction of the newest generation mp3 player, or unplanned, as in the immediate response of the government to shut down the airline industry immediately after the events of September 11, 2001. In both cases, there is a newness of the idea and a degree of uncertainty (Should we believe/buy it? What is it all about? Is there danger involved?). Diffusion also introduces a new social order because consequences can occur that influence the choice. For example, the peak in the epidemiologic occurrence of the H1N1 virus, which causes swine flu, led to the policy decision to enforce mandatory vaccination for key healthcare workers in New York State and in several hospitals. For many, there was great uncertainty about whether to be vaccinated, based on the side effects of the 1976 swine flu vaccination and the reported resistance of many healthcare workers to participate in vaccine programs (Tanner & Bauman, 2009).

Typically, combinations of strategies are applied simultaneously rather than one at a time. Figure 17-3 captures the deliberate selection of appropriate strategies to fit the ongoing needs and responses associated with leading change.

ROLES AND FUNCTIONS OF CHANGE AGENTS AND FOLLOWERS

Initiating change and managing its dynamics using linear and nonlinear approaches are key roles of change agents, with shared responsibilities by followers. Appropriate application of related functions, principles, and strategies can assist in meeting the challenges of any kind of change on the change continuum from low-complexity change to high-complexity change. The ultimate goal is a unified movement toward the adoption of something new or different. For example, nursing homes have experienced cultural changes that have positive outcomes (see the Research Perspective on p. 339). Anthony et al. (2005) indicate that retention is a key element of the professional role of nurse managers.

Effective followership requires that followers communicate constructively with the formal or informal change agent to offer information, suggestions, or concerns. Followers also benefit by actively seeking participation in change, staying flexible, tolerating ambiguity, and thoughtfully supporting change efforts. Lencioni (2002) suggests that the key

RESEARCH PERSPECTIVE

Resource: Mueller, C. (October 27-28, 2008). *Research in culture change in nursing homes.* Hartford Institute for Geriatric Nursing. New York University College of Nursing. Retrieved October 9, 2009, from http://hartfordign.org/uploads/File/issue_culture_change/Culture_Change_Background_Mueller.pdf.

Nursing home culture change is defined as the promotion of a resident-directed environment in which there is empowerment and control over one's living arrangements and day-to-day decision making. In this article, staff, resident, and organizational outcomes were reviewed over the past 20 years to understand the following:

1. How far has nursing home culture change penetrated current U.S. nursing homes?
2. Are there valid and reliable measures of nursing home culture change?
3. What evidence is there that nursing home culture change improves resident, staff, and organizational outcomes?
4. What is the extent of research on nursing homes and nursing home culture change?

Implications for Practice

The conclusion is that the change from the traditional, regulatory-oriented model of a nursing home to a more homelike residence where people may thrive in a manner consistent with their life path is slow. The author summarized the existing literature on nursing home culture change in this country and found that quality of life is improved, staff demonstrates increased work-related satisfaction, and organizations do not suffer more financially as a result of the culture change.

---

dysfunction of a team is lack of trust. Building trust, therefore, is critical for both leaders and followers.

Change agents use their personal, professional, and managerial knowledge and skills to lead or influence change and to build trust in the team. Staff members who are not officially in charge—possessing only informal power—can also fulfill important change agent functions. Through their early interest and expertise (early majority), informal leaders can model the new way of doing or thinking for others to emulate. Their positive attitudes toward integrating the change can positively influence staff participation and unity. The informal leader's close interaction with the formal change agent can lead to reinforcement with other staff members about changes in direction.

Brafman and Beckstrom, in *The Starfish and the Spider*, (2006) make the case that organizations that do not have a rigid, authoritarian leader actually have an advantage when they are confronted with the need for change. Their premise is that there are two types of leadership styles: one is exemplified by the starfish and the other by the spider. The spider is a creature with one central head and eight legs and serves as the metaphor for a centralized organization. The starfish, on the other hand, is a creature with redundancy throughout each arm and is a "neural network of cells" (p. 35). Therefore it exemplifies a decentralized system because there is no head and no central command. The authors illustrate these concepts through the examples of the Aztecs and the Apaches. When Spain attempted to raid the Aztec nation, it only took approximately 2 years for a society that had been in existence before the birth of Christ to collapse in ruins. Theirs was a culture that had one single decision maker who ruled by coercive power with many complex rules and regulations. They were the spiders. In contrast, the Apache tribe distributed political power throughout its complex network of individuals and had very little centralized leadership structure. Yet, for two centuries, the Apache nation was able to deter the strength of the Spanish invaders while the Aztecs were not. The reason lies in the characteristics of the starfish, of a decentralized organization in which there is flexibility, shared power, and ambiguity and in which there was truly no vocabulary word for the phrase, "you should." Individuals were free to follow the leader or to choose not to. When struck in battle, the Aztecs had nowhere to go but to collapse and die. When the Apaches were attacked, they simply abandoned their former homes and villages and moved on, taking their culture and their society with them. Seemingly, the starfish model means that power lies not in any central figure but, rather, in each one of the members.

Similarities may be drawn by examining the success of worldwide organizations such as Alcoholics Anonymous (AA), most definitely a starfish organization, in which there is no centralized leadership yet it is nearly always mutating and changing to address people's needs. For example, the 12-step program has transcended the combat of alcoholism as its focus. As our society has arrived at new definitions of addictions, such as gambling, food, and even shopping, AA members, to address these needs, have created specific 12-step programs. Our federal government, with its spider characteristics (for instance, in the wake of Hurricane Katrina in 2005), simply failed to be flexible enough to wield much effectiveness and failed to prepare adequately for a storm that everyone knew was coming.

In nursing, we have often bemoaned our lack of singularity and vision, perhaps believing that we should mimic the prevailing world view and seek to become a spiderlike organization. The authors of *The Starfish and the Spider* endorse a different approach, suggesting that we need to develop and endorse more starfish as well as spider qualities. Nursing leadership, when it embodies a starfish, might mean that we celebrate more innovation and diversity, decide to "break the rules" whenever possible, and embrace the contributions of everyone. Developing a shared understanding of the changes of which individuals are a part, understanding the business logic of the change, having the freedom to be part of adapting the change to the local level, and learning from failure and from the experiences of others are also critical to the achievement of change outcomes (Mohrman, 2008). Staff who share the creation of change that affects them directly and who trust the change agent usually are more receptive to change and integrate change more willingly. Giving and receiving information that includes clear explanations also encourages receptivity. Assertive communication projects self-confidence and a belief that the change will have some perceived benefit to both the individual and to the group at large. Persistence and persuasion can communicate the change agent's commitment to the change outcome.

Rewarding those at the local level who live through change and, in turn, rewarding the leaders who reward them makes good business sense. According to a study (Gunn, 2008) published in the *Harvard Business Review*, executives who embraced change and developed change leaders met or exceeded leadership's expectation and 62% of the executives were promoted. The fate of executives who did not embrace change had far-reaching implications. In such companies, a quarter of them left the organization entirely. This means that the executives most comfortable with taking risks and leading during times of uncertainty switched teams to go where behaviors are rewarded, because they accelerate leadership development and support change.

Having credibility, often as a result of their expertise and legitimate power, allows leaders to sometimes make independent decisions without negative responses. Leaders can role-model the change by actively participating in the change situation, which can translate into expectations for others to follow. For example, a manager who uses the new computerized medication dispenser may be more likely to earn the respect of the change participants.

EXERCISE 17-4

Recall a work or personal situation in which a particular individual tried to get you or a group to do something. What rationale supported the decision to cooperate or not? Was the idea worthwhile from your perception? Was the person making the suggestions known, understood, and trusted? Was the person making the suggestions aware of the real situation, an essential part of carrying out the idea, or had he or she not received official sanctioning to influence activities? Can you see that change agents need specific qualities and abilities to be trusted by others?

PRINCIPLES

Principles are assumptions and general rules that guide behavior and processes. Principles are useful for creating and leading change. Classic principles that characterize effective change implementation are provided in Box 17-2 (Harper, 2007).

EXERCISE 17-5

Prepare an actual or hypothetical change that is meaningful to you in your personal, work, or school life. Select a change that provides an opportunity to apply the linear (planned) and nonlinear principles of change. Draft a hypothetical or actual plan for change, drawing on the chapter content and paying particular attention to the array of change principles discussed. Share your plan and the rationale used with peers or a small group of other healthcare providers. Ask for their comments and suggestions. (If you need a hypothetical change to work with, consider this one: You are the assistant manager for a home health agency. The agency administrator just informed you by memorandum that in 1 month, because of new reimbursement rules, the agency will begin caring for patients receiving chemotherapy. How will you prepare for this change?)

Change is inevitable. Some change is formally planned, but much is not. Change involves specific steps to take as well as a positive attitude to embrace the concept of change. The follower is critical in raising issues to be addressed and in asking logical

---

BOX 17-2 **CLASSIC PRINCIPLES CHARACTERIZING EFFECTIVE CHANGE IMPLEMENTATION**

- Change agents within healthcare organizations use personal, professional, and managerial knowledge and skills to lead change.
- The recipients of change believe they own the change.
- Administrators and other key personnel support the proposed change.
- The recipients of change anticipate benefit from the change.
- The recipients of change participate in identifying the problem warranting a change.
- The change holds interest for the change recipients and other participants.

- Agreement exists within the work group about the benefit of the change.
- The change agents and recipients of change perceive a compatibility of values.
- Trust and empathy exist among the participants of the change process.
- Revision of the change goal and process is negotiable.
- The change process is designed to provide regular feedback to its participants.

Adapted from Harper, C.L. (2007). *Exploring social change* (5th ed.). Englewood Cliffs, NJ: Prentice Hall.

---

questions about proposed changes. These issues and questions are based on the distinctive view followers in an organization bring. Leaders are accountable for facilitating change that contributes to the vision and mission of the organization. It is the combined strength of these two groups that can effect powerful change for patients and their care and for the improvement of the workplace.

THE SOLUTION

The practice of hourly rounding was introduced to the staff—to both the nursing assistants and the professional nurses. We all developed an hourly rounding log, and it was decided that the unit secretary would announce at the top of every hour for the staff to begin hourly rounding. The nursing staff took to it immediately; the difficulty was coaching the nursing assistants in how to approach patients and anticipate their needs, using a prewritten script. My goal was to make it fun, so I involved other nurse managers to role-play being the patient so the staff could practice. Much focused staff education in the form of didactic lecture material was provided as well. After several months, the change was visible and had an immediate impact on patients and their families. In fact, the chief executive officer (CEO) of our system, along with the chief nursing officer (CNO), visited and thought at first that no patients were on the unit because of the peace and quiet. There were simply no more call bells ringing and no more intercom interruptions. My goal in managing this change was to maintain visibility, never losing sight of the goal and its associated requirements, and constantly praising the staff who were doing such a good job of rounding on the patients. Most of my change management strategies had to do with sitting down and asking the staff on all shifts about what worked and what didn't, being approachable, and addressing individual issues of concern before they became unit issues. I also draw the line when needed and have welcomed my assistant vice president when she rounds with one of my staff to coach them. If one of the staff is still not performing the essential elements of hourly rounding, after 3 to 6 months of intensive education and focus, then I will resort to the discipline process. Overall, I respect the work that the staff do everyday, and they know that about me. I think my strategy worked because I introduced hourly rounding first as a philosophy that would make the staff happy and more efficient. In fact, I made it a point to not tell them that hourly rounding was for patient satisfaction specifically, though it certainly has increased since we embraced it.

—*Sharon McEvoy*

Would this be a suitable approach for you? Why?

THE EVIDENCE

In the application of evidence to the change process, four steps identified by the Centre for Evidence Based Practice Australasia (CEBPA) are necessary (http://203.2.80.43/cebpa/):

1. Identifying the need for change
2. Developing a plan or proposal to ADDRESS the need
3. Implementing the proposal
4. Evaluating the results

NEED TO KNOW NOW

- Know how to recognize when change is needed and how to retrieve literature related to the change process.
- Understand how to be proactive and prepared for change regardless of how and when it occurs.
- Role-play with a friend or colleague some scenarios related to change so you know how you react.
- Expect people to respond differently to change, which may either keep movement toward the outcome on course or slow it down.

CHAPTER CHECKLIST

Change is an unavoidable constant in the rapidly transforming healthcare delivery system. As a result, uncertainty is an element in most healthcare institutions. Creating and leading change rather than merely reacting can promote overall organizational effectiveness.

The nature of accelerated change demands flexibility and prompt response to sometimes unpredictable environmental pressures as opposed to inflexible thinking and acting. Planned change as a linear approach to managing change can be useful for dealing with low-level, less-complex change. Nonlinear approaches offered by chaos and learning organization theories focus more on managing the dynamic elements of more-complex, high-level change situations.

- Characteristics of change include the following:
  - Is a natural social process
  - Involves individuals, groups, organizations, and society
  - Is constant and accelerates at various rates and intensities
  - Is inevitable and unpredictable
  - Varies from high complexity to low complexity
- Planned change occurs in sequential stages, according to planned change theorists:
  - Lewin:
    - Awareness of need for change
    - Experience of change
    - Integration of change
  - Havelock:
    - Building a relationship
    - Diagnosing the problem
    - Acquiring relevant resources
    - Choosing the solution

- Gaining acceptance
- Stabilizing the innovation and generating self-renewal
- Lippitt, Watson, and Westley:
  - Client system becomes aware of need for change
  - Relationship between client system and change agent
  - Change problem defined
  - Change goals set and options for achievement explored
  - Plan for change implemented
  - Change accepted and stabilized
  - Change entities redefine relationship
- Rogers:
  - Knowledge
  - Persuasion
  - Decision
  - Implementation
  - Confirmation
- Nonlinear change occurs in a different manner according to nonlinear change theorists:
  - Chaos theory:
    - Organizations as open systems
    - Non–human-induced, self-organizing patterns
    - Periods of stability interrupted with intense transformation
    - Small changes resulting in significant consequences
    - Conditions in one situation not recurring in the same pattern
  - Learning organization theory:
    - Emphasis on flexibility, responsiveness, and learning
    - Five disciplines interrelated by dialog

- Systems thinking:
  - Personal mastery
  - Mental models
  - Shared vision
  - Team learning
- Major change management functions:
  - Planning
  - Organizing
  - Implementing
  - Evaluating
  - Providing feedback/cybernetic theory
- The human responses to change manifest in various behavioral patterns that may help or hinder movement toward achievement of the change outcome:
  - Innovators
  - Early adopters
  - Early majority
  - Late majority
  - Laggards
  - Rejectors
- Multiple strategies are used selectively to promote involvement by the participants of change and to facilitate the overall change process:
  - Education and communication
  - Participation and involvement
  - Facilitation and support
  - Negotiation and agreement
  - Manipulation and cooptation
  - Coercion

- Information management
- Relationship facilitation
- Ongoing vision development
- Continuous learning
- Effective change agents, both formal and informal (those not in charge), exhibit the following characteristics in the change situation:
  - Display leadership
  - Possess excellent communication skills
  - Use observation skills
  - Know how groups work
  - Are perceptive about political issues
  - Are trusted by others
  - Establish positive relationships
  - Empower others
  - Are flexible
  - Manage conflict
  - Participate actively in change
  - Are respected, credible members of organization or community
  - Possess expert and legitimate power
  - Understand change process
  - Display appropriate timing
- Principles guide change:
  - Ownership of change
  - Anticipated benefits as change consequence
  - Negotiability between change agent and participants
  - Benefits of feedback to change process

TIPS FOR LEADING CHANGE

- Whether involved in planned (low-complexity) or nonlinear (high-complexity) change, create a group of outcome/goal scenarios with prospective actions to achieve.
- People cope and adapt better when they assume the role of continuous learner during accelerated change.
- People involved in change may assume the roles of followers or leaders and may emerge from both informal and formal or internal and external sources.
- Creating a detailed plan and rigidly adhering to it reduce opportunities to moderate the inevitable and changing aspects of a change process, especially in an accelerated change environment.
- Building ambiguity and flexibility into a plan and how it is managed promotes responsiveness and movement toward desired outcomes.

REFERENCES

Anthony, M. K., Standing, T. S., Glick, J., Duffy, M., Paschall, F., Sauer, M. R., Sweeney, D. K., Modic, M. B., & Dumpe, M. L. (2005). Leadership and nurse retention: The pivotal role of nurse managers. *Journal of Nursing Administration, 35*, 146-155.

American Organization of Nurse Executives (AONE). (2005). *AONE nurse competencies assessment tool.* Retrieved October 2009, from www.aone.org/aone/certification/ nurseexecassessment.html.

Ashby, W. R. (1957). *An introduction to cybernetics.* New York: John Wiley & Sons.

Begun, J. W., & White, K. R. (1995). Altering nursing's dominant logic: Guidelines from complex adaptive systems theory. *Complexity and Chaos in Nursing, 2*(1), 5-15.

Brafman, O., & Beckstrom, R. A. (2006). *The starfish and the spider.* New York: Penguin.

Cadwallader, M. L. (1959). The cybernetic analysis of change in complex social organizations. *The American Journal of Sociology, 65*, 154-157.

Dattee, B., & Barlow, J. (2010). Complexity and whole-system change programmes. *Journal of Health Services Research & Policy, 15*(Suppl. 2), 19-25.

Devereaux, M. W., Drynan, A. K., Lowry, S., MacLennan, D., Figdor, M., Fancott, C., & Sinclair, L. (2006). Evaluating organizational readiness for change: A preliminary mixed-model assessment of an interprofessional rehabilitation hospital. *Healthcare Quarterly, 9*(4), 66-74.

Gunn, R. W. (2008). The rewards of rewarding change. Harvard Business Review. Accessed May 11, 2010, from http:// hbr.org/product/the-rewards-of-rewarding-change/an/ F0804C-PDF-ENG?referral=00304.

Harper, C. L. (2007). *Exploring social change* (5th ed.). Englewood Cliffs, NJ: Prentice Hall.

Havelock, R. G. (1973). *The change agent's guide to innovation in education.* Englewood Cliffs, NJ: Educational Technology Publications.

Hirschhorn, L. (2002). Campaigning for change. *Harvard Business Review, 80*(7), 98-104.

Lakoff, G. (2004). *Don't think of an elephant! Know your values and frame the debate.* White River Junction, VT: Chelsea Green Publishing.

Lehman, K. L. (2008). Change management: Magic or mayhem? *Journal for Nurses in Staff Development, 24*(4), 176-184.

Lencioni, P. (2002). *The five dysfunctions of a team: A leadership fable.* San Francisco: Jossey-Bass.

Lewin, K. (1947). Frontiers in group dynamics: Concept, method, and reality in social science, social equilibria and social change. *Human Relations, 1*(1), 5-41.

Lippitt, R., Watson, J., & Westley, B. (1958). *The dynamics of planned change.* New York: Harcourt Brace.

Meyer, R. M., & O'Brien-Pallas, L. L. (2010). Nursing services delivery theory: An open system approach. *Journal of Advanced Nursing, 66*(12), 2828-2838.

Mohrman, S. A. (2008). Leading change: Do it with conversation. *Leadership Excellence, 25*(10), 5.

Mueller, C. (October 27-28, 2008). *Research in culture change in nursing homes.* Hartford Institute for Geriatric Nursing. New York University College of Nursing. Retrieved October 9, 2009, from http://hartfordign.org/uploads/File/issue_culture_ change/Culture_Change_Background_Mueller.pdf.

Rogers, E. M. (1995). *Diffusion of innovations* (4th ed.). New York: The Free Press.

Rogers, E. M. (2003). *Diffusion of innovations* (5th ed.). New York: The Free Press.

Salmela, S., Eriksson, K., & Fagerstrom, L. (2011). Leading change: A three-dimensional model of nurse leaders' main tasks and roles during a change process. *Journal of Advanced Nursing, 68*(2), 423-433.

Senge, P. M. (1990). *The fifth discipline.* New York: Doubleday.

Shanley, C. (2007). Management of change for nurses: Lessons from the discipline of organizational studies. *Journal of Nursing Management, 15*(5), 538-546.

Studer, Q. (2009). *Hardwiring excellence.* Gulf Breeze, FL: Fire Starter Publishing.

Tanner, L., & Bauman V. (2009). Health workers under pressure to get flu shots. *Sun Sentinel.* Retrieved May 11, 2010, from http://www.gosanangelo.com/news/2009/sep/08/ health-workers-under-pressure-to-get-flu-shots/.

Vicenzi, A. E., White, K. R., & Begun, J. W. (1997). Chaos in nursing: Make it work for you. *American Journal of Nursing, 97*(10), 26-31.

SUGGESTED READINGS

Chambers, C. & Ryder, E. (2011). Excellence in compassionate nursing care: Leading the change. *Journal of Holistic Healthcare, 8*(3), 46-49.

Mitchell, G. (2013). Selecting the best theory to implement planned change. *Nursing Management – UK, 20*(1), 32-37.

Needleman, J. (2010). Transforming care at the bedside. *PaceSetters, 7*(3), 10-13.

Nickitas, D. M. (2010). A vision for future health care: Where nurses lead the change. *Nursing Economics, 28*(6), 361-385.

Rantz, M., Zwygart-Stauffacher, M., Flesner, M., Hicks, L., Mehr, D., Russell, T., & Minner, D. (2012). Challenges of using

quality improvement methods in nursing homes that need improvement. *Journal of the American Medical Directors Association, 13*(8), 732-738.

Roussel, L., Dearmon, V., Buckner, E., Pomrenke, B., Salas, S., Mosley, A., & Brown, S. (2012). Change can be good. *Nursing Administration Quarterly, 36*(3), 203-209.

Williams, L. (2011). Organizational readiness for innovation in health care: Some lessons from the recent literature. *Health Services Management Research, 24*(4), 213-218.

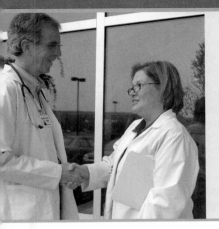

Building Teams Through Communication and Partnerships

Karren Kowalski

This chapter explains major concepts and presents tools with which to create and maintain a smoothly functioning team. Life requires that we work together in a smooth and efficient manner, communicate effectively, and develop relationships that produce partnerships. Many important team efforts occur in the work setting. Research has demonstrated that teams are critical to patient safety because they encourage frequent and ongoing communication and create a safety net for staff, a system in which safeguards and support are a part of the routine functioning of each team member. Such teams often include members with various backgrounds and educational preparation (e.g., physicians, nurses, administrators, allied health professionals, and support staff such as housekeeping and dietary staff members). Each team member has something valuable to contribute and deserves to be treated honorably and with respect. When teams are not working effectively, all team members must change how they communicate and interact within the team.

OBJECTIVES

- Evaluate the differences between a group and a team.
- Value four key concepts of teams.
- Demonstrate an effective communication interaction.
- Identify at least five communication pitfalls.
- Apply the guidelines for acknowledgment to a situation in your clinical setting.
- Compare a setting that uses the "rules of the game" with your current clinical setting.
- Develop an example of a team that functions synergistically, including the results such a team would produce.
- Discuss the importance of team to patient safety and quality.

TERMS TO KNOW

acknowledgment	dualism	synergy
active listening	effective communication	team
commitment	group	

Diane Gallagher, RN, MS
Director, Women's and Children's Services, Rush-
Presbyterian–St. Luke's Medical Center, Chicago, Illinois

An extensive "team" of people works together to care for the neonate in a neonatal intensive care unit (NICU). They include physicians, registered nurses, respiratory therapists, physical therapists, social workers, neonatal nurse practitioners, and ancillary staff. Occasionally, specialists are consulted for specific cardiac, neurologic, or gastrointestinal problems. These are intermittent "team" members who play a crucial role in the baby's care.

Recently, a new group of specialists joined our team. They were identified as a top-notch group who would, by virtue of their expertise and reputation, increase the census and revenues for the hospital. Our team was excited to have this opportunity to grow in an area in which we had infrequent experience. However, integration of these new team members did not go smoothly. There were clinical disagreements, communication breakdowns, and interpersonal conflicts. The experience evolved into mutual distrust and control issues.

As disagreements, insults, and complaints escalated on both sides, the situation came to a defining moment when the director of the specialty group said, "I'm never bringing any of our patients here. I'm sending them to the PICU." The response from the NICU team was, "Fine with us; we don't need you, your patients, or the hassle." It seemed reasonable not to work together because, in fact, functionally we were already not working together. This response was in direct conflict with our belief that we could provide a valuable service and make a difference for both the patients and their families. This posed a dilemma for the staff, but everyone felt the situation was hopeless.

No one believed we could function as a team, and therefore further efforts to work together were futile. We had tried and failed. Let's just cut our losses and move on. How does one create a team when no one believes it is possible and some believe it is not even necessary?

What do you think you would do if you were this nurse?

INTRODUCTION

As we experience changes such as cost-cutting and quality and safety issues in health care, teamwork becomes critical. The adage "If we do not all hang together, we will all hang separately" was never more true than now as we move through an era in which nursing is accountable for patient outcomes that affect reimbursement for care and the institutional financial bottom line. To create finely tuned teams, communication skills must improve. Each team member must focus on improving his or her own skills, as well as supporting other team members, to grow in effective communication. These skills will be increasingly important as teams negotiate an evolving healthcare system that includes accountable care organizations—an outcome of the 2010 Health Care Reform legislation.

In our society, in which so much emphasis is placed on the individual and individual achievement, teamwork is the quintessential contradiction. In other words, with all the focus on individuals, we still need individuals to work together in groups to accomplish goals and keep patients safe. Everybody knows and understands this, particularly individuals who spend their Sundays watching football or basketball. These

team sports are premier models of cooperation and competition. They are the model for teamwork for business today, and they represent a group following their respective leader or "coach" (Parcells, 2000).

GROUPS AND TEAMS

The definition of group is a number of individuals assembled together or having some unifying relationship. Groups could be all the parents in an elementary school, all the members of a specific church, or all the students in a school of nursing, because the members of these various groups are related in some way to one another by definition of their involvement in a certain endeavor. A team, on the other hand, is a number of persons associated together in specific work or activity. Not every group is a team, and not every team is effective.

A group of people does not constitute a team. A team is a group of people with a high degree of interdependence geared toward the achievement of a goal or a task (Dyer, Dyer, & Dyer, 2013). Often, we can recognize intuitively when the so-called team is not functioning effectively. We say things such as, "We need to be more like a team" or "I'd like to see more team players around here." Consequently, in the process of defining *team*, effective versus ineffective teams should be considered. Teams are groups that have defined objectives, ongoing positive relationships, and a supportive environment and that are focused on accomplishing a specific task. Teams are essential in providing cost-effective, high-quality health care. As resources are expended more prudently, patient care teams must develop clearly defined goals, use creative problem solving, and demonstrate mutual respect and support. Facilities with ineffective teams will find themselves out of business.

EXERCISE 18-1

Think of the last team or group of which you were a part. Think about what went on in that team or group. Specifically think about what worked for you and what did not work. Use the "Team Assessment Exercise" in Table 18-1 to assess aspects of your team more specifically. Address each of the identified areas and discover how well your team or group functioned. Think about roles, activities, relationships, and general environment. Consider examples of shared decision making, shared leadership, shared accountability, and shared problem solving. These are the concepts that can be used to evaluate the functioning of almost any team of which you are a member.

When a team functions effectively, a significant difference is evident in the entire work atmosphere, the way in which discussions progress, the level of understanding of the team-specific goals and tasks, the willingness of members to listen, the manner in which disagreements are handled, the use of consensus, and the way in which feedback is given and received. The original work done by McGregor (1960) sheds light on some of these significant differences, which are summarized in Table 18-2.

Ineffective teams are often dominated by a few members, leaving others bored, resentful, or uninvolved. Leadership tends to be autocratic and rigid, and the team's communication style may be overly stiff and formal. Members tend to be uncomfortable with conflict or disagreement, avoiding and suppressing it rather than using it as a catalyst for change. When criticism is offered, it may be destructive, personal, and hurtful rather than constructive and problem-centered. Team members may begin to hide their feelings of resentment or disagreement, sensing that they are "dangerous." This creates the potential for

---

TABLE 18-1   TEAM ASSESSMENT EXERCISE

ARE WE A TEAM?

Directions: Select a team with which you work. Place a checkmark beside each item that is true of your team. If the statement is not true, place no mark beside the item.

1. The language we use focuses on "we" rather than "you" or "I."
2. When one of us is busy, others try to help.
3. I know I can ask for help from others.
4. Most of us on the team could say what we are trying to accomplish.
5. What we are trying to accomplish on any given work day relates to the mission and vision of nursing and the organization.
6. We treat each other fairly, not necessarily the same.
7. We capitalize on people's strengths to meet the goals of our work.
8. The process for changing policies, procedures, equipment is clear.
9. Meetings are focused on the goals we are focused on.
10. Our outcomes reflect our attention to goals and efforts.
11. Acknowledgment is individual and goal-oriented.
12. Innovation is supported by the team and management.
13. The group makes commitments to each other to ensure goal attainment.
14. Promises are kept.
15. Kindness in communication is evident, especially when bad news is delivered.
16. Individuals can describe their role in the overall work of the group.
17. Other members of the team are seen as trustworthy and valued.
18. The group is cost-effective and time-effective in attaining goals.
19. No member is excluded from the process of decision making.
20. Individuals can speak highly of their team members.

Tally the number of checkmarks and multiply that number by 5. The resultant number is an assessment of how well your team is functioning. The higher the score, the better the functioning.

©The Wise Group, 2007, Lubbock, Texas.

---

later eruptions and discord. Similarly, the team avoids examining its own inner workings, or members may wait until after meetings to voice their thoughts and feelings about what went wrong and why.

In contrast, the effective team is characterized by its clarity of purpose, informality and congeniality,

TABLE 18-2	ATTRIBUTES OF EFFECTIVE AND INEFFECTIVE TEAMS	
ATTRIBUTE	**EFFECTIVE TEAM**	**INEFFECTIVE TEAM**
Working environment	Informal, comfortable, relaxed	Indifferent, bored, tense, stiff
Discussion	Focused Shared by almost everyone	Frequently unfocused Dominated by a few
Objectives	Well understood and accepted	Unclear, or many personal agendas
Listening	Respectful—encourages participation	Judgmental—much interruption and "grandstanding"
Ability to handle conflict	Comfortable with disagreement Open discussion of conflicts	Uncomfortable with disagreement Disagreement usually suppressed, or one group aggressively dominates
Decision making	Usually reached by consensus Formal voting kept to a minimum General agreement is necessary for action; dissenters are free to voice	Often occurs prematurely Formal voting occurs frequently Simple majority is sufficient for action; minority is expected to go along with opinion
Criticism	Frequent, frank, relatively comfortable, constructive Directed toward removing obstacle	Embarrassing and tension-producing; destructive Directed personally at others
Leadership	Shared; shifts from time to time	Autocratic; remains clearly with committee chairperson
Assignments	Clearly stated Accepted by all despite disagreements	Unclear Resented by dissenting members
Feelings	Freely expressed; open for discussion	Hidden; considered "explosive" and inappropriate for discussion
Self-regulation	Frequent and ongoing; focused on solutions	Infrequent, or occurs outside meetings

Adapted from McGregor, D. (1960). *The human side of enterprise*. New York: McGraw-Hill.

commitment, and high level of participation. The members' ability to listen respectfully to each other and communicate openly helps them handle disagreements in a civilized manner and work through them rather than suppress them. Through ample discussion of issues, they reach decisions by consensus. Roles and work assignments are clear, and members share the leadership role, recognizing that each person brings his or her own unique strengths to the group effort. This diversity of styles helps the team adapt to changes and challenges, as does the team's ability and willingness to assess its own strengths and weaknesses and respond to them appropriately.

The challenges encountered in today's healthcare systems are prodigious. Patient safety issues are at the forefront. Ongoing rounds of downsizing, budget cuts, declining patient days, reduced payments, and staff layoffs abound. Effective teams participate in effective problem solving, increased creativity, and improved health care. The effects of smoothly functioning teams on patient safety and the creation of a just culture are critically important, and one tool set to address these issues, including communication, can be found in the Literature Perspective on p. 349.

GENERATIONAL DIFFERENCES

It is not unusual today to have team members from four different generations of workers: Veterans, Baby Boomers, Generation X, and Generation Y. Because the workforce is aging, there may be a preponderance of Baby Boomers and Generation Xers in a work

📖 **LITERATURE PERSPECTIVE**

Resource: Kouzes, J. M., & Posner, B. Z. (2012). *The leadership challenge* (5th ed.). San Francisco: Jossey-Bass, John Wiley & Sons.

This model focuses on how leaders in all walks of life and all aspects of the workplace mobilize people to get extraordinary things done. Ordinary people such as novice nurses can guide others along pioneering journeys to phenomenal accomplishments. The research and work that Kouzes and Posner have done establish relationships as the core of leading any change or initiative. Five key aspects of establishing and maintaining relationships constitute the heart of this leadership model:

- **Model the Way**—Credibility is the foundation of leadership. It is established by consistently *Doing What You Say You Will Do* or by *Setting the Example* for the other team members.
- **Inspire a Shared Vision**—Imagine exciting and ennobling possibilities, and enlist others in these dreams through positive attitude, excitement, and hard work.
- **Challenge the Process**—Seek innovative ways to change, grow, and improve—experiment and take risks.
- **Enable Others to Act**—Foster collaboration by promoting cooperation and building trust. Create a sense of reciprocity or give and take. Establish a sense of "We're all in this together."
- **Encourage the Heart**—Novice leaders encourage their constituents to carry on. They keep hope and determination alive, recognize contributions, and celebrate victories.

Implications for Practice

When nurses use this model to approach leadership, they can strengthen their skills. Each of the examples above provides a way for new, emerging, and established leaders to remain committed to the team with which they work.

setting. Each generation, traditionally interpreted as a span of 20 years, grew up in a different era and was influenced by different historical events and cultural developments (Riggs, 2013). For example, Veterans live by the rules and do not question authority. Boomers lived through the Cold War and were influenced by the assassinations of President John F. Kennedy, Senator Robert Kennedy, and Martin Luther King, Jr.; the Civil Rights movement; and the Women's Rights movement. Generation X nurses were often the "latch-key kids" because both parents worked outside the home. Divorce was common, and job stability was no longer guaranteed. Generation Y nurses are the future of the profession and have grown up with

massive amounts of information and technology. They have experienced terrorism and natural disasters. They are culturally diverse and view education as the key to success. Efforts to understand and bridge these differences can be the difference between a dysfunctional and an effective team. Chapter 3 provides more detail about these differences.

COMMUNICATING EFFECTIVELY

Communication in the work environment is not only important to good working conditions that retain nurses but also is critical to reduction of medical errors (Brock et al., 2013). Because of such issues, new graduates go through a facility orientation that emphasizes communication skills. Many nurses view this as a waste of time that could be used to further technical skills; however, at evaluation time, communication skills are often seen as a significant area for improvement (Kramer et al., 2013). The only thing human beings do more often than communicate is breathe. Communication is the most important component of daily activities. It is essential to clinical practice, to building teams, and to leadership. A person cannot *not* communicate. Because communication consists of both verbal and nonverbal signals, humans are continuously communicating not just thoughts, ideas, and opinions but also feelings and emotions (Niedenthal & Brauer, 2012). Once the message is sent, it cannot be retracted; it can be amended, but the first impression of the communication usually is lasting. However, as important as this initial impression is, it is often an unconscious response or reaction.

How we communicate is also a reflection of self-worth: Once a human being has arrived on this earth, communication is the largest single factor determining what kinds of relationships she or he makes with others and what happens to each in the world (Satir, 1988). Self-worth is a major influence in all communication. Stress results whenever self-worth is threatened.

Communication is learned from watching others. A host of poor examples can be seen in movies and television. Poor communication leads to relationship breakdowns, misunderstandings, high levels of emotion, judgment, and an excess of drama. Nursing

Communication Rhythm

Sender ——— Receiver

Sender sends a message.   Receiver actively listens and receives.

Communication Non-rhythm

Sender ——— Sender

Both parties send simultaneously. Neither party is receiving.

Sender ——— No Receiver

Sender sends a message.   The receiver is preoccupied with another matter and is not attending.

No Sender ——— Receiver

The receiver awaits a message or response. The sender "clams up," refusing to speak or send a message.

Receiver ——— Receiver

When both parties are striving to receive and neither party sends a message (e.g., teacher questions what students know and gets no response), silence reigns.

FIGURE 18-1 Potential communication rhythms.

programs teach therapeutic communications with patients and their families. However, little focus is placed on effective communication in the workplace, although communication is essential to building and maintaining smoothly functioning teams.

A basic model of communication patterns between the sender and the receiver is found in Figure 18-1. Effective communication develops a rhythm in which messages are sent and received in a productive, respectful, and supportive manner (Nemeth, 2008). Communication begins to break down as the rhythm is disrupted. The sender-receiver pattern disintegrates into a non-rhythmic event, as described in Figure 18-1. When non-rhythmic patterns develop, the participants may feel disrespected, upset, and even fearful.

Stress

In her classic work, Satir (1988) identified the connection between stress and self-worth that can evolve as a result of a breakdown in communication. She defined stress as a threat to positive self-worth. Human beings tend to feel stress or anxiety whenever there is an unconscious linking of feelings, behaviors, or comments from others to a lowering of self-esteem or an attack on self-worth. A conscious effort ought to be made to relieve stress through activities such as ensuring specific/scheduled quiet time, requesting peer support, keeping a journal, treating yourself to something special, or going for a walk (Weiss, 2001).

Stress Response Model

When this threat is identified, the receiver often reacts using one of the five communication patterns: attribution of blame, placation, constrained cool-headedness, immaterial irrelevance, or congruence (Bradley & Edinberg, 1990; Satir, 1988). Each pattern interaction and the source of the interaction are described with examples of each pattern in Table 18-3. The pattern that produces effective communication, the one to strive for, is congruence. Congruent communication occurs when both the verbal and nonverbal actions fit the inner feelings of the sender and are appropriate to the context of the message. This communication pattern creates the kind of connection between the sender and the receiver that fosters respect, support, and the creation of a relationship.

Communication Barriers

In today's busy world, many interruptions and interferences to clear, focused, effective communication create breakdowns. According to Olen (1993), to be aware of these potential problems allows both sender and receiver to be prepared to minimize such barriers.

- *Distractions:* Distractions most commonly come through sensory perceptions, such as poor lighting or background noise, including music, talking, ringing phones, and interruptions by others. Papers, reports, and heavy workloads can also be distracting.
- *Inadequate knowledge:* The sender and receiver may be at different levels of knowledge, particularly in this time of highly specialized and

TABLE 18-3	COMMUNICATION PATTERNS		
PATTERN	**INTERACTION**	**SOURCE**	**EXAMPLE**
Attribution of blame	Sender blames receiver	Fault-finder dictator acts superior as camouflage for fear and low self-esteem	Mostly "you" messages; for example, "You really blew it!"
Placation	Sender placates receiver	Sender's low self-worth: puts herself/himself down	"I was wrong. I'm sorry. It's all my fault."
Constrained cool-headedness	Sender is correct and very reasonable without feeling or emotion	Feelings of vulnerability covered by cool analytical thinking	"Studies have shown that in 75% of cases, the patient is correct. I decided to use research data in coming to a solution."
Irrelevant	Sender is avoiding the issue, ignoring own feelings and feelings of the receiver	Fear, loneliness, and purposelessness	"Wait a minute. Let me tell you about …" (changes the subject)
Congruence	Sender's words and actions are congruent; inner feelings match the message	Any tension is decreased, and self-worth is at a high level	"For now, I feel concerned about the anger and hostility exhibited by Dr. X. I'm wondering what approach would de-escalate him."

Adapted from Satir, V. (1988). *The new peoplemaking.* Mountain View, CA: Science & Behavior Books; and Bradley, J., & Edinberg, M. (1990). *Communication in the nursing context* (3rd ed.). Norwalk, CT: Appleton & Lange.

technical knowledge bases. For multiple reasons, one person may not seek clarity from the other.

- *Poor planning:* The process of organizing, planning, and clearly thinking through what needs to be communicated is very helpful. If the interaction is more spontaneous, it can more easily fall into a non-rhythmic pattern.
- *Differences in perception:* Both the sender and the receiver have their individual mental filters—the way in which they see the world. Because of this individuality, no two filters are the same. Thus the same message is interpreted differently. Add to this, for example, sociocultural, ethnic, and educational differences, and it is easy to see how these differences can occur.
- *Emotions and personality:* Someone who is experiencing distress may not be able to receive another message or may have difficulty keeping his or her emotions out of an unrelated message. Most humans, at some point, bring distress or problems from home to the workplace. If these remain unconscious, they can influence the work setting in a negative or nonproductive way.

Communication Pitfalls

Effective communication suggests that the interaction is a rhythmic pattern that is respectful and clear, promotes trust, and encourages the expression of feelings and viewpoints. On the other hand, pitfalls in communication comprise actions, behaviors, and words that create distrust, are dishonoring, and decrease the feelings of self-worth in the receiver and can lead to poor outcomes for patients. Box 18-1 lists the major pitfalls of communication.

Communication Guidelines

Effective guidelines can be used when communicating. Such tools as SBAR are often used when conveying clinical information from one caregiver to another (Box 18-2). Most of these tools are used to facilitate a positive outcome and to create an environment in which the communicator can achieve the desired outcome. Unconscious use of any of the pitfalls will most likely result in thwarting the desired outcome. Box 18-3 lists effective guidelines for communication.

BOX 18-1 COMMUNICATION PITFALLS

1. Giving Advice

It is so tempting to give advice when a co-worker comes with an issue or problem. *Don't!* Most often what the person wants is to work through the issue by talking out loud. Just listen.

2. Making Others Wrong

When telling others "our" story of distress, the adversary is always "wrong." The telling of the story to a third party only reinforces how right "I" am and how wrong, bad, or terrible the other person is. If you have an issue or problem, take the problem to the person with whom you are upset. "Take the mail to the correct address." Don't gossip!

3. Being Defensive

Defensiveness occurs when you do not listen, are hostile or aggressive, or respond as if attacked when there was no attack. Look for a physiologic signal in your body so that you can identify your own distress. Stop. Breathe. Acknowledge that the message did not come out the way you intended, and begin again.

Also, defensiveness can occur when met with hostile, aggressive behavior from another. Rather than choose an emotional response or react to the attack, know that the other person's behavior has nothing to do with you personally but is the response chosen by that person in a moment of stress. Any one of a dozen other responses could have been chosen. Understand that the person is motivated by fear or hurt.

4. Judging the Other Person

Evaluating another person as "good" or "bad," as someone you like or do not like, or judging their actions or behavior as "stupid" or "crazy" or "inappropriate" is a reflection of how you judge yourself. Who is the hardest person on you? Of course, you are. Know

that you can have feelings about situations or behaviors without judging the other person in a negative way. Rather, you can feel compassion for his or her stress and fear, which often drives behavior. This is true particularly when a supervisor or physician is reprimanding you.

5. Patronizing

Speaking to others as though they are less than human or in need of custodial care fails to honor them as human beings. You do not have to be condescending or seek to humiliate in an overly sweet voice. These are merely other versions of judging or making the person wrong. Another approach is to question what is at issue for them in the moment.

6. Giving False Reassurance

One of the great temptations of nurses is to "fix" things and make them better, to rescue the situation or the person involved. To accomplish this goal, sometimes we reassure inappropriately. Know that you do not have to fix every situation. You can support people to work through situations themselves.

7. Asking "Why" Questions

When working in the team, refrain from asking "why" questions. These tend to create a defensive response in the other person. Instead, ask "What makes you think ..."

8. Blaming Others

Saying things such as "You make me so angry" is blaming the other person for your feelings, which you choose at any given time. In nearly every situation, the responsibility for communication breakdown is a joint responsibility. You can always choose your response, even if that response is to say, "I can't discuss this with you now. I would like to talk about this later when I am calmer."

BOX 18-2 SBAR COMMUNICATION

Miscommunication is the most commonly occurring cause of sentinel events and "near misses" in patient care. One of the most popular structured communication systems, created by professionals in the Colorado Kaiser Permanente System, focuses on a method to provide information that honors the system in which practitioners and medical providers learn to glean information and apply it to decision-making trees. SBAR is the system that honors the structured transfer of information.

Situation. The professional identifies the patient, the physician, the diagnosis, and the location of the patient. The nurse describes the patient situation that has instituted this SBAR communication.

Background. Next the nurse provides background information, which could include information relevant to the current situation, mental status, current vital signs (all of them), chief complaint, pain level, and physical assessment of the patient.

Assessment. The nurse offers an assessment of the chief problem and describes the seriousness of the situation. Any specific changes in the patient's condition should be described.

Recommendation. The nurse can make a request of the physician or suggest specific action such as a medication, laboratory work, or an x-ray examination. The nurse could also request that the physician come and evaluate the patient.

Modified from www.medleague.com/Articles/Newsletters/newsletter31.pdf. (Retrieved July 15, 2009.)

BOX 18-3 GUIDELINES FOR COMMUNICATION

- Approach each interaction as though the other person has no knowledge of effective communication. Assume responsibility for creating the sender-receiver rhythm.
- Share your thoughts and feelings. Be self-revealing.
- Use casual conversation or "small talk"; it can be important to relationships, particularly when it is light and humorous. It balances the deep, meaningful talk.
- Acknowledge, praise, and encourage the other person; doing so is supportive and brings life and energy to the relationship.
- Present messages in a way that the other person can receive them.
- Take responsibility for any problem or issue you have with another, and speak about it as your problem or issue also.
- Use language of equality even when position titles are not of the same level.

Adapted from Olen, D. (1993). *Communicating: Speaking and listening to end misunderstanding and promote friendship.* Germantown, WI: JODA Communications.

EXERCISE 18-2

In pairs or small groups, compare the effective guidelines for communication with the communication pitfalls. Give examples of each from your own recent personal experience. Hypothesize how you could have changed the pitfalls into a positive interaction.

KEY CONCEPTS OF TEAMS

In rare instances, a team may produce teamwork spontaneously, like kids in a schoolyard at recess. However, most management teams learn about teamwork because they need and want to work together. This kind of working together requires that they observe how they are together in a group and that they unlearn ingrained self-limiting assumptions about the glory of individual effort and authority that are contrary to cooperation and teamwork. Keys to the concept of team include the following:

- Conflict resolution
- Singleness of mission
- Willingness to cooperate
- Commitment

Conflict Resolution

When thinking about conflict, it is helpful to realize that conflict is fundamental to the human experience and is an integral part of all human interaction (Porter-O'Grady & Malloch, 2010)). Therefore the challenge is to recognize the breakdown in the communication process and to deal appropriately with it (Porter-O'Grady & Malloch, 2010). Conflict in nursing is most often viewed as a negative experience (Mahon & Nicotera, 2011). In contrast, communication experts view conflict as differences in perceptions about what is needed to accomplish common goals (Mahon & Nicotera, 2011). Hence, when a nurse recognizes upset and reaction between two nursing assistants with whom he or she is working, the following steps can be helpful (Sportsman, 2005):

- Identify the triggering event.
- Discover the historical context for each person.
- Assess how interdependent they are on each other.
- Identify the issues, goals, and resources involved in the situation.
- Uncover any previously considered solutions.

Assessing the level of working relationship between the conflicted parties is essential, particularly if they work together on a regular basis.

The word *team* is usually reserved for a special type of working together. This working together requires communication in which the members understand how to conduct interpersonal relationships with their peers in thoughtful, supportive, and meaningful ways. It requires that team members be able to resolve conflicts among themselves and to do so in ways that enhance rather than inhibit their working together. In addition, team members must be able to trust that they will receive what they need while being able to count on one another to complete tasks related to team functioning and outcomes. To communicate effectively, people must be willing to confront issues and to express openly their ideas and feelings—to use interactive skills to accomplish tasks. In nursing, constructive confrontation has not been a well-used skill. Consequently, if communication patterns are to improve, the onus is on each of us as individuals to change communication patterns. In essence, for things to change, each of us must change.

Singleness of Mission

Every team must have a purpose—that is, a plan, aim, or intention (see the Research Perspective on p. 364). However, the most successful teams have a number of common elements, all of which can be taught (Contratti, Ng, & Deeb, 2012). The more powerful and visionary the mission is, the more energizing it will be to the team. The more energy and excitement are engendered, the more motivated all members will be to do the necessary work (Pentland, 2012).

Willingness to Cooperate

Just because a group of people has a regular reporting relationship within an organizational chart, it does not mean the members are a team. Boxes and arrows are not in any way related to the technical and interpersonal coordination or the emotional investment required of a true team. In effective teams, members are required to work together in a respectful, civil manner. Most of us have been involved in organizations in which people could accomplish assigned tasks but were not successful in their interpersonal relationships. In essence, these employees received a salary for not getting along with a certain person or persons. Some of these employees have not worked cooperatively for years! Organizations can no longer afford to pay people to not work together. Personal friendship or socialization is not required, but cooperation is a necessity. Traditionally, these interpersonal skills were considered "soft" skills and difficult to coach people on or to hold them accountable. That is no longer the case. In most organizations, employees can now be terminated for a lack of willingness to work cooperatively with team members.

Commitment

Commitment is a state of being emotionally impelled and is demonstrated when there is a sense of passion and dedication to a project or event—a mission. Often, this passion looks a little crazy. In other words, people go the extra mile because of their commitment. They do whatever it takes to accomplish the goals or see the project through to completion. An example of commitment is discussed by Charles Garfield when he talks about being a part of the team that created the lunar landing module for the first man to walk on the moon. People did all kinds of things that looked crazy, including working extended hours and

shifts, calling in to see how the project was progressing, and sleeping over at their work station so as not to be separated from the project—all because everybody knew that he or she was a part of something that was much bigger than himself or herself. They were a part of sending a man to the moon, something that human beings had been dreaming about for thousands of years. It was a historical moment, and people were intensely committed to making it happen.

Many people go through their entire lives hating every single day of work. Needless to say, most of them are not committed. Because we spend an extensive amount of time in the work setting, it is critically important to both physical and mental well-being that we enjoy what we do. If this is not the case for you, then try to find a different job or profession—one you might love. Life is too short to do something that you hate doing every day. While you are moving into whatever you decide you love doing, commit to yourself to do your best at whatever you are now doing. Be 100% present wherever you are. Do the best work you are capable of doing. This honors you as a human being, and it honors your co-workers and patients.

EXERCISE 18-3

Box 18-4 contains eight questions. Spend at least 20 minutes in a quiet place thinking about and writing answers to these eight questions. Pay particular notice to question 7.

There are many examples of commitment, such as that of Jan Skaggs, the Vietnam veteran who was the driving force behind the building of the Vietnam War Memorial. He was a clerk in the Washington, DC, bureaucracy who attended a veterans' meeting and decided a memorial to those who lost their lives in Vietnam was needed—a memorial that had all 58,000 names inscribed on it. He had only a high school diploma and did not even own a suit, but 5 years and $7 million later, the wall was dedicated (Lopes, 1987). This demonstrates that one does not have to have a college degree to be committed. Sometimes a college degree can inhibit people from accomplishing their goals because they become diverted from a purpose, from a mission, or from life goals by, for example, good grades. Rather than understanding grades as a

BOX 18-4 **EXPLORING COMMITMENT**

The key to finding your compelling mission/passion that will lead you to success and peak performance is to ask yourself the right questions. Your answers to these questions will help you understand what you need to know about yourself. Read each question, then think carefully for a few minutes, and answer each question honestly. Do not censor or edit out anything, even if it seems impossible or unrealistic—allow yourself to be surprised. Let your imagination soar.

1. Am I deriving any satisfaction out of the work I am now doing?
2. If they did not reward (praise or pay) me to do what I now do, would I still do it?
3. What is it that I really love to do?
4. What do I want to pursue with my time and energy that is worthwhile?
5. What motivates me to reach out and do my best to excel?
6. What is it that only I can say to the world? What needs to be done that can best be done only by me?
7. If I won $10 million in the lottery tomorrow, how would I live? What would I do each day and for the rest of my life?
8. If I were to write my own obituary right now, what would be my most significant accomplishment? Is that enough?

Repeating this exercise often will give you additional insights and information about what you really want and love to do. If taken seriously, the exercise should help you have an understanding of why you selected this profession and whether you have the stamina to do whatever it takes to make a contribution and to make a difference in the practice of nursing.

tool of measurement, they see them as an end in themselves.

Almost anyone can be taught the technical aspects of what needs to be done in most patient care settings. Teaching people to love what they do or to care about patients and their families—even the most difficult and unique patients and families—is far more difficult.

TOOLS AND ISSUES THAT SUPPORT TEAMS

When individuals come together in a group, they spend considerable time in group process or social dynamics, which allows the group to advance toward becoming a team and completing a goal. Each person within the group struggles with three key questions

that must continually be re-evaluated and renegotiated. These three questions, according to Weisburg's classic work (1988), are as follows:

1. Am I in or out?
2. Do I have any power or control?
3. Can I use, develop, and be appreciated for my skills and resources?

"In" Groups and "Out" Groups

Most of us want to be valued and recognized by others as a part of the group, one who "knows" or understands. Most people want to be at the core of decision making, power, and influence. In other words, they want to be part of the "in" group, and researchers have demonstrated that those who feel "in" cooperate more, work harder and more effectively, and bring enthusiasm to the group. The more we feel we are not a part of the key group, the more "out" we feel and the more we withdraw, work alone, daydream, and engage in self-defeating behaviors. Often, intergroup conflict results when individuals who feel they are "out" and want to be "in" create a schism or a division that prohibits the team from accomplishing its goals.

Power and Control

Everybody wants at least some power, and everybody wants to feel he or she is in control. When faced with changes that we cannot influence, we feel impotent and experience a loss of self-esteem. Consequently, all of us want to feel that we are in control of our immediate environment and that we have enough power and influence to get our needs met. When a situation or an event arises that we cannot handle, we attempt to compensate for it in some way; most of these ways are not productive to smoothly functioning teams.

EXERCISE 18-4

Think about a time when you and a small group of classmates or co-workers wanted to change something, such as a scheduled time (a class or meeting), an assignment, or an outcome measure (grading curve of a test or a performance evaluation criterion), and the faculty or administration adamantly refused. How did you feel? What was the response? Did you engage in gossip to make others appear wrong? You may have been "right," but the sense of a loss of control or power is very uncomfortable, sometimes resulting in stress and fear. Mature behavior is required to maintain a positive, problem-solving approach.

Use, Develop, and Be Appreciated for My Skills and Resources

Each member of the team has unique skills and resources to bring to the goals and tasks to be accomplished by the team. The Gallup research is quite clear, in its evaluation of the work environment, that one of the most powerful indicators of a successful, supportive work environment can be predicted by the scores from the question "At work, do you have the opportunity to do what you do best every day?" When the score is low in this area, team members clearly do not feel their skills are recognized, well utilized, or appreciated. Making each team member feel that his or her skills are recognized, encouraged, and used and that his or her growth is encouraged requires a strong, knowledgeable *team leader*. Fewer than 20% of employees feel their strengths are used every day (Wagner & Harter, 2006). When nurses do not feel their skills are used, they are more prone to be in the "out group." This leads to being unengaged and even disengaged in the workplace. This is not supportive of a positive, creative work environment.

POSITIVE COMMUNICATION MODEL

Whenever human beings are in distress, unengaged, or disengaged or have an emotional reaction to a situation or the actions of another, a conditioned response is to move into one or all of the following: *blame, judgment,* or *demand.* These are depicted in the awareness model found in Figure 18-2. With effort and practice, it is possible to create a communication interaction that produces a significantly improved outcome.

When an individual is reacting at the feeling level, he or she tends to move unconsciously to blame. By taking accountability for these feelings, one can move out of blame and own one's feelings by stating, "I feel …"

Likewise, when an individual is trapped in distress or reaction at the thinking level, he or she most often turns to judgment. By thinking compassionately, one can dismantle the judgment and state what one thinks in a compassionate way: "I think …"

Finally, when in distress, we make demands that are often unreasonable. By calming oneself, one can

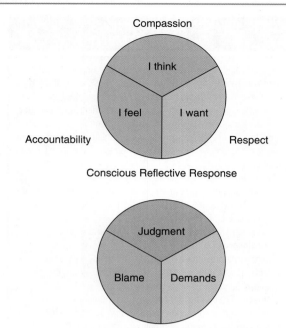

FIGURE 18-2 Awareness model: differentiating between conscious and unconscious responses.

find respect for the other human being and make a request: "I want …"

Most broken relationships are stuck in blame, judgment, and demand. Being accountable, compassionate, and respectful helps clarify what goes on inside each of us.

Everyone needs to feel as though his or her skills, tools, and contributions are needed and valued and that he or she is respected for what personal contributions are offered to the workplace, team, or group. Everyone has weaknesses, and there is no need to emphasize these or to spend time in ongoing correction. Rather, focus should be placed on people's strengths; specifically, acknowledging and emphasizing what people do well.

Part of focusing on people's strengths is being willing to acknowledge peers, faculty, and the other significant people in one's life (Uhm et al., 2012). In contrast, many role models focus on correction. Consequently, many of us spend a large portion of our time correcting others rather than appreciating them for all the wonderful things they are. Focusing on strengths rather than on weaknesses is far more

BOX 18-5 GUIDELINES FOR ACKNOWLEDGMENT

1. Acknowledgments must be specific. The specific behavior or action that is appreciated must be identified in the acknowledgment; for example, "Thank you for taking notes for me when I had to go to the dentist. You identified three key points that appeared on the test."
2. Acknowledgments must be "eye to eye," or personal. Look the person in the eye when you thank him or her. Do not run down the hall and say "Thanks" over your shoulder. Written appreciation also qualifies as "eye to eye."
3. Acknowledgments must be sincere, that is, from the heart. Each of us recognizes insincerity. If you do not truly appreciate a behavior or action, do not say anything. Insincerity often makes people angry or upset, thus defeating the goal.
4. Acknowledgments are more powerful when they are given in public. Most people receive pleasure from public acknowledgment and remember these occasions for a long time. For people who are shy and may prefer no public acknowledgment, this is an opportunity to work on a personal growth issue with them. Public acknowledgment is an opportunity to communicate what is valued.
5. Acknowledgments need to be timely. The less time that elapses between the event and the acknowledgment, the more powerful and effective it is and the more the acknowledgment is appreciated by the recipient.

EXERCISE 18-5

Within the next 3 days, find three opportunities to acknowledge a peer or acquaintance using the five guidelines for acknowledgment shown in Box 18-5. In addition, use the guidelines to accept at least one self-acknowledgment.

Group Agreements

One of the most helpful tools available is to have the team members come to an agreement about the ground rules concerning their relationships with one another. This can take place in various ways. Multiple types of guidelines or rules can even be used to set the context for how people relate. Many hospitals and facilities have service agreements that new employees accept when they are first hired. These are often in the employee handbook and must be used to hold people accountable for behaviors. One example of a set of guidelines can be found in Box 18-6. These are called the "Rules of the Game." They have gone through multiple transitions and redesign, but the basic tenets are essentially the same. People must agree on the goals and mission with which they are involved. They have to reach some understanding of how they will exist together. Tenets or rules such as "We will speak supportively" go a long way to avoid gossiping, backbiting, bickering, and misinterpreting others. As you review these group agreements, keep in mind that a part of this process is the willingness of members of the team to be accountable for upholding the agreements and to give feedback when the agreements have been violated. Without rules, people have implicit permission to behave in any manner they choose toward one another, including angry, hostile, hurtful, and acting-out behavior.

Trust

Trust is the basis by which leaders/managers facilitate the activities and the progress of the team. Kouzes and Posner (2012) conducted research on personal best leadership practices that mobilize others to get extraordinary things done. They focus on how leaders build high-performance teams through five key behaviors: modeling the way, inspiring a shared vision, challenging the process, enabling others to act, and encouraging the heart. Poorly performing teams show little evidence of these relational behaviors and,

productive and leads to excellence. Appreciative inquiry is one method for shifting from focusing on problems to highlighting successes (Trajkovski et al., 2013). If the focus is on improving our strengths, it is much easier to excel and then to be acknowledged for what we do well. Unfortunately, focusing on weaknesses tends to decrease the appreciation and thus the acknowledgments. Furthermore, we seem to believe that a finite number of available acknowledgments exist and we must not give out too many of them because they must be held in reserve for very important events. In addition, we do not always give acknowledgments in a way they can be received and valued. Box 18-5 can serve as a guide for giving acknowledgment.

To deal with the three personal issues discussed in this section, team members must learn how to state openly what is on their minds and be responsive and respectful as other members of the team do the same. In other words, team members must give and receive feedback constructively.

BOX 18-6   "RULES OF THE GAME" FOR WOMEN'S AND CHILDREN'S HOSPITAL, RUSH-PRESBYTERIAN–ST. LUKE'S MEDICAL CENTER

These "Rules of the Game" were adapted from a San Francisco real estate broker who was the founder and president of Hawthorne-Stone. Dr. Karren Kowalski proposes that we use them not only among ourselves but also with each new person who joins the organization, asking if we/they are willing and able to do the best we/they can to support the rules.

1. Be Willing to Support Rush's Purpose, Games, Rules, and Goals
By first asking if people will support the rules, we have their agreement that they can be held accountable for times when they violate the "rules of the game."

2. Speak Supportively
This means no swearing; if it does not serve, do not say it; if it does not support, do not say it; do not make other people wrong; you may choose not to say negative things. Language either empowers or limits people in terms of achieving their potential. How we speak about a colleague, the institution, our job, the workplace, and so forth does make a difference.

3. Correct Supportively
Dr. Kowalski says, "Make corrections without invalidation or correct without crucifixion."

4. Acknowledge that Whatever is Being Communicated is True for the Speaker at that Moment
Most of the time, people make comments because they believe them. Therefore it is important to not judge what is being said and to not misinterpret it but, instead, to listen so that we can understand what is being said. Emphasis is on active listening.

5. Complete Your Agreement
Make only agreements that you intend to and are willing to keep. This is especially important for those who (1) procrastinate and (2) say "yes" to everything. If you must break an agreement, communicate this information as soon as possible.

6. If a Problem Arises, First Use the System for Corrections and then Communicate the Problem with Optional Solutions to the Person Who Can Do Something About the Problem
This is another way to eliminate gossip, judgment, and self-righteousness.

7. Be Effective and Efficient

8. Optimize Every Event—Create More with Less
Items 7 and 8 go together. Look for value in every event. Focus on what can be learned or done; use "lateral thinking" to create effective options.

9. Have the Willingness to Win and to Allow Others to Win
"Win/lose" is a "zero sum game." Effective problem solving allows everyone to win—to get his or her needs met.

10. Focus on What Works
The corollary is, get beyond what isn't working. Be willing to try something new. When it's broke, fix it!

11. When in Doubt, Check Out Feelings
When there seem to be blocks to communication or progress, they are often related to how people are feeling. Check this out; ask the person/people in question. Get the feelings out in the open where they can be checked out, tested, and responded to.

12. Agree to Disagree Until Reaching Consensus
Commit to working together toward mutually agreeable solutions. This keeps things in a forward motion without judgment. It keeps things hopeful.

13. Tell the Truth from the Point of View of Personal Responsibility
Always begin with the pretence that you are willing to assume 50% of the responsibility. This eliminates "you, you, you" messages and allows you to work with others toward a solution, not toward blame.

Adapted from Thurber, M. (1973). *Rules of the game.* San Francisco: Hawthorne-Stone Real Estate.

consequently, trust is low for the leader and for each other.

Trust is also a major issue among group members, and one of the first questions to come up in the group concerns is whom one can trust or not trust. In the early days of organizational development, McGregor (1967) defined *trust* in the following way:

Trust means: "I know that you will not— deliberately or accidentally, consciously or unconsciously—take unfair advantage of me." It means, "I

can put my situation at the moment, my status and self-esteem in this group, relationship, my job, my career, even my life, in your hands with complete confidence." (p. 163)

One can see from this description how critical trust is within a team (Appreciative inquiry is one method for shifting from focusing on problems to highlighting successes (Trajkovski et al., 2013)). The leader models trust through behaviors such as setting the ground rules/agreements by which the team will function and holding team members accountable for adhering to the rules. Trust is probably the most delicate aspect within relationships and is influenced far more by actions than by words. In other words, what people do is more powerful than what they say. Trust is a fragile thread that can be severed by one act. Once destroyed, trust is more difficult to re-establish than its initial creation.

QUALITIES OF A TEAM PLAYER

For students, it soon becomes clear that working in teams is important. Understanding what is required of a strong teammate becomes clear as students are assigned teams for various projects. Most people have participated in teams that did not work and in those that worked very well. Maxwell (2002) identified 17 characteristics that make a good team player:

1. **Adaptable**—Inflexibility does not work in teams. Being rigid in thinking or behavior is destructive to both the individual and to the team.
2. **Collaborative**—Collaboration is more than cooperation. It means each person brings something to the project that adds value to the team and supports the creation of synergy.
3. **Committed**—Commitment is a passion in the face of adversity to take action and make things happen. It is the passion to do whatever it takes to accomplish the team objectives.
4. **Communicative**—Communication should happen early and often. Frequency of interaction with other team members, talking with them and sharing thoughts, ideas, and experiences—these are the activities that support teamwork.
5. **Competent**—Competence translates as someone who is quite capable and highly qualified and does the job well.
6. **Dependable**—Team members who are dependable follow through and do what they have agreed to do well, without prodding or delay.
7. **Disciplined**—Discipline is doing what you really do not want to do so you can accomplish the goals you really want and includes paying attention to the details in thinking, in emotions, and in the actions you take.

8. **Enlarging**—Helping a teammate advance or grow into a better person or team player; helping teammates advance the team; believing in your teammates before they believe in themselves are examples of value-added.
9. **Enthusiastic**—Enthusiasm focuses on becoming a highly energetic team member who has a positive attitude and believes that the team, together, can be better than anyone dreamed they could.
10. **Intentional**—The team and its members have a purpose for themselves and for the team. Every action counts and is meaningful. The focus is on doing the right things in each moment and following through with these actions to their logical conclusion.
11. **Mission Conscious**—Each team member has a sense of purpose and mission that drives all thoughts, ideas, and actions to do what is best for their team and their cause.
12. **Prepared**—Being prepared translates as preparation for every meeting and event and begins with a thorough assessment of what is needed, aligning the appropriate work with the appropriate effort, addressing the mental aspects of the right attitude, and being ready to take action.
13. **Relational**—The ability to be connected to other members of the team, to be in a relationship with them, is the core of being relationship-oriented. These relationships and the mutual respect upon which they are built create cohesiveness on the team.
14. **Self-Improving**—As a team member, you strive to continually grow and reflect, both routinely and periodically, on how well each venture of assignment went and what you could have done better. This is a process of self-reflection.
15. **Selfless**—Putting others on the team ahead of yourself through being generous to team members, avoiding "playing politics," showing loyalty toward team members, and valuing interdependence among team members over the American value of being independent are all examples of selflessness.
16. **Solution-Oriented**—Do not be consumed with all of the problems associated with the

endeavor; rather, focus on finding the solutions; think about what is possible.

17. **Tenacious**—Being tenacious means giving your all, with determination, and refusing to stop until the goal has been accomplished.

EXERCISE 18-6

Think about the last team project in which you participated. What worked about the team? What did not work about the team? Was there a member who did not carry his or her share of the work? Was there a team member who was a "know it all"? How did you handle the situation? Was there a person on the team who took the lead? How many of the qualities of a good team player do you possess? Be honest. What are areas in which you could improve? What are your strengths; that is, where do you shine?

CREATING SYNERGY

Teams function with varying levels of effectiveness. The interesting part of this is that effectiveness can be created systematically. Truly effective teams are ones in which people work together to produce extraordinary results that could not have been achieved by any one individual. This phenomenon is often described as synergy. In the physical sciences, synergy is found in metal alloys. Bronze, the first alloy, was a combination of copper and tin and was found to be much harder and stronger than either copper or tin separately; the tensile strength of bronze cannot be predicted by merely adding the tensile strength of tin and of copper. It is far greater than simple addition.

We see the same properties of synergy in human endeavors; an example is the 1980 U.S. Olympic hockey team. Many people remember the hockey game, in which the Americans defeated the Russians. The team consisted of a group of college kids, none of whom could establish a celebrated successful career in the National Hockey League. However, for 2 weeks they were the best hockey team in the world—and they were the best because they knew how to work together to produce extraordinary results. Working cooperatively, an effective team produces extraordinary results that no one team member could have achieved alone. To create synergy consistently, certain basic rules must be followed:

- Establish a clear purpose.
- Use active listening.
- Be compassionate.
- Tell the truth.
- Be flexible.
- Commit to resolution.

Establish a Clear Purpose

Creative synergy requires a clear purpose. Each member of the team must understand the reason the team is together, determine what he or she wishes to accomplish (as delineated by defined goals and objectives), and express his or her belief in both the value and feasibility of the goals and tasks. Teams function best when the members cannot only tell others about their purpose but also define and operationalize succinctly the meaning and value of this purpose.

Use Active Listening

Active listening means that you are completely focused on the individual who is speaking. It means listening without judgment. It means listening to the essence of the conversation so that you can actually repeat to the speaker most of the speaker's intended meaning. It means being 100% present in the communication. (For guidelines for active listening, see Box 18-7.)

It does not mean developing a defensive response or argument in your head while the other person is still speaking. To listen actively, a person must be absorbing words, posture, tone of voice, and all the clues accompanying the message so that the intent of the communication can be received. Specific purposes used in active listening, including examples, are found in Table 18-4.

Be Compassionate

To be compassionate means to have a sympathetic consciousness of another's distress and a desire to alleviate the distress. Consequently, it is inappropriate to focus time and energy on making the other person wrong, especially when your perspective differs from his or hers. It means listening from a caring perspective—one that is focused on understanding the viewpoint of the other person rather than insisting on the "rightness" of one's own point of view.

Tell the Truth

To tell the truth means to speak clearly to personal points and perspectives while acknowledging that

BOX 18-7   GUIDELINES FOR ACTIVE LISTENING

1. Slow down your internal processes and seek data. Do not interrupt the speaker.
2. The more information you acquire through listening, the less interpretation you do (making up the missing pieces or motivations). The less information you have, the more interpretation you do.
3. Realize that the first words from the other person are not necessarily representative of inner thoughts and feelings. Be patient.
4. When listening, suspend your own beliefs and views and judgments, at least temporarily. Attempt to understand the perspective of the other person, particularly if it is different from yours.
5. Realize that any judgments or "labels" strongly influence the manner in which you listen to the other person.
6. Appreciate the difference between understanding other people's perspective and agreeing with them. First strive to understand. Then you may agree or disagree.
7. Effective listening is based on an inner desire to learn about another's unique experience of the world.

Adapted from Olen, D. (1993). *Communicating: Speaking and listening to end misunderstanding and promote friendship.* Germantown, WI: JODA Communications.

TABLE 18-4   ACTIVE LISTENING

USE OF ACTIVE LISTENING	EXAMPLES
To convey interest in what the other person is saying	I see! I get it. I hear what you're saying.
To encourage the individual to expand further on his or her thinking	Yes, go on. Tell us more.
To help the individual clarify the problem in his or her own thinking	Then the problem as you see it is …
To get the individual to hear what he or she has said in the way it sounded to others	This is your decision, then, and the reasons are … If I understand you correctly, you are saying that we should …
To pull out the key ideas from a long statement or discussion	Your major point is … You feel that we should …
To respond to a person's feelings more than to his or her words	You feel strongly that … You do not believe that …
To summarize specific points of agreement and disagreement as a basis for further discussion	We seem to be agreed on the following points … But we seem to need further clarification on these points …
To express a consensus of group feeling	As a result of this discussion, we as a group seem to feel that …

they are, merely, personal perspectives. If an observation is made about the tone or behavior of a speaker that affects the ability of others to hear the message, feedback can be provided in a way that does not make the speaker wrong. This is accomplished in an objective rather than subjective manner using neither a cynical nor a critical tone of voice. To be effective, one must own—be responsible for—personal opinions and attitudes.

Be Flexible

Flexibility and openness to another person's viewpoint are critical for a team to work well together. No single person has all the right answers. Therefore acknowledging that each person has something to contribute and must be heard is important. Flexibility reflects a willingness to hear another team member's point of view rather than being committed to the "rightness" of a personal point of view.

Commit to Resolution

To commit to resolution means that one can agree to disagree with someone even when that perspective is different. Rather than assuming the person is wrong, this is a commitment to hear his or her perspective, listen to the real message, identify differences, and creatively seek solutions to resolve the areas of differences so that there can be a common understanding and shared commitment to the issue. Both parties need to then agree that they feel heard and agree to the resolution. This differs greatly from compromise and majority vote seen in the democratic process. When compromise exists, there is acquiescence or relinquishing of a significant portion of what was desired. This generally leaves both parties feeling negative about themselves or the agreement. Consequently, most compromises must be reworked at some future date. Working on conflict and its resolution (Table 18-5) is time-consuming but

TABLE 18-5	ASPECTS OF CONFLICT

DESTRUCTIVE	CONSTRUCTIVE
• Diverts energy from more important activities and issues	• Opens up issues of importance, resulting in their clarification
• Destroys the morale of people or reinforces poor self-concepts	• Results in the solution of problems
• Polarizes groups so they increase internal cohesiveness and reduce intergroup cooperation	• Increases the involvement of individuals in issues of importance to them
• Deepens differences in values	• Causes authentic communication to occur
• Produces irresponsible and regrettable behavior such as name-calling and fighting	• Serves as a release for pent-up emotion, anxiety, and stress
	• Helps build cohesiveness among people sharing the conflict, celebrating in its settlement, and learning more about each other
	• Helps individuals grow personally and apply what they learn to future situations

Adapted from Hart, L.B. (1980). *Learning from conflict*. Reading, MA: Addison-Wesley.

essential to effectively functioning teams (Eisenhardt, Kahwajy, & Bourgeois, 1997). Commitment to resolution is integral to the needs of the team. One team member may disagree with another team member, but the successful work of the team is at stake in this conflict. Without commitment to resolution for the sake of the team, individuals often have less impetus to seek a common ground or to agree to disagree (Dechurch, Mesmer-Magnus, & Doty, 2013).

Synergy cannot occur when one team member becomes a self-proclaimed expert who has the "right" answer. Nor can synergy occur when people refuse to speak. Each team member has good ideas, and these need to be shared. They are not shared, however, when someone feels uncomfortable in the team. It is difficult to speak up and appear wrong or inadequate. The challenge each person faces is to push through discomfort and become a full participant in problem identification and resolution for the overall benefit of the team.

Our society tends to be dualistic in nature. Dualism means that most situations are viewed as right or wrong, black or white. Answers to questions are often reduced to "yes" or "no." As a result, we sometimes forget there is a broad spectrum of possibilities. Exercising creativity and exploring numerous possibilities are important. This allows the team to operate at its optimal level.

We have all known people who were self-proclaimed experts, to whom it was critically important that they be right and acknowledged as right and who become judgmental of others whose perspectives and opinions differ from theirs. Consequently, being able to tell the truth to one's synergistic team and to encourage team members to stretch and look at different ways of functioning is vital. This requires strong skills in good negotiation and conflict resolution, something for which few of us have been trained. If self-proclaimed experts think we are judging them, they will not hear the questions, the observations, or the "truth" because the message seems to be making them wrong rather than originating from compassion. The most valuable contribution an individual can make to an organization is a passionate commitment to the creation of synergistic teams.

INTERDISCIPLINARY/ INTERPROFESSIONAL TEAMS

Interprofessional teams are essential to quality patient care. Nurses, physicians, dietitians, social workers, case managers, pharmacists, and physical therapists, to name but a few, must work together to achieve cost-effective care while achieving the highest quality of care in the healthcare setting. This means there must be efforts to understand the various roles and backgrounds of each discipline. At the same time, nurses are frequently leading teams comprising licensed practical/vocational nurses and technicians or assistants of various kinds. Here again, it is critical to understand everyone's role and job description as well as his or her background and who he or she is as an individual and human being. In addition, the collaboration needed in interdisciplinary teams cannot be created without mutual trust and respect among the members (Contratti, Ng, & Deeb, 2012).

Several additional aspects of interdisciplinary work are crucial to creating and maintaining these teams. Coyne (2005) emphasizes *the importance of understanding each situation,* which includes clarifying misperceptions and inaccurate information about others within the team including any assumptions that one professional group is favored over another. *Noticing professional expectations and unwritten processes* and cultures of the various professions within the team is also critical to working together seamlessly. It is helpful for nurses to note how other groups talk and behave and to note the special language they use. *Encourage the different disciplines to learn* from each other. For example, in comparing the different codes of ethics, it is quite amazing to discover similarities as opposed to the differences. Most are focused on the patient. The team leader must *set a positive tone.* If the leadership expects interdisciplinary teamwork and verbalizes and models positive and upbeat attitudes, the various disciplines will work together smoothly.

Frequency of interaction of the team members can create ongoing interactions and familiarity with one another. Team members who are in a professional relationship with one another are more apt to work together smoothly. There may be a weekly patient care meeting in which patients with significant needs or problems are reviewed and each profession addresses issues from the specific area of expertise. *Keep communication open* includes telling the truth in a way that it can be heard and understood. If an aspect of care is governed by regulations, it is helpful when a knowledgeable member of the team speaks to the issue or regulation, always remembering to phrase the information in a way that facilitates hearing and understanding. At all times the interdisciplinary team must *focus on the patient.* When the deliberations are focused on the delivery of best patient care for the specific patient, mutual respect can be developed and open sharing of ideas and problem solving occurs.

THE VALUE OF TEAM-BUILDING

The value of team-building is to enhance functioning in any one or all of the following processes (Coyne, 2005; Herman & Reichelt, 1998):
- The establishment of goals and objectives
- The allocation of the work to be performed

- The manner in which a group works: its processes, norms, decision making, and communication patterns
- The relationships among the people doing the work

When things are not going well in an organization and there are problems that need to be resolved, the first intervention people think of is "team-building." Naturally, for teams (a collection of people relying on each other) to be effective, they must function smoothly and communicate effectively to create the best possible work environment (Taplin, Foster, & Shortell, 2013). The difficulty is that when organizations are feeling stress and facing difficulties, they generally do not have teams whose members function well together. Team-building can address any one of the aforementioned activities, depending on the available time and other resources. A team-building consultant can teach a team how to set goals and priorities; help a team analyze the distribution of the workload using various team members' strengths; examine a team's process, norms, decision-making processes, and communication patterns; and promote resolution of interpersonal conflicts or problems within the team.

Regardless of which areas are problematic, appropriate assessment of the team is essential. The problems may be in priority or goal-setting, allocation of the work, team decision making, or interpersonal relationships among the members (see the Research Perspective on p. 364). The success of the team depends on its members and its leadership.

Druskat and Wolff (2001) build a strong case for dealing constructively with building an underlying foundation for teams. They believe that three major components of smoothly functioning teams must be created:
- Mutual trust among the members
- A strong sense of team identity (that the team is unique and worthwhile)
- A sense of team efficacy (that the team performs well and its members are synergistic in their manner of working together)

At the heart of these components are the emotions we often work so hard to keep out of the workplace. However, as human beings, we function in the same way in both work and personal lives. Mutual trust can be developed only when each team member tells the

RESEARCH PERSPECTIVE

Resource: Klein, C., Granados, D., Salas, E., Huy Le, C., Burke, S., Lyons, R., & Goodwin, G. (2009). Does team building work? *Small Group Research, 40*(2), 181-222.

This article reports an extensive meta-analysis of team-building research that focuses on four specific components of teams: goal-setting, interpersonal relationships, problem solving, and role clarification. This analysis includes 103 articles published between 1950 and 2007 and expands the original work of this same group and the analysis conducted in 1999. Previous team-building reviews are also summarized. The outcomes that were measured were cognitive, affective, process, and performance based. The results suggest that team-building activities have a moderately positive effect across all team outcomes, whereas the strongest effect existed for goal-setting and role clarification. The size of the team can also be important, and teams of 10 or fewer members seem to have more success.

This means that most work teams need to be limited in size (fewer than 10 members per group) and that the focus when forming the team is on clarifying the goals of the team and the role of each team member.

Implications for Practice
The Institute of Medicine has set the expectation that all health-care providers function as a patient-centered team, yet not all curricula prepare practitioners to do so. Using the knowledge about the outcomes of these key components helps practitioners perform more effectively in teams.

BOX 18-8   INTERVIEW QUESTIONS FOR TEAM-BUILDING

1. What do you see as the problems currently facing your team?
2. What are the current strengths of your institution or work group? What are you currently doing well?
3. Does your boss do anything that prevents you from being as effective as you would like to be?
4. Does anybody else in this group do anything that prevents you from being as effective as you would like to be?
5. What would you like to accomplish at your upcoming team-building session? What changes would you be willing to make that would facilitate a smoother-functioning team and accomplishment of the team goals?

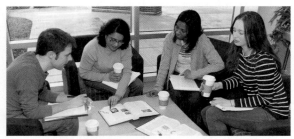

Teams can form strong relationships external to the work environment.

truth about feelings, thoughts, and wants and listens and supports other members of the team to do likewise. Every person yearns to be a part of something bigger than himself or herself—to do something important that makes a difference. Well-functioning teams allow this to happen. Developing such teams can increase nursing job satisfaction and group cohesiveness, as well as decrease nurse turnover rates (DiMeglio et al., 2005).

Understandable anxiety exists concerning the safety of being vulnerable and exposed if personal issues are revealed. That is why it is helpful for the team-building facilitator to make a thorough assessment of major issues and the willingness on the part of members to work on issues. One approach is to interview members of the team individually to discover what the critical issues are. The types of questions that might be asked are found in Box 18-8. This kind of tool gives the facilitator some sense of what

the major issues are within the group so that he or she has a better understanding of how to work with the group.

MANAGING EMOTIONS

Probably one of the greatest fears in team-building exercises is that people will become emotional, that they will lose control of themselves or the environment, or that they will appear weakened or vulnerable. Men have a particularly difficult time with this fear, but many women also want to appear strong and are hesitant to be open and vulnerable. Although many people acknowledge that we are all thinking and feeling persons, management/leadership is usually more willing to deal with the "thinking" side than the "feeling" side of individuals within the team.

Because people spend such a large percentage of their time in the work setting, it would be un-realistic to believe that they continually appear in an unemotional and controlled state. Human beings simply do not function that way. What is observed are people's aspirations, their achievements, their hopes, and their social consciousness; they are observed falling in love; falling in hate and anger; winning and losing; and being excited, sad, fearful, anxious, and jealous. Consequently, these "feelings" are important components of organizational life and do much to undermine work effectiveness. Most of us know of situations in which, because of an emotional disagreement, two individuals have avoided each other for years. Because of the power of emotions and the inevitability of their presence, their effect on interpersonal relationships, and their influence on productivity, the quality of work, and the safety of patients, emotions should be a high priority when examining the functioning of the team. Fortunately, research addresses the importance of emphasizing the "emotional intelligence" of individuals and teams when working in teams (Ferrazzi, 2012). Those teams that address these issues are much more successful and create a positive work environment.

According to Bocialetti (1988), people are sensitive to what happens when emotions are revealed. When people yell or get angry or upset and when goals, objectives, and tasks are disputed, employees see the following:

- A member intimidating and frightening others within the group
- Embarrassment
- A member overstating or exaggerating another's view to appear right
- Provocation of defensive and hostile responses
- Over-concern with oneself—self-absorption
- Gossip
- Loss of control
- A member distracting others from "real work"
- Disruption or termination of relationships within a group

These are behaviors that destroy any hope of creating a smoothly functioning team, one that supports its members to grow and learn and provide quality patient care. On the other hand, the cost of suppressing emotions or "feelings" includes the following:

- Physical and psychological stress
- Withdrawal from participation
- Loss of energy and depression
- Reduction of learning
- Hiding of important data because of fear

- Festering problems and emotions
- Prevention of others from being acknowledged
- Decreased motivation
- Weakening of the ability to receive constructive feedback
- The loss of one's influence

These types of outcomes lead to the conclusion that suppressing emotions at work is neither healthy nor constructive for team members.

When emotions are handled appropriately within the team, there are several positive outcomes for the work setting. One creates a sense of internal comfort with the workings of the team and the organization. When stress is lowered and kept at lower levels on average, problems are much more easily resolved. This phenomenon is similar to releasing steam slowly with a steam valve rather than having the gasket blow. Interpersonal relationships on the team are more stable, and people have a sense of closer ties and collegiality when emotions are addressed. Fewer negative relationships or interactions develop, which results in more effective and pleasant working relationships all around.

Work group effectiveness improves when the team is functioning smoothly and emotions and "feelings" are being addressed on a routine basis rather than waiting for a volcanic eruption. Problems of withdrawal, boredom, and frustration are much less likely to overwhelm the team and lead to its breakdown (Turpin, 2000). The skills and tools previously discussed (e.g., speaking supportively) are the basic tools one needs to handle the emotional aspects of the team. Choosing to cope with emotional upset must be a conscious choice, one that requires practice to improve the skill.

REFLECTIVE PRACTICE

The process of reflective practice consists of the active, careful consideration of a belief or knowledge and can derive from "learning from experience." It is an internal learning process in which an issue of concern is closely examined (Freshwater, Taylor, & Sherwood, 2008). Through this reflective process, the nurse may come to see the world differently and, as a result of these new insights, see the work world differently, which can translate to acting differently. Thus, upon reflection of how an interaction progressed with a complex patient, the nurse can examine how this event unfolded compared with how he or she might have wanted the event to occur. This is an opportunity to learn experientially from what works and what does not work as well. Many of us think about what happened during our shift or day as we travel home. The major area for growth is when we identify specific behaviors to do differently and make a commitment to actually do them differently. Bringing issues to the conscious level is the first step in personal/professional growth.

THE ROLE OF LEADERSHIP

Teams usually have a leader. In addition, teams function within large organizations that have leaders. Without the approval and the support of the leader, team-building, which can be a costly endeavor in terms of consultation fees as well as work time and resources of the team, is difficult to undertake and of questionable effectiveness. Although very strong teams may be able to educate themselves regarding some of the issues, such as establishing goals and priorities or clarifying their own team process, addressing any kind of relationship issue among team members without a more objective outside party facilitating the process is exceedingly difficult.

Because leadership is such a pivotal part of smoothly functioning teams, it is illuminating to examine leaders more carefully. Truly progressive leaders understand that leadership and followership are not necessarily a set of skills; rather, these are qualities of character, a manifestation of a person's own being (Tracey & Hinkin, 1998). On speaking specifically to leadership, we are not talking about "putting on a role." In actuality, leaders realize their capacity for influence, risk taking, and decision making more fully. Leadership, and to some degree followership, is as much about character and development as it is about education. According to Peter Vaill (1991), leadership is concerned with bringing out the best in people. For a leader who believes this, team-building is a natural outgrowth. This type of leader understands that the best in a person is tied intimately to the individual's deepest sense of himself or herself—to one's spirit. The efforts of leaders must touch the spiritual aspect in themselves and others. Warren Bennis (2009) once said that leaders simply care about more people. Consequently, this caring manifests itself in doing whatever it takes to improve team functioning. This may imply involving oneself in team-building with the team. The risk in such an endeavor is that the team leader is open to being vulnerable, to being judged by others, and to being wrong. However, if the leader has been a role model for the "rules of the game" and has held people to these rules, the team-building exercise will not degenerate into judging and placing blame.

If true leadership is about character development as much as anything, then character development is also beneficial for followers—that is, members of the team. The areas of character development often addressed include communication, particularly those aspects of speaking supportively that avoid placing blame and justifying and enhance understanding the other person's message. Box 18-9 highlights an example of character development from personal experience.

Leaders understand the multiple aspects of the issue of control. They take control of their lives rather than being at the mercy of others—rather than being victims. They have clarity regarding their own control issues. They focus time and energy primarily and almost exclusively on those issues, events, and behaviors over which they have control. Their activities are thus focused primarily on areas relating directly to them—not on world events or other happenings over which they have neither influence nor control.

Confidence, which loosely translates as faith or belief that one will act in a correct and effective way, is a key aspect of character. Thus it follows that confidence in oneself can be closely tied to self-esteem, which is satisfaction with oneself. The greatest deterrent to self-esteem and self-confidence is fear. Fear is described by some as "false evidence appearing real." Susan Jeffers (2006) believes the core fear—the one that rules our lives—is one of "I can't handle it." So, the core of our fears is "I can't handle it," and it is exactly the opposite of being confident or holding oneself in high esteem. Working on self-confidence requires an attitude of belief, of confidence, of I "CAN DO" whatever is required (see Box 18-9).

BOX 18-9   THE "CAN DO" BRIGADE: AN ARMY NURSE'S STUDY IN CHARACTER DEVELOPMENT

As life events are reviewed, important or pivotal learning can be identified. One life event that significantly affected me was the year I spent as an Army Nurse Corps officer in South Vietnam. This was the first time I remember an awareness and understanding of confidence in the face of incredible obstacles. I had spent the first 10 months of my nursing career in labor and delivery at Indiana University before volunteering for a guaranteed assignment to Vietnam. I went to Fort Sam Houston for 6 weeks of basic training, where they taught me really important things like how to salute, how to march, and how many men are in a battalion. No one ever asked me if I could start an IV or draw a tube of blood. This was important because Indiana University had the largest medical school class in the United States at that time and nurses did nothing that interfered with medical education. Therefore I had never started an IV or drawn blood. When I arrived in Saigon, they put me in a sedan with another nurse and sent me up to the Third Surgical Hospital, one not unlike the one in MASH. We even had a Major Burns—that was not his name but it was his function. Surgical hospitals receive only battle casualties; their purpose is to stabilize and to transport.

The Third Surgical Hospital was located in the middle of the 173rd Airborne Brigade, whose job it was to defend the Bien Hoi Air Base, where all the sorties in the south were flown during the war. We were stopped at the gate by an MP who stepped up and saluted very snappily. He knew that a staff car must contain either a very-high-ranking officer or, if it was his lucky day, females.

When I was in Vietnam, 500 American women and 500,000 American men were there. The MP looked in the window, saluted snappily, and said "Afternoon, ma'am!" He wanted to know where we were going; he talked to us for a few minutes and assured us that if there was anything he could do for us, we should just give him a call. He saluted us and said, "CAN DO." I didn't understand because I did not know that there are units with very high esprit de corps who attach snappy little sayings at the end of things like salutes, phone conversations, memos, and so forth. The 173rd was the "CAN DO" brigade.

When we got to the hospital and met the chief nurse, she took us down to the mess hall and introduced us to all the doctors and nurses. We were sitting and having coffee when the field phone rang in the kitchen and the mess sergeant yelled out, "Incoming wounded." Everybody got up and started to leave for the preop area. I just sat there until the chief nurse said, "Come on." I said, "You don't understand, I deliver babies." She was not impressed! She took me by the arm and led me to preop.

When we got there, we discovered there were not just a few incoming wounded, there were more than 30, and some were very seriously injured. She immediately told the sergeant to call headquarters battalion of the 173rd Airborne and tell them that the Third Surg needed blood. She turned to me and said, "Lieutenant, you are responsible for drawing 50 units of fresh whole blood." I was shocked! I had never drawn a tube of blood, but I found in the back section of preop a Specialist 4th class who was already setting up "saw horses" and stretchers, putting up IV poles, and hanging plastic blood sets. I started to help, and soon I heard trucks out back. I opened the door and looked outside. There were two huge Army trucks, and kids—17, 18, 19, and 20 years old—were jumping out. They were covered with red mud from the bottom of their boots to the tops of their helmets. I looked at them, and I looked at the clean cement floor, and in an instant, my mother came to me. I put my hand on my hip and said, "Where have you boys been?" One PFC stepped forward and saluted me very snappily and said, "Ma'am, we just came in this afternoon from 30 days in the field, we have been out in the rice paddies chasing the Viet Cong, we have not had a hot meal, and we've not had a shower but Sergeant Major said the Third Surg needs blood!" He saluted smartly and said, "CAN DO!" They were very clear. After 30 days of chasing and being chased by the Viet Cong, giving a unit of blood was easy. "CAN DO!" They were confident. They were kids who had looked into the face of death. At that moment, I knew if they CAN DO, I Can Do! Life requires confidence. With confidence, you can make your dreams come true!

False
Evidence
Appearing
Real

Simply caring about more people translates into a willingness to focus time and energy on members of the team. From one perspective, caring is risking being with someone and sharing both suffering and joy. Healing often emerges from caring. Behaviors that demonstrate caring include giving of oneself in terms of warmth and love and particularly giving one's time. The second aspect of caring is truly listening to team members and hearing and understanding them. The third aspect includes being 100% present for them. The fourth is to honor the other person—to see his or her wholeness, possibilities, hopes, and dreams.

Leading the team is clearly not the easiest thing to do, but neither is being an active, fully participating member of the team. Both require taking risks, including being in a relationship. Being in a team-building experience and hearing those things that have not worked for people in their interactions with peers and the leader can be scary but worthwhile. It requires a focus on personal and professional growth. It requires building character.

THE SOLUTION

The first question that needed to be asked was, "Were we committed to providing the most optimal care for the neonate?" In other words, why would teamwork be important in this situation? What's the vision or mission? After achieving agreement among the NICU team, we strategized on how to create a "team" with the specialists. Making our intent clear was very important. A meeting with the director of the specialty team, the NICU medical director, and nursing leadership was arranged. We discovered that we shared a common goal: to provide the best care possible for the baby. Keeping that goal as the focus, we then identified areas of mutual respect. From there, both sides were willing to listen to each other's concerns. Care guidelines could be identified, as well as areas of responsibility. Ideas on how to improve the communication process were also discussed. A plan based on patient needs, complete with agreements, was implemented.

Were we a team yet? The answer is "no." There was still a little skepticism and reserve. Everyone seemed to have a "wait-and-see" attitude. The first big chance was identified when the specialty group insisted that a patient of theirs be admitted to the NICU because they believed it was the best place for the baby to be.

Another measurable outcome was having the agreements honored. This reinforced to everyone that his or her concerns had been heard and respected. Mutual trust was building, and a collegial relationship began. A year later, it is hard to imagine that this situation ever occurred. There is enthusiasm for this specialty's physicians and their patients. It is certainly a change in attitude.

There are many components to team-building, but the most important component is to be clear about your mission and intentions when working with potential team members. The intention to provide the best care possible assisted each one of us to be more open, creative, and trusting. These are all necessary components of team-building. Remember, teams are made up of individuals. Ask yourself if you are willing to accept responsibility for your response and actions. Be the change that you want to see.

—Diane Gallagher

Would this be a suitable approach for you? Why or why not?

THE EVIDENCE

TeamSTEPPS is an integrated program created through the auspices of Health and Human Services Agency for Healthcare Research and Quality (AHRQ) and the Department of Defense (DOD) Health Care Team Coordination Program; it stresses teamwork and communication among physicians, nurses, and other healthcare personnel to increase patient safety (Brock et al., 2013). Multiple projects and evidence have been accrued regarding the use and implementation of TeamSTEPPS, as well as the outcomes produced from this program. The goal is to produce highly effective interdisciplinary teams that achieve the best outcomes for patients. The tools and strategies used include leadership that coordinates the team and initiates planning, problem solving, and process improvement. Also, situation monitoring is employed. This tool focuses on the ability of the nurse to actively scan behaviors and actions of co-workers; it also fosters mutual respect and team accountability, which creates a safety net for the team and patient. Specific skills are taught that increase the ability of each team member to support other team members by accurately assessing their workload and helping them. These skills protect the team from work overload that might reduce effectiveness and increase risk to patients. The last skill set focuses on communication that highlights clear, accurate information exchange among team members including SBAR, Call-out, and Handoff. The TeamSTEPPS teaching manual, including PowerPoints and teaching videos, is available from the DOD Patient Safety Program for minimal cost.

NEED TO KNOW NOW

- Remember that team members are your friends.
- Practice effective communication tools such as SBAR.
- View physicians as colleagues and team members who want only the best possible care for patients.

CHAPTER CHECKLIST

Nurse managers must help build teams. Although the manager does not have to lead the team, he or she must ensure that the group can function effectively as a team. The team members must be able to communicate with each other effectively, share a single mission, be willing to cooperate with each other, and be committed to achieving their objectives. Successful teamwork requires leadership, trust, and willingness to take risks.

- A team is a highly interdependent group of people that has the following characteristics:
  - Has defined goals and objectives
  - Communicates effectively with one another
  - Has an ongoing relationship
  - Is focused on accomplishing a task
- Attributes of effective teams include the following:
  - Clarity of purpose
  - Informality
  - Effective communication
  - Participation
  - Listening
  - Civilized disagreement
  - Consensus decisions
  - Clear roles and work assignments
  - Shared leadership
  - Diversity of styles
  - Self-assessment and self-regulation
- Each team member deals continually with three questions:
  - Am I in the "in" group or the "out" group?
  - Do I have any power or control?
  - Can I use, develop, and be appreciated for my skills and resources?

- Focusing on team members' strengths and acknowledging what they do well are two of the keys to team-building.
- To be effective, acknowledgments must be the following:
  - Specific
  - Personal
  - Sincere
  - Timely
  - Public
- One of the most helpful tools for teams is a set of ground rules that govern how members will interact with each other.
- Trust is essential for successful teamwork.
- Synergy allows a team to produce results that could not have been achieved by any one individual. Creating it requires the following:
  - Active listening
  - Compassion
  - Honesty
  - Flexibility
  - Commitment to resolution of conflicts
- Managing emotions is a key strategy in team-building.
- Leadership is a pivotal part of a smoothly functioning team.
  - Leadership relies on personal character development as much as on education.
  - Confidence is a key aspect of the leader's character.
- A "can do" attitude is one of the most important confidence-building strategies a leader can adopt.
- Taking a risk and experimenting with a new behavior is the most effective way to change behavior.

TIPS FOR TEAM-BUILDING

- Commit to the purpose of the team.
- Develop team relationships of mutual respect.
- Communicate effectively, and actively listen.
- Create and adhere to team agreements concerning function and process.
- Build trust.

REFERENCES

Bennis, W. (2009). *On becoming a leader*. Reading, MA: Addison-Wesley.

Bocialetti, G. (1988). Teams and management of emotion. In W. B. Reddy & K. Jamison (Eds.), *Team building blueprints for productivity and satisfaction* (pp. 62-71). Alexandria, VA: NTL Institute for Applied Behavioral Sciences; and San Diego: University Associates.

Bradley, J., & Edinberg, M. (1990). *Communication in the nursing context* (3rd ed.). Norwalk, CT: Appleton & Lange.

Brock, D., Abu-Rish, E., Chiu, C. R., Hammer, D., Wilson, S., Vorvick, L., Blondon, K., Schaad, D., Liner, D., & Zierler, B. (2013). Interprofessional education in team communication: Working together to improve patient safety. *BMJ Quality and Safety, 22*(5), 414-423.

Contratti, F., Ng, G., & Deeb, J. (2012). Interdisciplinary teams traning: Five lessons learned. *American Journal of Nursing, 112*(6), 47-52.

Coyne, C. (2005). Strength in numbers: How team building is improving care in a variety of practice settings. *PT— Magazine of Physical Therapy, 13*(6), 40-51.

Dechurch, L. A., Mesmer-Magnus, J. R. & Doty, D. (2013). Moving beyond relationship and task conflict: toward a process-state perspective. *Journal of Applied Psychology*, June 3, PMID: 23731027.

DiMeglio, K., Padula, C., Piatek, C., Korber, J., Barrett, A., Ducharme, M., et al (2005). Group cohesion and nurse satisfaction: Examination of a team-building approach. *The Journal of Nursing Administration, 35*(3), 110-120.

Druskat, V., & Wolff, S. (2001). Building the emotional intelligence of groups. *Harvard Business Review, 79*(3), 81-91.

Dyer, W. G., Dyer, J. H., & Dyer, W. G. (2013). *Team building: Proven strategies for improving team performance* (5th ed.). San Francisco, CA: Jossey-Bass.

Eisenhardt, K., Kahwajy, J., & Bourgeois, L. (1997). How management teams can have a good fight. *Harvard Business Review, 75*, 77-85.

Ferrazzi, K. (2012). Candor, criticism, teamwork. *Harvard Business Review, 90*(1/2), 40.

Freshwater, D., Taylor, B., & Sherwood, G. (2008). *Reflective practice in nursing*. Chichester, UK: Blackwell Publishing.

Herman, J., & Reichelt, P. (1998). Are first line nurse managers prepared for team building? *Nursing Management, 29*(10), 68-72.

Jeffers, S. (2006). *Feel the FEAR and DO IT anyway*. NewYork: Ballantine Books.

Klein, C., Granados, D., Salas, E., Huy Le, C., Burke, S., Lyons, R., et al. (2009). Does team building work? *Small Group Research, 40*(2), 181-222.

Kouzes, J. M., & Posner, B. Z. (2012). *The leadership challenge* (5th ed.). San Francisco: Jossey-Bass, John Wiley & Sons.

Kramer, M., Maguire, P., Halfer, D., Brewer, B. & Schmalenberg, C. (2013). Impact of residency programs on professional socialization of newly licenses registered nurses. *Western Journal of Nursing Research, 35*(4), 459-496.

Lopes, S. (1987). *The wall*. New York: Collins.

Mahon, M. M. & Nicotera, A. M. (2011). Nursing and conflict communication: Avoidance as preferred strategy. *Nursing Administration Quarterly, 35*(2), 152-163.

Maxwell, J. (2002). *The 17 essential qualities of a team player*. Nashville, TN: Thomas Nelson Publishers.

McGregor, D. (1960). *The human side of enterprise*. New York: McGraw-Hill.

McGregor, D. (1967). *The professional manager*. New York: McGraw-Hill.

Nemeth, C. P. (2008). *Improving healthcare team communication: Building on lessons from aviation and aerospace*. Aldershot, UK. Ashgate Publishing.

Niedenthal, P. M. & Brauer, M. (2012). Social functionality of human emotion. *Annual Review of Psychology, 63*, 259-283.

Olen, D. (1993). *Communicating: Speaking and listening to end misunderstanding and promote friendship*. Germantown, WI: JODA Communications.

Parcells, B. (2000). The tough work of turning around a team. *Harvard Business Review, 78*(6), 179-184.

Pentland, A. (2012). The new science of building great teams. *Harvard Business Review, 90*(4), 60-70.

Porter-O'Grady, T., & Malloch, K. (2010). *Quantum leadership* (3rd ed.). Sudbury, MA: Jones & Bartlett.

Riggs, C. (2013). Multiple generations in the nursing workplace: Part I. *The Journal of Continuing Education in Nursing, 44*(3), 105-106.

Rath, T. (2007). *Strengths Finder 2.0*. New York, NY: Gallup Press.

Roman, M. (2001). Teams, teammates, and team building. *MedSurg Nursing, 10*(4), 161-165.

Satir, V. (1988). *The new peoplemaking*. Mountain View, CA: Science & Behavior Books.

Sportsman, S. (2005). Build a framework for conflict assessment. *Nursing Management, 36*(4), 12-40.

Taplin, S. H., Foster, M. K. & Shortell, S. M. (2013). Organizational leadership for building effective health care teams. *Annals of Family Medicine, 11*(3), 279-281.

Tracey, J., & Hinkin, T. (1998). Transformational leadership or effective managerial practices? *Group & Organizational Management, 23*(3), 220-237.

Trajkovski, S., Schmied, V., Vickers, M. & Jackson, D. (2013). Implementing the 4D cycle of appreciative inquiry in health care: A methodological review. *Journal of Advanced Nursing, 69*(6), 1224-1234.

Turpin, C. (2000). Creating winning teams. *Nephrology Nursing Journal, 27*(2), 171.

Uhm, S., Liabo, K., Stewart, R., Rees, R. & Oliver, S. (2012). Patient and public perspectives shaping scientific and medical research: Panels for data, discussions, and decisions. *Patient Intelligence, 4*, 1-10.

Vaill, P. (1991). *Managing as a performing art*. San Francisco: Jossey-Bass.

Wagner, R., & Harter, J. (2006). *12: The elements of great managing.* New York: Gallup Press.

Weisburg, M. (1988). Team work: Building productive relationships. In W. B. Reddy & K. Jamison (Eds.), *Team building blueprints for productivity and satisfaction.* Alexandria, VA: NTL Institute for Applied Behavioral Sciences; and San Diego: University Associates.

Weiss, W. (2001). Attitude: A major managerial challenge. *Supervision, 62*(6), 3-7.

SUGGESTED READINGS

Ahmann, E. & Dokken, D. (2012). Strategies for encouraging patient/family member partnerships with the health care team. *Pediatric Nursing, 38*(4), 232-235.

Castner, J., Foltz-Ramos, K., Schwartz, D. G. & Ceravolo, D. J. (2012). A leadership challenge: Staff nurse perceptions after an organizational TeamSTEPPS initiative. *Journal of Nursing Administration, 42*(10), 467-472.

Huis, A., Hulscher, M., Adang, E., Grol, R., van Achterberg, T. & Schoonhoven, L. (2013). Cost-effectiveness of a team and leaders-directed strategy to improve nurses' adherence to hand hygiene guidelines: A cluster randomized trial. *International Journal of Nursing Studies, 50*(4), 518-526.

Johnson, J. E. (2013). Working together for the best interest of patients. *Journal of American Board of Family Medicine, 26*(3), 241-243.

Kalisch, B. J., Russell, K. & Lee, K. H. (2013). Nursing teamwork and unit size. *Western Journal of Nursing Research, 35*(2), 214-225.

Leach, L. S. & Mayo, A. M. (2013). Rapid response teams: Qualitative analysis of their effectiveness. *American Journal of Critical Care, 22*(3), 198-210.

Timmermans, O., Van Linge, R., Van Petegem, P., Van Rompaey, B. & Denekens, J. (2013). A contingency perspective on team learning and innovation in nursing. *Journal of Advanced Nursing, 69*(2), 363-373.

White, D. E., Straus, S. E., Stelfox, H. T., Holrowd-Leduc, J. M., Bell, C. M., Jackson, K., Norris, J. M., Flemons, W. W., Moffatt, M. E. & Forster, A. J. (2011). What is the value and impact of quality and safety teams? A scoping review. *Implementation Science, 23*(6), 97.

Collective Action

Denise K. Gormley

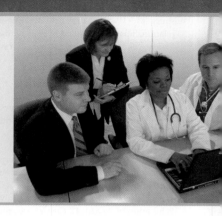

Today's nurses expect and, in some situations, demand a greater voice in decisions involving their work life. These decisions involve both the context and the content of their work. Policy, education, and experience influence professional nurses to actively participate in decision making about work environment issues. Specifically, participation in decisions regarding practice is an appropriate expectation of a professional nurse. Collective action is one mechanism available to achieve that participation. Understanding collective action is critical if nurses' efforts to shape the practice environment are to be successful. The manager can capitalize on collective action to accomplish positive outcomes.

OBJECTIVES

- Evaluate how key characteristics of selected collective action strategies apply in the workplace through shared governance, workplace advocacy, and collective bargaining.
- Distinguish between the rights of individuals included in collective bargaining contracts and the rights of at-will employees.
- Compare the factors that contribute to nurses' decisions to be represented for the purpose of collective bargaining and the decision for no representation.
- Evaluate decision-making strategies for their effectiveness within diverse workplace environments.
- Evaluate how participation of staff nurses in decision making relates to job satisfaction and improved patient outcomes.
- Analyze the influence of culture on the selection of a governance model or model of care delivery.

TERMS TO KNOW

at-will employee	culture	role model
Centers for Disease Control and Prevention (CDC)	empowerment	shared governance
	followership	subculture
collective action	governance	whistleblower
collective bargaining	mentor	workplace advocacy

THE CHALLENGE

Ann Evans, BSN, RN
Nurse Manager, Medical-Surgical Nursing Services, Garvin
Community Hospital, Garvin, Tennessee

I had previously worked in a large urban hospital system in Knoxville, Tennessee, as a staff nurse. When I moved to Garvin, I took a staff nurse position in medical-surgical nursing at the community hospital and was promoted to nurse manager within the first year. Care on my units was disjointed and ineffective, and patient and nurse satisfaction scores were low. After several months of assessing the unit, I determined that I would like to redesign how care was delivered on the medical-surgical units that I managed. Patient-centered care was a model of care that I was familiar with at the large city hospital where I previously worked but was not a model that had been used at the community hospital.

What do you think you would do if you were this nurse?

INTRODUCTION

The excitement of beginning a career in nursing or assuming the position of a manager is balanced by events taking place in health care and the effect of these events on nursing, nurses, and health systems. The knowledge gained in your profession provides a background for considering issues within health care and factors that promote or inhibit the achievement of professional nursing practice.

Nurses are deeply involved in the complex clinical problems of individuals, families, and communities because nursing practice requires the acquisition, synthesis, and retrieval of knowledge to provide competent nursing care. Having the time and resources to engage in high-level preparation for quality, competent care can be achieved through the collective actions of nurses.

Collective Action

Collective action is defined as activities that are undertaken by a group of people who have common interests. Collective action is a benign phrase; it refers to many aspects of daily life, including work. When parishioners contribute to a mission, that is the result of collective action. When nurses work to achieve Magnet™ status, that is the result of collective action. When patient care is delivered in hospitals 24 hours per day, that is the result of the collective action of shifts of nurses. Collective action aids nurses in advocating for patients, families, and communities in the healthcare and political arenas.

The collective action of nurses requires a level of independence during the shift and interdependence among shifts and with other healthcare professionals.

Nurses learn quickly to rely on their colleagues but have been less comfortable with formal collectives than some other occupational groups. Several factors may contribute to this discomfort. Chief among those factors are gender, career focus, and view of power. Women have had less experience in working and playing within a team structure than have men. Before Title IX (before 1972), few girls participated in competitive team sports. In addition, many women, including nurses, viewed employment as a job rather than a career. For those individuals, the time to work with others to achieve common goals deprived them of personal time.

Women have not always perceived themselves to be powerful, but understanding power and learning how to use it are essential if nurses expect to influence practice and their work environments (Ponte et al., 2007). Nursing has been characterized as an "oppressed group" (Roberts, 2000). The "good" nurse was considered obedient. The Nightingale Pledge reinforced obedience: "With loyalty will I endeavor to aid the physician in his work …" (Dock & Stewart, 1920). This obedience or acquiescence to authority appears to have been transferred to other authority figures, including but not limited to hospital administrators.

Minarik and Catramabone (1998) described four main purposes of collective participation for nurses: (1) to promote the practice of professional nursing, (2) to establish and maintain standards of care, (3) to allocate resources effectively and efficiently, and (4) to create satisfaction and support in the practice environment. Collective action helps define and sustain individual nurses in achieving these purposes. In the absence of collective action, the average individual has limited influence in achieving his or her purpose. Many children learned the strength and value of collective action early in life as siblings banded together to make a request to their parents. The same strategy has probably served in an organization when, together, a group of peers makes a point or pleads a case. Nurses have identified practice concerns and have joined together to bring about change in numerous practice settings.

The strategies for developing networks, developing a collective voice, and cultivating a collective require strong leaders and a broad followership. Leaders and followers have separate and distinct roles. Those roles are complementary—each requires the other. The relationship is interdependent. Followers and leaders also share many characteristics. Successful people move easily between the roles of follower and leader. Though the knowledge and skills of followers may differ from those of the leader, they are not less. Leaders and followers are knowledgeable of the context and content of their practice. Followers are active, involved participants committed to an agreed-upon agenda. They are loyal and supportive to the individual who is setting the pace and the agenda. Good leaders will need good followers to accomplish goals. The nurse who becomes a leader finds that the absence of followers is personally painful.

EXERCISE 19-1

Identify two groups in which you have been a leader (e.g., school, church, sports, clubs, and work). Identify two groups in which you have been a follower. How did your role as a leader differ from your role as a follower? List the skills you used in each role.

Changes in an initiative or an agenda may result in today's leader being tomorrow's follower. The opposite may also be applicable: today's follower may be tomorrow's leader. The change may result from the context of the situation. In the operating room, the surgeon is the acknowledged leader and the anesthesiologist follows that lead with respect to the extent of the anesthesia. If the patient's condition changes, the anesthesiologist becomes the leader and the surgeon may simply step away from the table, an overt act that demonstrates a change in leadership. As healthcare consumers and participants, we salute the clarity.

BOX 19-1   TRAITS OF A GOOD FOLLOWER

- Trustworthy
- Dependable
- Excellent Communicator and Listener
- Team Player
- Courage of Convictions
- Collaborator
- Questioner

From Kouzes, J.M., & Posner, B.Z. (2007). *The leadership challenge* (4th ed.). San Francisco: Jossey-Bass.

Informed followers are not submissive participants blindly following a cultist personality. They are effective group members, not "groupies." They are skilled in group dynamics and accountable for their actions. They are willing and able to question, debate, compromise, collaborate, and act. Box 19-1 lists the traits of a good follower.

Collective action provides a mechanism for achieving professional practice through greater participation in decision making. The governance structure provides the framework for participation. Participation in decision making regarding one's practice is an appropriate expectation for professional nurses, provides for greater autonomy and authority over practice decisions, contributes to supporting the professional nurse, and is a major component of job satisfaction (Kramer et al., 2008; Pittman, 2007). The privilege and the obligation to participate are inherent in the discipline of nursing. Consistent with the *Code of Ethics for Nurses* (American Nurses Association [ANA], 2005), members of the discipline participate based on their competence. Although nurses are expected to be informed, active participants, not all nurses wish to participate in decisions. For these nurses, going to work and doing their assigned job may fulfill their expectations. They may not perceive themselves as being in a subordinate position, or if they do, it is not a concern for them. Their orientation is to serve the care recipient and to be loyal to the organization. For these individuals, asserting the right and responsibility to participate in decisions may be considered disrespectful to the organization's policies and to the physician, or they may be energy-draining. However, for the professional nurse, participation in practice-related decisions is critical to quality patient care, is expected by society, and is essential to autonomy for nursing. Today's healthcare environment demands that nurses exercise the four key historical concepts identified by Lewis and Batey (1982): responsibility, authority, autonomy, and accountability.

Responsibility

The history of nursing provides evidence of nurses accepting responsibility or the "charge to act." Historically, this charge took the form of unquestioningly and meticulously following the physician's orders and hospital procedures. The "good" nurse rendered disclosure at the convenience of the physician and management. Today, healthcare organizations achieving Magnet™ recognition are characterized by the control of nursing practice by nurses (Kramer & Schmalenberg, 2004). Nursing and individual nurses must have the power to control practice. The recognition of credentialing, especially certification, has contributed to the exercise of expert power by nurses.

Authority

Authority based on preparation and experience suggests a departure from the tradition of delegating authority to individual nurses based on the physician's or nurse manager's knowledge of the nurse—knowledge that too often was based on personal characteristics, not clinical competence. That statement does not denigrate the collegial relationship between and among nurses and physicians, relationships that are based on mutual respect and trust. There is evidence that patient care improves when these relationships exist. Authority suggests that nurses use the power of their professional status to act in behalf of the best interest of patients.

Autonomy

Autonomy, the freedom to make independent decisions exceeding the standard nursing practice and that are in the best interest of the patient (Kramer & Schmalenberg, 2004), is critical to the control of nursing practice. To maximize the clinical effectiveness of registered nurses (RNs), they must have autonomy consistent with their scope of practice. Multiple studies demonstrate that a healthcare organization that provides a climate in which nurses have authority and autonomy has better patient outcomes, retains nurses at a higher rate, is more cost-effective, and has evidence of greater patient satisfaction than an organization in which such a climate does not exist (Aiken, Clarke, Sloane, Sochalski, & Silber, 2002; Dunton, Gajewski, Klaus, & Pierson, 2007; Kramer & Schmalenberg, 2004). According to Kennerly (2000), the future depends on designing delivery models and implementing freedom in decision making to create and sustain positive work environments in nursing. Nurse involvement in decision making contributes to higher levels of job satisfaction for the nurse and higher levels of satisfaction with care for the patient and positively influences health outcomes.

Autonomy encourages innovation and increases productivity. A lack of autonomy and advocacy for standards frequently results in organizational silence and marginalization of nurses (Duchscher & Cowin, 2004; Hascup, 2003). Nurse managers have influence in this area of working with staff. Mrayyan (2004) found that nurses in an international study reported that the three most important variables in increasing nurse autonomy were supportive management, education, and experience. Specific managerial actions were defined as elements of interactions with others, especially when conflict was involved. Helping nurses communicate and supporting them in dealing with conflict help nurses describe themselves as having more autonomy. According to the U.S. Department of Health & Human Services (1988):

> Failure on the part of healthcare delivery organizations, physicians, and policy-making bodies to fully recognize the decision-making abilities of RNs has contributed to problems in recruiting and retaining nurses, hindered the development of a career orientation in professional nursing, and limited the efficiency and effectiveness of patient care delivery. (p. vii)

This statement was accurate when written and has become more important as the delivery of and payment for health care evolves and healthcare reform becomes a reality.

Although automobile manufacturing is a highly mechanized process, management has learned that it is cost-effective to give the employee on the shop floor the autonomy to "stop the line" when the potential for error is detected. Stopping errors before they occur is more efficient than recalling items and retrofitting and is more humane than causing injury and perhaps death. Unlocking minds by providing greater autonomy and diversifying tasks decreases fear, specifically fear of ridicule, fear of punishment, and fear of job loss. The Institute for Healthcare Improvement (IHI) (2006) took the concept of change to the nursing unit level with its "Protecting 5 Million Lives from Harm" campaign. By supporting unit-level change without complex organizational structure approvals, change will occur more quickly and efficiently and patients will benefit.

Accountability

Accountability focuses the organization and all its members on the purposes and the outcomes of their collective activities. Accountability requires ownership. Porter-O'Grady and Malloch (2002) assert, "Accountability is always internally generated. It rests first and foremost within" (p. 261). Although Porter-O'Grady and Malloch (2010) make many points about accountability, the following are six critical considerations in shared governance:

- Defined by the person in the role
- Defined by role, not job or task
- Based on outcomes
- Set in advance
- Linked to results
- Has observable processes

The value of process is determined by the extent to which individuals observe a particular protocol while accomplishing a goal. Accountability focuses on the achievement of the specified outcome. This shift in thinking has had a tremendous effect on healthcare reimbursement. An example of the shift is evident in patient education. Initialing a form to indicate that patient teaching has occurred is no longer acceptable. The criteria now expect that the patient's behavior has changed. Porter-O'Grady and Malloch (2002) call this the *Age of Accountability;* work is viewed in terms of outcomes. To achieve positive outcomes within an organization, shared accountability is critical. "When responsible adults refuse to share accountability, it poisons human relationships, corrupts professions, and makes self-esteem impossible" (Kupperschmidt, 2004, p. 115).

> **EXERCISE 19-2**
> Review the American Nurses Association's (ANA) position statement on "Take Action on Safe Staffing" on *www.nursingworld. org.* From the perspective of a staff nurse, how do you feel about your professional organization's call to action regarding safe staffing? As a nurse manager, do you have the same perspective? Why or why not?

GOVERNANCE

Nursing governance is the methodology or system by which a department of nursing controls and directs the formulation and the administration of nursing policy. Organizational structure provides a framework for fulfilling the organization's mission. Organizational charts show the relationship among and between roles. The structure of the organization and the relationship among the components of the structure are influenced by the individuals selected to interpret and implement the organization's philosophy. A particular form of governance evolves from the mission and values of the organization and the relationships among and between its components. Thus managers and leaders who enact the mission and values on a daily basis support nursing more openly. To paraphrase an adage, behavior speaks louder and has more clout than organizational charts.

Nurses have multiple strategies to achieve collective action at their disposal; three prevalent ones are shared governance, workplace advocacy, and collective bargaining. These strategies are not mutually exclusive. As noted, governance is influenced by the context within which the organizational culture is embedded. Often the culture itself dictates the avenue of collective action.

The culture of the geographic area influences the organizational culture and the selected governance structure. For example, in right-to-work states, collective bargaining may be tolerated more than supported by nurses and administration. Although mobility and the mass media have diluted the "purity" of geographic cultures, it is prudent to acknowledge how deeply embedded these cultural influences are within the fabric of American society.

When a subculture is clearly rooted in the mission of the organization (e.g., delivery of quality care in a cost-effective environment), the possibility of genuine negotiation or problem solving is enhanced. A subculture has its own unique and distinctive features, even as other features overlap with those of the larger culture. Members may adhere to values that are specific to their group while espousing values of the larger society. The presence of congruent subcultures supports healthy relationships. Healthy relationships are an important variable in the development of a strong internal governance structure capable of supporting a professional practice environment that works well for everyone involved.

Nurses and administrators are often members of separate subcultures. This phenomenon should not be given a negative connotation. Several factors may increase the distinct ideologies of the two groups, including the existence of a distant corporate structure and the presence of a union. Both factors may be considered external tensions. By tradition, decision making in the United States has been centralized at the top administrative level. There is a tendency to increase the concentration of decision making during economic downturns and the pressures inherent in maintaining a healthy "bottom line." Actions are taken to avoid risk. However, history shows that broader input, not less, is important during these times.

When efforts have been made to address nurses' perceptions about job satisfaction, the relationship between nursing and the top administration of a hospital has been affected. Work environment factors that have a direct impact on nurses' job satisfaction and the ability to influence patient care include supervisory support in patient care decisions and the provision of adequate staffing to provide quality care, positive working relationships with physicians and nurses, and a clear philosophy of nursing; all of these factors are influenced by the relationship between nurses and administration (Cummings et al., 2008; Manojlovich, 2005; Mrayyan, 2004).

EXERCISE 19-3

Identify four factors in your practice (experience) that contribute to job satisfaction. Compare your responses with those of three practicing nurses who are not supervisors and three practicing nurses who are supervisors. Are your factors similar to the responses of others? Are you surprised by the responses?

In the past, nurses experienced practice environments and working conditions controlled by the medical profession and hospital administration. In today's work environment, nurses expect a motivating, satisfying work environment that includes a role in decision making. Many nurses today are unwilling to remain outside the decision-making loop. Work redesign efforts to increase productivity and lower costs have contributed to increased tension regarding the role of nursing and nurses in decision making. Evolving or creating a system that incorporates others in the decision-making process may be difficult for many individuals in upper-management positions. High-performing organizations that provide quality health care create climates that provide for participation by all stakeholders. Each stakeholder shares responsibility and risk, and that requires optimism and trust.

Contractual models allow nurses to form an organization and contract with the healthcare organization to provide nursing services. A contractual model can be characterized as a self-governance model as opposed to shared governance. Nurses become contract providers instead of employees. Historically, nurses were direct contractors as private-duty nurses before becoming hospital employees. Free agency may be the contractual model for the future (Manion, 2000).

Shared Governance

Shared governance is described as a democratic, egalitarian concept; it is a dynamic process resulting from shared decision making and accountability (Porter-O'Grady, 2009). According to Porter-O'Grady, Hawkins, and Parker (1997), basic principles of shared governance include partnerships, equity, accountability, and ownership. It is more accurate to say that shared governance *demands* participation in decision making rather than *provides for* participation. Characteristics of self-governance that empowered nurses were career ladders, access to power, participation in decision making, recognition of accomplishments, and evidence-based practice (Kramer et al., 2008) (see the Research Perspective on p. 378).

Through numerous reports and stories about organizations that have experienced the Magnet™ journey, staff nurses have praised the quality of their

RESEARCH PERSPECTIVE

Resource: Kramer, M., Schmalenberg, C., Maguire, P., Brewer, B. B., Burke, R., Chmielewski, L., Cox, K., Kishner, J., Krugman, M., Meeks-Sjostrom, D., & Waldo, M. (2008). Structures and practices enabling staff nurses to control their practice. *Western Journal of Nursing Research, 30*(5), 539-559.

This research study used interviews, participant observations, and the CWEQII empowerment questionnaire to examine the characteristics and components of self-governance structures that enabled nurses to control their practice (control over nursing practice [CNP]). The strategic sampling of eight study hospitals all had Magnet™ designation resulting in high CNP scoring. The characteristics that enabled the high CNP scoring, based on both quantitative and qualitative data, were structural components of self-governance and career ladders, as well as the attributes of access to power, participation, recognition, accomplishments, and evidence-based practice initiatives. Findings suggest that self-governance structures are effective in enabling nurses to have control over their practice regarding issues of importance to the nurse, the patient, and the organization.

Implications for Practice

Nurse managers should include nurses in decision making regarding issues pertaining to the role of the nurse and the quality and safety of patients. Managers should support and encourage nurses to participate actively in unit and department councils and should recognize accomplishments and achievements of staff.

---

direct involvement through shared governance. In addition, nurses favor work and learning (consistent with the Institute of Medicine [IOM] report [2003]) that is interdisciplinary and patient focused.

Some organizations mislabel their governance structures. Although structures may be called "shared governance," they possess few of the characteristics outlined by those who are recognized as experts on the topic. In addition, many organizations have developed thinly veiled mechanisms designed to preclude nurses from participating in collective action. In today's competitive environment, it is critical that nurses are informed of potential implications of various approaches. Professional-practice climates recognize individual and team performance. Increasingly, nurses are seeking organizations that provide professional-practice climates, ones that have effective activities, not just effective documents. Thus, when filling any new, non-entry position, it is wise to include nurses within the organization among those being considered.

Workplace Advocacy

Workplace advocacy is an umbrella term encompassing activities within the practice setting. The choice of advocacy to reflect the framework in which nurses control the practice of nursing is consistent with the goals of the profession. Workplace advocacy includes an array of activities undertaken to address the challenges faced by nurses in their practice settings. The focus of these activities is on career development, employment opportunities, terms and conditions of employment, employment rights and protections, control of practice, labor-management relations, occupational health and safety, and employee assistance. The objective of workplace advocacy is to equip nurses to practice in a rapidly changing environment. Advocacy occurs within a framework of mutuality, facilitation, protection, and coordination.

Gadow's (1990) historic discussion of the manifestations of advocacy is relevant to a discussion of today's workplace advocacy. These manifestations include (1) ensuring relevant information, (2) enabling the selection of information, (3) disclosing a personal view, (4) providing support for making and implementing decisions, and (5) helping determine personal values.

Ensuring Relevant Information

Nurses must have relevant information to support their practice. Access to information is the basis for initiatives, full participation, and sharing information. Clinical nursing practice demands that nurses begin with patient information. The use of clinical data is necessary for patient well-being. However, patient information is the beginning of data gathering, not the end. It is equally important for nurses to have information related to how decisions are made for determining nurse staffing, occupational health and safety issues, equal employment opportunity information, professional liability, and labor law information.

Enabling the Selection of Information

Just as healthcare patients must have relevant information to make good decisions, nurses must be able to select information that is relevant to their practice. Nurses have an obligation to know about the organization in which they work. A good way to begin is by learning the mission of the organization and becoming knowledgeable of the culture. Becoming acquainted with nurses who practice in the organization is important. The time and effort devoted to this will be well spent. Many nurses and other individuals spend more time making decisions about the cars they drive than about a potential employment site. Think about a time when you were deciding about a car. You probably checked various makes and models and determined price; you may have visited a website or visited the dealership; you may have visited the service department and talked with those who had purchased a car from the dealership; you may have, literally or figuratively, kicked the tires. A similar process is appropriate in selecting a place of employment. Data regarding the workplace inform nurses of the history of the workplace and help them make decisions about employment.

Disclosing a Personal View

Nurses and managers must disclose their views on issues related to the work environment. Disclosure of management's perspective is important. The failure to build a trusting relationship jeopardizes the achievement of outcomes. Similarly, when nurses do not disclose their perspective, the relationship is at risk.

Risk takes many forms. For example, healthcare organizations constitute one of the most unsafe work environments in the United States. Violence toward healthcare personnel continues to increase. Risk is greater in emergency departments and psychiatric settings. Evidence reveals that many incidents are not reported. Identified toxins in the workplace are also a risk factor. Latex is a particular problem. Disinfectants, sterilants, antineoplastic agents, radiation, and noise are constants. The organization has a responsibility to ensure a safe environment for staff and patients. Nurses need to be involved in addressing workplace safety by voicing their concerns. Occupational health nurses provide expert consultation in the identification of potential hazards and suggestions for change, yet many healthcare organizations do not seek such experts. Box 19-2 describes two key sources of environmental support.

Providing Support for Making and Implementing Decisions

The support needed to make and implement decisions is achieved through role models, mentors, and empowerment. Role models may include the nurse

BOX 19-2   SAFETY IN THE WORKPLACE

The **Occupational Safety and Health Act** of 1970 requires employers to provide a safe and healthy environment. Fire protection, construction, maintenance of equipment, worker training, machine guarding, and protective equipment are specified. Employers are required to familiarize themselves with applicable standards.

The **Centers for Disease Control and Prevention (CDC)** guidelines assume that all patients are infectious for human immunodeficiency virus (HIV) and other bloodborne pathogens. Although the CDC is not an enforcement agency, its guidelines are adopted as professional practice standards.

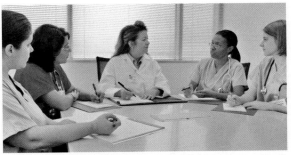

The support needed to make and implement decisions is achieved through role models, mentors, and empowerment.

who has excellent clinical skills in assessment. Similarly, observing someone who is skilled in assertive communication, transforming an explosive situation into a positive interaction, is impressive. The implementation of a primary mentorship program for nurses may contribute to the development of these and other skills. Mentoring is a unique dynamic relationship between two individuals, usually in a professional setting (Pinkerton, 2003). A mentoring relationship is an ongoing "hands-on" process. Individuals who have experienced a successful mentorship have identified positive, frequently occurring behaviors that characterized their mentor. These behaviors include trust and the opportunity to make decisions that derive from that trust. The value to the individual is professional growth (Restifo & Yoder, 2004). The value to the organization is in the outcome: the individual will make better decisions that will well serve the organization, the nurse, and the patient.

EXERCISE 19-4

List the characteristics that you would want a mentor to possess. If you have identified a person you would want as a mentor, ask if he or she is willing to mentor you. Identify factors that are contributors and barriers to your seeking a mentorship relationship with the individual. Consider ways that you can address these factors.

RESEARCH PERSPECTIVE

Resource: Armstrong, K., Laschinger, H., & Wong, C. (2009). Workplace empowerment and Magnet hospital characteristics as predictors of patient safety climate. *Journal of Nursing Care Quality, 24*(1), 55-62.

This study was conducted to examine the variables of workplace empowerment and Magnet™ hospital characteristics as predictors of patient safety climate. The framework used to guide the study was Kanter's theoretical model of workplace empowerment in nursing that has linked empowerment in nursing to control over practice, job satisfaction, work productivity, burnout, and organizational commitment. Three hundred randomly selected registered nurses employed in acute care hospital organizations were surveyed about conditions of work effectiveness, practice environment, and safety climate. Results showed moderate to strong correlations between empowerment and Magnet™ hospital characteristics, empowerment and patient safety climate, and Magnet™ characteristics and patient safety climate. The findings support the Kanter theoretical model of workplace empowerment in nursing and suggest that nurses who feel empowered in their workplace will perceive the patient safety climate as positive.

Implications for Practice

Nurses who feel empowered to make decisions and implement patient care strategies may feel that the care environment on the unit is safer and more effective and have higher ratings of job satisfaction. Nurse managers should support nurses to make decisions over their practice and include nursing staff in unit-based plans and activities that affect the work and practice environment.

Empowerment, or supporting other nurses, is a complex process. Nurses generally want to work hard, continue to learn, perform well, and be involved in the decision-making process. Managers and administrators who support these efforts are empowering nurses and enhancing professionalism and autonomy. An example of empowering nurses involves the act of documenting an unsafe assignment. Accepting an unsafe assignment or refusing an assignment is difficult for nurses—both those nurses at the beginning of their careers and those who are experienced. Critical elements to note are date, unit, assignment, staff available, rationale for objections, and documentation of notification of supervisor. Accurate, concise, and clear documentation can assist the nurse manager by providing a source of data necessary to support the preparation of their budgets and to support the documenters of such occurrences. Many assignments are classified as unsafe because of a lack of personnel and a lack of training of the existing personnel; therefore nurses need to be prepared to respond when an assignment is inappropriate (see the Research Perspective at right).

Empowering nurses is important. Powerless nurses feel more depersonalization in the work environment and are less satisfied with their jobs (Laschinger, Finegan, Shamian, & Wilk, 2004; Leiter & Laschinger, 2006). Manojlovich (2007) states that nurses' power develops from an organizational structure that promotes empowerment, a psychological conviction in the ability to be empowered and the acknowledgement that power is present in the relationships and the caring that nurses provide.

Helping Determine Personal Values

Professional values evolve through education in classroom settings, clinical assignments, and interactions with other nurses. "Professional values are beliefs and ideologies that are generally held in common by members of the profession and are used to guide professional practice" (Chinn & Kramer, 2008, p.49). Nurses have an opportunity to solidify their own values as skilled mentors guide practice and assist more novice nurses to engage in value clarification. Inherent in professional values are ethical codes, standards of practice, standards for protecting participants, and a willingness to challenge social traditions, cultural mores, and priorities for allocating resources (Chinn & Kramer, 2008).

Determining personal values increases an individual's value to an organization because the individual is then empowered to make decisions within his or her scope of practice. This situation is both simple and complex. Empowerment requires redefining the managerial role and a change in behavior by nurses and administrators. The behavior change is one in which trust replaces distrust and respect replaces disrespect. How will the beginning nurse determine individual values within various types of decisions if there are inadequate guided opportunities to practice decision making?

Organizational patterns may segment the responsibility for the provision of care and the management of resources for that care. It is in the best interest of healthcare consumers for nurses to participate in decisions regarding the provision of care and resources. The involvement of nurses can vary from none whatsoever to a high degree of input by nurses in virtually every decision affecting the conditions of employment and their practice. Nurses must be prepared and willing to participate.

EXERCISE 19-5

Identify three factors that you consider most empowering in a governance model. Would the presence of one or more of these factors influence you to practice in such an environment? Identify three factors that you would consider least empowering in a governance model. Would the presence of one or more of these factors influence you to avoid practicing in this environment?

Collective Bargaining

Collective bargaining is the performance of the mutual obligation of the employer and representatives of the employees to meet at reasonable times and confer in good faith with respect to wages, hours, and other terms and conditions of employment or the negotiation of any agreement or any question arising from those terms and conditions. The purpose of collective bargaining or unionization by nurses (Box 19-3) is to secure reasonable and satisfactory conditions of employment, including the right to participate in decisions regarding their practice. Although it is possible to bargain collectively without a union, the union model is commonly used.

Changes in labor law have had a direct impact on the level of union activity in the healthcare sector. The federal role in labor relations is a dynamic, evolving one. The 1935 Wagner Act (National Labor Relations Act) established election procedures for employees to be able to choose their collective bargaining representatives freely. Two years later, the ANA included provisions for improving nurses' work and professional lives. The 1947 Taft-Hartley Act placed curbs on some union activity and excluded employees of not-for-

---

BOX 19-3   UNIONIZATION

In non-healthcare industries, unionization is acknowledged as a usual and expected business practice. Improved communication and goodwill cannot eliminate the gap between labor and management. Cooperation between management and labor will remain an illusion unless or until there is sharing of responsibility, power, and profits (Levitan & Johnson, 1983). If cooperation and trust exist between the union and the company, the members of the union will understand when the company is experiencing financial difficulties and management will understand when members of the union experience difficulties. In 1996, the Malden Mills continued to assist employees from company funds when the company could not produce popular Polartec items because of a fire. In 2001, unions representing 1200 workers voted to accept a reduction in pay and benefits in an effort to keep Freightliner in Portland, Oregon (Hunsberger, 2001).

Heckscher (1996) suggests that the union model is outdated because of trends that have made the public-policy framework of unionization less useful. In nursing, Porter-O'Grady (2001) takes a much different perspective: "The union isn't the enemy; it's a new reality for nurse leaders." He suggests that, through partnering, the formal requirements of the union contract "advances the practice of managing well and maintains the foundation of good management" (p. 32). Union activity in nursing and in health care has grown in the past 20 years and has been stimulated by healthcare reorganization, work redesign, and changes in patient care delivery models. Some of the major issues that have led to increased union activity in nursing are as follows:

- Lack of professional autonomy and professional practice models
- Inadequate staffing and unqualified caregivers
- The absence of procedures for the reporting of unsafe work environments and poor quality care
- Mandatory overtime and work overload
- Low wages and poor benefits

---

profit hospitals from coverage. The Labor Management Reporting and Disclosure Act of 1959, the Landrum-Griffin Act, provides greater internal democracy within unions. The 1974 amendments to the Taft-Hartley Act removed the exemption of not-for-profit hospitals, and employees of these types of organizations have the same rights as industrial workers to join together and form labor unions. The removal of the exemption for not-for-profit hospitals created a frenzy of activity as traditional industrial unions targeted healthcare facilities. The National Labor Relations Board (NLRB) administers the National Labor Relations Act. State laws further define labor law.

Why is there an increase in organizing nurses and other healthcare professionals? Health care is a "hot" topic at the state and federal levels. Pittman (2007) found that nurses, both represented by collective bargaining and not represented, were generally satisfied with their work, but represented nurses were more satisfied with regard to compensation (see the Literature Perspective below). The morning newspaper, nightly news, and a continuous parade of news magazines have featured countless articles related to health and illness. One may paraphrase Willie Sutton when he was asked why he robbed banks: "That is where the money is." Why organize nurses and other healthcare workers? Because that is where potential members are.

As technology replaces unskilled workers, a smaller pool of workers is available for trade-union organizing. Declining union membership has been the catalyst for unions to explore other membership bases. In 2007, the number of wage and salary workers belonging to a union rose to 15.7 million (U.S. Bureau of Labor Statistics, 2009). Union members accounted for only 12.1% of employed wage and salary workers, essentially unchanged from 12.0% in 2006. With numerous groups seeking to represent nurses, nurses seeking collective bargaining should carefully consider the representing agent. (See Box 19-4 for suggested screening criteria.)

Traditional industrial unions are increasingly seeking opportunities to represent nurses for the purpose of collective bargaining and to speak for nursing with boards of nursing, regulatory agencies, and legislatures. Organizing nurses and other healthcare workers for the purpose of collective bargaining is very attractive because of the large numbers of people involved and the decrease in organizing in other sectors. In addition, nurses and other healthcare workers have a low rate of unionization. In 2006, only 10% of workers in health care were members of unions, compared with 13% for all other industries (U.S. Bureau of Labor Statistics, 2009), and the nursing profession is viewed as a prime target for membership growth. The United American Nurses (UAN) estimates that approximately 20% of nurses are represented by a collective bargaining unit (UAN, 2009).

Historically, nurses were reluctant to be identified with unions; however, that view has changed. Working together in a cooperative, collaborative manner is important for the safety and quality of care, especially when strain occurs between management and nurses. Nurses have a legal right to bargain. The American Hospital Association has spent millions of dollars

 ## LITERATURE PERSPECTIVE

Resource: Pittman, J. (2007). Registered nurse job satisfaction and collective bargaining unit membership status. *Journal of Nursing Administration, 37*(10), 471-476.

This study examined the differences in job satisfaction between registered nurses who were members of a nursing collective bargaining unit and nurses who were not. This study was a descriptive secondary analysis of data from the Minnesota Registered Nurse Workforce Study that included a stratified sample of 3645 registered nurses. Overall, all nurses reported high levels of job satisfaction. The study found that nurses in collective bargaining units were significantly more satisfied with wages than were non–collective bargaining unit nurses, but non–collective bargaining unit nurses were significantly more satisfied with the image of nursing, professional relationships, work activity and setting, supervision, and patient care. The study demonstrated that nurses who were members of collective bargaining units had an overall lower level of job satisfaction than non-member nurses.

Implications for Practice
Nurse managers in organizations that are unionized and in organizations that are not must be aware of issues that affect job satisfaction in nursing staff and employ strategies that allow nurses to participate in implementation of the practice and work environment concerns. Nurses are more satisfied with their work setting when included in decision making regarding issues pertaining to the role of the nurse and the quality and safety of patients. Managers should serve as professional role models for their staff.

BOX 19-4	SUGGESTED CRITERIA FOR SELECTING A BARGAINING UNIT

- A strong commitment to nursing practice, legislation, regulation, and education
- A well-prepared practice, policy, and labor staff; a minimum of a bachelor's degree in nursing
- Representative of those the bargaining unit represents in both gender and ethnic makeup
- National scope and local implementation
- Control by individual members over bargaining unit activities

challenging the appropriateness of all-RN bargaining units or a unit separate from other organized employees. In a 1991 unanimous opinion, the U.S. Supreme Court upheld the NLRB's ruling that provides for RN-only units. This decision was critical for nursing. At stake was the ability of nurses to control nursing practice and the quality of patient care. Employees, including nurses, must be accorded workplace rights and the protection that allows them to practice. Nurses must have the freedom to do what the profession and their licensure status require them to do.

Labeling all RNs as supervisors is a second challenge to the right of nurses to organize. RNs monitor and assess patients as a part of their professional practice, not as a statutory supervisor within the definition of the National Labor Relations Act. A 1996 NLRB ruling held that RNs were not statutory supervisors and were protected by federal labor law; the decision was upheld in 1997 by the U.S. Court of Appeals for the Ninth Circuit (Nguyen, 1997). However, a 2001 Supreme Court decision (*National Labor Relations Board v. Kentucky River Community Care, Inc.*, 2001) upheld a lower court's decision to classify RNs as supervisors, though this decision was later appealed.

Nurses as Knowledge Workers

The change from producing a product to providing a service has many implications for management and labor. In the past, employees in manufacturing were treated like interchangeable cogs: when a cog was broken, it was replaced. A large pool of unskilled workers was available to step forward in the steel mill, the coal mine, and the shop floor. The move from an industrial model in society requires a "knowledge worker." The unskilled worker of yesterday did not have a high school diploma. Today, knowledge workers may have multiple college degrees and certifications. When knowledge workers unionize, they develop organizations that are more similar to associations than traditional industrial unions. They become involved in activities such as lobbying and coalition building. Today's nurses are knowledge workers. The tools of knowledge workers differ from those of the workers of the past. As the knowledge content of the work increases, the practice of the worker (nurse) is guided more by science than by procedure. Nurses may ask, "Why be represented for collective bargaining?" A collective bargaining contract requires management to bargain, a requirement not present in noncontract organizations. Several factors influence nurses to seek collective bargaining, such as (1) working conditions, including mandatory overtime, nurse-patient ratios, and limited opportunities to participate in decision-making; and (2) the successes that have been achieved by nurses in other healthcare organizations. In addition, many nurses identify the lack of good communication and a decrease in the quality of care as major factors in their decision to seek representation for the purposes of collective bargaining (Budd, Warino, & Patton, 2004).

Union or At-Will

The fear of arbitrary discipline and dismissal may be the catalyst for nurses to seek ways to protect themselves from what are perceived to be arbitrary actions. Nurses are seeking assistance from external sources in an effort to balance the assistance available to the organization's administrative personnel. A collective bargaining contract typically alters a balance of power. The discipline structure provided by contract treats all employees in the same manner and may decrease the manager's flexibility in designing or selecting discipline. Although there is whistleblower legislation (Box 19-5), the current environment in health care places the at-will employee who voices concern about the quality of care in a vulnerable position. Managers of at-will employees have greater latitude in selecting disciplinary measures for specific infractions. State and federal laws do provide a level of protection; however, an at-will employee may be terminated at

---

BOX 19-5 WHISTLEBLOWER PROTECTION

Whistleblowing "*refers to a warning issued by a current or former employee of an* organization to the public about a serious wrongdoing or danger created or concealed within the organization" (Hunt, 1995, p. 155). The 1989 Whistleblower Protection Act protects federal workers. The law does not cover the private sector. Some states have specific laws. It is imperative that the whistleblower understand the consequences of action, and inaction, as the shield is an imperfect one (Solomon, 2004). Whistleblowing is often a result and symptom of organizational failure (Fletcher, Sorrell, & Silva, 1998).

any time for any reason except discrimination. At-will employees, in essence, work at the will of the employer. An at-will "employee can be terminated … for any reason as long as the reason is not unlawful" (Wright, 2004, p. 17). It is critical for nurses to know their rights regarding discipline and termination (Smith, 2002).

Union contract language requires management to follow "due process" for represented employees. That is, management must provide a written statement outlining disciplinary charges, the penalty, and the reasons for the penalty. Management is required to maintain a record of attempts to counsel the employee. Employees have the right to defend themselves against charges and the opportunity to settle disagreements in a formal grievance hearing. They have the right to have their representative with them during the process. Management must prove that the employee is wrong or in error. Management maintains the record of counseling. The commitment to nursing requires the manager to be clear about the charge. Although all disciplinary charges are important, those directly related to patient care have a more critical dimension. Clarity in describing the situation is important because it affects patient care, the individual nurse, and nurse colleagues. In a non-union environment, the burden of proof is generally on the employee.

Many nurses continue to be intimidated by those individuals who charge that "unions are unprofessional." A labor contract, a collective bargaining agreement/union contract, is unrelated to being professional. Sociologists have characterized the responsibilities of the professional as a respect for the duty to perform, respect for the duty to learn, respect for the public interest, and preservation and enhancement of the image (Moore, 1970). Many physicians and many faculty members have collective bargaining contracts. Why? They want to have greater control of their practice, improve working conditions, and influence their compensation. Contracts are a usual part of our current environment. It is ironic that a contract between an employer and employee is considered unusual. Replacing the adversarial system should be the goal of efforts to redesign the workplace. A new social order in the workplace must be based on a spirit of genuine cooperation between management and nurses.

Selecting a Bargaining Agent

The ANA represents the interests of the profession, nurses, and health care at the state, federal, and international levels. In 1999, the House of Delegates of the ANA created the UAN to ensure that nurses had a meaningful access to collective bargaining. In less than 10 years the ANA and UAN terminated their agreement, and the UAN became a freestanding organization. In 2009, the UAN joined other nursing unions to form the National Nurses United (NNU). The collective bargaining program of the UAN, an affiliate of the AFL/CIO, is designed to implement strategies that maintain or attain improvement in nursing practice in addition to addressing the economic issues. Also, nurses may be represented by more traditional unions, including the Service Employees International Union; the American Federation of State, County and Municipal Employees; and the American Federation of Teachers.

EXERCISE 19-6

If you practice in a setting with a collective bargaining agreement, secure a copy. Identify the articles of this contract. Are they practice issues or economic issues? What is the relationship between the two? If you work in a setting that does not have a collective bargaining agreement, secure dispute resolution policies. Identify the areas that may be disputed. Are they practice issues or economic issues? What is the relationship between the two?

Not all nurses are eligible to participate in collective bargaining. The nurse who is a statutory supervisor is excluded. Statutory supervisors are those nurses who have the authority to act in the interest of the employer, including the power to hire, terminate, reward, and discipline. These functions are stipulated in the statute (the law). These acts differ from those of nonsupervisory nurses, who act in the interest of the patient. Supervisory nurses share a concern for working conditions, practice standards, and the care delivery environment with nonsupervisory nurses. Many supervisory nurses may think that they are unnecessarily placed in an adversarial relationship with nonsupervisory nurses in the hospital who are represented by the union.

CONCLUSION

Nurses practice in multiple settings; some have collective bargaining (union) contracts, and others do not. Collective bargaining and non–collective bargaining environments espouse safe, quality care. Both environments exist within the context of state and federal laws. Professional practice models may exist in both environments. Nurses may feel valued in both environments, but there is a critical difference. A contract requires the employer to negotiate within a legally binding framework. Non–collective bargaining environments do not provide that structure.

The future may hold new relationships, and public policy may continue to include provisions that were formally negotiated through contracts. Nurses practice in highly competitive environments. Decision making is at the core of nursing practice. Nurse involvement in decision making contributes to higher levels of job satisfaction for the nurse and higher satisfaction with care for the patient, and it also has a positive influence on health outcomes. Nurses and those they serve benefit from collective action that uses a wide range of strategies.

THE SOLUTION

When planning any new change, and particularly a major change, it is important to always include all of the stakeholders in the planning process. All of the staff on the unit, and particularly the nurses, needed to have a voice in the decision-making and planning process for a change in the care delivery system on the units that would affect all of them and the patients on the service. I opened up the discussion about changing the care delivery system on the units at numerous meetings and elicited input from all of the nurses and other staff about their feelings and concerns and ideas regarding the change. I then formed several task forces to develop ideas on the assessment, planning, implementation, and evaluation of a patient-centered care delivery system. I believe that the only way to effectively implement any new idea is to include everyone in the decision-making, planning, and change processes.

—*Ann Evans*

Would this be a suitable approach for you? Why?

THE EVIDENCE

- Collective action by nurses in organizations that seek Magnet™ designation has been demonstrated effectively.
- Nurses involved in collective action in organizations in which unions are present describe their gains as positive and their losses as minimal.
- Nurses who experience a sense of empowerment in the workplace perceive those organizations as providing safer care.

NEED TO KNOW NOW

- Validate if the organization has a collective bargaining agreement.
- Know your individual rights as a registered nurse.
- Seek clarity from the state law and rules and regulations governing nursing about whistleblower protection.

CHAPTER CHECKLIST

Collectively, nurses possess the knowledge, skills, abilities, and numbers to influence decisions. Collective action may take many forms. Geographic and organizational contexts influence the formal and informal structures in which nurses participate. An organization's structure establishes the parameters for participation in decision making. Managers establish the context for participation. The decision to organize for the purpose of collective bargaining is important for nurses and for the organization in which they practice. A level of tension exists when an external group becomes a part of an organization's decision-making processes. External groups may enter as a new management consultant, as a part of a merger, as a new owner, or as a union representing registered nurses. The acceptance and appreciation of the external group are influenced by understanding the rationale for the group's entry and by the respect between the constituencies.

- The purposes of collective participation by nurses are to do the following:
  - Promote the practice of professional nursing
  - Establish and maintain standards of care
  - Allocate resources effectively and efficiently
  - Create satisfaction and support in the practice environment
- Increased autonomy and diversification decrease the following:
  - Fear of ridicule
  - Fear of punishment
  - Fear of job loss
- Governance strategies dictate levels of participation. The type and level of participation in decision making influence job satisfaction.

- Shared governance is characterized by partnerships, equity, accountability, and ownership.
- The framework for advocacy includes mutuality, facilitation, protection, and coordination. The manifestations of advocacy are as follows:
  - Ensuring relevant information
  - Enabling the selection of information
  - Disclosing a personal view
  - Providing support for making and implementing decisions
  - Helping determine personal values
- The goal of workplace advocacy is to equip nurses to practice in a rapidly changing environment.
- Collective bargaining is an effective, legal mechanism used by nurses to obtain the right to participate in decisions regarding their practice.
- Represented nurses are supported by the resources of the union. Unrepresented nurses do not have these resources.
- Representation for the purpose of collective bargaining (belonging to a union) is neither professional nor unprofessional.
- Nurses who are statutory supervisors are excluded from representation.

TIPS FOR COLLECTIVE ACTION

- Staff nurses and managers both need to be cognizant of the issues related to collective action and collective bargaining for both the individuals involved and the organization.
- Some states have laws that are more supportive of whistleblowing than others.
- Nurses interested in collective bargaining at their organizations need to be fully aware of what each union organization brings to the bargaining table

and how aware each union organization may or may not be of workplace issues for nurses.
- An understanding of the culture and the organization's approach to any collective action strategy is important for managers and staff.
- Where collective bargaining is the appropriate strategy, develop criteria for the selection of the appropriate collective bargaining agent.

REFERENCES

American Nurses Association (ANA). (2005). *The code of ethics for nurses with interpretive statements.* Washington, DC: Author.

Aiken, L. H., Clarke, S. P., Sloane, D. M., Sochalski, J., & Silber, J. H. (2002). Hospital nursing staffing and patient mortality, nurse burnout and job dissatisfaction. *Journal of American Medical Association, 288*, 1987-1993.

Armstrong, K., Laschinger, H., & Wong, C. (2009). Workplace empowerment and Magnet hospital characteristics as predictors of patient safety climate. *Journal of Nursing Care Quality, 24*(1), 55-62.

Budd, K. W., Warino, L. S., & Patton, M. E. (2004). Traditional and non-traditional collective bargaining: Strategies to improve the patient care environment. *Online Journal of Issues in Nursing, 9*(1). Retrieved October 1, 2009, from www.nursingworld.org/MainMenuCategories/ANAMarketplace/ANAPeriodicals/OJIN/TableofContents/Volume92004/No1Jan04/CollectiveBargainingStrategies.aspx.

Chinn, P., & Kramer, M. (2008). *Integrated theory and knowledge development in nursing* (7th ed.). St. Louis: Mosby.

Cummings, G. G., Olson, K., Hayduk, L., Bakker, D., Fitch, M., Green, E., Butler, L., & Conlon, M. (2008). The relationship between nursing leadership and nurses' job satisfaction in Canadian oncology work environments. *Journal of Nursing Management, 16*, 508-518.

Dock, L., & Stewart, A. (1920). *A short history of nursing.* New York: Putnam & Sons.

Duchscher, J., & Cowin, L. (2004). The experience of marginalization in new nursing graduates. *Nursing Outlook, 52*(6), 289-296.

Dunton, N., Gajewski, B., Klaus, S., & Pierson, B. (2007). The relationship of nursing workforce characteristics to patient outcomes. *OJIN: The Online Journal of Issues in Nursing, 12*(3). Retrieved December 12, 2008, from www.medscape.com/viewarticle/569394.

Fletcher, J., Sorrell, J., & Silva, M. (1998). Whistleblowing as a failure of organizational ethics. *Online Journal of Issues in Nursing, 3.* Retrieved September 30, 2009, from http://medscapenursing.com/viewarticle.

Gadow, S. (1990). Existential advocacy: Philosophic foundations of nursing. In T. Pence & J. Cantrell (Eds.), *Ethics in nursing: An anthology.* New York: NLN.

Hascup, V. (2003). Organizational silence: The threat to nurse empowerment. *Journal of Nursing Administration, 33*(11), 562-563.

Heckscher, D. (1996). *The new unionism: Employee involvement in the changing corporation.* Cornell University Press.

Hunsberger, G. (October 1, 2001). *Freightliner union approves reduced pay.* The Oregonian.

Hunt, G. (1995). *Whistleblowing in the health service: Accountability, law and professional practice.* London: Edward Arnold.

Institute for Healthcare Improvement (IHI). (2006). Protecting 5 million lives from harm. Retrieved December 20, 2008, from www.ihi.org/IHI/Programs/Campaign/Campaign.htm.

Institute of Medicine (IOM). (2003). *Health professions education: A bridge to quality.* Washington, DC: The National Academies.

Kennerly, S. (2000). Perceived worker autonomy: The foundation for shared governance. *Journal of Nursing Administration, 30*(12), 611-617.

Kramer, M., & Schmalenberg, C. (2004). Development and evaluation of essentials of Magnetism tool. *Journal of Nursing Administration, 34*(7/8), 365-378.

Kramer, M., Schmalenberg, C., Maguire, P., Brewer, B. B., Burke, R., Chmielewski, L., Cox, K., Kishner, J., Krugman, M., Meeks-Sjostrom, D., & Waldo, M. (2008). Structures and practices enabling staff nurses to control their practice. *Western Journal of Nursing Research, 30*(5), 539-559.

Kupperschmidt, B. R. (2004). Making a case for shared accountability. *Journal of Nursing Administration, 34*(3), 114-116.

Laschinger, H. K. S., Finegan, J., Shamian, J., & Wilk, P. (2004). A longitudinal analysis of the impact of workplace empowerment on work satisfaction. *Journal of Organizational Behavior, 25*(1), 527-545.

Levitan, S. & Johnson, C. (1983). Labor and management: The illusion of cooperation. *Harvard Business Review. 61,* 8-16.

Leiter, M. P., & Laschinger, H. K. S. (2006). Relationships of work and practice environment to professional burnout. *Nursing Research, 55*(2), 137-146.

Lewis, F., & Batey, M. (1982). Clarifying autonomy and accountability in nursing service, Part 2. *Journal of Nursing Administration, 12*(10), 10-15.

Manion, J. (2000). Emergence of the free agent nurse workforce. *Nursing Administration Quarterly, 26*(5), 68-78.

Manojlovich, M. (2005). The effect of nursing leadership on hospital nurses' professional practice behaviors. *Journal of Nursing Administration, 35*(7/8), 363-371.

Manojlovich, M. (2007). Power and empowerment in nursing: Looking backward to inform the future. *OJIN: Online Journal of Issues in Nursing, 12*(1). Retrieved October 1, 2009, from www.nursingworld.org/MainMenuCategories/ANAMarketplace/ANAPeriodicals/OJIN/TableofContents/Volume122007/No1Jan07/LookingBackwardtoInformtheFuture.aspx.

Minarik, P., & Catramabone, C. (1998). Collective participation in workforce decision-making. In D. Mason, D. Talbot, & J. Leavitt (Eds.), *Policy and politics for nurses: Action and change in the workplace, government, organizations and community* (3rd ed.). Philadelphia: Saunders.

Moore, W. (1970). *The professions: Roles and rules.* New York: Russell Sage Foundation.

Mrayyan, M. T. (2004). Nurses' autonomy: Influence of nurse managers' actions. *Journal of Advanced Nursing, 45*(3), 326-336.

National Labor Relations Board v. Kentucky River Community Care, Inc., 121 S. Ct. 1861; No. 99-1815 (Argued February 21, 2001; decided May 29, 2001).

Nguyen, B. (1997). Long-awaited Providence ruling upholds right of charge nurses to bargain. *The American Nurse, 29,* 1, 14.

Pinkerton, S. E. (2003). Mentoring new graduates. *Nursing Economic$, 21*(4), 202-203.

Pittman, J. (2007). Registered nurse job satisfaction and collective bargaining unit membership status. *Journal of Nursing Administration, 37*(10), 471-476.

Ponte, P. R., Glazer, G., Dann, E., McCollum, K., Gross, A., Tyrrell, R., Branowicki, P., Noga, P., Winfrey, M., Cooley, M., Saint-Eloi, S., Hayes, C., Nicolas, P. K., & Washington, D. (2007). The power of professional nursing practice: An essential element of patient and family-centered care. *OJIN: The Online Journal of Issues in Nursing, 12*(1). Retrieved January 5, 2009, from www.medscape.com/viewarticle/553405.

Porter-O'Grady, T. (2001). Collective bargaining: The union as partner. *Nursing Management, 32,* 30-32.

Porter-O'Grady, T. (2009). *Interdisciplinary shared governance: Integrating practice, transforming health care* (2nd ed.). Boston: Jones & Bartlett Publishers.

Porter-O'Grady, T., Hawkins, M., & Parker, M. (1997). *Whole systems shared governance: Architecture for integration.* Gaithersburg, MD: Aspen.

Porter-O'Grady, T., & Malloch, K. (2002). *Quantum leadership: A textbook of new leadership.* Gaithersburg, MD: Aspen.

Porter-O'Grady, T., & Malloch, K. (2010). *Innovation leadership: Creating the landscape of healthcare.* Boston: Jones & Bartlett.

Restifo, R., & Yoder, L. (2004). Partnership: Making the most of mentoring. *Nurseweek, 4,* 30-33.

Roberts, S. J. (2000). Development of a positive professional identity: Liberating oneself from the oppressor within. *Advances in Nursing Science, 22*(4), 71-82.

Smith, M. (2002). Protect your facility and staff with effective discipline and termination. *Nursing Management, 33*(7), 15-16.

Solomon, D. (October 4, 2004). Risk Management: For financial whistle-blowers, new shield is an imperfect one. *The Wall Street Journal.*

United American Nurses (UAN). (2009). The RN union difference. Retrieved October 1, 2009, from www.uannurse.org/organize/organize.html.

U.S. Bureau of Labor Statistics. (2009). Union members summary. Retrieved October 1, 2009, from www.bls.gov/news.release/union2.nr0.htm.

U.S. Department of Health & Human Services. (1988). *Secretary's commission on nursing: Final report.* Washington, DC: U.S. Government Printing Office.

Wright, L. (2004). Employer-employee dynamics for nurses. *The American Nurse, 36*(6), 17.

SUGGESTED READINGS

Budd, K. W., Warino, L. S., & Patton, M. E. (2004). Traditional and non-traditional collective bargaining: Strategies to improve the patient care environment. *Online Journal of Issues in Nursing, 9*(1). Retrieved October 1, 2009, from www.nursingworld.org/MainMenuCategories/ANAMarketplace/ANAPeriodicals/OJIN/TableofContents/Volume92004/No1Jan04/CollectiveBargainingStrategies.aspx.

Collins, J. (2001). *Good to great: Why some companies make the leap … and others don't.* New York: Harper Business.

Fisher, R., Ury, W., & Patton, B. (1991). *Getting to yes: Negotiating agreement without giving in.* New York: Penguin Books.

Kouzes, J. M., & Posner, B. Z. (2007). *The leadership challenge* (4th ed.). San Francisco: Jossey-Bass.

Kramer, M., Schmalenberg, C., Maguire, P., Brewer, B. B., Burke, R., Chmielewski, L., Cox, K., Kishner, J., Krugman, M., Meeks-Sjostrom, D., & Waldo, M. (2008). Structures and practices enabling staff nurses to control their practice. *Western Journal of Nursing Research, 30*(5), 539-559.

Perlow, L., & Williams, D. (2003). Is silence killing your organization? *Harvard Business Review, 81,* 52-58.

Pittman, J. (2007). Registered nurse job satisfaction and collective bargaining unit membership status. *Journal of Nursing Administration, 37*(10), 471-476.

WEBSITES

National Nurses Organizing Committee (NNOC). National RN movement. Website: www.calnurses.org/nnoc/.

United American Nurses, AFL-CIO (UAN). Website: www.uannurse.org/.

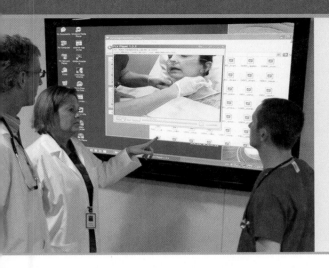

Managing Quality and Risk

Victoria N. Folse

This chapter explains key concepts and strategies related to quality and risk management. All healthcare professionals, including nurses, must be actively involved in the continuous improvement of patient care.

OBJECTIVES

- Apply quality management principles to clinical situations.
- Use the six steps of the quality improvement process.
- Practice using select quality improvement strategies to do the following:
  - Identify customer expectations.
  - Diagram clinical procedures.
  - Develop standards and outcomes.
  - Evaluate outcomes.
- Incorporate roles of leaders, managers, and followers to create a quality management culture of continuous readiness.
- Apply risk management strategies to an agency's quality management program.

TERMS TO KNOW

benchmarking
continuous quality improvement (CQI)
failure mode and effects analysis (FMEA)
near miss

never event
nursing-sensitive outcome
patient-care outcome
performance improvement (PI)
quality assurance (QA)
quality improvement (QI)

quality management (QM)
risk management
root-cause analysis
sentinel event
total quality management (TQM)

THE CHALLENGE

Kathleen M. Hoff, RN, BSN
Staff Nurse, Infant Special Care Unit, Evanston Hospital,
NorthShore University HealthSystem, Evanston, Illinois

Medical errors are one of the most common issues discussed among quality care and risk management healthcare professionals and are of great concern to me as a new graduate. The Institute of Medicine brought the issue of medical errors to the forefront of healthcare awareness with its landmark report *To Err is Human: Building a Safer Health System*, but the concern existed in hospitals long before that publication and, without further intervention, will continue to be an issue in years to come. Many policies and procedures have been put into place to try to decrease the rate of medical errors in hospitals, such as electronic bar coding. With hospitals growing in capacity and with increasing demands placed on nurses, it is critical that individual units address what they can do to foster quality care and prevent errors.

What do you think you would do if you were this nurse?

INTRODUCTION

Healthcare agencies and health professionals strive to provide the highest quality, safest, most efficient, and cost-effective care possible. The philosophy of quality management and the process of quality improvement need to shape the entire healthcare culture and provide specific skills for assessment, measurement, and evaluation of patient care. The goal of an organization committed to quality care is a comprehensive, systematic approach that prevents errors or identifies and corrects errors so that adverse events are decreased and safety and quality outcomes are maximized. Leadership must acknowledge safety shortcomings and allocate resources at the patient care and unit levels to identify and reduce risks (Pronovost, Rosenstein, et al., 2008). Quality management and risk management are focused on optimizing patient outcomes and emphasize the prevention of patient care problems and the mitigation of adverse events. Hospital leaders, including nurses, must sharpen their expertise in healthcare quality and patient safety, and staff at all levels must be empowered to act on nursing performance data (Kurtzman & Jennings, 2008).

QUALITY MANAGEMENT IN HEALTH CARE

Healthcare systems that demand quality recognize that survival and competitiveness are built on improved patient outcomes. Success depends on a philosophy that permeates the organization and values a continuous process of improvement. It is essential to integrate patient safety and risk management into broader quality initiatives. Nurses must be prepared to continuously improve the quality and safety of healthcare systems within which they work and must focus on the six competencies identified by Quality and Safety Education for Nurses (QSEN): patient-centered care, teamwork and collaboration, evidence-based practice, quality improvement, safety, and informatics (Cronenwett et al., 2007). Quality necessitates maintaining safety in patient care, with a continual focus on clinical excellence from the entire multidisciplinary team. Patient safety is a key component of quality improvement and clinical governance. Moreover, the prevention of adverse events is paramount to improved patient outcomes.

The terms quality management (QM), quality improvement (QI), performance improvement (PI), total quality management (TQM), and continuous quality improvement (CQI) are often used interchangeably in health care. Quality-related terminology continues to evolve.

In this chapter, *quality management* refers to a philosophy that defines a healthcare culture emphasizing customer satisfaction, innovation, and employee involvement. Similarly, *quality improvement* refers to an ongoing process of innovation, prevention of error, and staff development that is used by institutions that adopt the quality management philosophy. Nurses maintain a unique role in quality management and quality improvement because of the amount of direct patient care provided at the bedside and because they have an understanding of the day-to-day issues and "real world" nursing involved in delivery of care. Involvement of nurses in patient care improvement efforts (e.g., patient flow problems, safe delivery of care during low staffing or high census and high acuity times, communication problems associated with complex patients, improving medication safety) can not only promote quality and safety of patient care but also positively affect job satisfaction and improve the work environment (Hall, Moore, & Barnsteiner, 2008).

BENEFITS OF QUALITY MANAGEMENT

Healthcare systems employing a comprehensive QM program benefit in a number of ways. First, greater efficiency and proactive planning may overcome some of the resource constraints, including limited reimbursement imposed by prospective payment plans and key staff shortages. Second, successful malpractice suits could be reduced with quality care because QM is based on the philosophy that actions should be right the first time and that improvement is always possible. Third, job satisfaction could be enhanced because QM involves everyone on the improvement team and encourages everyone to contribute. This style of participative management makes employees feel valued as team members who can really make a difference.

PLANNING FOR QUALITY MANAGEMENT

Multidisciplinary planning is integral to the quest for quality. Issues are examined from various perspectives using a systematic process. Planning takes time and money; however, the price of poor planning can be very expensive. Costs of inadequate planning might involve correcting a patient care error, resulting in extended length of stay and added procedures. In turn, this increases the risk of liability for what was originally done, it risks a negative public image, and it magnifies employee frustration and turnover. The costs of errors and ineffective nursing actions are avoidable costs.

EVOLUTION OF QUALITY MANAGEMENT

Non-healthcare industries have excelled in focusing on process improvement as part of their core operating strategies. Numerous business management philosophies have been expanded and modified for use in healthcare organizations. For example, Six Sigma, a data-driven approach targeting a nearly error-free environment, empowers employees to improve processes and outcomes. As healthcare organizations "go lean," nurses are challenged to eliminate unnecessary steps and reduce wasted processes (saving time and money) to improve quality and the patient experience (de Koning, Verver, van den Heuvel, Bisgaard, & Does, 2006). To achieve this, Six Sigma uses a five-step methodology known as *DMAIC,* which stands for **d**efine opportunities, **m**easure performance, **a**nalyze opportunity, **i**mprove performance, and **c**ontrol performance to improve existing processes.

Define opportunities
Measure performance
Analyze opportunity
Improve performance
Control performance

In health care, emphasis is placed in the areas of patient safety and patient and employee satisfaction. Leadership development is fostered. The role of the leader or manager in this TQM method is to enable the team, remove barriers, and instill accountability.

Within healthcare systems, QI combines the assessment of *structure* (e.g., adequacy of staffing, effectiveness of computerized charting, availability of unit-based medication delivery systems), *process* (e.g., timeliness and thoroughness of documentation, adherence to critical pathways or care maps), and *outcome* (e.g., patient falls, hospital-acquired infection rates, patient satisfaction) standards. These three factors are usually considered interrelated, and research has been conducted to determine the characteristics of effective structures and processes that would result in better outcomes. The Literature Perspective on p. 392 expands the classic Donabedian model of the structure, process, and outcome framework in promoting quality in healthcare organizations.

Recognizing the relationship between quality patient care and nursing excellence, the American Academy of Nursing undertook a study that resulted

LITERATURE PERSPECTIVE

Resource: Glickman, S. W., Baggett, K. A., Krubert, C. G., Peterson, E. D., & Schulman, K. A. (2007). Promoting quality: The health-care organization from a management perspective. *International Journal for Quality Health Care, 19*(6), 341-348.

Although agreement exists about the need for quality improvement in health care, the best approach to measuring and achieving quality has not been identified. Avedis Donabedian developed the structure, process, and outcome framework in 1966 to measure quality initiatives, and the Donabedian model continues to be used today. Structural indicators are based on an assessment of an organization's features or staff characteristics that may affect an organization's performance and quality. Examples might include factors that contribute to The Joint Commission accreditation or Magnet™ status designation such as the leadership climate and staff governance structure. Process standards are based on evidence relating to the quality of the staff's work behaviors and include rates of nosocomial infections and medication errors. Outcome standards relate to performance measures that can be attributed to the quality of services performed and include patient satisfaction and patient health status.

The focus in most healthcare arenas has been on process and outcomes, but a need exists to increase the understanding of structure's role in quality initiatives. An updated view of the Donabedian's conceptualization of structure emphasizes five key elements that define structure in today's healthcare arena: executive management, culture, organizational design, incentive structures, and information exchange and technology.

Implications for Practice
The updated Donabedian framework can be used to enhance organizational performance and quality. Healthcare leaders must attend to these core structural components to transform quality improvement initiatives and to actively involve direct care providers to improve the quality and safety of care they deliver to patients.

BOX 20-1   PRINCIPLES OF QUALITY MANAGEMENT AND QUALITY IMPROVEMENT

1. Quality management operates most effectively within a flat, democratic, organization structure.
2. Managers and workers must be committed to quality improvement.
3. The goal of quality management is to improve systems and processes, not to assign blame.
4. Customers define quality.
5. Quality improvement focuses on outcomes.
6. Decisions must be based on data.

and influential nurse executives) and process factors (e.g., professional autonomy and decision making, ongoing professional development/education). Organizations that have not pursued Magnet™ status can implement strategies (e.g., introducing a clinical ladder program, facilitating professional certification, assisting with evidence-based projects, enhancing the new graduate nurse orientation program) to promote a professional practice environment for staff nurses and improve organizational outcomes (Lacey et al., 2008).

QUALITY MANAGEMENT PRINCIPLES

The combination of QI ideas from theory and research is sometimes referred to as *total quality management (TQM)* or, more simply, *quality management (QM)*. The basic principles of QM are summarized in Box 20-1 and are developed further in the next section of this chapter.

Involvement

Leaders, managers, and followers must be committed to QI. Top-level leaders and managers retain the ultimate responsibility for QM but must involve the entire organization in the QI process. Although some healthcare organizations have achieved significant QI results without systemwide support, total organizational involvement is necessary for a culture transformation. If all members of the healthcare team are to be actively involved in QI, clear delineation of roles within a nonthreatening environment must be established (Table 20-1).

in the distinction known as *Magnet™*. The American Nurses Credentialing Center (ANCC) created a process called the *Magnet Recognition Program®*. The term *Magnet™ hospital* was chosen to describe a hospital that attracts and retains nurses even in times of nursing shortages. Magnet™ hospital research has examined the characteristics of hospital systems that impede or facilitate professional practice in nursing and also promote quality patient outcomes. Common organizational characteristics of Magnet™ hospitals include structure factors (e.g., decentralized organizational structure, participative management style,

TABLE 20-1   ROLES/RESPONSIBILITIES IN QUALITY IMPROVEMENT PLAN

ROLE OF SENIOR LEADER	ROLE OF NURSE MANAGER	ROLE OF FOLLOWER
• Leads culture transformation • Sets priorities for house-wide activities, staffing effectiveness, and patient health outcomes • Builds infrastructure, provides resources, and removes barriers for improvement • Defines procedures for immediate response to errors involving care, treatment, or services and contains risk • Assesses management and staff knowledge of quality management process regularly, and provides education as needed • Implements and monitors systems for internal and external reporting of information • Defines and provides support system for staff who have been involved in a sentinel event	• Is accountable for quality and safety indicator performance within areas of responsibility • Communicates performance priorities and targets to staff • Meets regularly with staff to monitor progress and help with improvement work • Uses data to measure effectiveness of improvement • Works with staff to develop and implement action plans for improvement of measures that do not meet target • Provides time for unit staff to participate in quality improvement measures • Directly observes staff and coaches as needed • Consults quality management team (e.g., Six Sigma) or risk management team as appropriate • Writes and submits to senior leaders periodic action plan including performance measures and plans for improvement • Shares information and benchmarks with other units and departments to improve organization's performance	• Follows policies, procedures, and protocols to ensure quality and safe patient care • Remains current in the literature on quality and safety specific to nursing; promotes evidence-based practice standards • Communicates with and educates peers immediately if they are observed not following quality and safety standards • Reports quality and safety issues to supervisor/manager • Invests in the process by continually asking self, "What makes this indicator important to measure?" "What has been done to improve it?" "What can I do to improve it?" • Participates actively in the quality improvement activities

To work effectively in a democratic, quality-focused corporate environment, nurses and other healthcare workers must accept QI as an integral part of their role. Nurses have a direct impact on patient safety and healthcare outcomes (Kurtzman & Jennings, 2008). Nursing must be recognized and empowered to mobilize performance improvement knowledge and practice measures throughout the organization. When a separate department controls quality activities, healthcare managers and workers often relinquish responsibility and commitment for quality control to these quality specialists. Employees working in an organizational culture that values quality freely make suggestions for improvement and innovation in patient care. Exercise 20-1 may help nurses make QI suggestions.

> **EXERCISE 20-1**
> Think of something that can be improved in your work setting. Define the problem, using as many specific facts as possible. List the advantages to the staff, patients, and agency of improving this problem. Describe several possible solutions to the problem. Decide whom you would contact about these suggestions.

Goal

The goal of QM is to improve the system, not to assign blame. Managers strive to provide a system in which workers can function effectively. To encourage commitment to QI, nurse managers must clearly articulate the organization's mission and goals. All levels of employees, from nursing assistants to hospital administrators, must be educated about QI strategies.

Communication should flow freely within the organization. When healthcare professionals understand each other's roles and can effectively communicate and work together, patients are more likely to receive safe, quality care (Hall et al., 2008). Because QM stresses improving the system, detection of employees' errors is not stressed; and if errors occur, re-education of staff is emphasized rather than imposition of punitive measures. When patient safety indicators are used to examine hospital performance, the focus of error analysis shifts from the individual provider to the level of the healthcare system (Glance, Li, Osler, Mukamel, & Dick, 2008).

Customers

Customers define quality. Successful organizations measure the factors that are most important to customers and focus their energies on enhancing quality in these areas. As patients become more sophisticated and view themselves as "consumers" who can take their business elsewhere, they want input into treatment decisions. Although typical patients may not be knowledgeable about a specific treatment, they know if they were satisfied with their experience with the healthcare provider.

Every nurse and healthcare agency has internal and external customers. Internal customers are people or units within an organization who receive products or services. A nurse working on a hospital unit could describe patients, nurses on the other shifts, and other hospital departments as internal customers. External customers are people or groups outside the organization who receive products or services. For nurses, these external customers may include patients' families, physicians, managed care organizations, and the community at large. Some customers (e.g., physicians, patient families) could be either internal or external customers depending on the actual care environment. Managers and staff nurses can use Exercise 20-2 to identify their internal and external customers.

EXERCISE 20-2

For one week, list every person with whom you interact as a nurse. The internal customers are those people who work for or receive care in your organization. External customers come from outside the organization. What is the best method to obtain feedback from each of these customers?

Public reporting of quality and risk data is changing the way customers make decisions about health care and is intended to improve care through easily accessed information. For example, Hospital Compare (U.S. Department of Health and Human Services, 2009) allows customers to (1) find information on how well hospitals care for patients with certain medical conditions or surgical procedures and (2) access patient survey results about the quality of care received during a recent hospital stay. This information allows customers to compare the quality of care hospitals provide. Hospital Compare was created through the efforts of the Centers for Medicare & Medicaid Services (CMS), the Department of Health & Human Services (DHHS), and other members of the Hospital Quality Alliance (HQA). The information on this website comes from hospitals that have agreed to submit quality information for Hospital Compare to make public.

Consumer satisfaction with health care can be assessed through the use of questionnaires, interviews, focus group discussions, or observation. Patients' perspectives should be a key component of any quality improvement initiative. However, patients cannot always adequately assess the competence of clinical performance, and therefore patient feedback and patient satisfaction surveys must serve as only one data source for QI initiatives.

Focus

QI focuses on outcomes. Patient outcomes are statements that describe the results of health care. They are specific and measurable and describe patients' behavior. Outcome statements may be based on patients' needs, ethical and legal standards of practice, or other standardized data systems. Healthcare organizations that implement nursing-sensitive performance measures value nurses and have a strong commitment to patients and a goal to outperform competitors (Kurtzman & Jennings, 2008).

Decisions

Decisions must be based on data. The use of statistical tools enables nurse managers to make objective decisions about QI activities. It is imperative that data are not merely collected to support a preconceived idea. Quality information must be gathered and analyzed without bias before improvement suggestions and recommendations are made.

THE QUALITY IMPROVEMENT PROCESS

QI involves continual analysis and evaluation of products and services to prevent errors and to achieve customer satisfaction. The work of continuous QI never stops because products and services can always be improved.

The QI process is a structured series of steps designed to plan, implement, and evaluate changes in healthcare activities. Many models of the QI process exist, but most parallel the nursing process and all contain steps similar to those listed in Box 20-2. The six steps can easily be applied to clinical situations. In the following example, staff at a community clinic use the QI process to handle patient complaints about excessive wait times.

A community clinic receives a number of complaints from patients about waiting up to 2 hours for scheduled appointments to see a licensed practitioner. The clinic secretary and staff nurses suggest to the clinic manager that scheduling clinic appointments be investigated by the QI committee, which is composed of the clinic secretary, two clinic nurses, one physician, and one nurse practitioner. The clinic manager agrees to the staff's suggestion and assigns the problem to the QI committee. At their next meeting, the QI committee uses a flowchart to describe the scheduling process from the time a patient calls to make an appointment until the patient sees a physician or nurse practitioner in the examining room. Next, the committee members decide to gather and analyze data about the important parts of the process:

the number of calls for appointments, the number of patients seen in a day, the number of cancelled or missed appointments, and the average time each patient spends in the waiting room. The committee discovers that too many appointments are scheduled because many patients miss appointments. This overbooking often results in long waiting times for the patients who do arrive on time. The QI committee also gathers information on clinic waiting times from the literature and through interviews with patients and colleagues. A measurable outcome is written: "Patients will wait no longer than 30 minutes to be seen by a licensed practitioner." After a discussion of options, the team recommends that appointments be scheduled at more reasonable intervals, that patients receive notification of appointments by mail and by phone, and that all clinic patients be educated about the importance of keeping scheduled appointments. The committee communicates its suggestions for improvement to the manager and staff and monitors the results of the implementation of their improvement suggestions. Within 3 months, the average waiting room time per patient decreases to 90 minutes, and the number of missed patient appointments decreases by 20%. Because the desired outcome has not been met, the QI committee will continue the QI process.

Identify Consumers' Needs

The QI process begins with the selection of a clinical activity for review. Theoretically, any and all aspects of clinical care could be improved through the QI process. However, QI efforts should be concentrated on changes to patient care that will have the greatest effect. To determine which clinical activities are most important, nurse managers or staff nurses may interview or survey patients about their healthcare experiences or may review unmet quality standards. The results of the research study in the Research Perspective on p. 396 identify prevention of errors during hand-off.

Assemble a Team

Once an activity is selected for possible improvement, a multidisciplinary team implements the QI process. QI team members should represent a cross section of workers who are involved with the problem. To maximize success, team members may need to be educated about their roles before starting the QI process.

BOX 20-2	STEPS IN THE QUALITY IMPROVEMENT PROCESS

1. Identify needs most important to the consumer of healthcare services.
2. Assemble a multidisciplinary team to review the identified consumer needs and services.
3. Collect data to measure the current status of these services.
4. Establish measurable outcomes and quality indicators.
5. Select and implement a plan to meet the outcomes.
6. Collect data to evaluate the implementation of the plan and the achievement of outcomes.

RESEARCH PERSPECTIVE

Resource: Berkenstadt, H., Haviv, Y., Tuval, A., Shemesh, Y., Megrill, A., Perry, A., Rubin, O., & Ziv, A. (2008). Improving handoff communications in critical care. *Chest, 134*(1), 158-162.

This study was conducted in response to a patient event on a medical step-down unit where the patient experienced severe hypoglycemia caused by an infusion of a higher-than-ordered insulin dose. This adverse event might have been prevented if the insulin syringe pump was checked during the nursing shift hand-off. Follow-up included direct observations of nursing shift hand-offs, which led to the development and implementation of a hand-off protocol and the incorporation of hand-off training including simulation-based teamwork and communication work-shop. The intervention demonstrated improved communication of crucial information during hand-off including patient's name, events that occurred during the previous shift, and treatment goals for the next shift. However, no change occurred in the incidence of checking and adapting the monitor alarms, checking the mechanical ventilator, or checking medications being admin-istered by continuous infusion.

Implications for Practice
Even minor incidents can reveal safety gaps and needed changes within the healthcare system to prevent future occurrences. Reflecting the importance of the hand-off process for safe patient care, hand-off was introduced by The Joint Commission Interna-tional Center for Patient Safety as a national patient safety goal aimed at improving the effectiveness of communication among caregivers. This means that every organization must define, com-municate to staff, and implement a process in which information about patient care is communicated in a consistent manner. Also, organizations must provide opportunities to ask clarifying ques-tions and to receive answers in a time frame that is consistent with having complete and accurate information available to the patient's caregivers when they are providing the care. Improving hand-off communication, including when to use certain tech-niques (e.g., Situation-Background-Assessment-Recommendation [SBAR] or repeat-back), is needed to address time pressures, work overload, and conflicting demands of nurses.

EXERCISE 20-3
Ask yourself the following questions about your department:
1. Is communication between nurses and other professionals promoted? If so, how?
2. Could the communication process be improved in any way?
3. Does your system encourage nurses to act as a team?
4. Are other disciplines/departments included in team activities?
5. Can the team focus be improved in any way?

Collect Data

After the multidisciplinary team forms, the group col-lects data to measure the current status of the activity, service, or procedure under review. Various data tools may be used to analyze and present this information. These data tools include flowcharts, line graphs, his-tograms, Pareto charts, and fishbone diagrams. The use of empirical tools to organize QI data is an essen-tial part of the QI process, and although many nurses lack formal training in the use of QI tools, being familiar with those used most frequently in quality improvement work is important (Hughes, 2008).

A detailed flowchart is used to describe complex tasks. The flowchart is a data tool that uses boxes and directional arrows to diagram all the steps of a process or procedure in the proper sequence. Sometimes, just diagramming a patient-care process in detail reveals gaps and opportunities for improvement. The flow-chart in Figure 20-1 depicts the process of a home health agency receiving a new patient referral.

Line graphs present data by showing the connec-tion among variables. The dependent variable is usually plotted on the vertical scale, and the indepen-dent variable is usually plotted on the horizontal scale. In QI, this technique is often used to show the trend of a particular activity over time, and the result may be called a *trend chart*. The line graph in Figure 20-2 illustrates the number of referrals a home health agency receives during a year.

The histogram in Figure 20-3 illustrates the number of home health referrals that come from five different referral sources during a selected year. A histogram is a bar chart that shows the frequency of events.

A bar chart that identifies the major causes or components of a particular quality control problem is called a *Pareto chart*. It differs from a regular bar

---

To develop effective unit-based quality councils, the workplace environment must promote teamwork. Some departments within healthcare facilities are more open to teamwork than are others. Nurse leaders and managers can use Exercise 20-3 to decide whether their clinical unit is ready for a unit-based QI team.

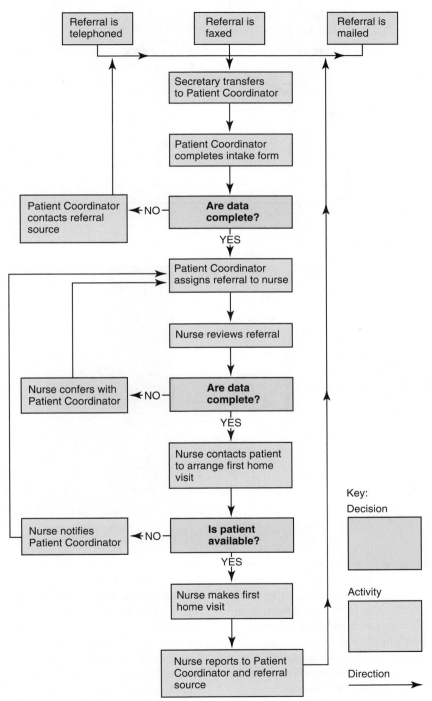

FIGURE 20-1 Steps in a flowchart diagramming process of a new patient referral, starting with the time a home health referral is made and ending with the first home visit.

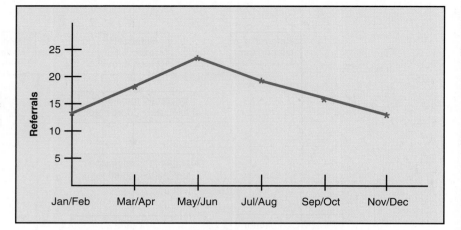

FIGURE 20-2 Line graph depicting the number of home health referrals received during 1 year.

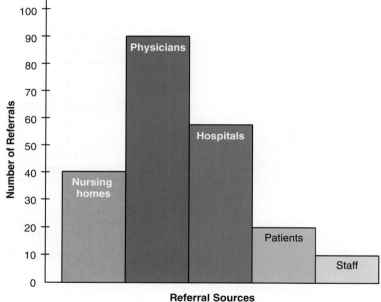

FIGURE 20-3 Histogram depicting the number of home health referrals received from five sources during 1 year.

graph in that the highest frequencies of occurrence of a factor are designated in the bar at the left, with the other factors appearing in descending order. Used often in QI, the Pareto chart helps the QI team determine priorities, allowing the most significant problem to be addressed first. The Pareto chart in Figure 20-4 demonstrates that, on a medical-surgical unit over a 1-month period, omission of vital signs was the most common type of documentation error.

The fishbone diagram is an effective method of summarizing a brainstorming session. A specific problem or outcome is written on the horizontal line. All possible causes of the problem or strategies to meet the outcome are written in a fishbone pattern. Figure 20-5 uses a fishbone diagram to present possible causes of patients' complaints about extended waits for clinic appointments.

Although QI teams should be able to use these basic statistical tools, analysis that is more complex is sometimes necessary. In this situation, a statistical expert could be included on the QI team or the team may consult a statistician.

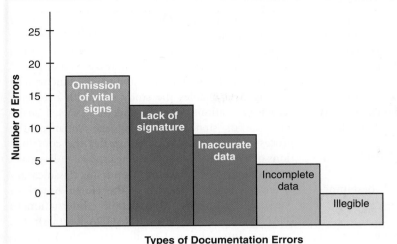

FIGURE 20-4 Pareto chart presenting major types of documentation errors that occurred on a medical/surgical unit over a 1-month period.

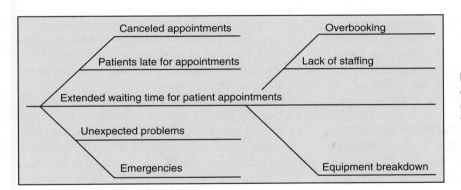

FIGURE 20-5 Fishbone diagram showing possible causes of extended waiting time for clinic patients.

Establish Outcomes

After analyzing the data, the team next sets a goal for improvement. This goal can be established in a number of ways but always involves a standard of practice and a measurable patient-care outcome or nursing-sensitive outcome. Nursing-sensitive indicators reflect the structure, process, and outcomes of nursing care. The structure of nursing care is indicated by the supply of nursing staff, the skill level of the nursing staff, and the education/certification of nursing staff. Process indicators measure aspects of nursing care such as assessment, intervention, and RN job satisfaction. Patient outcomes that are determined to be nursing sensitive are those that improve if there is a greater quantity or quality of nursing care (e.g., pressure ulcers, falls, intravenous [IV] infiltrations). Some patient outcomes are more highly related to other aspects of institutional care, such as medical decisions and institutional policies (e.g., frequency of primary cesarean sections, cardiac failure) and are not considered nursing sensitive. The multidisciplinary team should use accepted standards of care and practice whenever possible. Clinical practice guidelines and standards should reflect evidence-based practice and should be updated as new research emerges. Sources that establish these standards include the following:

1. American Nurses Association (ANA) standards of nursing practice
2. State nurse practice acts
3. Accrediting bodies such as The Joint Commission (TJC) or recognition bodies such as the American Nurses Credentialing Center (ANCC)
4. Governmental bodies such as the Agency for Healthcare Research and Quality (AHRQ), the Centers for Medicare & Medicaid Services

(CMS), the Centers for Disease Control and Prevention (CDC) Division of Healthcare Quality Promotion (DHQP), and the National Institute for Occupational Safety and Health (NIOSH)

5. Healthcare advisory groups such as the Institute of Medicine (IOM), the National Quality Forum (NQF), and the Quality & Safety Education of Nurses (QSEN)
6. Nationally recognized professional organizations
7. Nursing research/evidenced-based, best practice standards
8. Internal policies and procedures
9. Internal or external performance measurement data such as patient satisfaction surveys, employee opinion surveys, safety assessment surveys, and patient or employee rounding

Although individual healthcare organizations may have unique patient needs related to their specific population or environment, many targeted outcomes are similar. One way to evaluate the quality of outcomes is to compare one agency's performance with that of similar organizations. In a process called benchmarking, a widespread search is conducted to identify the best performance against which to measure others. Through this process of comparing the best practices with your practice and process, your organization learns to identify desired standards of quality performance. Available data include all reported hospital-acquired infection rates in other institutions as well as specific data, such as postoperative infection rates in adult surgical intensive care units of similar-size institutions.

However, recent mandates in select states to publicly disclose nosocomial infection rates highlight potential issues with disclosure of data. Specifically, simply reporting hospital infection rates is not enough to promote hand-hygiene practices and may do little to improve outcomes and reduce hospital-acquired infections. Unfortunately, the usefulness of the information from other institutions continues to be hampered by differences in terminology. Information technology plays a vital role in QI by increasing the efficiency of data entry and analysis. A consistent information system that trends high-risk procedures and systematic errors would provide a useful database regarding outcomes of care and resource allocation.

The purpose of the NQF is designed to standardize measures so that true comparisons can be made.

Nursing has been a leader in the information system field by developing standardized nursing classification systems. The availability of standardized nursing data enables the study of health problems across populations, settings, and caregivers. Consistent use of standardized language enhances the process of QI and also demonstrates the contributions of nursing to lawmakers, healthcare policymakers, and the public. Three leading nursing classification systems have been identified: the North American Nursing Diagnosis Association International's (NANDA-I) nomenclature (NANDA-I, 2008); the Nursing Intervention Classification (NIC) system (Bulechek, Butcher, & Dochtermann, 2008); and the Nursing Outcomes Classification (NOC) system (Moorhead, Johnson, Maas, & Swanson, 2008). The use of standardized nursing terminologies like NANDA-I, NIC, and NOC provides a means of collecting and analyzing nursing data and evaluating nursing-sensitive outcomes.

Each classification system focuses on one component of the nursing process. Nursing diagnoses can be labeled using NANDA-I. These diagnosis labels represent clinical judgments about actual or potential health problems. Each diagnosis contains a definition, major and minor defining characteristics, and related factors. Accurate nursing diagnoses guide the selection of nursing interventions to achieve the desired treatment effects, determine nursing-sensitive outcomes, and ensure patient safety (NANDA-I, 2008).

The NIC system consists of interventions that represent both general and specialty nursing practice. Each intervention includes a label, a definition, and a set of activities that nurses perform to carry it out. For example, pain management is defined and specific activities are listed to alleviate pain or reduce the pain to a level that is acceptable to the patient (Bulechek et al., 2008).

The NOC system consists of outcomes that focus on the patient and include patient states, behavior, and perceptions that are sensitive to nursing interventions. Each outcome includes a definition, a five-point scale for rating outcome status over time, and a set of specific indicators to be used in rating the outcomes (Moorhead et al., 2008). Clinical testing for validation and refinement has occurred in various settings, and the standardization of terms continues to develop to reflect current knowledge and changes in nurses' roles and the structure of healthcare systems. The consistency of terms is essential in providing a large database across healthcare settings to predict resource requirements and establish outcomes of care.

The National Database of Nursing Quality Indicators (NDNQI) is a national nursing quality measurement program from the ANA that provides hospitals with unit-level performance reports with comparisons with national averages and percentile rankings (ANA, 2009). All indicator data are collected and reported at the nursing unit level, which is valuable for unit-based quality initiatives. NDNQI's nursing-sensitive indicators reflect the structure, process, and outcomes of nursing care. NDNQI's mission is to aid the nursing provider in patient safety and quality improvement efforts by providing research-based national comparative data on nursing care and the relationship to patient outcomes. Many of the NDNQI indicators are NQF-endorsed measures and are part of NQF's nursing-sensitive measure set (e.g., falls with injuries, nosocomial infections, restraint prevalence, nursing hours per patient day, staff mix). However, the NDNQI allows additional comparisons of indicators such as nurse job satisfaction, RN education and certification, and pressure ulcer, psychiatric patient assault, and pediatric IV infiltration rates.

Discuss Plans

The team discusses various strategies and plans to meet the new outcome. One plan is selected for implementation, and the process of change begins. Because QM stresses improving the system rather than assigning blame to employees, change strategies emphasize open communication and education of workers affected by the new standard and outcome. QI is impossible without continual education of all managers and followers.

Policies and procedures may need to be written or rewritten during the QI process. Policies should be reviewed frequently and updated so that they reflect best practice standards and do not become barriers to innovation. Communication about the change or improvement is essential.

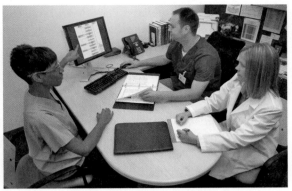

Diagramming a patient-care process in detail can reveal gaps and opportunities for improvement.

Evaluate

As the plan is implemented, the team continues to gather and evaluate data to document that the new outcomes are being met. If an outcome is not met, revisions in the implementation plan are needed. Sometimes improvement in one part of a system presents new problems. For example, nurses implemented screening for suicide risk in adolescents and adults presenting to the emergency department. A result of this improvement in care was a greatly increased number of referrals for counseling, which overwhelmed the existing hospital and community resources. The interprofessional team may need to reassemble periodically to handle the inevitable obstacles that develop with the implementation of any new process or procedure. Furthermore, individuals outside the medical center (external customers) may need to be included in the process. The example that follows also illustrates this idea.

A hospital is implementing a pneumatic tube system to dispense medications. A multidisciplinary team is assembled to discuss the process from various viewpoints: pharmacy, nursing, pneumatic tube operation managers, aides who take the medications from the pneumatic tube to the patient medication drawers, administrators, and physicians. The tube system is implemented. A nurse on one unit realizes that several patients do not have their morning medications in their medication drawers. The nurse borrows medications from another patient's drawer and orders the rest of the medications "stat" from pharmacy. Other nurses on that unit and other units have the same problem and are taking the same or similar actions. Several problems are occurring—some of the medications are being given late, nurses waste precious time by searching other medication drawers, the pharmacy charges extra for the stat medications and is overwhelmed with stat requests, and the situation increases the nurses' frustration level. In some cases, patients suffer because of late administration of medications. QM principles would encourage the nurses to report the problems to the nurse manager or appropriate team member. The pneumatic tube team could compile data such as frequency of missing medications, timing of medication orders, and nursing units involved. The problems are analyzed with a system perspective to solve the late medication problem effectively.

In some organizations, when a change is implemented successfully, the QI team disbands. One of the crucial tasks of the nurse manager is to publicize and reward the success of each QI team. The nurse manager must also evaluate the work of the team and the ability of individual team members to work together effectively.

Some organizations that have used the QM philosophy for several years establish permanent QI teams or committees. These QI teams do not disband after implementing one project or idea but, rather, may meet regularly to focus on improvements in specific areas of patient care. The use of permanent QI teams or the adoption of a culture driven by QM can provide continuity and prevent duplication of efforts within the quality teams.

QM organizations stress system-level change and the evaluation of outcomes. However, in recent years, the need for process/performance improvement, including individual performance appraisal, has re-emerged within healthcare organizations. Peer review and self-evaluation are performance-assessment methods that fit within the QM philosophy.

Any nurse can use the six steps of the QI process to self-evaluate and improve individual performance. For example, a nurse on a medical unit who wants to improve documentation skills might study past entries on patient records; review current institution policies, professional standards, and literature related to documentation; set specific performance-improvement goals after consultation with the nurse manager and expert colleagues; devise strategies and a timeline for achieving performance goals; and after implementing the strategies, review documentation entries to see whether self-improvement goals have been met.

QUALITY ASSURANCE

Although QI is a comprehensive process to prevent problems, it is naive to suggest the total abandonment of periodic inspection. One method used to monitor health care is quality assurance (QA) programs, which ensure conformity to a standard. QA focuses on clinical aspects of the provider's care, often in response to an identified problem. Many QA activities focus on process standards (e.g., documentation, adherence to practice standards). The focus may be asking questions such as "Did the nurse document the response to the pain medication within the required time period?" instead of "Did the patient receive adequate pain relief postoperatively?" In contrast, QI may examine process, structure, and outcome standards. The similarities and differences between QI and QA are summarized in Table 20-2.

One of the methods most often used in QA is chart review or chart auditing. Chart audits may be conducted using the records of active or discharged patients. Charts are selected randomly and reviewed by qualified healthcare professionals. In an internal audit, staff members from the same hospital or agency that generated the records examine the data. External auditors are qualified professionals from outside the organization who conduct the review. An audit tool containing specific criteria based on standards of care is applied to each chart under review. For example, auditors might compare documentation related to use of restraints for medical-surgical purposes with the criterion "Licensed independent practitioner evaluates patient in person within 4 hours of application." Auditors note compliance or lack of compliance with each audit criterion and report a summary of these findings to the appropriate manager or committee for corrective action.

Because the focus of the chart audit is on detecting errors and determining the person responsible for them, many staff members tend to view QA negatively. The nurse manager must reinforce that QA is not intended to be punitive but, instead, is an opportunity to improve patient care at the unit level. For example, to reinforce the importance of documentation, providing the standard of care for

TABLE 20-2   COMPARISON OF TRADITIONAL QUALITY ASSURANCE AND QUALITY IMPROVEMENT PROCESSES

	QUALITY ASSURANCE (QA) PROCESS	QUALITY IMPROVEMENT (QI) PROCESS
Goal	To improve quality	To improve quality
Focus	Discovery and correction of errors	Prevention of errors
Major tasks	Inspection of nursing activities Chart audits	Review of nursing activities Innovation Staff development
Quality team	QA personnel or department personnel	Multidisciplinary team
Outcomes	Set by QA team with input from staff	Set by QI team with input from staff and patients

documentation and assisting the RN in reviewing several charts is an appropriate educational tool to reinforce policies and procedures or standards regarding documentation. It is the responsibility of the manager to communicate the importance of daily QA activities and how unit-based monitoring ties into the overall quality improvement program. Moreover, many institutions incorporate both the participation in and the results of QA into annual performance appraisals or clinical ladders.

RISK MANAGEMENT

QM and risk management are related concepts and emphasize the achievement of quality-outcome standards and the prevention of patient-care problems. Risk management also attempts to analyze problems and minimize losses after an adverse event occurs. These losses include incurring financial loss as a result of malpractice or absorbing the cost of an extended length of stay for the patient, negative public relations, and employee dissatisfaction. Moreover, the inclusion of safety standards in TJC guidelines further emphasizes the importance of risk management. See Box 20-3 for the 2009 National Patient Safety Goals, as an example. The TJC website carries the most up-to-date patient safety goals, which are revised annually.

The risk management department has several functions, which include the following:
- Defining situations that place the system at some financial risk, such as medication errors or patient falls

BOX 20-3   2009 NATIONAL PATIENT SAFETY GOALS FOR HOSPITALS

- Improve the accuracy of patient identification.
- Improve the effectiveness of communication among caregivers.
- Improve the safety of using medications.
- Reduce the risk of healthcare-associated infections.
- Accurately and completely reconcile medications across the continuum of care.
- Reduce the risk of patient harm resulting from falls.
- Encourage patients' active involvement in their own care as a patient safety strategy.
- The organization identifies safety risks inherent in its patient population.
- Improve recognition and response to changes in a patient's condition.
- The organization meets the expectations of the Universal Protocol.

From The Joint Commission. Retrieved January 20, 2009, from www.jointcommission.org/patientsafety/nationalpatientsafetygoals.

- Determining the frequency of occurrence of those situations
- Intervening and investigating identified events
- Identifying potential risks or opportunities to improve care

Each individual nurse is a risk manager and has the responsibility to identify and report unusual occurrences and potential risks. Active involvement in quality and risk management by direct caregivers, however, is a challenge complicated by staffing issues and increased demands on the nurse. Increased nursing staffing in hospitals is associated with better care outcomes. Consistent evidence shows that an increase in RN-to-patient ratios is associated with a reduction in hospital-related mortality, failure to rescue, and other nursing-sensitive outcomes, as well as reduced length of stay (Kane, Shamliyan, Mueller, Duval, & Wilt, 2007). Similarly, favorable patient care environments are associated with lower rates of serious complications or adverse events (Aiken, Clarke, Sloane, Lake, & Cheney, 2008). Findings from the Aiken et al. (2008) and Kane et al. (2007) studies are combined in The Evidence section on pp. 406-407 to reflect the current knowledge about nursing and the patient care environment.

Another barrier to improving patient safety is fear of punishment, which inhibits people from acknowledging, reporting, or discussing errors. One way to minimize errors is to monitor threats to patient safety continually and to recognize that individual errors often reflect organizational and system failures. For example, targeting nurse-to-patient load and work schedules, including 12-hour shifts and overtime, can reduce potential errors from human factors such as fatigue, stress, and distractions. Rotating shifts may have a negative effect on nurses' stress levels and job performance, and working longer hours may have a negative impact on patient outcomes and safety (Kane et al., 2007).

Both risk management and quality management deal with changing behavior, prevention, focus on the customer, and attention to outcomes. The following clinical examples illustrate how quality management and risk management complement each other. First, the implementation of lift teams reduces employee injuries associated with lifting heavy or fully dependent patients and simultaneously, for the patient, decreases adverse events associated with difficult transfers. The implementation of lift teams reflects managing both quality and risk. Second, adherence to the universal safety verification known as "time out" before the beginning of a surgical procedure ensures perioperative safety within a TQM framework. Although nursing managers would prefer that all staff intrinsically embrace risk management practices aimed at patient and staff safety, accountability for safety can be one aspect of performance evaluations. Active involvement of staff in risk management activities is key to prevention of adverse events. Nurse managers should conduct safety rounds and praise employees for employing safe practice as part of best practice standards. This philosophy reinforces that risk management not only benefits the patient but also works to keep individual employees safe in the workplace.

Adverse-event reduction is a key strategy for reducing healthcare mortality and morbidity because patients who suffer adverse events are more likely to die or suffer permanent disability. Nurses have always played a pivotal role in the prevention of adverse events and can reduce negative outcomes with a focus on accurate assessment, early identification, and correction of potentially adverse situations. Also, adherence to best practice standards and ensuring quality standards for high-risk/high-volume practices (e.g., restraint use, medication reconciliation) can reduce adverse events. The NQF and CMS define never events as errors in medical care that are clearly identifiable, preventable, and serious in their consequences for patients and that indicate a real problem in the safety and credibility of a healthcare facility. Examples of never events include surgery on the wrong body part, foreign body left in a patient after surgery, mismatched blood transfusion, major medication error, severe pressure ulcer acquired in the hospital, and preventable postoperative deaths. Now that many third-party payers are following the CMS lead in withholding payment for preventable complications of care, no member of the healthcare team can fail to recognize the implications of quality care in their organization's overall success (Pronovost, Goeschel, & Wachter, 2008).

A comprehensive quality and risk program would proactively identify and reduce risks to patient safety through completion of a failure mode and effects analysis (FMEA) on select high-risk situations as advanced by TJC. If an adverse event occurs, nurses should also be able to recognize near misses and sentinel events and participate with a multidisciplinary team in the root-cause analysis. A sentinel event is a serious, unexpected occurrence involving death or physical or psychological harm, such as inpatient suicide, infant abduction, or wrong-site surgery. Similarly, a near miss may have resulted in no harm but highlights an imminent problem that must be corrected and can provide useful lessons in terms of risk analysis and reduction. TJC calls for voluntary

BOX 20-4	MOST COMMON HEALTHCARE SENTINEL EVENTS

- Wrong-site surgery
- Suicide
- Operative/postoperative complications
- Medication error
- Delay in treatment
- Patient fall
- Assault/rape/homicide
- Unintended retention of foreign body
- Patient death/injury in restraints
- Perinatal death/loss of function
- Transfusion error
- Medical equipment–related event
- Infection-related event
- Anesthesia-related event
- Patient elopement
- Fire
- Maternal death
- Ventilator-related death/injury
- Abduction
- Utility systems–related event
- Infant discharge to wrong family

From The Joint Commission. Retrieved January 20, 2009, from www.jointcommission.org/SentinelEvents/Statistics/.

self-reporting of sentinel events by both inpatient institutions and home health agencies. See Box 20-4 for the most common sentinel events reported in the healthcare arena. After a sentinel event is identified, a root-cause analysis is performed by a team that includes those directly involved in the event and those in leadership positions. A root-cause analysis is very similar to the QI process described in this chapter except that the root-cause analysis is a retrospective review of an incident to identify the sequence of events with the goal of identifying the root causes. The root-cause analysis leads to the development of specific risk-reduction strategies, and in certain situations, the plan must be reported to TJC.

Whereas reporting to TJC illustrates external reporting to regulatory or accrediting agencies, an internal method of communicating risks or adverse events is through electronic safety reporting systems or through incident reporting. Incident reports are kept separate from the patient's medical record and should serve as a means of communicating an inci-

dent that did cause or could have caused harm to patients, family members, visitors, or employees. Aggregated incident reports should be used to improve quality of care and decrease future risk. Trending data can illuminate systems issues that need to be modified to reduce risk and achieve quality patient care. Although an incident report may not be warranted for a unit-specific problem or an interdepartmental issue in which no adverse event occurred (e.g., delay in diagnosis or treatment), communication at the appropriate chain of command is essential to improve quality. Nurse managers are often responsible for investigating and remedying each identified hazard, which can result in safety being approached in a reactionary way (Pronovost, Rosenstein, et al., 2008). The resources to develop, implement, and evaluate a comprehensive patient safety program require investing in an infrastructure for patient safety that includes a sufficient number of qualified clinicians to provide care and an adequate number of qualified individuals to focus on safety initiatives (Pronovost, Rosenstein, et al., 2008).

Evaluating Risks

In gathering data about unusual occurrences, the risk management team may involve perspectives from numerous disciplines to discover underlying problems that a single discipline might miss. Risk managers also use multiple data sources, data collection techniques, and perspectives to collect and interpret the data. Quantitative methods such as questionnaire or records of medication administration can be combined with qualitative methods such as open-ended question interviews. Actionable plans for reducing the incidence of common preventable adverse events such as medication administration errors (wrong patient, time, dose, drug, or mode of delivery) could result from assessment and analysis of both quantitative and qualitative data. Quality and risk strategies aimed at targeting high-volume and high-risk occurrences are essential. Moreover, accountability for quality efforts to third-party payers, including the federal government, on programs such as pay-for-performance, in which healthcare systems receive additional payment incentives if specific quality targets are achieved, and public reporting, in which quality data are made available for comparison, has significant implications for nurses. Opportunities include participation on quality improvement teams, data collection, and involvement in the implementation of quality initiatives (Bodrock & Mion, 2008).

However, recognizing errors does not always translate into reporting errors. The lack of agreement as to what constitutes error influences the willingness of healthcare professionals to report errors and subsequently affects whether they develop strategies that could reduce future risk. A lack of consensus exists regarding whether patients and families should be informed about healthcare errors.

EXERCISE 20-4

Describe an error that occurred in the agency where you practice that resulted in harm to the patient and one that did not. What would you suggest to avoid a reoccurrence? Decide under what circumstances you would inform the patient and family and under what circumstances you would withhold the information.

Approaches to patient safety and risk management require healthcare providers to challenge their attitudes that errors are an unfortunate but inevitable part of patient care. Diminished resources and challenges in the work environment have the potential to compromise communication among providers and to contribute to an environment in which unsafe practices are overlooked or excused. For example, communication errors between nurses and other healthcare providers may result from hurried exchanges in crowded hallways or in the midst of a busy nursing station. Poorly designed medication rooms make uninterrupted medication preparation difficult; finding a physical space to take a break can be impossible because the nursing lounge is often used for shift report and meetings (Stichler, 2007). A team approach to quality and risk management is needed to promote optimal outcomes. Nurses have a responsibility to provide quality care and thus must serve in leadership roles to ensure a culture of integrated quality management and risk management.

THE SOLUTION

"Nursing M&Ms" is a new program our unit has implemented to encourage nurses to feel comfortable discussing medical errors, near misses, and good catches. Nurses who have made medical errors are encouraged to share their experience at one of our monthly meetings and address what steps they or the hospital could have taken to prevent the mistake from happening. Situations that occurred that were "good catches or near misses" are shared too, such as a laboratory order that was questioned by a nurse and found to be incorrect or a medication double-checked by another nurse who noted the dosage to be wrong. This meeting allows nurses to share with their co-workers strategies and techniques to improve the quality and safety of care. Minutes are recorded and provided to anyone unable to attend the meeting so that he or she, too, can learn from others' experiences. In this way, we can work together as a team to prevent future medical errors from occurring.

—*Kathleen M. Hoff*

Would this be a suitable approach for you? Why?

THE EVIDENCE

A strong correlation has been established between nurse practice environments and patient outcomes. Aiken et al. (2008) added to an established program of research and analyzed data from 10,184 nurses and 232,342 surgical patients in 168 Pennsylvania hospitals to determine the effects of nurse practice environments on nurse and patient outcomes. Outcomes included nurse job satisfaction, burnout, intent to leave, and reports of quality of care including mortal-

ity and failure to rescue patients. This large multisite study reinforces findings from the systematic review of 94 research studies examining the relationship of nurse staffing to patient outcomes in hospitals for the Agency of Healthcare Research and Quality (AHRQ) published in 2007 by Kane et al.

Kane et al. showed that increased nurse staffing was associated with reduced patient mortality, reduced failure to rescue, and decreased length of stay, whereas Aiken et al. advanced that nurses reported more positive job experiences and fewer concerns about quality care and that patients had a significantly lower risk of death and failure to rescue in hospitals with better care environments. Specifically, surgical mortality rates were more than 60% higher in poorly staffed hospitals with the poorest patient care environments than in hospitals with better care environments, the best nurse staffing levels, and the most highly educated nurses. The number of patient deaths that could be avoided by improved care environments, nurse staffing, and nurse education is estimated to be approximately 40,000 per year. Nurse leaders have several options for improving nurse retention and patient outcomes including improving RN staffing, moving to a more educated nurse workforce, and improving the care environment. Hospitals (e.g., Magnet™ designation) whose practice environment includes investment in staff development, quality management, frontline managerial ability, and good nurse-physician relations are associated with better nurse and patient outcomes.

NEED TO KNOW NOW

- Know how to access clinical practice guidelines and standards for quality and safety using sources including Agency for Healthcare Research and Quality (AHRQ), Institute of Medicine (IOM), The Joint Commission (TJC), and National Quality Forum (NQF).

- Identify nursing-sensitive outcomes most pertinent to your practice area, and identify evidence-based practice literature addressing managing quality and risk.
- Know how to address any patient care issue using the six steps of the quality improvement process.

CHAPTER CHECKLIST

Many healthcare organizations are in the process of transforming their system to QM. Greater efficiency with improved quality is the goal of this approach. Effective QI includes identifying consumer expectations, planning, using a multidisciplinary approach, evaluating outcomes, and changing the system to provide an environment in which employees can perform their best.

- The main principles of QM and QI are as follows:
  - QM operates most effectively within a flat, democratic, organizational structure.
  - Leaders and followers must be committed to QI.
  - The goal of QM is to improve systems and processes without assigning blame.
  - Customers define quality.
  - QI focuses on outcomes.
  - Decisions must be based on facts.

- QM strives to prevent errors. Initial planning requires both time and money, but QM contributes to the bottom line in the long run.
- The major steps in the continuous QI process to evaluate and improve patient care are as follows:
  - Identify needs most important to the consumer of healthcare services.
  - Assemble a multidisciplinary team to review the identified consumer needs and services.
  - Collect data to measure the current status of these services.
  - Establish measurable outcomes and quality indicators.
  - Select and implement a plan to meet the outcomes.
  - Collect data to evaluate the implementation of the plan and the achievement of outcomes.
- Any process can be improved.

- Risk management focuses on ensuring safety and on minimizing loss after a patient-care error occurs.

- QA is the responsibility of all nurses and provides an opportunity to improve patient care at the unit level.

◼ TIPS FOR QUALITY MANAGEMENT

- QM is based on data; anything measured and recorded can be improved.
- Concentrate QI energies on factors that are most important to patient quality and safety.

- Working together to prevent problems is more effective than fixing problems after they occur.

REFERENCES

Aiken, L., Clarke, S. P., Sloane, D. M., Lake, E. T., & Cheney, T. (2008). Effects of hospital care environment on patient mortality and nurse outcomes. *Journal of Nursing Administration, 38*(5), 223-229.

American Nurses Association. (2009). National database of nursing quality indicators. Retrieved October 2009, from www.nursingquality.org.

Berkenstadt, H., Haviv, Y., Tuval, A., Shermesh, Y., Megrill, A., Perry, A., Rubin, O., & Ziv, A. (2008). Improving handoff communications in critical care. *Chest, 134*(1), 158-162.

Bodrock, J. A., & Mion, L. C. (2008). Pay for performance in hospitals: Implications for nurses and nursing care. *Quality Management in Health Care, 17*(2), 102-111.

Bulechek, G. M., Butcher, H. K., & Dochtermann, J. M. (2008). *Nursing interventions classification (NIC)* (5th ed.). St. Louis: Mosby.

Cronenwett, L., Sherwood, G., Barnsteiner, J., Disch, J., Johnson, J., Mitchell, P., Sullivan, D. T., & Warren, J. (2007). Quality and safety education for nurses. *Nursing Outlook, 55*(3), 122-131.

de Koning, H., Verver, J. P., van den Heuvel, J., Bisgaard, S., & Does, R. J. (2006). Lean Six Sigma in healthcare. *Journal for Healthcare Quality, 28*(2), 4-11.

Glance, L. G., Li, Y., Osler, T. M., Mukamel, D. B., & Dick, A. W. (2008). Impact on date stamping on patient safety measurement in patients undergoing CABG: Experience with AHRQ patient safety indicators. *BMC Health Services Research, 8*, 176.

Glickman, S. W., Baggett, K. A., Krubert, C. G., Peterson, E. D., & Schulman, K. A. (2007). Promoting quality: The health-care organization from a management perspective. *International Journal for Quality Health Care, 19*(6), 341-348.

Hall, L., Moore, S., & Barnsteiner, J. (2008). Quality and nursing: Moving from a concept to a core competency. *Urologic Nursing, 28*(6), 417-425.

Hughes, R. (2008). Tools and strategies for quality improvement and patient safety. In *Patient safety and quality: An evidence-*

based handbook for nurses. AHRQ Publication No. 08-0043. Rockville, MD: Agency for Healthcare Research and Quality.

Kane, R. L., Shamliyan,T., Mueller, C., Duval, S., & Wilt, T. (2007). *Nursing staffing and quality of patient care. Evidence report/technology assessment No. 151.* (Prepared by the Minnesota Evidence-based Practice Center under Contract No. 290-02-0009.) AHRQ Publication No. 07-E005. Rockville, MD: Agency for Healthcare Research and Quality.

Kurtzman, E. T., & Jennings, B. M. (2008). Capturing the imagination of nurse executives in tracking quality of nursing care. *Nursing Administration Quarterly, 32*(3), 235-246.

Lacey, S. R., Teasley, S. L., Henion, J. S., Cox, K. S., Bonura, A., & Brown, J. (2008). Enhancing the work environment of staff nurses using targeted interventions of support. *The Journal of Nursing Administration, 28*(7/8), 336-340.

Moorhead, S., Johnson, M., Maas, M., & Swanson, E. (2008). *Nursing outcomes classification (NOC)* (4th ed.). St. Louis: Mosby.

North American Nursing Diagnosis Association International (NANDA-I). (2008). *Nursing diagnoses: Definitions and classifications, 2009-2011.* Indianapolis: Wiley-Blackwell.

Pronovost, P. J., Goeschel, C. A., & Wachter, R. M. (2008). The wisdom and justice of not paying for "preventable complications." *The New England Journal of Medicine, 299*(18), 2197-2199.

Pronovost, P. J., Rosenstein, B. J., Paine, L., Miller, M., Haller, K., Davis, R., Demski, R., & Garrett, M. R. (2008). Paying the piper: Investing in infrastructure for patient safety. *The Joint Commission Journal on Quality and Patient Safety, 34*(6), 342-348.

Stichler, J. (2007). Nurse executive leadership competencies for health facility design. *Journal of Nursing Administration, 37*(3), 109-112.

U.S. Department of Health and Human Services. (2009). Hospital Compare. Retrieved October 2009, from www. hospitalcompare.hhs.gov.

SUGGESTED READINGS

Finkelman, A., & Kenner, C. (2007). *Teaching IOM: Implications of the Institute of Medicine reports for nursing education*. Silver Springs, MD: American Nurses Association.

Institute of Medicine. (2000). *To err is human: Building a safer health system*. Washington, DC: National Academies Press.

Institute of Medicine. (2001). *Crossing the quality chasm: A new health system for the 21st century*. Washington, DC: National Academies Press.

Institute of Medicine. (2003). *Keeping patients safe: Transforming the work environment of nurses*. Washington, DC: National Academies Press.

Institute of Medicine. (2007). *Preventing medication errors*. Washington, DC: National Academies Press.

The Joint Commission. (2007). *Improving hand-off communication*. Oak Brook, IL: Joint Commission Resources, Inc.

The Joint Commission. (2007). *Must-have information for nurses about quality and patient safety*. Oak Brook, IL: Joint Commission Resources, Inc.

The Joint Commission. (2007). *Front line of defense: The role of nurses in preventing sentinel events*. Oak Brook, IL: Joint Commission Resources, Inc.

The Joint Commission. (2002). Health care at the crossroads: Strategies for addressing the evolving nursing crisis. Oak Brook, IL: Joint Commission Resources, Inc.

WEBSITES

Agency for Healthcare Research and Quality: www.ahrq.gov/.

Centers for Disease Control and Prevention's Division of Healthcare Quality Promotion: www.cdc.gov/ncidod/dhqp/.

Institute of Medicine: www.iom.edu/.

The Joint Commission: www.jointcommission.org/.

National Institute for Occupational Safety and Health: www.cdc.gov/NIOSH/.

National Quality Forum: www.qualityforum.org/.

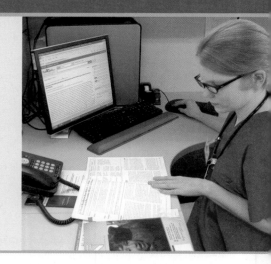

The importance of research in the development of the scientific basis for nursing practice is described in this chapter. The role of the nurse as a follower, manager, and leader of a healthcare organization in applying research to practice is delineated in the context of twenty-first century demands for providing health care based on the best available scientific evidence. The practical aspects of evaluation and utilization of research, the development of evidence-based practice in nursing, and practice-based evidence are described. Strategies for translating research into practice that can be used by the individual nurse as a follower, leader, and manager in the context of the organization are outlined.

OBJECTIVES

- Value the individual nurse's obligation to use research in practice.
- Analyze the differences among research utilization, evidence-based practice, and practice-based evidence.
- Formulate a clinical question that can be searched in the literature.
- Evaluate resources for the best available evidence.
- Identify resources for critically appraising evidence.
- Assess organizational barriers to and facilitators of the implementation of research findings.
- Identify strategies for translating research into practice within the context of an organization.

TERMS TO KNOW

clinical guidelines	practice-based evidence	research
diffusion of innovation	practice-based research network	research utilization
evidence-based practice (EBP)	(PBRN)	translating research into practice
meta-analysis	randomized controlled trial	(TRIP)
outcomes	(RCT)	

Holly Olsen, BSN, RN, CCRN
Staff Nurse, LifeFlight®, Miami Children's Hospital, Miami, Florida

I had been a staff nurse in neonatal intensive care units for 10 years, first in Miami and then Dallas, before returning to my hometown of Miami. I have been a member of the neonatal/pediatric transport team for LifeFlight®, which transports critically ill infants from the outlying community hospitals in Florida, as well as some international hospitals, back to our medical center. I was concerned about the care that we were able to provide to these fragile neonates. During the emergency of establishing an airway at the referral hospitals, using the correct endotracheal tube size and tube place-

ment were not always done according to the Neonatal Resuscitation Program (NRP) guidelines. Sometimes we would need to reinsert a tube, wasting precious time. We knew that not selecting an appropriate-size endotracheal tube for extremely-low-birth-weight (ELBW) infants could possibly lead to complications. We were not confident that everyone was familiar with best practices regarding neonatal resuscitation. I felt strongly that there had to be a way that we could improve on what we were doing.

What do you think you would do if you were this nurse?

INTRODUCTION

If you or a loved one required nursing care, you would want that care to be based on the best research evidence available. For example, if a family member needed to be on a ventilator, you would want to be sure that the nurses providing the care were using best practices to prevent ventilator-associated pneumonia. You would want to know that communication is good among nurses and physicians on the clinical unit where your family member has been placed, because you know that research demonstrates that teamwork and collaboration lead to lower mortality and fewer errors. If that family member also had a central venous catheter, you would want to be sure that the nurse who removes that catheter is using an established procedure that minimizes the risk for introducing an air embolism into the circulation. And, when that family member is discharged, you would want to know that the nurses are using well-tested strategies to help that person transition to home, recover from his or her illness, and manage that illness. As a follower, leader, and manager, you should be concerned about incorporating research not only into clinical practices but also into the management of systems of care. The challenge is how to (1) find the best research evidence, (2) incorporate the best evidence into practice in a meaningful manner, and (3) motivate nurses, nursing leadership, and organizational leadership to care about using evidence in practice in the midst of all the other challenges faced in delivering high-quality nursing care.

Research is an integral part of professional practice. Research is the "diligent, systematic inquiry or investigation to validate and refine existing knowledge and generate new knowledge" (Burns & Grove, 2009, p. 2). Nurses, as professionals, have an obligation to society that involves rights and responsibilities as well as a mechanism for accountability. These obligations are outlined in *Nursing's Social Policy Statement: The Essence of the Profession* developed by the American Nurses Association (ANA, 2010) and includes: "To refine and expand nursing's knowledge base, nurses use theories that fit with professional nursing's values of health and health care that are relevant to professional nursing practice. Nurses apply research findings and implement the best evidence into their practice ... (p. 13).

The *Code of Ethics for Nurses* (ANA, 2001, p. 22) directs that the "nurse participates in advancement of the profession through contributions to practice, education, administration and knowledge development." Furthermore, the global importance of nursing research is illustrated by an International Council of Nurses' (ICN) position statement indicating support for "national nurses' associations in their efforts to enhance nursing research, particularly through improving access to education which prepares nurses to conduct research, critically evaluate research outcomes and promote appropriate application of research findings to nursing practice" (2007, p. 3). Nursing research is designed to refine and expand the scientific foundation for nursing, which is defined as the "protection, promotion, and optimization of health and abilities, prevention of illness and injury, alleviation of suffering through the diagnosis and treatment of human response, and advocacy in the care of individuals, families, communities, and population" (ANA, 2003, p. 6). The practice of nursing draws on nursing science and the physical, economic, biomedical, behavioral, and social sciences (ANA, 2010). Therefore all nurses need to apply findings of nursing research and research conducted by members of other disciplines that have relevance for their own practice.

The translation of research into practice involves all healthcare disciplines. The National Institutes of Health (NIH) created a roadmap to harness scientific discovery to improve the health of all people. The roadmap has three major themes: (1) new pathways to discovery, (2) research teams of the future, and (3) re-engineering the clinical research enterprise (NIH, n.d.). The focus of new pathways to discovery is on new strategies for diagnosing, treating, and preventing disease. It includes building blocks, biologic pathways and networks, molecular libraries and imaging, structural biology, bio-informatics and computational biology, and nanomedicine. The research teams of the future focus on high-risk research, interdisciplinary teams, and public-private partnerships. Re-engineering the clinical research enterprise focuses on clinical research networks, policy analysis and coordination, dynamic assessment of patient-reported chronic disease outcomes, and translational research. The emphasis is getting research into the hands of practitioners who use it to better patient care.

The oft-quoted statistic of taking 17 years to apply research discoveries to clinical practice (Balas & Boren, 2000) suggests that healthcare professionals need to accelerate the integration of research with practice. Research indicates that adults in the United States receive only 54.9% of recommended care (Asch et al., 2006). We might believe that once a research study is published in a journal, clinicians read it immediately and then nurses and/or policymakers use it to improve practice. Often, that is not the case. For example, Norma Metheny has been researching techniques for testing nasogastric tube placement for many years. She and her colleagues demonstrated that relying on listening to the "swoosh" sound with a stethoscope to determine correct placement could be dangerous. Her recommendation is to test gastric contents for pH, with a pH of 0 to 4 indicating gastric placement. When the pH is greater than 4, additional testing of the aspirate for bilirubin or pepsin at the bedside is recommended. Yet, many nurses may not be familiar with the technique, nor do they have access to point-of-care testing methods (Metheny & Titler, 2001). The American Association of Critical-Care Nurses (AACN) practice alert (2005) draws heavily on Metheny's work, recommending radiographic confirmation for the initial indicator of placement. Metheny's research has also been incorporated into recommendations for enteral nutrition (Bankhead et al., 2009). EBP promotes the use of effective strategies to help patients and helps nurses stop the use of ineffective strategies that might harm patients.

Research provides the foundation for nursing practice improvement. Examples include preoperative teaching, pain management, child development assessment, falls prevention, pressure-ulcer risk detection, incontinence care, and family-centered care in critical care units. Nurses need to systematically evaluate nursing studies to decide what interventions should be implemented to improve the outcomes of care. Practices that were once thought to be the standard of care may quickly become outdated. Some practices may have been carried out for many years without ever being examined for their scientific basis or effectiveness. The latest research findings need to be incorporated into procedures using an evidence-based model when they are being updated by an organization. The Evidence section on pp. 430-431 illustrates how research can be incorporated into organizational practices.

EXERCISE 21-1

Identify a common activity that is part of your nursing practice, and determine whether any research supports that particular intervention or nursing care activity.

Nursing research designs can be categorized in several ways, such as basic versus applied, qualitative versus quantitative, cross-sectional versus longitudinal, experimental versus descriptive, and retrospective versus prospective. Regardless of the design, some research is ready for implementation and some research may not yet be ready to warrant a change in practice. Some decisions should not be based on the results of quantitative research alone but, instead, should be integrated with data from qualitative research when applied to a particular practice situation. The quality of care and the quality of the outcomes of care can be dramatically improved with the implementation of EBP. Patients, those entrusted to our care, are deserving of practices that are based on the best available evidence. Examining the evidence for a particular practice generally needs to go beyond examining the results of a single study. A single, well-designed study might be adequate for recommending and implementing a practice change at times. However, developing an EBP requires the development of a clearly written clinical question and a more thorough search of the literature, the review of single studies, meta-analyses, meta-syntheses, critically appraised topics, systematic reviews, and clinical guidelines.

Also, the evidence must be appraised and placed in the context of patient, family, and community values. Nurse managers/leaders may not necessarily be the ones actually conducting research, evaluating research evidence, or developing evidence-based guidelines, but they will be facilitating the application of research findings in practice. Key concepts for facilitating improved nursing outcomes include research utilization, evidence-based practice (EBP), practice-based evidence, diffusion of innovations, translation of research into practice (TRIP), evaluation of evidence, organizational strategies (for translating research into practice), and issues for nurse leaders and managers faced with implementing these processes.

RESEARCH UTILIZATION

Research utilization is the process of synthesizing, disseminating, and using research-generated knowledge to influence or change existing practices (Burns & Grove, 2009). Research utilization is different from, but complementary to, research. Although individual nurses may apply research findings to their own practice, nurses' broader responsibility to society includes activating the change process in translating research into practice. Research use can be in a variety of forms: enlightenment, implementation of a research-based protocol, or the widespread adoption of stan-

dards based on research findings. Ultimately, multiple factors influence how a particular research finding is adopted, translated into practice, and sustained in practice.

Nurse researchers have a distinguished record of facilitating research utilization in clinical practice that has gone beyond dissemination through publication in research journals. In the 1970s, three major federally funded projects facilitated research utilization: the Western Interstate Commission on Higher Education in Nursing (WICHEN) project, 1975; the Conduct and Utilization of Research in Nursing (CURN) project at the University of Michigan, 1976; and the Nursing Child Assessment Satellite Training (NCAST), 1976 to 1985. These early initiatives spawned the growth of many demonstration projects in an effort to implement research findings in practice, as well as research studies conducted to identify factors that facilitate or create barriers to research utilization. The NCAST program illustrates the far-reaching and enduring effect of research utilization. This program, developed by Kathryn Barnard in 1976, is widely used today by home health nurses and public health departments across the country and even internationally (NCAST Programs, 2007). More than 21,000 healthcare professionals have been trained in the use of the NCAST assessment materials, with 200 of them actively providing education at any given time.

Many research utilization models in nursing were developed in the 1970s and 1980s. One of the first was the Stetler-Marram model developed in 1976, which now includes the facilitation of EBP (Stetler, 2001). Other models developed by nurses are listed in Table 21-1.

Originally, research utilization consisted of evaluating research and determining its applicability to practice. In the 1990s, the focus changed to finding a research-based solution to a problem. Large healthcare institutions began to use research and began to evaluate the changes instituted. The forerunner of the federal Agency for Healthcare Research and Quality (AHRQ) issued consensus-based clinical guidelines for common healthcare problems, such as acute pain, incontinence, pressure ulcers, depression, and human immunodeficiency virus (HIV) prevention. Professional associations and other groups also began to issue clinical guidelines. The *National Guideline*

TABLE 21-1	RESEARCH UTILIZATION MODELS
MODEL	**SELECTED SOURCE**
Dracup-Breu (WICHEN Project)	Dracup, K.A., & Breu, C.S. (1978). Using nursing research findings to meet the needs of grieving spouses. *Nursing Research, 27,* 212-216.
Goode Research Utilization Model	Goode, C.J., Lovett, M.K., Hayes, J.E., & Butcher, L.A. (1987). Use of research-based knowledge in clinical practice. *Journal of Nursing Administration, 17*(12), 11-18.
Quality Assurance Model Using Research	Watson, C.A., Bulecheck, G., & McCloskey, J. (1987). QAMUR: A quality assurance model using research. *Journal of Nursing Quality Assurance, 2*(1), 21-27.
University of North Carolina Model	Funk, S.G., Tornquist, E.M., & Champagne, M.T. (1989). A model for improving the dissemination of nursing research. *Western Journal of Nursing Research, 11*(3), 361-372.
Multidimensional Framework of Research Utilization	Kitson, A., Harvey, G., & McCormack, B. (1998). Enabling the implementation of evidence based practice: A conceptual framework. *Quality in Health Care, 7,* 149-158.
Change to Evidence-Based Practice Model	Rosswurm, M.A., & Larrabee, J.H. (1999). A model for change to evidence-based practice. *Image: Journal of Nursing Scholarship, 31,* 317-322.
Iowa Model of Evidence-Based Practice to Promote Quality of Care	Titler, M.G., Kleiber, C., Steelman, V.J., Rakel, B.A., Budreau, G., Everett, L.Q., Buckwalter, K.C., Tripp-Reimer, T., & Goode, C.J. (2001). The Iowa model of evidence-based practice to promote quality care. *Critical Care Nursing Clinics of North America, 13,* 497-509.
Collaborative Research Utilization Model	Dufault, M. (2004). Testing a collaborative research utilization model to translate best practices in pain management. *Worldviews on Evidence-Based Nursing, 1*(3), S26-S32.
Ottawa Model of Research Use	Graham, K., & Logan, J. (2004). Using the Ottawa model of research use to implement a skin care program. *Journal of Nursing Care Quality, 19,* 18-24.
Promoting Action on Research Implementation in Health Services (PARIHS)	Rycroft-Malone, J. (2004). The PARIHS Framework: A framework for guiding the implementation of evidence-based practice. *Journal of Nursing Care Quality, 19,* 297-304.

Clearinghouse for clinical guidelines was created on the Web by the AHRQ in partnership with the American Medical Association and the American Association of Health Plans. The AHRQ guidelines, as well as guidelines developed by other groups, are included. Now, researchers and clinicians are collaborating to solve particular problems and advance health care. For example, health maintenance organizations are developing strategies to facilitate patients' adherence to screening guidelines, such as patients who have diabetes having a hemoglobin A1c test or the newer estimated average glucose (eAG) test every 3 months. Voluntary organizations providing support

services for individuals not covered by health insurance are attempting to strengthen the research foundation—that is, the evidence for the types of services they fund—to more effectively meet community needs.

Stetler's research utilization model (2001) provides direction for an individual and for group members. It has implications for nurses in leadership roles responsible for patient care management. According to Stetler, the preparatory steps of research utilization sustain EBP. Stetler's model consists of five phases: preparation, validation, comparative evaluation/decision making, translation/application, and evaluation

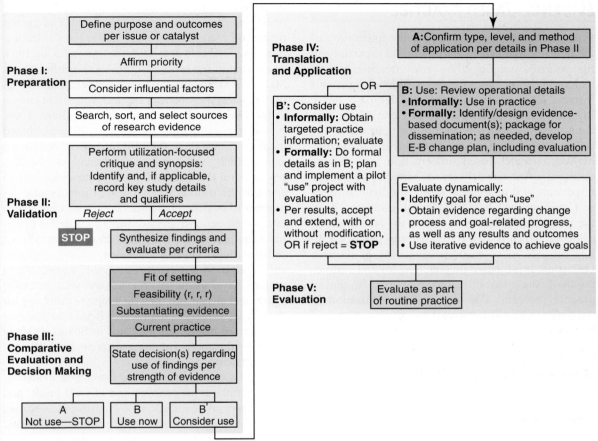

FIGURE 21-1 Stetler's model. *Feasibility (r,r,r),* Evaluation of **r**isk factors, need for **r**esources, and **r**eadiness of others involved.

(Figure 21-1). The preparatory phase involves searching, sorting, and selecting sources of evidence, defining external factors influencing the application of a research finding, and defining internal factors diminishing objectivity. The second phase, validation, focuses on utilization with an appraisal of study findings rather than the critique of a study's design. This phase includes completing review tables to facilitate understanding each study and to facilitate decision making. The third phase, comparative evaluation and decision making, involves making a decision about the applicability of the studies by synthesizing cumulative findings; evaluating the degree and nature of other criteria, such as risk, feasibility, and readiness of the finding; and actually making a recommenda-

tion about using the research. The fourth phase, translation and application, involves practical aspects of implementing the plan for translating the research into practice at the individual, group, department, or organizational level. Multiple strategies are recommended for the implementation of change. It is important to be sure that translating the research finding into practice does not exceed what the evidence warrants. The last phase includes an evaluation, which can be informal or formal and may include a cost-benefit analysis. Evaluation can include whether the research innovation was implemented as intended and goal achievement. Stetler's model focuses heavily on the change process to facilitate the successful translation of research into practice.

EVIDENCE-BASED PRACTICE

Evidence-based practice (EBP) is the integration of the best research evidence with clinical expertise and the patient's unique values and circumstances in making decisions about the care of individual patients (Straus, Richardson, Glasziou, & Haynes, 2005). Ingersoll (2000, p. 151) developed one of the first definitions for evidence-based nursing practice: "the conscientious, explicit, and judicious use of theory-derived, research-based information on making decisions about care delivery to individuals or groups of patients and in consideration of individual needs and preferences." In EBP, clinical problems drive the search for solutions based on the best available evidence, which is then translated into practice. EBP is a broader, more encompassing view of research utilization. It is focused on searching for and evaluating the best evidence to address a particular clinical practice problem. The role of the organization in implementing evidence-based practice is illustrated by Brown (2008) in the Literature Perspective below.

EBP, including evidence-based medicine, is derived from the work of Archie Cochrane. He described the lack of knowledge about healthcare treatment effects and advocated for the use of proven treatments. Subsequently, the Cochrane Collaboration was established at Oxford University in 1993. About that time, Gordon Guyatt and his colleagues at McMaster University authored a series of articles in the *Journal of the American Medical Association* known as the *Users' Guides to the Medical Literature*. These provided a foundation for teaching evidence-based medicine. Since then, the EBP movement has grown exponentially with the establishment of centers, resources on the Web, and grants given specifically to advance the translation of research into practice. A number of evidence-based nursing centers have been established around the world. The Joanna Briggs Institute, based in Australia, has a network of collaborating centers and evidence-based synthesis and utilization groups around the world. These centers have teams of researchers who critically appraise evidence and then disseminate protocols for the use of evidence in practice. Resources for evidence-based health care are listed in Box 21-1. Many nursing education programs incorporate EBP into their curricula.

Various organizations have developed evidence-based standards of practice and clinical guidelines. The American Association of Neuroscience Nurses (2007) developed a series of practice guidelines, including one about the nursing management of adults with severe traumatic brain injury. Guidelines developed by the American Society of PeriAnesthesia Nurses have been tested for their cost-effectiveness and efficiency (Berry, Wick, & Magons, 2008). The Oncology Nursing Society and the Registered Nurses Association of Ontario have developed toolkits for EBP. The American Heart Association's Council on Cardiovascular Nursing participates in interdisciplinary teams for guideline development. Many of these guidelines produced by evidence-based centers and other professional groups are available either online on the organization's website or through the *National Guideline Clearinghouse*.

Societal factors, such as the rising cost of health care, quality improvement initiatives, and the pressures to avoid errors, have resulted in an increased emphasis on research as a basis for practice decisions. Nurses and other healthcare professionals are called

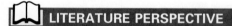

LITERATURE PERSPECTIVE

Resource: Brown, S. J. (2008). Time to move on: Definitions of evidence-based practice. *Journal of Nursing Care Quality, 23,* 201.

Using a definition of evidence-based practice (EBP) based on definitions of evidence-based medicine is limiting in that they do not accommodate EBP as it is practiced in clinical settings in which nurses work. Evidence-based medicine focuses on individual clinicians using research evidence for individual patients, whereas nurses typically practice within an organizational context and are part of a multidisciplinary team. Many nurses providing direct care have not had the educational preparation for the use of EBP. Workplace pressures may also affect the use of EBP.

Implications for Practice
EBP models in nursing need to include a broader-based organizational approach that more accurately reflects the use of evidence-based standards of care for patient populations and the nurse's use of research evidence for patient care decisions.

BOX 21-1   RESOURCES FOR EVIDENCE-BASED HEALTH CARE

Agency for Healthcare Research and Quality (AHRQ) evidence-based practice: www.ahrq.gov/clinic/epcix.htm

Centre for Evidence-Based Medicine (CEBM): www.cebm.net

The Cochrane Collaboration: www.cochrane.org

Cochrane Database of Systematic Reviews (CDSR): http://mrw.interscience.wiley.com/cochrane/cochrane_clsysrev_articles_fs.html

Centre for Evidence-Based Medicine Toronto: www.cebm.utoronto.ca

Centre for Reviews and Dissemination (CRD): www.york.ac.uk/inst/crd

Database of Abstracts of Reviews of Effects (DARE)

Health Technology Assessment (HTA) Database

NHS Economic Evaluation Database (EED)

Guidelines International Network: www.g-i-n.net/

National Guideline Clearinghouse: www.guideline.gov

National Institute for Health and Clinical Excellence: www.nice.org.uk

National Institute of Clinical Studies: http://www.nhmrc.gov.au/nics/

Scottish Intercollegiate Guidelines Network (SIGN): www.sign.ac.uk/

BOX 21-2   RESOURCES FOR EVIDENCE-BASED NURSING

Arizona State University College of Nursing Center for the Advancement of Evidence-Based Practice (CAEP): http://nursing.asu.edu/caep

Centre for Evidence Based Nursing at the University of York (UK): www.york.ac.uk/healthsciences/centres/evidence/cebn.htm

Gerontological Nursing Interventions Research Center (GNIRC), University of Iowa: www.nursing.uiowa.edu/excellence/nursing_interventions/index.htm

The Joanna Briggs Institute: www.joannabriggs.edu.au/about/home.php

The Sarah Cole Hirsch Institute for Best Nursing Practices Based on Evidence: http://fpb.case.edu/Centers/Hirsh/

Oncology Nursing Society Evidence-Based Practice Resource Area (EBPRA): http://onsopcontent.ons.org/toolkits/evidence/

The Registered Nurses Association of Ontario Nursing Best Practice Guidelines: www.rnao.org/bestpractices/

University of Texas Health Science Center at San Antonio's Academic Center for Evidence-Based Practice (ACE): www.acestar.uthscsa.edu/

upon to use evidence in practice in the midst of an exponentially expanding scientific knowledge base. The Institute of Medicine calls for all healthcare professionals to be educated in EBP. Specifically, professionals should be able to do the following (Greiner & Knebel, 2003):

- Know where and how to find the best possible sources of evidence
- Formulate clear clinical questions
- Search for relevant answers to those questions from the best possible sources, including those that evaluate or appraise evidence for its usefulness with respect to a particular patient or population
- Determine when and how to integrate those findings into practice

Nursing research exists on a continuum, and not all research is ready for, or of a quality that is appropriate for, implementation, or it may not be ready for implementation in a particular setting. However, the quality of care and the quality of the outcomes of care can be dramatically improved with the implementation of evidence-based nursing practices. Nurses are heeding the call to develop evidenced-based practices. Nurse leaders and managers have a critical responsibility in promoting the use of the best evidence for practice. Resources for evidence-based nursing are listed in Box 21-2.

EXERCISE 21-2

Select a clinical guideline appropriate for implementation in your clinical setting (see *National Guideline Clearinghouse [www.guideline.gov]*). Identify as many strategies as possible for disseminating the guideline's key points to staff nurses at your facility or a facility where you have your clinical experiences. Compare your list of strategies with that of a colleague.

PRACTICE-BASED EVIDENCE

With the growth of large databases, the use of electronic health records, and sophisticated statistical techniques, it is increasingly possible to examine practices in real-world situations and evaluate the comparative effectiveness of interventions. **Practice-based evidence**—clinical practice improvement

(PBE-CPI) is a research methodology that helps inform practice decisions by examining outcomes in the real world in which patients may not be similar and the actual application of an intervention may have multiple variations. A PBE-CPI project will (1) compare clinically relevant interventions, (2) include diverse study participants, (3) use heterogeneous practice settings, and (4) collect data on a broad range of health outcomes (Horn & Gassaway, 2007). The National Pressure Ulcer Long-term Care Study (NPULS) used this methodology at 95 facilities to identify interventions associated with decreased likelihood of pressure ulcer development (Bergstrom et al., 2005). Subsequently, the interventions were refined and implemented consistently. This resulted in a 65% decrease in the development of new pressure ulcers. Similarly, the National Database of Nursing's Quality Indicators® established by the ANA (n.d.) collects quarterly data on nursing quality indicators

and annually surveys nurse job satisfaction and work environment. Hospitals receive comparative reports and can design evidence-based practice improvement projects with outcomes measured using a standard methodology. These methodologies used together with results of clinical trials can be used to enhance patient care.

DIFFUSION OF INNOVATIONS

The now classic theory of diffusion of innovations (Rogers, 2003) describes how innovations spread through society, occurring in stages: knowledge, persuasion, decision, implementation, and confirmation. This theory, highlighted in the Theory Box below, provides a useful model in planning for the integration of evidence into practice over time.

An innovation might be continued because of the positive reinforcement received when outcomes are

---

THEORY BOX

Rogers' Diffusion of Innovations Theory

STAGE	KEY IDEA	ACTIVITIES
Knowledge	Exposure to an innovation and how it functions	The process includes seeking and analyzing information. Literature reviews are focused on addressing practice problems. Information can be disseminated through journals, conferences, educational programs, audiovisual or electronic media, journal clubs, and/or other outlets.
Persuasion	Development of attitudes about an innovation through psychological involvement and selective perception	Informal communication networks are used to facilitate change. Positive or negative attitudes can develop. An event or activity can be used to spark interest in moving from a favorable attitude to behavior change.
Decision	Commitment to adoption	The innovation can be adopted, adopted and then discontinued, rejected outright, or not even considered by the organization at this stage.
Implementation	Putting the innovation into practice	Change agents provide support for the implementation process. Behavior changes as the innovation is adopted. Key features of an innovation are identified to evaluate its effectiveness. Problems with implementing the innovation are addressed. Change and modification (reinvention) occur to use the innovation in a particular practice environment. Reinvention facilitates the sustainability of the innovation.
Confirmation	Evaluating the innovation	A decision is made about continuing or discontinuing the innovation. The innovation, if adopted, is integrated into the organization's practices.

Data from Rogers, E. (2003). *Diffusion of innovations* (5th ed., pp. 171-195). New York: Free Press.

favorable. An innovation also might be discontinued—for example, when a better idea is adopted or when disenchantment occurs because of dissatisfaction with the process or outcome.

An intervention's characteristics can influence its adoption. These include the relative advantage (whether it is better than what it replaces), compatibility (consistency with values, experiences, needs), complexity (difficulty in understanding its use), trialability (the degree to which it can be easily tested), and observability (the ease of seeing the results) (Rogers, 2003).

Widespread media attention to a particular finding can be instrumental in the adoption of a practice change. Extensive publicity accompanied the publication of a study about family presence during emergency procedures and resuscitation (Meyers et al., 2000). Publication of the study was accompanied by press releases and television news stories. Since then, the research was replicated and expanded to other settings (Smith, Hefley, & Anand, 2007), thus strengthening the scientific basis for the innovation and facilitating the practice of allowing families to be present during resuscitation. Hatfield, Gusic, Dyer, and Polomano (2008) found that the administration of oral sucrose to babies receiving their 2-month and 4-month immunizations reduced their pain scores. Their study received wide publicity in media outlets. Thus parents were alerted about the importance of asking that this simple pain management strategy be implemented for their infants when being immunized.

Nurse researchers write clinical articles in addition to research articles. Many journals that are directed toward clinicians provide nurses with easy-to-understand summaries of studies from the general healthcare and nursing research literature. Nursing schools develop press releases when researchers publish studies, which are then used by the media for their news articles. For example, Rachel Jones (2008) conducts research on the use of urban soap opera videos delivered on a handheld device to convey messages about HIV risk reduction in young adult urban women. Publicity in various media outlets in the community, her receipt of a *New York Times* award, and a website (*www.stophiv.newark.rutgers.edu/*) increase visibility of this important public health problem.

EXERCISE 21-3

Locate a research column in a clinical nursing journal. Identify one study that has implications for your practice. Retrieve the original article to learn more about the patient population, details of the study design, and results.

The translation of research into practice requires that nurse leaders and managers understand group dynamics, individual responses to innovation and change, and the culture of their healthcare organization. Rogers (2003) categorizes people according to how quickly they are willing to adopt an innovation. Box 21-3 describes these categories. Understanding the characteristics of innovation adopters is critical when planning to introduce new practices based on research evidence.

Nursing as a profession has an obligation to the public to condense the 17-year typical time frame from discovery to the adoption of a research finding. Those committed to the EBP movement in nursing have attempted to speed the adoption of innovations. Rogers' (2003) theory of diffusion of innovations is useful in helping us understand how research can be disseminated to the larger community. It also provides guidance on how to take advantage of organizational dynamics to accelerate the process.

BOX 21-3   CHARACTERISTICS OF INNOVATION ADOPTERS

Type	Characteristics
Innovators	Active in seeking new information. Organization's visionaries.
Early adopters	Organization's opinion leaders who learn about an innovation and apply it to their practice. Can be effective in communicating the value of an innovation.
Early majority	Will not bring forth an innovation but will readily adopt it when brought forth by others.
Late majority	Skeptics who do not adopt something unless there is pressure. Feel safe when there is limited uncertainty.
Laggards	Most secure in holding on to the past. Most comfortable when an idea cannot fail.

Data from Rogers, E. (2003). *Diffusion of innovations* (5th ed.). New York: Free Press.

The diffusion of an innovation does not necessarily follow a linear path. External factors may sometimes contribute to the adoption of an innovation. These may include the development of standards regarding the practice that are widely disseminated, cost-effectiveness studies, changes in the products or technology, the publication of clear and compelling evidence, and changes in staff members and leadership at an institution. The Women's Health Initiative (WHI) demonstrated a higher rate of heart disease and breast cancer in women who had estrogen plus progestin therapy (Rossouw et al., 2002). Women learning about the study's findings rushed to their healthcare providers' offices and discontinued their use of estrogen replacement therapy. Genuis (2006) examined the impact of the WHI study on medical and consumer articles and found that they are not neutral communication vehicles but, instead, provide information, reinforce knowledge, and produce and shape meaning.

A meta-analysis of the use of saline and the elimination of a low-dose heparin flush solution for capped angiocatheters is a well-known example of compelling evidence for innovation diffusion (Goode et al., 1991). A meta-analysis statistically combines the results of similar studies to determine whether the aggregated findings are significant. Although some institutions continued to use heparin flushes for a number of years, their use became less common and all but disappeared in the late 1990s. This was considerably later than one would expect, given the compelling nature of the evidence. This example illustrates the particular challenges in implementing an EBP when more than one discipline is involved. The innovation needed to be communicated to nurses. Nurses also needed to convince physicians and the institutional hierarchy that using heparin was no longer appropriate. For some institutions, it was not until the costs were analyzed and concerns were raised about complications from small doses of heparin that the transition to saline flushes was finally accomplished. This research has been extended to central line catheters in adults and capped peripheral and central line catheters in children and neonates. A systematic review of heparin use in peripheral intravenous catheters in neonates indicated that because of variations in the neonates' clinical conditions and treatments, a recommendation to use heparin could

not be made (Shah, Ng, & Sinha, 2005). The American Society of Health-System Pharmacists (2006) concurs about the lack of clarity in using heparin in intravenous catheters placed in children and neonates. Unfortunately, heparin's continued use has led to several widely publicized serious and deadly errors. Thus, careful analysis of research results, the timely implementation of important findings, and ongoing clinical research are critical to the nurse's role in promoting patient safety.

Another example of innovation diffusion is a review of the evidence for intramuscular injection technique conducted by Malkin (2008). The practice of administering intramuscular injections for pain management to adults in acute care settings has virtually disappeared with the use of the intravenous and epidural routes. Malkin rightfully emphasizes that nurses learn the technique in their initial nursing program but may never subsequently question their practice in using this technique. Intramuscular injections are widely used in many settings throughout the world to deliver long-acting antibiotics; biologicals such as immune globulins, vaccines, and toxoids; and hormonal agents. The use of the dorso-gluteal site is no longer recommended, yet we do not know what proportion of nurses continue to use this technique. This review provides nurses with an evidence-based standard that takes on even more significance because of wide variation among nurses in injection technique.

Madsen et al. (2005) questioned the practice of listening to the bowel sounds of abdominal surgery patients to assess the return of gastrointestinal motility. They concluded that the presence or absence of bowel sounds was not associated with any interventions. The authors recommend that problems experienced by patients after abdominal surgery that indicate absent bowel motility (e.g., nausea, abdominal distention) can be treated with interventions such as administering an antiemetic or inserting a nasogastric tube. A practice guideline was developed and evaluated by the research team outlining the steps in gastrointestinal assessment. Astute practitioners should observe for the subsequent adoption of these guidelines by nurses in other healthcare facilities and whether textbooks continue to mention the assessment of bowel sounds for patients after abdominal surgery.

Fetzer's (2002) meta-analysis of 20 studies demonstrated that the pain of venipuncture and intravenous line insertion could be reduced in 85% of the population (adults and children) with the use of eutectic mixture of local anesthetics (EMLA) cream. This practice has not been widely adopted; this was illustrated by a study conducted in a large urban pediatric setting that indicated that minor procedures are commonly performed without pain management (MacLean, Obispo, & Young, 2007). A stumbling block described by practitioners is the length of time required for the EMLA to take effect. This is also indicative of the relative value placed on patient comfort and patient satisfaction and the challenge in using research to change pain management practices.

TRANSLATING RESEARCH INTO PRACTICE

The science of how research is adopted is known as *translation science,* the science of translating research into practice (TRIP). Translation research has different meanings to researchers, including harnessing scientific discovery for the treatment of disease as well as ensuring that new treatments reach patients (Woolf, 2008). Translation research is the "scientific investigation of methods and variables that affect adoption of evidence-based healthcare practices by individual practitioners and healthcare systems to improve clinical and operational decision-making.... This includes testing the effects of strategies to promote and sustain evidence-based practices." (Titler, 2004, p. 38).

Research takes a long time to be translated into practice. This is illustrated by the classic example of scurvy. Lancaster demonstrated that lemon juice supplements eliminated scurvy in sailors in 1601, and Lind replicated that finding in 1747. However, it was not until 1795 that the British navy added a citrus-juice supplement to the diet of its sailors (Brown, 2005). In nursing, medication tickets or small cards were first used in 1910 to facilitate the administration of medications. One hundred years later, some institutions are still using these tickets as reminders for some aspects of their medication-administration and/or treatment-administration systems despite evidence of the potential for error through their loss or duplication. This issue is indicative of a much broader problem related to the limited use of electronic health records. According to Geibert (2006, p. 132), "technology is the bridge to integrating EBP [evidence-based practice] into patient care."

Although interest in research utilization in nursing paralleled the development of nursing as a research-based discipline, the actual translation of research into practice has not been as rapid. The seminal work of Funk, Champagne, Wiese, & Tornquist (1991) in categorizing barriers to research utilization according to the research itself, the nurse, the setting or organization, and presentation demonstrated that nurses perceived the most significant barrier to be organizational support, particularly time to use and conduct research. Nearly 10 years later, barriers to using research in Australia included access to research, anticipated outcomes of research use, organizational support, and support from others (Retsas, 2000). Some of these same barriers exist today.

The conceptual structure of research utilization includes direct, indirect, and persuasive aspects of research utilization (Estabrooks, 1999). An example of direct research utilization consists of actually using recommended interventions to prevent ventilator-associated pneumonia. An indirect research utilization example is when a nurse reads a research report and then has greater understanding of a person's response to diabetic teaching. An example of persuasive research utilization is when nurses work to implement an institutional change in practice such as using pH paper to test nasogastric tube placement. Different strategies should be used to achieve different research utilization goals.

When planning to translate a research finding into practice, nurses need to know what types of strategies have been most successful. It is also helpful to know how much time commitment was involved, how often the strategy was used, how long the treatment lasted, and whether the results were sustainable. Nurses are now testing the effectiveness of specific interventions within an organizational context and evaluating adherence to the EBP. For example, although results may be good from a particular protocol used in a randomized controlled trial to decrease ventilator-associated pneumonia, those same results may not be as dramatic when the protocol is implemented at institutions with varying resources and degrees of commitment to implementing the protocol. Nurses need to pay careful attention to the development of a clinical protocol or an evidence-based guideline and also address the implementation process. For example, implementation of EBPs with regard to pain management continues to be challenging. The implementation of an EBP pain management protocol for older adults with hip fractures not only improves the quality of pain management for these patients but also reduces hospital costs (Brooks, Titler, Ardery, & Herr, 2009; Titler et al., 2009). This EBP protocol used multifaceted strategies including practitioners' review and "reinvention" of the EBP guideline, quick reference guides, and clinical reminders. In addition, the use of opinion leaders and change champions, a 3-day train-the-trainer educational program, and educational outreach for physicians and nurses was incorporated into the protocol. The intervention had a strong effect on nurse practice but had less effect on physician practices (Titler et al., 2009).

Dobbins, Ciliska, Estabrooks, and Hayward (2005) evaluated the strength of the research evidence for various strategies that promote behavioral change among health professionals. Consistently effective strategies included academic detailing or educational outreach visits (providing healthcare providers with accurate information in face-to-face visits), reminders, multifaceted interventions, and interactive education meetings and workshops. Strategies having mixed effects included audit and feedback, local opinion leaders, local consensus processes, and patient-mediated interventions. Strategies having little or no effect included the distribution of educational materials and didactic educational programs. The key point here is that active involvement leads to greater success. In a systematic review of interventions to increase nurses' research use, only four studies met inclusion criteria (Thompson, Estabrooks, Scott-Findlay, Moore, & Wallin, 2007). Educational meetings led by an opinion leader and formation of multidisciplinary committees were effective at increasing research use. Clearly, such limited evidence illustrates the need for additional research to examine best practices in increasing nurses' use of research.

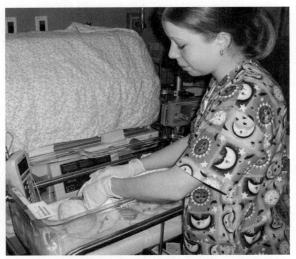

The purpose of gathering and analyzing evidence is to improve patient care.

According to Ferlie and Shortell (2001), the translation of research into practice operates at four levels: the individual healthcare professional, healthcare groups or teams, organizations, and the larger healthcare system or environment. They go on to describe strategies for change that are appropriate at each level, such as protocol and guideline development at the individual and team level, knowledge management at the organizational level, and the establishment of EBP centers at the systems level. This implies a multifaceted approach to disseminating EBPs and the responsibility to the larger healthcare community in fostering EBP. Various funding agencies support TRIP projects designed to evaluate the effectiveness of strategies to implement research findings because of the societal need for the timely implementation of scientific findings. TRIP science has the potential to speed up the adoption of innovations and sustain their use over time.

For research to be translated into practice, it needs to reach the nurse, nurse leaders, nurse managers, and administrators in an institution, as well as policymakers who can provide the infrastructure and support necessary for the implementation of research results. Reaching the nurse also involves understanding how nurses make decisions to use scientific information (Bucknall, 2007). Changing widespread practices can be very challenging. For example, Brooten et al. (2002) have consistently demonstrated that interventions by advanced practice registered nurses have improved patient outcomes and reduced healthcare costs for very-low-birth-weight (VLBW) infants; women with unplanned cesarean births, high-risk pregnancies, and hysterectomies; and older adults with cardiac medical and surgical diagnoses. However, this research was being conducted and disseminated during the same period that hospitals were eliminating clinical nurse specialist positions! The public and government agencies will increasingly expect that research findings be implemented, particularly when patient outcomes and cost savings improve significantly.

Evidence-based nursing involves a fundamental shift in philosophy. Rather than relying on nurses, be they clinicians, managers, or administrators, to read the research and apply it to practice, they are now called upon to analyze practice problems and identify the research that will help them answer questions about how they should go about delivering care. Translation science takes EBP a step further in accountability for using evidence-based strategies to implement scientifically based practices.

EVALUATING EVIDENCE

Evidence is best evaluated with a systematic process. The EBP steps are illustrated in Box 21-4. The first steps in the implementation of EBP are creating a spirit of inquiry and identifying the problem so that the relevant information can be obtained. The clinical question should be put into the widely used PICOT format of *patient, intervention, comparison intervention or group, outcome,* and *time* to facilitate searching for the appropriate evidence (Melnyk, Fineout-Overholt, Stillwell & Williamson, 2010; Thabane, Thomas, Ye, & Paul, 2009). These steps are illustrated in Box 21-5.

Identifying the question may be the most challenging part of the process. Different strategies can be used to identify practice problems. For example, one might conduct a survey of staff members or use a focus group methodology. Conducting a staff survey would necessitate that staff members have sufficient knowledge of research and EBP to understand what is desired. The data from surveys or focus groups, or

---

BOX 21-4   STEPS OF EVIDENCE-BASED PRACTICE

0. Cultivate a spirit of inquiry.
1. Ask the burning clinical question in PICOT (patient, intervention, comparison, outcome, and time frame) format.
2. Search for and collect the most relevant best evidence.
3. Critically appraise the evidence (i.e., rapid critical appraisal, evaluation, and synthesis).
4. Integrate the best evidence with one's clinical expertise and patient preferences and values in making a practice decision or change.
5. Evaluate outcomes of the practice design or change based on evidence
6. Disseminate the outcomes of the EBP (evidence-based practice) decision or change.

From Melnyk, B.M., Fineout-Overholt, E. (2011). Making the case for evidence-based practice and cultivating a spirit of inquiry. In Melnyk, B.M., & Fineout-Overholt, E. (Eds.), *Evidence-based practice in nursing and healthcare: A guide to best practice* (pp. 3-24). Philadelphia: Lippincott, Williams & Wilkins.

BOX 21-5   ASKING THE RIGHT QUESTION: THE PICOT FORMAT

Patient population	What is the patient population or the setting? This could be adults, children, or neonates with a certain health problem; or home care versus an acute care setting.
Intervention/ Interest Area	What is the intervention? This can be an intervention or a specific area of interest (e.g., postoperative complications, the experience of postoperative pain).
Comparison	What is a comparison intervention? This is what the intervention might be compared with, such as a treatment, or the absence of a risk factor.
Outcome	What are the results? There might be multiple strategies to measure the results, such as complication rate, satisfaction, a nursing diagnosis, or a nursing quality indicator.
Time	What is the time frame for this intervention? Is time a relevant factor for this particular evaluation? For example, are you interested in short-time or long-term outcomes?

Adapted from Thabane, L., Thomas, T., Ye, C., & Paul, J. (2009). Posing the research question: Not so simple. *Canadian Journal of Anaesthesia, 56*(1), 71-79.

even informal interviews with staff, can be examined along with patient outcome data for a particular setting to address relevant practice problems. Collaborating with nurses and extending that to collaboration with members of other disciplines to identify desired outcomes will enhance the ultimate success of an evidence-based project. This is because the staff members who will eventually be involved in implementing the practice are involved in its design and conception. Once the clinical question has been identified, writing it down will help in moving on to the next step of gathering evidence.

EXERCISE 21-4

Develop a clinical question using the PICOT (patient, intervention [interest], comparison, outcome, and time) format. Do a search in *PubMed* with the key PICOT terms.

The third step of the process is searching for evidence. A number of databases are available to search for evidence. Some databases contain preprocessed evidence, such as abstracts of studies and systematic reviews of evidence. Others contain citations for original single studies. Commonly used databases are listed in Box 21-6. Obtaining a librarian's assistance to navigate the databases is helpful because the databases are constantly being upgraded with new features. Several of the suggested readings include more detailed information on locating research evidence. Preprocessed evidence can also be located in the evidence-based resources listed in Boxes 21-1 and 21-2.

The evidence for a particular practice problem can come from a single research study, an integrative review of the literature, a meta-analysis, a metasynthesis, a clinically appraised topic, a clinical guideline, or a systematic review. Sometimes a single research study might be appropriate for application to a particular problem. For other clinical questions, there might be multiple guidelines from different organizations on essentially the same clinical problem with slightly different recommendations. DiCenso, Ciliska, and Guyatt (2005) describe a hierarchy for

---

BOX 21-6	COMMONLY USED DATABASES AND SEARCH PLATFORMS FOR NURSING
CANCERLIT www.cancer.gov/search/cancer_literature/	Bibliographic database with over a million citations and abstracts related to cancer. Includes proceedings of meetings, government reports, selected monographs, and theses.
CINAHL Cumulative Index to Nursing and Allied Health Literature www.ebscohost.com/cinahl/	A comprehensive nursing and allied health abstract database that includes some full-text material such as state nursing journals, nurse practice acts, research instruments, government publications, and patient education material from 1982 to the present.
EMBASE www.embase.com	Biomedical and pharmaceutical studies. By institutional subscription.
EBSCO www.ebscohost.com	A search platform for a variety of databases including CINAHL and MEDLINE. By institutional subscription.
MEDLINE http://www.nlm.nih.gov/databases	The largest component within PubMed, indexing over 5200 journals according to medical subject headings, MeSH. Free through PubMed.
OVID www.ovid.com	A search platform for a variety of databases including CINAHL and MEDLINE. By institutional subscription and individual pay-per-view.
PsycINFO www.apa.org/psycinfo/	Abstract database of the behavioral sciences and mental health literature from the 1800s to the present. By institutional subscription or individual article purchase.
PubMed www.ncbi.nlm.nih.gov/entrez	The abstract database of the National Library of Medicine, providing access to over 15 million citations from the 1950s to the present. Links to publishers' websites for many articles. Free.

rating the strength of evidence for treatment decisions as follows:

1. Unsystematic clinical observations
2. Physiologic studies (e.g., blood pressure, bone density)
3. Single observational study addressing important patient outcomes
4. Systematic review of observational studies addressing important patient outcomes
5. Randomized trial
6. Systematic review of randomized trials

A hierarchy of preprocessed evidence (i.e., evidence from a single research study to systems that integrate and regularly update EBP) originally developed by Haynes (2001) and adapted by Collins, Voth, DiCenso, and Guyatt (2005) is illustrated in Figure 21-2. Researchers examining evidence and developing guidelines use a variety of different rating systems that include a hierarchy and key quality domains. Rating evidence is a rapidly growing field. No single established method of rating evidence is best for all situations. Ultimately, whoever conducts the analysis will have to make some decisions about the strength of the evidence and whether it can be applied to a particular patient population. What is important is that once the evidence has been located, an appropriate and systematic method for rating or appraising the evidence is used. This rating system should include an analysis of whether the evidence can be applied to a particular clinical situation.

Appraisal tools exist for evaluating different types of evidence from a single qualitative study, qualitative meta-syntheses, descriptive studies, and randomized clinical trials to systematic reviews. The suggested readings provide examples. These appraisal tools generally include a series of steps for evaluating the quality of the research that is specific to the study design, type of review or guideline, or strategy for determining the applicability of the evidence to one's practice. The *AGREE Collaboration* (2001) provides a tool for evaluating clinical guidelines. Key elements of such appraisal tools include an assessment of the reliability and validity of the evidence.

Much of the EBP literature has been devoted to evaluating randomized clinical trials. A randomized controlled trial (RCT) includes at least two groups and the random assignment of study participants to one group or another either by a coin toss or by some other strategy to test a treatment's effectiveness. Generally, it is preferable that such studies are double-

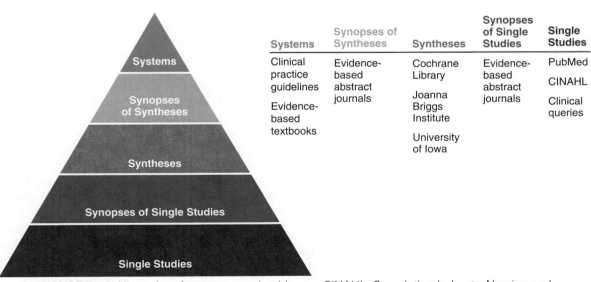

Systems	Synopses of Syntheses	Syntheses	Synopses of Single Studies	Single Studies
Clinical practice guidelines	Evidence-based abstract journals	Cochrane Library	Evidence-based abstract journals	PubMed
Evidence-based textbooks		Joanna Briggs Institute		CINAHL
		University of Iowa		Clinical queries

FIGURE 21-2 Hierarchy of preprocessed evidence. *CINAHL,* Cumulative Index to Nursing and Allied Health Literature.

blinded, meaning that the participants and those who are evaluating the outcomes do not know who has received the treatment. Although this design is generally considered the gold standard in terms of ranking individual studies, the number of RCTs conducted in nursing has been limited. Also, in certain clinical trials, blinding the recipients to a nursing intervention may be difficult to accomplish. An RCT is not always an appropriate design for answering a particular research question. Hence it is important that the appraisal method examine the rigor or the quality of the research in accordance with standards for that type of study.

Once the evidence has been appraised, this information needs to be integrated with clinical expertise and the preferences and values of patients, families, and communities in making the change. For example, in evaluating a research-based protocol for teaching oncology patients about preparing for a bone marrow transplant, the amount and type of information that would be desired by the patient need to be considered. In this instance, a qualitative research study might provide guidance for decision making. For certain types of interventions, the inclusion of patient preferences might not be appropriate, as in the example of implementing a protocol for the reduction of ventilator-associated pneumonia. Determining patient preferences depends on the nature of the intervention or change that is proposed.

The sheer quantity and complexity of information available indicate that nurses in direct practice need to collaborate with researchers. Nurses bring their clinical expertise, their assessment of clinically relevant questions, and their understanding of the patient population. Researchers bring their capacity to appraise evidence to facilitate its application to the clinical setting. Together, nurses and researchers can forge a partnership in the development of an evidence-based solution to a clinical practice problem, which can then be systematically evaluated and disseminated to the wider community.

ORGANIZATIONAL STRATEGIES

The partnership between nurses and researchers needs to be extended to top leaders and stakeholders within an organization. To implement EBPs, an organization needs to be committed to the process. Staff and management need to partner with researchers to identify the appropriate evidence. Key decision makers within the organization then need to receive the evidence in a usable format. For example, in deciding whether it is best for nurses to administer pre-procedure sedation or for parents to administer sedatives to children before their arrival in a department for a procedure, one needs to consider the evidence, the safety of the procedure, and the risks of unmonitored or parent-administered sedation, particularly if the child is being transported to the procedure in the back seat of a car. Providing key organizational decision makers with evidence regarding the safety of such a practice would be critical for decision making.

Nurse leaders and managers need to understand the organizational context for using research evidence. Lomas (2004) identifies the specific characteristics and competencies for creating the demand for research knowledge:

- Ability to understand the research and the decision-making environment
- Ability to find and assess relevant research
- Mediation and negotiation skills
- Communication skills
- Credibility

He recommends that healthcare organizations place themselves on the mailing lists for key alerts from agencies concerned with healthcare quality improvement, such as the AHRQ, distribute easy-to-read summaries to key decision makers, and have researchers brief senior management and board members directly.

The Registered Nurses Association of Ontario (2002) developed a comprehensive toolkit to assist nurses in the implementation of evidence-based guidelines. The toolkit describes strategies for working with key stakeholders and stresses their early involvement because of their understanding of the extent of the problem, unmet needs, and motivation required to address the problem. An environmental assessment included in the toolkit appears in Box 21-7. Stetler (2003) emphasizes that to sustain EBP in an organization, the leadership needs to support a research culture, the organization needs capacity to engage in EBP, and an infrastructure needs to be created to facilitate EBP. The latter includes integrating research into key documents, creating

BOX 21-7   IMPLEMENTATION OF CLINICAL PRACTICE GUIDELINES (CPG): ENVIRONMENTAL READINESS ASSESSMENT WORKSHEET

Element	Question	Facilitators	Barriers
Structure	To what extent does decision-making occur in a decentralized manner? Is there enough staff to support the change process?		
Workplace culture	To what extent is the CPG consistent with the values, attitudes and beliefs of the practice environment? To what degree does the culture support change and value evidence?		
Communication	Are there adequate (formal and informal) communication systems to support information exchange relative to the CPG and the CPG implementation processes?		
Leadership	To what extent do the leaders within the practice environment support (both visibly and behind the scenes) the implementation of the CPG?		
Knowledge, skills, and attitudes of target group	Does the staff have the necessary knowledge and skills? Which potential target group is open to change and new ideas? To what extent are they motivated to implement the CPG?		
Commitment to quality management	Do quality improvement processes and systems exist to measure results of implementation?		
Availability of resources	Are the necessary human, physical, and financial resources available to support implementation?		
Interdisciplinary relationships	Are there positive relationships and trust between and among the disciplines that will be involved or affected by the CPG?		

Reprinted with permission from Registered Nurses Association of Ontario. (2002). *Toolkit: Implementation of clinical practice guidelines.* Toronto, Canada: Author. Available online at www.rnao.org/bestpractices.

expectations and roles, and providing recognition and technical support.

EXERCISE 21-5

Use the environmental readiness assessment in Box 21-7 to assess the capacity of your agency to implement an evidence-based guideline. Identify one strategy to address a specific barrier to implementation.

The Magnet Recognition Program® was developed by the American Nurses Credentialing Center (ANCC) to recognize excellence in nursing services. As more hospitals seek Magnet™ designation, greater emphasis will be placed on the integration of research with the delivery of nursing care. Research on the revised Magnet™ model is expected to include evidence of redesign, new models of care, application of new evidence to guide practice, and visible contributions to the science of nursing (Wolf, Triolo, & Ponte, 2008).

The adoption of EBPs ultimately depends on a complex interaction of individual and organizational factors. Outside of nursing, factors associated with the adoption of innovation include larger organizational size, presence of a research champion, less traditionalism, and uncommitted organizational resources. Organizational determinants that positively influence research utilization by nurses include staff development, opportunity for nurse-to-nurse collaboration, staffing and support services; less research utilization was associated with increased emotional exhaustion and higher rates of patient and nurse adverse events (Cummings, Estabrooks, Midodzi, Wallin, & Hayduk, 2007). Nurse managers and administrators are increasingly called upon to support individual nurses, implement strategies to enhance individuals' use of evidence, and create an organizational infrastructure that promotes EBP.

ISSUES FOR NURSE LEADERS AND MANAGERS

Some of the issues faced by nurse leaders and managers include a lack of resources, limited expertise of staff members with respect to EBP, lack of knowledge about nursing research, and limited time for planning. Not all organizations can hire a full-time nurse researcher. Some organizations may not employ clinical nurse specialists. This is shortsighted in view of the potential benefits of improved patient outcomes and cost savings because of a reduction in adverse outcomes. However, this resource limitation is a reality faced in many organizations. Regardless, it is important to remember that using the best available evidence can be most successful in a partnership model.

Therefore working with nurse researchers at a local college or university could be valuable. An example of a partnership between second-degree nursing students and clinicians facilitated by Patricia Stone at Columbia University is illustrated in Box 21-8. New graduates who have recently completed research courses can use this model to partner with experienced nurses, thus demonstrating leadership skills and strengthening mentorship bonds. Faculty can partner with staff in a facility to provide consultation for a specific patient care problem, and agencies can partner together to address a specific practice problem.

Collaboration is a critical organizational attribute ensuring that evidence-based practices are incorporated into nursing care. Collaboration within the

---

BOX 21-8   COLLABORATION IN DEVELOPING AN EVIDENCE-BASED PROTOCOL FOR KANGAROO CARE

Clinician Perspective

We discovered there was interest in, but not common practice of, kangaroo care for premature babies. Many of the staff members in our facilities have a wealth of clinical experience. But, they really did not have the chance to learn about evidence-based practice in school. The students came to us to talk about our needs. When they finished their work, they presented their findings about the evidence for kangaroo care and thermoregulation at our regional perinatal center nursing leadership retreat. Initially, they were intimidated about presenting to a group of such experienced nurses. However, it was rewarding to see them become more confident about their work.

Since the student presentation, we have had an upsurge of interest in providing kangaroo care. It has helped us in overcoming resistance to its use. We are now working on how to most effectively implement kangaroo care because it takes concerted work and staff time to teach and prepare the parents. One of our hospitals is using the poster developed by the students as a training tool. I enjoyed working with the students in a way that produced a tangible outcome for everyone involved. Learning how to conduct research for evidence-based practice gave the students a skill that they will have as new nurses and can offer as a complement to their more experienced nursing colleagues as they begin their professional careers.

Sally Girvin, MPH, BS, RN, NP
Coordinator, New York Presbyterian Regional Perinatal Centers, New York

Student Perspective

The eight of us who worked on this project were in the middle of our accelerated nursing program when it was assigned to us. We had to come up with an answerable clinical question, but due to our lack of clinical experience, we had only a vague idea of what to ask. We were able to develop our question after we talked with Sally and listened to her needs. We had spent some time in the neonatal intensive care unit and realized how hard it would be for the already busy nurses to take on this project. As students, we had the time.

When we went to the retreat to present our project, we thought no one would be interested in what we had done, that it might not be applicable, or that we had discovered something they already knew. The response was incredible. Our presentation created open debate. Some hospitals had kangaroo-care policies, some did not, some had them and did not follow them, and some people were unsure what they had in place. It really prompted people to look at their practices. It was a great experience to work with Sally and her colleagues and to see that what we did had an influence on policy. It was an experience that we can take with us wherever we go.

Elizabeth K. Kelly, BS, RN
Student at Columbia University School of Nursing, New York, when this project was developed

organization should involve the interdisciplinary healthcare team. For example, the adoption of suctioning guidelines should include all members of the healthcare team involved in suctioning including nurses, pulmonologists, hospitalists, and respiratory therapists. Ideally, documentation is integrated and focused on patient outcomes in order to improve practice. Collaboration also can take place through a practice-based research network (PBRN). Originally formed to address research issues in primary care, PBRNs are being used increasingly in large healthcare organizations having the capability of integrating systems across multiple practice sites. PBRNs in nursing exist for primary care, community nursing centers, and school nurses (Deshefy-Longhi, Swartz, & Grey, 2008; Vessey et al., 2007; Anderko, Lundeen, & Bartz, 2006). These networks facilitate answering research questions that require larger samples and can draw upon the depth of the group's practice and research expertise. They also have the potential for expansion into other settings such as home care, hospice, rehabilitation, and long-term care. The U.S. Department of Veterans Affairs (VA) established the *Quality Enhancement Research Initiative (QUERI)* to improve health care by translating research into practice. Its efforts are focused on heart failure, diabetes, HIV/hepatitis, heart disease, mental health, polytrauma, stroke, and substance use disorders (VA, n.d.). In addition, numerous informal groups have been established to address specialized needs and common concerns (e.g., researchers at Magnet™-accredited facilities).

Another organizational issue is that many nurses might not have had research and/or statistics courses in their basic nursing education. Or nurses may have had research courses many years ago and have not since used their research knowledge. Even if they did have a course, nurses, nurse managers, and administrators might not be familiar with the critical appraisal of evidence. Nurses on a clinical unit might not be familiar with reading research or with using advanced search strategies for locating evidence for a particular practice problem. This might be especially true for nurses who have been out of school for a long time and have not had the opportunity to develop computer literacy skills. Information on evidence-based nursing as an approach has only recently been incorporated into nursing research textbooks. Therefore a first step in developing the capacity to evaluate evidence for practice can be facilitated by starting a journal club that meets once a month. This involves reading a relevant research article and discussing how it might be applied to the practice situation. Although there are a number of general and specialty nursing research journals, *Evidence-Based Nursing* and *Worldviews on Evidence-Based Nursing* are specifically devoted to evidence-based nursing practice. *Implementation Science* is a journal devoted specifically to the examination of strategies to promote the incorporation of research findings into routine health care. The resulting discussion at a journal club can be used as a springboard for the identification of clinical practice problems. Even small hospitals have libraries and perhaps a part-time librarian who can assist with gathering information and identifying useful articles for the journal club's agenda. Nurses returning to school for advanced education have access to a university library, as do nurses who are employed as adjunct faculty in nursing programs.

When translating research into practice, conduct an evaluation to document outcomes. It is preferable to collect outcomes data before implementing a protocol in order to have a basis for comparison. This is especially important when it is not possible to carry out an experimental design in which the intervention is implemented in one setting but not another. This may be the case because of sample size considerations or staff of different units casually talking with one another about the intervention. It is also important to consider whether the implementation of an evidence-based practice will turn into a research project. Research is usually considered to be the generation of new knowledge. Quality improvement activities and the adoption of evidence-based practices might not meet the standards for a research project, and the results might not be generalizable to other settings (Newhouse, 2007). Regardless, nurses preparing to engage in a project that might be considered research should consult with the organization's institutional review board early in the planning phase regardless of whether data are collected directly from patients, medical records, or staff members.

Nurses, other healthcare professionals, and the public might not be familiar with nursing research or evidence-based nursing. Therefore it is important to publicize key nursing research findings. When nursing research is publicized in the media or through news alerts, be sure to communicate these findings to organizational key decision makers. Sending e-mails, posting articles, and providing people with the resources help others learn for themselves. Joining a professional association and a specialty association and signing up for alerts from key agencies provide nurses with access to the latest news, research, and standards. Research has a much better chance of being implemented if key stakeholders have the opportunity to understand its relevance. It may be necessary to introduce concepts related to translating research into practice in small increments. For example, a first step might be incorporating research into the revision of procedures and agency guidelines as they come up for review. Subsequently, nurses and key stakeholders can be asked to identify clinical practice problems that create challenges in providing care in order to develop an evidence-based solution. Multiple strategies are needed to implement research findings. Multiple strategies are needed to change a culture to one that is driven by research and evidence-based standards for practice Finally, if one should have the opportunity to implement an EBP, as much consideration needs to be given to planning for implementation as protocol development (see Chapter 17). Advance planning should include a thorough and frank discussion of the barriers and facilitators, as well as how to minimize the barriers and maximize the facilitators. Also, strategies to sustain the adoption of the practice over time need to be considered. Although the implementation of EBP is a very complex process, the increased emphasis on the use of scientifically based evidence creates an exciting opportunity for nurses to demonstrate the value of nursing in improving patient care and healthcare outcomes.

THE SOLUTION

I began by working with a team that included a fellow staff nurse, a nurse researcher, and a nurse practitioner. We reviewed the literature and found that guidelines for selecting an appropriate-size endotracheal tube for ELBW infants were unclear. We also decided to do a retrospective chart audit to determine what, if any, were the effects of size variations of the endotracheal tube and the depth of endotracheal tube placement on oxygen saturation and carbon dioxide levels upon intubation. We used guidelines from the NRP.

Conducting research is not without its challenges. I have not had much experience with data collection. It was also difficult to get the time to do the study. However, we really wanted to carry out this project. Sometimes, we would take our laptop on transport with us and do data entry during the "dead leg" (on the way to get the patient), as well as during our down times between transports. We shared the results with the staff at our hospital and with our community partners. Subsequently, we made large charts to be used by everyone who would be involved in neonatal resuscitation. We had a very positive response. I believe that the work we did was really important in improving the quality of care provided by the staff of our transport team and our outlying community hospitals for these tiny, fragile babies.

—*Holly Olsen*

Would this be a suitable approach for you? Why?

▌THE EVIDENCE

Dufault et al. (2008) describe the strategy used by a collaborative team consisting of university nurse researchers, a Magnet™ coordinator, a staff nurse, and a librarian to examine the research evidence for the assessment of peripheral vascular circulation by checking capillary refill. The literature search yielded eight studies meeting their criteria. Students at the local universities provided an in-depth critique of each study. The authors used staff nurse–led roundtables at the local hospital to further examine each study's scientific merit, clinical applicability, usefulness, and potential for translation into best practice to supplement the analysis provided by the critiques. In addition, three independent reviewers assessed each study's quality with two-thirds agreement required for the study's endorsement. Despite being unable to locate clinical trials comparing assessment of capillary refill with newer techniques, the authors concluded that no evidence supported the use of capillary refill assessment in clinical practice. It was further noted that no nursing interventions are based solely on capillary refill assessment.

NEED TO KNOW NOW

- Identify the most common practice problems in a clinical setting.
- Update practice by using the latest evidence.
- Work together with fellow nurses, key stakeholders, and colleagues across disciplines to adopt an evidence-based practice.

- Evaluate the results of a practice change.
- Communicate successes to colleagues, patients, families, and the public.

CHAPTER CHECKLIST

Society increasingly demands that health care be based on the best available evidence. Nurses have a societal obligation to use practices that are based on sound scientific evidence. The time from scientific discovery or publication of research to implementation in practice is lengthy and needs to be shortened. Nurses can speed this process by using scientifically based strategies to facilitate the translation of research into practice. The nurse manager needs to understand the organizational context for the implementation of evidence-based protocols. Multiple strategies need to be developed to enhance the use of evidence as the foundation for nursing care delivery.

- Research is an integral part of professional nursing practice and part of every nurse's obligation under the *Code of Ethics for Nurses* (ANA, 2001).
- Research utilization is critical to an organization:
  - Synthesis, dissemination, and use of research are three distinct efforts.
  - Nurse researchers have a long history of developing demonstration projects to enhance research utilization.
  - A number of research utilization models have been developed in nursing.
  - The Stetler model (2001) incorporates elements of EBP and focuses heavily on the change process to facilitate translation of research into practice. The model's steps include preparation, validation, comparative evaluation and decision making, translation/application, and evaluation.

- Evidence-based nursing practice is the driving force in today's healthcare approaches:
  - Research-based information is used to make decisions.
  - Patient needs and preferences need to be considered.
  - EBP is broader in scope in that it involves appraising the evidence to address a specific clinical practice problem, whereas research utilization involves applying the findings from a particular study in practice.
- Rogers' diffusion of innovations theory (2003) is a useful framework for understanding how innovations are diffused throughout an organization. The phases of the innovation adoption process include knowledge, persuasion, decision, implementation, and evaluation.
- According to Rogers (2003), innovation adopters can be classified in the following categories: innovators, early adopters, early majority, late majority, and laggards.
- The science of how research is adopted is the science of translating research into practice (TRIP). Once an evidence-based protocol has been developed, research-based methods need to be used to enhance its implementation and sustain its adoption over time.
- Evaluating research evidence should be done in a systematic manner:
  - Asking the relevant clinical question
  - Searching for the evidence

- Appraising the evidence
- Integrating the evidence with clinical expertise; patient, family and community preferences; and values
- Evaluating the outcomes
- Developing a relevant clinical question is enhanced by using the PICOT format:
  - Patient population
  - Intervention/interest
  - Comparison
  - Outcome
  - Time
- An organizational assessment of the capacity for EBP will facilitate the translation of research into practice. An organization assessment includes the following:
  - Access to resources for evidence
  - Capacity to appraise evidence
  - Adaptability in providing key leaders with summarized evidence
- Capacity to demonstrate applicability of the evidence to key leaders
- Practice-based evidence is a strategy to answer clinical practice questions in real-world settings.
- Skills required for translating research into practice include the following:
  - Ability to understand the research and decision-making environment
  - Ability to find and assess relevant research
  - Mediation and negotiation skills
  - Communication skills
  - Credibility
  - Collaboration
- Strategies to enhance individuals' abilities in using evidence, support for individual nurses' efforts to use research, as well the establishment of an organizational infrastructure, will promote the use of EBPs.

TIPS FOR DEVELOPING SKILL IN USING EVIDENCE

- Make a personal commitment to read research articles.
- Complete an online tutorial in EBP.
- Use your clinical experiences to develop relevant clinical questions.
- Obtain assistance from researchers, advanced practice registered nurses, and nurse leaders.
- Use the Patient, Intervention, Comparison, Outcome, and Time (PICOT) format to search for evidence on a clinical practice problem.
- Use a journal club to encourage your colleagues to join you in learning about EBP and evaluating research evidence.

REFERENCES

The AGREE Collaboration. (2001). Appraisal of guidelines for research & evaluation (AGREE) instrument. Retrieved April 6, 2010, from www.agreecollaboration.org.

American Association of Critical-Care Nurses (AACN). (2005). AACN clinical practice alert: Verification of feeding tube placement. Aliso Viejo, CA: Author. Retrieved October 2009, from www.aacn.org.

American Association of Neuroscience Nurses. (2007). Nursing management of adults with severe traumatic brain injury. Glenview, IL: Author. Retrieved April 4, 2010 from http://www.aann.org/pubs/guidelines.html.

American Nurses Association (ANA). (2001). Code of ethics for nurses with interpretive statements. Washington, DC: Author.

American Nurses Association (ANA). (2003). Nursing's social policy statement (2nd ed.). Silver Spring, MD: Author.

American Nurses Association (ANA). (2010). Nursing's social policy statement: The essence of the profession. Silver Spring, MD: Author.

American Nurses Association (ANA). (n.d.). National database of nursing's quality indicators. Silver Spring, MD: Author.

American Society of Health-System Pharmacists. (2006). ASHP therapeutic position statement on the institutional use of 0.9% sodium chloride injection to maintain patency of peripheral indwelling intermittent infusion devices. American Journal of Health-System Pharmacy, 63, 1273-1275.

Anderko, L., Lundeen, S., & Bartz, C. (2006). The Midwest Nursing Centers Consortium Research Network: Translating research into practice. Policy, Politics & Nursing Practice, 7, 101-109.

Asch, S. M., Kerr, E. A., Keesey, J., Adams, J. L., Setodji, C. M., Malik, S., & McGlynn, E. A. (2006). Who is at greatest risk for receiving poor-quality health care? New England Journal of Medicine, 354(11), 1147-1156.

Balas, E., & Boren, S. (2000). Managing clinical knowledge for health care improvement. In J. vanBemmel & A. McCray

(Eds.), *Yearbook of medical informatics 2000: Patient-centered systems* (pp. 65-70). Stuttgart, Germany: Schattauer.

Bankhead, R., Boullata, J., Brantley, S., Corkins, M., Guenter, P., Krenitsky, J., Lyman B., Metheny, N. A., Mueller, C., Robbins, S., Wessel, J. & A.S.P.E.N. Board of Directors. (2009). Enteral nutrition practice recommendations. *JPEN Journal of Parenteral and Enteral Nutrition, 33*(2), 122-167.

Bergstrom, N., Horn, S. D., Smout, R. J., Bender, S. A., Ferguson, M. L., Taler, G., Sauer, A. C., Sharkey, S. S., & Voss, A. C. (2005). The National Pressure Ulcer Long-Term Care Study: Outcomes of pressure ulcer treatments in long-term care. *Journal of the American Geriatrics Society, 53*, 1721-1729.

Berry, D., Wick, C., & Magons, P. (2008). A clinical evaluation of the cost and time effectiveness of the ASPAN Hypothermia Guideline. *Journal of Perianesthesia Nursing, 23*, 24-35.

Brooks, J. M., Titler, M., Ardery, G., & Herr, K. (2009). Effect of evidence-based acute pain management practices on inpatient costs. *HSR: Health Services Research, 44*, 245-263.

Brooten, D., Naylor, M. D., York, R., Brown, L. P., Munro, B. H., Hollingsworth, A. O., Cohen, S. M., Finkler, S., Deatrick, J., & Youngblut, J. M. (2002). Lessons learned from testing the quality cost model of advanced practice nursing (APN) transitional care. *Journal of Nursing Scholarship, 34*(4), 369-375.

Brown, S. R. (2005). *Scurvy: How a surgeon, a mariner, and a gentlemen solved the greatest medical mystery of the age of sail.* New York: St. Martin's Press.

Brown, S. J. (2008). Time to move on: Definitions of evidence-based practice. *Journal of Nursing Care Quality, 23*, 201.

Bucknall, T. (2007). A gaze through the lens of decision theory in translation science. *Nursing Research, 56*(4 Suppl. 1), 560-566.

Burns, N., & Grove, S. K. (2009). *The practice of nursing research: Conduct, critique, and utilization* (6th ed.). St. Louis: Saunders.

Collins, S., Voth, T., DiCenso, A., & Guyatt, G. (2005). Finding the evidence. In A. DiCenso, G. Guyatt, & D. Ciliska (Eds.), *Evidence-based nursing: A guide to clinical practice* (pp. 20-43). St. Louis: Mosby.

Cummings, G. G., Estabrooks, C. A., Midodzi, W. K., Wallin, L., & Hayduk, L. (2007). Influence of organizational characteristics and context on research utilization. *Nursing Research, 56*(Suppl. 4), S24-S39.

Deshefy-Longhi, T., Swartz, M. K., & Grey, M. (2008). Characterizing nurse practitioner practice by sampling patient encounters: An APRNet study. *Journal of the American Academy of Nurse Practitioners, 20*, 281-287.

DiCenso, A., Ciliska, D., & Guyatt, G. (2005). Introduction to evidence-based nursing. In A. DiCenso, G. Guyatt, & D. Ciliska (Eds.), *Evidence-based nursing: A guide to clinical practice* (pp. 3-19). St. Louis: Mosby.

Dobbins, M., Ciliska, D., Estabrooks, C., & Hayward, S. (2005). Changing nursing practice in an organization. In A. DiCenso, G. Guyatt, & D. Ciliska (Eds.), *Evidence-based nursing: A guide to clinical practice* (pp. 172-200). St. Louis: Mosby.

Dufault, M. (2004). Testing a collaborative research utilization model to translate best practices in pain management. *Worldviews on Evidence-Based Nursing, 1*(3), S26-S32.

Dufault, M., Davis, B., Garman, D., Hehl, R., Henry, J., Lavin, M., Barnes-Mullaney, J., & Stout, P. (2008). Translating best practices in assessing capillary refill. *Worldviews on Evidence-Based Nursing, 5*(1), 36-44.

Estabrooks, C. A. (1999). The conceptual structure of research utilization. *Research in Nursing and Health, 22*, 203-216.

Ferlie, E. B., & Shortell, S. M. (2001). Improving the quality of health care in the United Kingdom and the United States: A framework for change. *Milbank Quarterly, 79*, 281-315.

Fetzer, S. J. (2002). Reducing venipuncture and intravenous insertion pain with eutectic mixture of local anesthetic: A meta-analysis. *Nursing Research, 51*, 119-124.

Funk, S. G., Champagne, M. T., Wiese, R. A., & Tornquist, E. (1991). Barriers: The Barriers to Research Utilization Scale. *Applied Nursing Research, 4*, 39-45.

Funk, S. G., Tornquist, E. M., & Champagne, M. T. (1989). A model for improving the dissemination of nursing research. *Western Journal of Nursing Research, 11*(3), 361-372.

Geibert, R. C. (2006). The journey to evidence: Managing the information infrastructure. In K. Malloch & T. Porter-O'Grady (Eds.), *Introduction to evidence-based practice in nursing and health care* (pp. 125-148). Boston: Jones & Bartlett.

Genuis, S. K. (2006). Exploring the role of medical and consumer literature in the diffusion of information related to hormone therapy for menopausal women. *Journal of the American Society for Information Science and Technology, 57*(7), 974-988.

Goode, C. J., Lovett, M. K., Hayes, J. E., & Butcher, L. A. (1987). Use of research-based knowledge in clinical practice. *Journal of Nursing Administration, 17*(12), 11-18.

Goode, C. J., Titler, M., Rakel, B., Ones, D. S., Kleiber, C., Small, S., & Triolo, P. K. (1991). A meta-analysis of effects of heparin flush and saline flush: Quality and cost implications. *Nursing Research, 40*, 324-330.

Graham, K., & Logan, J. (2004). Using the Ottawa model of research use to implement a skin care program. *Journal of Nursing Care Quality, 19*, 18-24.

Greiner, A. C., & Knebel, E. (Eds.), Board on Health Care Services, Committee on the Health Professions Summit, Institute of Medicine. (2003). *Health professions education: A bridge to quality.* Washington, DC: National Academies Press.

Hatfield, L. A., Gusic, M. E., Dyer, A. M., & Polomano, R. C. (2008). Analgesic properties of oral sucrose during routine immunizations at 2 and 4 months of age. *Pediatrics, 121*, 327-334.

Haynes, R. B. (2001). Of studies, syntheses, synopses, and systems: The "4S" evolution of services for finding current best evidence. *ACP Journal Club, 134*(2), A11-A13.

Horn, S., & Gassaway, J. (2007). Practice-based evidence study design for comparative effectiveness research. *Medical Care, 45*(Suppl. 2), S50-S57.

Ingersoll, G. (2000). Evidence-based nursing: What it is and what it isn't. *Nursing Outlook, 48*, 151-152.

International Council of Nurses (ICN). (2007). Nursing research (position statement). Retrieved October 2009, from www.icn.ch/PS_B05_Nsg%20Research.pdf.

Jones, R. (2008). Soap opera video on handheld computers to reduce young urban women's HIV sex risk. *AIDS Behavior, 12*, 876-884.

Kitson, A., Harvey, G., & McCormack, B. (1998). Enabling the implementation of evidence based practice: A conceptual framework. *Quality in Health Care, 7*, 149-158.

Lomas, J. (2004). It takes two to tango: The importance of joint knowledge production for research use. *Canadian Health Services Research Foundation.* Presentation at the Ministerial Summit on Health Research and Global Forum, Mexico City, Mexico, November 2004.

MacLean, S., Obispo, J., & Young, K. D. (2007). The gap between pediatric emergency department procedural pain management treatments available and actual practice. *Pediatric Emergency Care, 23*, 87-93.

Madsen, D., Sebolt, T., Cullen, L., Folkedahl, B., Mueller, T., Richardson, C., & Titler, M. (2005). Listening to bowel sounds: An evidence-based practice project. *American Journal of Nursing, 105*(12), 40-49.

Malkin, B. (2008). Are techniques used for intramuscular injection based on research evidence? *Nursing Times, 104*(50/51), 48-51.

Melnyk, B. B., Fineholt-Overholt, E., Stillwell, S. B., & Williamson, K. M. (2010). Evidence-based practice: Step-by-step: The seven steps of evidence-based practice. *American Journal of Nursing, 110*(1), 51-53.

Metheny, N. A., & Titler, M. G. (2001). Assessing placement of feeding tubes. *American Journal of Nursing, 101*(5), 36-46.

Meyers, T. A., Eichhorn, D. J., Guzzetta, C. E., Clark, A. P., Klein, J., Taliaferro, E., & Calvin, A. (2000). Family presence during invasive procedures and resuscitation: The experience of family members, nurses, and physicians. *American Journal of Nursing, 100*(2), 32-43.

National Institutes of Health (NIH). (n.d.). NIH roadmap; Accelerating medical discovery to improve health. Retrieved April 15, 2006, from http://nihroadmap.nih.gov.

NCAST Programs. (2007). *History.* Seattle, WA: Author. Retrieved April 4, 2010 from www.ncast.org/about_us.html.

Newhouse, R. (2007). Diffusing confusion among evidence-based practice, quality improvement, and research. *Journal of Nursing Administration, 37*, 432-435.

Registered Nurses Association of Ontario. (2002). *Toolkit: Implementation of clinical practice guidelines.* Toronto, Canada: Author. Retrieved April 6, 2010, from www.rnao.org/bestpractices.

Retsas, A. (2000). Barriers to using research evidence in nursing practice. *Journal of Advanced Nursing, 31*, 599-606.

Rogers, E. (2003). *Diffusion of innovations* (5th ed.). New York: Free Press.

Rossouw, J. E., Anderson, G. L., Prentice, R. L., LaCroix, A. Z., Kooperberg, C., Stefanick, M. L., Jackson, R. D., Beresford, S. A., Howard, B. V., Johnson, K. C., Kotchen, J. M., & Ockene, J.; Writing Group for Women's Health Initiative Investigators. (2002). Risks and benefits of estrogen plus progestin in healthy postmenopausal women: Principal results from the Women's Health Initiative randomized control trial. *Journal of the American Medical Association, 288*, 321-333.

Rosswurm, M. A., & Larrabee, J. H. (1999). A model for change to evidence-based practice. *Image: Journal of Nursing Scholarship, 31*, 317-322.

Shah, P. S., Ng, E., & Sinha, A. K. (2005). Heparin for prolonging peripheral intravenous catheter use in neonates. *Cochrane Database of Systematic Reviews*, CD002774.

Smith, A. B., Hefley, G. C., & Anand, K. J. (2007). Parent bed spaces in the PICU: Effect on parental stress. *Pediatric Nursing, 33*, 215-221.

Stetler, C. B. (2001). Updating the Stetler model of research utilization to facilitate evidence-based practice. *Nursing Outlook, 49*(6), 272-279.

Stetler, C. B. (2003). Role of the organization in translating research into evidence-based practice. *Outcomes Management, 7*(3), 97-103.

Straus, S. E., Richardson, W. S., Glasziou, P., & Haynes, R. B. (2005). *Evidence-based medicine: How to practice and teach EBM* (3rd ed.). Edinburgh: Churchill Livingstone.

Thabane, L., Thomas, T., Ye, C., & Paul, J. (2009). Posing the research question: Not so simple. *Canadian Journal of Anaesthesia, 56*(1), 71-79.

Thompson, D. S., Estabrooks, C. A., Scott-Findlay, S., Moore, K., & Wallin, L. (2007). Interventions aimed at increasing research use in nursing: A systematic review. *Implementation Science, 2*, 15.

Titler, M. G. (2004). Methods in translation science. *Worldviews on Evidence-Based Nursing, 1*, 38-48.

Titler, M. G., Herr, K., Brooks, J. M., Xie, X. J., Ardery, G., Schilling, M. L., et al. (2009). Translating research into practice intervention improves management of acute pain in older hip fracture patients. *Health Services Research, 44*, 265-287.

Titler, M. G., Kleiber, C., Steelman, V. J., Rakel, B. A., Budreau, G., Everett, L. Q., Buckwalter, K. C., Tripp-Reimer, T., & Goode, C. J. (2001). The Iowa model of evidence-based practice to promote quality care. *Critical Care Nursing Clinics of North America, 13*, 497-509.

U.S. Department of Veterans Affairs. (n.d.). VA Quality Enhancement Research Initiative. Retrieved April 6, 2010, from www.queri.research.va.gov/.

Vessey, J. A., & Founding Oversight Board Members of MASNRN. (2007). Development of the Massachusetts School Nurse Research Network (MASNRN): A practice-based research network to improve the quality of school nursing practice. *Journal of School Nursing, 23*, 65-72.

Watson, C. A., Bulecheck, G., & McCloskey, J. (1987). QAMUR: A quality assurance model using research. *Journal of Nursing Quality Assurance, 2*, 21-27.

Wolf, G., Triolo, P., & Ponte, P. R. (2008). Magnet Recognition Program: Next generation. *Journal of Nursing Administration, 38*, 200-204.

Woolf, S. (2008). The meaning of translational research and why it matters. *JAMA, 299*, 211-213.

SUGGESTED READINGS

Ackley, B. J., Ladwig, G. B., Swan, B. A., & Tucker, S. J. (2008). *Evidence-based nursing care guidelines: Medical-surgical interventions*. St. Louis: Mosby.

Bakken, S., Currie, L. M., Lee, N. J., Roberts, W. D., Collins, S. A., & Cimino, J. J. (2008). Integrating evidence into clinical information systems for nursing decision support. *International Journal of Medical Informatics, 77*, 413-420.

Brown, S. J. (2008). *Evidence-based nursing: The research practice connection*. Boston: Jones & Bartlett.

Dunton, N., & Montalvo, I. (Eds). (2009). *Sustaining improvement in nursing quality: Hospital performance on NDNQI indicators, 2007-2008*. Silver Spring, MD: American Nurses Association.

Fawcett, J., & Garrity, J. (2009). *Evaluating research for evidence-based nursing*. Philadelphia: F.A. Davis.

Houser, J., & Bokovy, J. (2006). *Clinical research in practice: A guide for the bedside scientist*. Boston: Jones & Bartlett.

Kleinpell, R. (2009). *Outcome assessment in advanced practice nursing* (2nd ed.). New York: Springer.

Melnyk, B., & Fineout-Overholt, E. (Eds.). (2010). *Evidence-based practice in nursing and healthcare: A guide to best practice* (pp. 3-24). Philadelphia: Lippincott.

PART 4

Interpersonal and Personal Skills

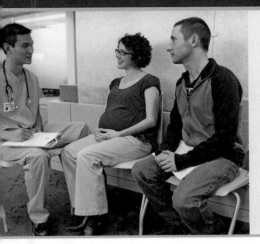

Consumer Relationships

Margarete Lieb Zalon

This chapter explores the changes that have altered consumer relationships with healthcare providers and looks specifically at nurses' responsibilities to the consumer. Nurses set the tone for effective staff-patient interaction. Because nurses are the healthcare providers who spend the most time with the consumer, this chapter provides concepts and strategies to assist in developing effective nurse-consumer relationships.

OBJECTIVES

- Categorize health consumers' interactions into three relationship structures.
- Interpret the results of selected changes that have influenced consumer relationships in health care.
- Examine the importance of a service-oriented philosophy to the quality of the nurse-consumer relationship.
- Apply the four major responsibilities of nursing—service, advocacy, teaching, and leadership—to the promotion of successful nurse-consumer relationships.

TERMS TO KNOW

advocate	healthcare consumer	patient satisfaction
consumer focus	healthcare provider	quality indicator
cultural competence	high tech	service
gatekeeper	high touch	service recovery
health literacy	medical home	

THE CHALLENGE

Suzanne Freeman, RN, MBA
President of Carolinas Medical Center, Charlotte, North Carolina

Customer satisfaction is the number-one goal in our healthcare facilities. The hospital board officially acknowledged this goal, and systems were set in place to measure, monitor, and improve customer satisfaction. The staff ultimately defined principles to illustrate their commitment to this goal: teamwork, integrity, caring, commitment, and communication. Each individual would be treated with dignity and as a valued member of a "family."

The husband of a patient seen in the emergency department (ED) some time ago called the nurse manager a few days after his wife's visit. When she arrived at the ED, her chief complaint was intermittent chest pain for 2 days. She had indicated that she did not have pain upon arrival to the ED and was ultimately admitted to the hospital with the diagnosis statement "Chest pain, rule out MI [myocardial infarction]."

The husband complained that his wife had been required to "sign herself in," even though he had asked the nurse to have his wife seen immediately. He thought that the nurse had not taken his wife's complaints seriously and that the resulting delay had caused her condition to worsen. He attributed this issue to the fact that his wife required coronary artery bypass surgery the following day.

The nurse manager immediately met with the triage nurse involved. They talked through the encounter and examined the documentation. The triage nurse thought that her assessment of "nonemergent" was valid. She noted that the patient was registered by the patient registration personnel and that the physician saw her within 30 minutes of her arrival. The triage nurse's assessment indicated "Vital signs stable, no history of heart disease, right-sided chest pain × 2 days." The pain scale records indicated "No pain now." The assessment made by the triage nurse appeared valid to the nurse manager. The nurse manager also noted that the nurse's competency in assessing patients for triage was historically reliable. The triage nurse did not recall the husband asking for his wife to be seen immediately.

The nurse manager visited the patient and her spouse in the coronary care unit. She apologized for their expectations not being met during the triage process. She assured the couple that their concerns were taken seriously and offered her sincerest apologies. Her words seemed to be well received by the couple. Each thanked her for her concern and visit.

Apparently, the couple was not satisfied, however, because the husband called the vice president for patient services that same day. He related the story, including the nurse manager's visit. He added that he had recently viewed a news report about how women were undertreated and misdiagnosed with regard to chest pain. The vice president listened carefully and promised to follow up quickly with a response.

What do you think you would do if you were this nurse? The staff nurse? The nurse manager? The vice president?

INTRODUCTION

Consumer relationships in healthcare delivery refers to the multitude of encounters between the consumer (client, patient, or customer) and healthcare system representatives. Who are the consumers of health care, and what do they expect from providers? What are their likes and dislikes, and how do they evaluate their health care?

Today, hospitals and other healthcare organizations are concerned with protecting consumer rights and are actively engaged in assessing patient/consumer satisfaction as a strategy to improve quality, enhance market share, and meet regulatory and/or accreditation requirements. The role of nurses as trusted professionals in the development of consumer relationships in healthcare organizations is increasingly recognized for its importance.

Consumers hold nurses in high regard. They view nurses as knowledgeable, worthy of respect, concerned for others, honest, caring, confidential, friendly, hardworking, and especially trustworthy. Nurses are perceived by 52% of Americans as having very great prestige (Harris Interactive, Inc., 2008). Nurses top the list in the 2009 Gallup poll of the public's ratings of honesty and ethical standards of various professions with 83% of Americans believing nurses' honesty and ethical standards are "high" or "very high" (American Nurses Association [ANA], 2009). Nurses have been at the top of the list in all but one year since they were added to the annual survey in 1999. Nurses, by virtue of this favorable status with the public, occupy positions of influence and can foster and promote successful consumer relationships across healthcare settings.

We are all consumers of health care—friends, neighbors, families, people like us, and people very different from us. Consumers are diverse culturally, ethnically, socially, physically, and psychologically. Consumers are indeed becoming better connoisseurs of health care than they were in the past. One sure sign of the healthcare industry's response to that fact is direct marketing of pharmaceuticals and other health-related products. Between 1996 and 2005, the annual spending on direct-to-consumer advertising for prescription drugs in the United States grew from $11.2 billion to $29.9 billion (Donohue, Cevasco, & Rosenthal, 2007). Chronic health conditions require that consumers take an active role in managing their health. Chronic illnesses account for 60% of global mortality and one third of the world's disease burden, with 80% of chronic disease deaths occurring in low-income and middle-income countries (World Health Organization, 2008). Employers view consumerism as a vehicle for reducing healthcare costs and for improving quality by empowering employees to make more appropriate choices about healthcare services while improving health care. The Leapfrog Group, a consortium of more than 160 employers and organizations that buys health care, is working to prevent mistakes in health care and improve the quality and affordability of health care. Its focus is on making leaps in hospital quality, safety, and affordability by implementing computerized physician order entry, referring patients to appropriate facilities for high-risk surgeries and conditions, staffing intensive care units with intensivists, and implementing practices to improve safety (Leapfrog Group, 2009). According to a survey conducted by Parks Associates, 20 million U.S. households do not have Web access, half of the people who do not use the Web are older than 65 years, and 56% of those without Web access do not have education beyond high school (Smith, 2008). Despite this digital divide, individuals with chronic conditions are more likely to use the Web for health information than those without a chronic condition, and the uninsured, particularly those with chronic conditions, are more likely to use the Web to search for health-related information (Bundorf, Wagner, Singer, & Baker, 2006). Although these data have implications for access to healthcare information, they also reflect changes that affect the nature of the relationship between consumers and nurses, consumers and other healthcare providers, and consumers and healthcare organizations.

Consumers have access to limitless amounts of information about health; however, such access may vary to some degree by ethnicity and socioeconomic status. Although some information that is available from the Internet and other resources might not be valid, healthcare consumers tend to be better informed now more than they ever have been. Numerous government agencies and voluntary organizations provide consumers with guidance in managing chronic conditions, making decisions about health, and preventing harm from lapses in patient safety. Publicity about medical errors and the nursing shortage and information campaigns directed toward consumers to promote safety have heightened consumer awareness being involved in all aspects of one's health care. Consumers question providers regarding the care they receive or do not receive, and they ask, "Why are you doing that?" "Where can I get the best care?" "Why did my nurse do that differently yesterday?" and "How do I know what is the best decision for me?"

RELATIONSHIPS

The Consumer Focus

Consumer relationships are constantly changing and thus affect the providers of health services: primary care and public health services, managed care organizations, hospitals, home health agencies, and long-term care facilities, as well as individual providers such as nurses and physicians. As inpatient services have become more complex and outpatient services have grown, competition for patients becomes fiercer. This has resulted in a shift in focus from healthcare providers to healthcare consumers. As noted in "The Challenge" at the beginning of the chapter, consumers drive what happens in our healthcare settings. Healthcare processes are being redefined with the consumer as the center. How consumers view and value their care is important data. Consumers enter into distinct relationships to meet their healthcare needs, including relationships with healthcare agencies, insurers or payers, nurses, physicians, and allied health providers. Changes in access, insurance coverage, nurses' roles and responsibilities, physician services, communication technology, pay-for-performance, and globalization are just a few factors influencing these relationships.

Health Literacy

Consumers rely on information from a variety of sources to make healthcare decisions. The relationships that consumers develop with their healthcare providers, including nurses, are important in helping them navigate the healthcare system. However, nearly half of America's adults—that is, 90 million people—have difficulty understanding and using health information (Nielson-Bohlman, Panzer, & Kindig, 2004). The definition of health literacy used by the federal government is "the degree to which individuals have the capacity to obtain, process, and understand basic health information and services needed to make appropriate health decisions" (U.S. Department of Health and Human Services, 2008).

Understanding consumers' health-literacy needs goes beyond examining reading ability. The first component of its definition is the *capacity to obtain*. This accessibility is also influenced by global aging, climate change, war and terrorism, and life-extending medical and technologic advances (Perlow, 2010). Health literacy is important because research has demonstrated that people with low health literacy do not understand health information very well and tend to get less preventive health care, which in turn may affect their health (Nielson-Bohlman et al., 2004). Promoting health literacy involves education, consideration of the context, and sociocultural factors. For example, a nurse who is an expert clinician in a specialty practice area, when diagnosed with a serious chronic illness, may not have the appropriate background to make informed healthcare decisions. Promoting health literacy is an important component of health care because individuals with limited literacy are vulnerable. They are more likely to be sicker when they enter into the healthcare system and are more likely to use more healthcare services.

Healthcare Provider–Consumer Relationships

Healthcare provider–consumer relationships have changed as physicians' typical mode of practice moved from a single, private enterprise to multigroup practices that also include nurse practitioners, certified nurse-midwives, certified registered nurse anesthetists, clinical nurse specialists, registered nurse first assistants, physician assistants, and other healthcare professionals. Some group practices are incorporated into health maintenance organizations (HMOs), managed care programs, physician-hospital organizations or the emerging accountable care organizations. When consumers visit a group practice, they might

not have the option of selecting a specific healthcare provider. Patients no longer know their healthcare providers as they did in the past, and providers may be less familiar with their patients, resulting in decreased opportunity for the development of mutual respect and trust. Furthermore, many hospitals now use hospitalists and there is some evidence that the coordination of care and accountability for the quality of care after discharge are more challenging (Pham, Grossman, Cohen, & Bodenheimer, 2008). However, trust still is an important component of consumer relationships. Trust is influenced by the healthcare provider's competence but also is linked to interpersonal caring attributes (Hupcey & Miller, 2006). Older adults are interested in caring, respectful, and educational relationships with their healthcare providers and perceive nurses as authority figures who provide reliable information to help them with treatment decisions (Calvin, Frazier, & Cohen, 2007). Patients want and expect attentiveness to their concerns and respectful treatment.

Rural healthcare consumers have seen local hospitals close, and therefore they need to seek care in regional health centers. They may not have relationships with their new healthcare providers. This often leads consumers to be more critical and less accepting of their care. They may feel alienated and insecure in unfamiliar circumstances, even if they are receiving the best care. Patients' perceptions are an increasingly valued outcome of care. Consumers may be caught in the middle without a healthcare provider when physicians leave communities because of malpractice premiums, when insurance companies limit access to certain types of healthcare providers, or when the providers change their healthcare facility affiliations. Furthermore, sicker patients are less satisfied with the quality of health care they receive than are their healthier counterparts (Wolff & Roter, 2008). It is incumbent upon healthcare practitioners to be sensitive to the needs of patients with complex conditions requiring expert intervention.

Agency-Consumer Relationships

Healthcare consumers may have been accustomed to receiving acute care in an inpatient setting. This option is no longer available for many. Patients may be angry and frightened at the thought of being on their own or receiving very limited services from home health agencies. The type of insurance coverage and the insurance carrier will probably dictate the specific hospital or healthcare agency used. Managed care options require that the consumer use particular and specific healthcare facilities or be responsible for all or a larger portion of the bill.

Patients discharged from emergency departments are often ill-prepared to manage their care at home because they do not understand discharge instructions (Engel et al., 2008). Nurses in acute care settings have limited time to provide complex discharge instructions. Home health nurses may not be able to make a sufficient number of visits to enable patients to successfully manage a chronic illness. Care options are decreasing, and costs are increasing. Most insurance plans have included a copayment or a deductible clause requiring the consumer to meet a certain dollar amount before the insurance companies will pay their 60% to 90% of the bill. In some instances, workers with entry-level jobs have had health plans requiring deductibles of $2000 to $5000, making preventive health services largely prohibitive. Medicare and Medicaid recipients also find themselves in the midst of changes in terms of how healthcare costs are managed. Understanding the Medicare prescription drug benefit is a daunting task for many seniors. As the 2010 Health Care Reform laws unfold, some of these challenges may be minimized.

Consumer-directed healthcare plans generally have had high deductibles with the goal of reducing healthcare costs by providing consumers with information about choices, risks, benefits, and costs. The goal has been to have greater emphasis on case management, disease management, and patient education. These plans use report cards, risk assessments, nurse-help telephone lines, websites, and an array of other consumer education materials. Consumers will be comparison-shopping for healthcare services just as they might comparison-shop for prescription drugs. Despite this growth in consumer awareness, the impact of consumer-directed healthcare plans on patient satisfaction and healthcare costs is unknown. Critics of consumer-directed healthcare plans indicate that these plans shift costs to consumers without any true reductions in healthcare spending. People enrolled in a high-deductible health plan were more likely to start forgoing medical care to save money (Dixon, Greene, & Hibbard, 2008). Furthermore, as the number of chronic illnesses among family members increases, the more likely they are to switch to using a high-deductible healthcare plan (Naessens et al., 2008).

Many healthcare organizations are still operating under an outmoded paradigm with only the needs of physicians and third-party payers driving the agency's priorities. In increasingly competitive healthcare markets, there is greater application of information-sharing services known as *Web 2.0* (allowing users to interact with and alter content), the potential for open-source electronic health records, and the use of digital media and mobile computing (Gardiner, 2008). New services include self-monitoring with technology in the home, videoconferencing, text messaging and instant messaging with healthcare providers, and clinics staffed by nurse practitioners in grocery stores. These changes will require that healthcare organization leaders focus efforts on relationships with patients who are more knowledgeable and demanding.

Nurse-Consumer Relationships

Nurses spend a lot of time with the consumer, and these encounters are generally personal and intensely meaningful. Nurses are in a distinct position to influence and promote positive consumer relationships. The nurse manager sets the tone for effective staff-patient interactions centered on the patient.

Changes from hospital or nursing home care to outpatient and in-home care have particularly altered the nurse-consumer relationship. Nurses are taking leadership roles as primary care providers (e.g., nurse practitioners, midwives), teachers and educators, and home healthcare managers and advocates, particularly in compensation and insurance areas. Nurses are emerging as the gatekeepers of the healthcare system, the liaisons between the consumer and a complex healthcare market. Ensuring that patients receive well-coordinated care across all providers, settings, and levels of care has been recognized as integral to the quality of care by the National Priorities Partnership (2008), a coalition of 28 major healthcare organizations including the American Nurses Association (ANA). The nurse manager is a key position to facilitate care coordination by working with case managers and members of the interdisciplinary healthcare team. The nurse in the gatekeeper or care coordinator role can be an influential advocate for consumers who could receive less-than-desired care in a complicated healthcare system. This group typically has included those who receive no care and need it most, such as those who are homeless, uninsured, or underinsured persons, persons who abuse drugs or alcohol, children of poverty, migrant workers, and people with acquired immunodeficiency syndrome (AIDS). Some institutions and private corporations capitalize on the case-management skills of nurses by developing the "nurse navigator" or "patient navigator" roles, which are designed to assist patients through a complex healthcare system or with healthcare decisions. Policymakers are examining the role of "medical homes" in facilitating the integration of care across systems. A medical home is a patient-centered, multifaceted source of personal primary health care (Rosenthal, 2008). The concept was originally focused on children and adolescents and includes having a usual source of health care. People with a usual source of health care are more likely to get health care (Robert Graham Center, 2007). Although discussions have focused on physician-directed care, advanced practice nurses provide an integral safety net for patients who are uninsured or underinsured or who have chronic health conditions and need to be included in policy decisions about medical homes.

Nursing has long recognized the value of the integral nature of the nurse-patient relationship and the value of caring as an element of that relationship. The *Code of Ethics for Nurses* holds that the "nurse's primary commitment is to the patient" with an expectation that the nurse involves patients in planning for care (ANA, 2001, pp. 9-10). Patient-centered care includes alleviating vulnerabilities, both physiologic and interpersonal; it also includes therapeutic engagement and developing a relationship in a manner that is reinforced by the information practices of a particular setting (Hobbs, 2009). Wylie and Wagenfeld-Heintz (2004) describe the evidence for nurses' receptiveness to mutuality and reciprocity in relationships that honor all persons. Mutuality balances power and respect and promotes productive communication.

Nurses have four major responsibilities in promoting successful consumer relationships, as follows:

1. Service
2. Advocacy
3. Teaching
4. Leadership

EXERCISE 22-1

List as many clinical situations as you can think of in which the nurse might carry out the four aforementioned responsibilities. Compare your list with those of your peers.

SERVICE

A service orientation responds to the needs of the customer. In "The Challenge" at the beginning of the chapter, activities centered on the patient and family, including how nursing care and all other services are delivered so that patient care is holistic. The National Priorities Partnership's goals (2008), in addition to the previously mentioned care coordination, include engaging patients and their families in managing their health and making decisions about their care, improving the health of the population, improving the safety and reliability of America's healthcare system, guaranteeing appropriate and compassionate care for patients with life-limiting illnesses, and eliminating overuse.

The patient must be at the center of care to achieve these goals. Healthcare professionals, including nurses, want to deliver patient-centered care. However, assessing how well that is accomplished in an organization is challenging. The Picker Institute, a nonprofit organization, has done extensive research on the evaluation of care from the patient's perspective. Its model of patient-centered care, no matter where the services are delivered, focuses on the consumer's perspective, as illustrated in Box 22-1. Each dimension is an important part of the consumer's interaction with the healthcare system and provides guidance in promoting consumer relationships.

Even with an increasing emphasis on customer service, most healthcare facilities are not as "customer-friendly" as they might be; that is, they are built and organized in a manner that best serves the organization, not the consumer. They are compartmentalized, with each department having specialized functions. Patients are transported to departments to receive services. They risk loss of privacy, excessive exposure, and increased discomfort and fatigue during the transfer and waiting episodes. On an

BOX 22-1   SEVEN PRIMARY DIMENSIONS OF PATIENT-CENTERED CARE

- **Respect for patient's values, preferences, and expressed needs:** includes attention to quality of life, involvement in decision making, preservation of patient's dignity, and recognition of patient's needs and autonomy
- **Coordination and integration of care:** involves clinical care, ancillary and support services, and "front-line" patient care
- **Information, communication, and education:** includes information on clinical status, progress, and prognosis; information on processes of care; and information and education to facilitate autonomy, self-care, and health promotion
- **Physical comfort:** considers pain management, help with activities of daily living, and hospital environment
- **Emotional support and alleviation of fear and anxiety:** demands attention to anxiety over clinical status, treatment, and prognosis; anxiety over the effect of the illness on self and family; and anxiety over the financial impact of the illness
- **Involvement of family and friends:** recognizes the need to accommodate family and friends and involve family in decision making; to support the family as caregiver; and to recognize family needs
- **Transition and continuity:** addresses patient anxieties and concerns about information on medication, treatment regimens, follow-up, danger signals after leaving the hospital, recovery, health promotion, and prevention of recurrence; coordination and planning for continuing care and treatment; and access to continuity of care and assistance

From Gerteis, M., Edgman-Levitan, S., Daley, J., & Delbanco, T.L. (2002). *Through the patient's eyes: Understanding and promoting patient-centered care.* San Francisco: Jossey-Bass.

the *service* is a measure of perception of what matters to the patient (Doucette, 2003).

EXERCISE 22-2
List five examples of what you think are not consumer-friendly practices or situations in your nursing setting. (Example: Patients being asked to repeat information several times to different staff members such as admissions clerks, nurses, and radiograph technicians.) Identify at least two strategies to help address each problem.

Providing satisfying and meaningful service is not easy. Every consumer is different, and every situation is different. How things are done and how needs are met vary. Service is not a prescribed set of rules and regulations. Service is a multidimensional concept and means placing a premium on the design, development, and delivery of care. For example, a home care patient needs intravenous (IV) antibiotic therapy. Inserting the IV catheter is the task-oriented, production part of the care. The service aspect involves considering the patient's specialized needs, such as placing the needle in the left arm so that he can continue to use a cane with his right arm or using a local anesthetic before inserting the needle to reduce discomfort.

Delivering nursing care includes both service and product characteristics. In the context of health care, a service involves interaction between a consumer and the healthcare system related to the provision of needs, whereas a product is a tangible item with physical characteristics. Some nursing actions require clearly prescribed rituals—the actual physical act of production, such as insertion of a Foley catheter. In performing this act, certain physical characteristics are apparent and the outcome is predictable. At the same time, no two patients are alike; human interaction alters the situation, and unforeseen variables demand spontaneity. Caring, concern, and respect for the individual are intangible characteristics that affect the ultimate success or failure of the nursing action. Quality nursing care must be both clinically correct and satisfying to the customer. "Clinically correct" is the product aspect, and "satisfying to the consumer" is the service orientation. Each individual nurse is responsible for being competent and providing quality patient care that is clinically correct and satisfying. The nurse manager is accountable for the overall quality of care delivered to patients.

average day, a seriously ill hospitalized patient may have encounters with 50 or more personnel in the course of receiving care and treatment. This approach is not "service-oriented." A service orientation means delivering services in a manner that is least disruptive. When possible, services should come to the patient and should be as easy, comfortable, pleasant, and effective as possible. Meeting the emotional, psychosocial, and spiritual needs of the patient is important. The consumer is interested in high-quality care that is technologically advanced and compassionate (Doucette, 2003). The *quality of care* refers to the outcomes of care in relation to a standard, whereas

Healthcare agencies must be sensitive to whether the agency milieu is indeed a healing environment that supports and reinforces the actual quality of clinical care. The challenge in the busy, unpredictable, cost-constrained healthcare environment is to provide care that has a consumer focus by meeting or exceeding customer expectations. Nurses, as leaders, need to recognize the economic value of their services as well as the economic value of improving the quality of the patient experience. Linking a satisfactory patient experience with positive outcomes depends on identifying patient preferences (Ervin, 2006). This is illustrated in the Literature Perspective below in Kerfoot's description of the signature experience.

Organizations desiring to have a competitive edge strive for a standardized signature experience—the ideal experience for a patient that is its hallmark (Kerfoot, 2007). The nurse leader and the nursing staff members need to partner in developing that experience and focusing on its achievement for all patients and their families. People are looking for an environment that meets their needs for safety and security, support, and psychological and physical comfort.

📖 LITERATURE PERSPECTIVE

Resource: Kerfoot, K. (2007). Patient satisfaction and high reliability organizations: What's the connection? *Nursing Economic$*, *25*, 119-120.

Organizations desiring to have a competitive edge strive for a standardized signature experience, the ideal experience for a patient that is its hallmark. The emphasis needs to be on the development of that experience and focusing on its achievement for all patients and their families. Drawing upon the work of theorists and examples from industry, Kerfoot recommends that healthcare organizations identify a vision of the ideal experience, develop educational programs to help staff understand how to apply the signature experience in different situations and scenarios, and then measure the patients' perceptions of that experience. Furthermore, efforts need to be made to intervene promptly to eliminate negative experiences.

Implications for Practice

Nurse managers are critical to the successful development of signature experiences for patients. When employees are involved in creating the signature experience for patients, the employees are engaged, performance is improved, and patients are satisfied.

Hospital leaders value the role of the Magnet Recognition Program® in terms of promoting competent care and a service orientation. Magnet™ designation demonstrates excellence of nursing care through transformational leadership; structured empowerment; exemplary professional nursing practice; and new knowledge, innovations, and improvement, which lead to empirical quality outcomes (Wolf, Triolo, & Ponte, 2008). These attributes cannot be achieved without excellence in a consumer service orientation. This culture of excellence must be exemplified in every aspect of the organization, from the chief executive officer, to the chief nursing officer, to the nurse manager for nurses at the front lines of care to feel empowered to promote excellence in consumer service.

A service orientation is consumer-driven and consumer-focused, and it places the emphasis on the quality of the nurse-patient relationship. The importance of relationships is reflected in current nursing theory in the caring philosophy. Caring has been described as the essence of nursing. It denotes a special concern, interest, or feeling capable of fostering a therapeutic nurse-patient relationship. Caring is important, but simply caring is not enough. The ability to think critically and take appropriate, timely action must be a part of the therapeutic process. The nurse must do the right thing right at the right time.

The concept of nursing as a caring service is seen in the reality of "high tech–high touch." High tech denotes a mechanistic perspective, whereas high touch denotes a caring, humanistic perspective. Caring for patients is challenging in an environment driven by technology. At the same time, patients depend on nurses to deliver high-tech care in a caring, humanistic manner. The more high technology is used in health care, the more the patient wants and needs high touch—someone who is trusted and respected and who will add human touch to the experience. The quality of these human contacts becomes the measure by which the consumer forms perceptions and judgments about nursing and the health agency. In health care, consumers frequently cannot judge or evaluate the quality of interventions but they always can evaluate the quality of the relationship with the person delivering the service.

Patient satisfaction ratings, along with measurable healthcare outcomes, are important data used by healthcare organizations to provide quality care and to maintain a competitive edge. Nurses, because of their 24-hour accountability for patient care, are integral to high patient-satisfaction ratings. Healthcare organizations collect patient satisfaction data and want high ratings, so much so that they advertise their ratings in the community. Standard-setting organizations, such as The Joint Commission and the National Quality Forum include patient satisfaction as a quality indicator. The patient's satisfaction and perception of the quality of care are affected by patient-centered care which focuses on individual needs and preferences (Wolf, Lehman, Quinlin, Zullo, & Hoffman, 2008).

Hospitals and other healthcare organizations contract with vendors to measure patient satisfaction or use their own instruments. Very often, patient-satisfaction ratings are clustered together at the high end of the scale, making it difficult to interpret results and make improvements. One needs also to consider the range and the depth of the information that is collected. For example, some hospitals collect data only on the hotel amenities, such as the cleanliness of the room and data required by government or regulatory organizations. Other hospitals collect more specific data on satisfaction with nursing care, including such elements as how promptly the call light was answered and whether patients were satisfied with a specific aspect of nursing care, such as pain management. The National Database of Nursing Quality Indicators (NDNQI®) is a national repository for unit-based quality data that can be used by organizations to benchmark their outcomes against those of other institutions (ANA, n.d.). Unit-based quality indicators, including satisfaction with nursing care, are a key feature of the NDNQI®, enabling nurse managers and nurses to make improvements.

Nurses have a responsibility to exercise critical thinking and decision making with respect to patient satisfaction with nursing care. For example, postoperative patients may not want to cough and deep breathe, yet we know that failure to do so can result in pneumonia. National survey data indicate that pain management is suboptimal (Jha, Orav, Zheng, & Epstein, 2008). One of the challenges in providing effective pain management is that research demonstrates that patients can be quite satisfied with pain management yet still experience severe postoperative pain (Sauaia et al., 2005). This paradox illustrates the responsibility that nurses have for (1) advocating on behalf of their patients, (2) ensuring that their patients' pain is relieved, (3) correcting patient misconceptions, and (4) implementing pain-management strategies that are consistent with established standards. Reviewing and analyzing patient satisfaction survey results are invaluable tools to improve consumer relationships.

A service recovery program needs to be put into place in order for an organization to be responsive to its customers. Service recovery is a strategy for identifying complaints and rectifying service failures to retain or "recover" dissatisfied customers. Axioms for service recovery are listed in Box 22-2. Effective service recovery includes encouraging healthcare providers, rather than just hospital administrators, to talk with patients about a serious error. In the past, healthcare organizations have been concerned with the potential risk for liability when the person making an error talks with the patient or family about it. However, research suggests that the content of the message has a significant effect on how the person feels about an error. Messages containing both an apology and an effort to address the problem in the future are the most productive (Kiger, 2004). Patients want to be treated with fairness and respect, want a change in hospital performance as a result of the complaint, and are more interested in an explanation than an apology (Friele & Sluijs, 2006). Consideration must be given to deciding which person in the

---

BOX 22-2   AXIOMS OF SERVICE RECOVERY

1. All customers have basic expectations related to reliability, assurance, tangibles (e.g., cleanliness of a unit), empathy, and responsiveness.
2. Successful recovery is psychological as well as physical.
3. Working with customers in a spirit of partnership in problem solving and based on needs improves healthcare experiences.
4. Customers react more strongly to "fairness mistakes" than "honest mistakes."
5. Effective recovery is a planned process.

Adapted from Agency for Healthcare Research and Quality (AHRQ). (October 27, 2008). *The CAHPS improvement guide: Practical strategies for improving the patient care experience.* Adapted from Zemke, R., & Bell, C. (2000). *Knock your socks off service recovery.* New York: American Management Association. Retrieved May 6, 2010, from www.cahps.ahrq.gov.

organization is the most appropriate to offer an apology as well as planning its content. A nurse making a medication error that did not harm a patient is the best person to make the disclosure and apology. However, if a patient's discharge is delayed by a day because of an omission or error in preparation for a diagnostic test, then the nurse manager and/or nurse administrator might be the more appropriate person to initiate discussion with the patient. Nurse managers can work with staff to help patients have their concerns addressed. Some organizations use scripts for use with situations in which care has not gone as planned. For example, when there is an excessive delay in the emergency department, staff training on when and how to use a script for this situation can help a patient or family member feel less distressed.

EXERCISE 22-3

Make a "what-if" list of actions that would enhance services to the consumers of health care. (Example: What if every single nurse would ask each patient at the beginning of the shift about the patient's most important concern that day.)

ADVOCACY

Nurses practice in a healthcare environment that is dominated by unrest and insecurity. Some of these forces are shown in Box 22-3. Such forces bring about ethical and moral questions: Who gets care? Where do they get care? How much care? Who has the right to die? Who has the right to live? Who makes the decisions? Differing values and beliefs, along with economic constraints and limited resources, affect decisions that are made.

Consumers have basic rights that need to be protected—the right to individualized care; the right to their own values, beliefs, and cultural ways; and the right to be informed and participate in care decisions. Unresolved within the healthcare system is the issue of two levels of care that are based on economics but tend to result in racial-cultural discrimination. Not only has care been on a two-tiered basis but also minorities and women have been significantly underrepresented in health-related research; this results in additional healthcare disparities because less information is available for decision making.

BOX 22-3 **FORCES OF UNREST AND INSECURITY IN THE HEALTHCARE ENVIRONMENT**

1. Increased costs
2. Shift to outpatient services
3. Complex social problems (AIDS, violence, poverty, global climate change)
4. Decreased access to health care
5. Aging population (increasing life span)
6. Technologic and genetic advances
7. Shortage of nurses and other healthcare professionals
8. Culturally and ethnically diverse work/consumer groups
9. Underrepresentation of women and ethnic groups in health-related research
10. Economic instability
11. Increase in regulatory and reporting requirements
12. Uncertainty and divisiveness about implementation of healthcare reforms.

Who in the healthcare system is in a position to be the guardian of consumer rights? The nurse is! The nurse acts as the primary person to be alert to circumstances that may prevent a successful outcome for the patient and to intervene on the patient's behalf. The nurse is in the position to address the issues of cultural, ethnic, and racial sensitivity. The nurse is concerned with addressing the individualized needs and wants of the patient.

The definition of *nursing* includes advocacy in the care of individuals, families, communities, and populations (ANA, 2003b). Nurses, in accordance with the ANA *Code of Ethics for Nurses,* have the responsibility to promote, advocate, and strive to protect the health, safety, and rights of the patient (2001). Patient advocacy includes (1) safeguarding patients' autonomy, (2), acting on behalf of patients, and (3) championing social justice in the provision of health care (Bu & Jezewski, 2007). An **advocate** is one who does the following:

- Defends or promotes the rights of others
- Changes systems to meet the needs of others
- Empowers and promotes self-determination in others
- Promotes autonomy of diverse cultures and social groups
- Ensures respect, equality, and dignity for others
- Cares for the humaneness of all

BOX 22-4	RACIAL AND CULTURAL DIFFERENCES

A young adult African-American male, shot while running from the police, had been hospitalized for more than 3 weeks. A psychiatric clinical nurse specialist made the following assessment:

PERSPECTIVE OF NURSING STAFF	**PERSPECTIVE OF PATIENT OF COLOR**
1. No one wants to take care of this patient. Avoiding him is common. His call light goes unanswered.	1. Patient feels isolated and forgotten. His room is at the end of the hall. He infrequently sees nurses and physicians, has little information about his gunshot wounds, and fears he is never going to walk again. He fears dying in his room and no one will know.
2. The patient is loud and rude and uses vulgar language.	2. Patient speaks loudly and uses vulgar talk to emphasize his concerns.
3. Nursing staff suspects that sexual activity is occurring between the man and his girlfriend in the hospital.	3. Patient makes comments with sexual overtones and spends hours with his girlfriend when she visits; he seeks comfort and affirmation through sexuality.
4. Nurses feel physically and sexually threatened when trying to provide care.	4. Patient's family comes only on weekends and then in large numbers.

Summary: Stereotypes about black males were operational on the unit. The staff members avoided the patient because of the sexual overtones and withheld information regarding his condition. Overt and covert battles of will with the patient resulted in further patient isolation.

Modified from Malone, B.L. (1993). Caring for culturally diverse racial groups: An administrative matter. *Nursing Administration Quarterly, 17*(2), 21-29.

Nursing practice involves interacting with consumers who are culturally, economically, and socially diverse. Diversity encompasses more than differences in nationality or ethnicity and may include a variety of ways that patients are different from their healthcare providers. Nurses are responsible for assisting consumers in accessing and participating in the healthcare system. Some patients enter the healthcare system much like immigrants entering a foreign country. Patients who enter a system with a set of values, beliefs, behaviors, and language unlike their own may experience culture shock. Patients who speak little or no English and those who may have low health literacy are vulnerable for poor health outcomes. Nurses need to recognize the culture of their work setting, realizing that it may differ markedly from the culture of the consumer, and move beyond ethnocentrism to provide culturally competent care. Cultural competence brings together attitudes, behaviors, and policies within an organization in such a way that allows people to work effectively in cross-cultural situations (National Alliance for Hispanic Health, 2000). It includes cultural knowledge, actively learning about a community; cultural sensitivity—valuing and respecting beliefs, norms, and practices of the people being served—and collabora-

tion within a community (Flaskerud, 2007). Cultural competence is critical to reducing the potential impact of healthcare disparities and providing consumer service.

The advocate role requires the nurse to perceive and be comfortable with conflict and then mediate, negotiate, clarify, explain, and intervene. The nurse can advocate by being a liaison between the consumer and the system. The nurse's role is to interpret the rules and customs of the agency to the consumer. The role is also to negotiate changes when the consumer and agency differ in values and beliefs. An example is shown in Box 22-4.

To provide culturally appropriate care, the nurse must possess knowledge about various culturally diverse groups (see Chapter 9). It takes time to develop cultural sensitivity and awareness. Some guidelines that are useful in learning to appreciate and value diversity are the following:

- Avoid stereotyping.
- Avoid making assumptions.
- Learn by observing interactions of minority group members.
- Adjust expectations to be culturally sensitive.
- Create a more level playing field—modify your behavior to accommodate diversity.

Powerlessness or an imbalance in power between the consumer and the system can result in value systems being forced on the recipient of care. Consumers who lack economic means by being uninsured, underinsured, or undocumented often become powerless in the healthcare delivery system. They are at the mercy or will of those who control the power and the money. These consumers (described earlier) may be denied access to care, or if they achieve access, they may not receive equal care.

Consumers interacting with our healthcare systems, regardless of their status, have a right to know about their eligibility for services and care. The nurse must be willing to ensure that economic constraints do not prevent consumers from receiving what they need. Some advocacy for the recipients of inequality in our healthcare system is done on the here-and-now level—initiating a referral to a social agency when a patient does not have transportation to his home or appealing to the ethics committee when a patient's wishes for end-of-life decisions are not being followed. On a broader scale, advocacy means becoming involved professionally and politically to change the systems and policies to provide healthcare access and equality.

EXERCISE 22-4

Using the scenario in Box 22-4, determine how the culturally competent nurse can mediate the cultural differences between the staff and the patient.

Race and ethnicity as factors in health and health care have been the subject of concern; however, people very often may erroneously assume that members of a particular minority group have the same beliefs, attitudes, and values about health when, in fact, there is extraordinary diversity.

The Census Bureau predicts that by 2040, more than half the U.S. population will comprise ethnic minorities. Currently, residents of the United States speak at least 329 languages (Agency for Healthcare Research and Quality [AHRQ], 2001)! It is most useful to define diversity broadly, to include not only race and ethnicity but also age, gender, socioeconomic status, religion, sexual orientation, physical characteristics, and disability. Thus cultural compe-

tence will play an increasingly important role in nurse-consumer relationships. In addition, an organization that creates a culture of mutual respect, recognizing the contributions of all its employees, will be much more effective in providing culturally competent health care.

The following are some of the keys to becoming a successful nurse advocate:

- Developing networking systems within work agencies
- Being involved in professional associations to enhance awareness of issues affecting practice and, thus, consumers
- Acquiring the knowledge needed to access systems
- Learning about community resources and support networks
- Developing skill in referring and engaging patients

A patient advocate's ultimate aim is to empower patients (i.e., the consumers of health care) to help them use their own abilities to promote health. Patient empowerment is a critical component of health care today and is seen as integral to the error reduction. Patient participation in nursing practice refers to an established relationship between nurse and patient, surrendering of some power or control by the nurse, shared information and knowledge, and active engagement in intellectual and/or physical activities (Sahlsten, Larsson, Sjöström, & Plos, 2008). Nurses must be sensitive to patient preferences for information and decision making, as illustrated in the Research Perspective on p. 451.

EXERCISE 22-5

Using the model described in the Research Perspective, ask patients in your clinical setting about the two things that they need the most help with from nurses.

The nurse manager should keep in mind the most basic element of empowerment—helping people assert control. Support for patients and their families is critical when a hospitalized patient suffers an illness requiring major transition in roles and responsibilities. Cameron and Gignac (2008) identified a "Timing it Right" framework for family caregiver support

RESEARCH PERSPECTIVE

Resource: Tea, C., Ellison, M., & Feghali, F. (2008). Proactive patient rounding to increase customer service and satisfaction on an orthopaedic unit. *Orthopaedic Nursing, 27*, 233-240.

This study assessed staff responsiveness to needs and requests of patients at four hospitals. After analyzing inpatient satisfaction data from over 2500 patients who had joint replacements, the authors used the Plan-Do-Check-Act (PDCA) methodology to address timely responsiveness. The goals were to learn about the meaning of timely response to patients, which staff members are considered exemplary in timely response, the most common needs experienced, processes used to meet needs, and root causes of inadequate responsiveness. The most common needs of patients undergoing orthopaedic procedures were (1) bathroom/toileting, (2) mobility/positioning needs, (3) pain needs, and (4) having things in reach. The *I Care Rounding* model was developed to help staff anticipate patient needs. The leadership team supported staff changes through role-playing, daily verbal reminders, reference cards, staffing meeting emphasis, role-modeling, and staff recognition. Significant improvement was made in timely response to requests, staff anticipation of needs, staff rounding hourly, and staff asking if there was anything else is to be done (n = 4362). Some improvement was made in registered nurses sitting with patients to discuss goals and needs. In addition, calls using the call bell system on one unit decreased from 3591 over a 2-week period to 2509 calls.

Implications for Practice

Timely staff responsiveness is an important component of patient satisfaction. This study illustrates the value of determining the specific needs of patients and understanding what is happening in a patient care environment. Nurse managers need to be proactive in guiding and supporting the staff in implementing changes in order to improve consumer relationships.

useful across the continuum of care that includes the (1) event/diagnosis, (2) stabilization, (3) preparation, (4) implementation, and (5) adaptation. This is a helpful guide to tailoring interventions according to the changing needs of patients and their families.

Nurses can evaluate the consumer's quality of care by comparing it with quality indicators or critical pathways in the quality-review process. For example, if patient care standards indicate patients with a particular bronchial condition need a chest radiograph examination on day 2 and another on day 5, all patients should receive this same level of care. In agencies using critical pathways to prescribe the plan of care, patients who cannot pay for services should not be denied treatment, therapy, or tests if the pathway requires specific action. Organizations examine nurse-sensitive quality indicators as important outcomes. For example, pressure ulcers and nosocomial infections, such as hospital-acquired pneumonia, are indicators of the quality of nursing care. The NDNQI® is a resource that can be used by hospitals to track nurse-sensitive outcomes on a unit basis (Montalvo, 2007). Nurse managers are in a distinct position to ensure that all patients receive appropriate care. The tone set by the manager signals staff to report and document discrepancies and omissions.

Nurse managers must acknowledge and respect the legal, ethical, and moral responsibilities of the staff to advocate for patients. For example, if a patient receives the wrong medication just before being discharged, the patient needs to be informed and this information needs to be included in the patient's record. Therefore, if the patient has an adverse reaction and needs to return to the emergency department, a record exists that would aid in diagnosis and facilitate the institution of an appropriate treatment promptly. In Pennsylvania, written notification to consumers is required for serious errors. Although efforts have been made to increase error reporting to facilitate the institution of system changes to decrease errors, the use of blame hinders the staff in disclosing medication errors to the leadership of an organization (Scott-Cawiezell et al., 2006). This situation represents a major challenge for nurse managers who are attempting to identify problematic practices in order to reduce error and promote patient safety. In addition, nurses in leadership positions also are obligated legally and ethically to report unacceptable or questionable clinician and organizational practices. As Yoder-Wise (2010) points out, having the courage to advocate for patients can sometimes impose personal risks, as it did in the case known nationally as the "Winkler County Nurses." Nurses such as Vickilyn Galle and Anne Mitchell reported their concerns about a physician's practices to the medical board; they became their patients' heroes—and ours as well.

The savvy manager knows that the way in which consumers define quality may not always match the way "experts" define it. However, patient-centered care is related to higher patient satisfaction ratings and higher ratings of care quality (Wolf, Lehman, Quinlin, Zullo, & Hoffman, 2008). Quality health care and quality nursing care do not depend on the ability to pay or social acceptance. Good care occurs irrespective of the economic circumstance of the consumer. Nurses are the guardians of that right for consumers. Nurses have historically been the champions for the poor and the underserved. It is no different today.

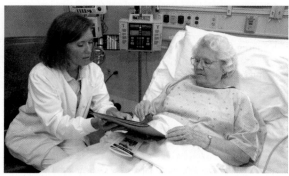

Education empowers consumers to exercise self-determination.

TEACHING

Consumers of health care have a right and a need to know how to care for their own health needs. Nurses have an obligation to teach the consumer. Patient teaching is included in the standards of nursing practice (ANA, 2003a) and is often included in the definitions of professional nursing found in state nurse practice acts. The model for the Magnet Recognition Program® includes five components: transformational leadership, exemplary professional practice, new knowledge, innovations, and improvements, all of which lead to quality outcomes (Wolf, Triolo & Ponte, 2008). Exemplary professional practice includes the role of nurses as teachers. Consumers are demanding information about their health status and plan of care. They are entitled to information regarding health concerns, to participate in caring for their health needs, and to contribute to finding solutions to their health problems. Education empowers consumers to exercise self-determination. It allows them to have greater control over what happens, to make informed decisions, and to choose wisely from options. Knowledge is power. Sharing knowledge means sharing power. Health-related education needs also to consider patient preferences for information and decision making. For example, in a study of preferences of patients with diabetes for telephone support, group medical visits, or Internet support, patient preferences varied by race/ethnicity, language proficiency, and self-reported health literacy (Sarkar et al., 2008). Nurses must understand the unique needs of the communities served by a healthcare facility, as well as assess the individual patient's preferences.

Healthcare delivery systems affect the ways nurses teach consumers. Short hospital stays and care provided in outpatient and transitional settings require effective use of time and resources. Patients need to be able to manage their own health care earlier and more independently. Hands-on, technical training is needed in many instances. Nurses' perceptions of their patients' understanding of post-discharge treatment plans differ from the perceptions of patients themselves. Nurses often perceive patients to be much more knowledgeable than the patients themselves report. Teaching prevention and health promotion will increase the consumer's quality of life. Three *P's* for a successful consumer education focus are shown in Box 22-5.

BOX 22-5 THREE P'S FOR A SUCCESSFUL CONSUMER EDUCATION FOCUS

1. **Philosophy**—Patient education is an investment with a significant positive return. Money invested in teaching is money well spent. Time and energy invested are time and energy well spent.
2. **Priority**—Education is important. Quality nursing care always has an educational component. Informed consumers want to participate and look to nurses to teach them.
3. **Performance**—Clinical teaching excellence is a required nurse competency. Nurses must be skilled in using a variety of techniques and methods to meet the needs of the diverse consumers served.

Nurses need to be sensitive to the teaching needs of those at risk for disparities in health care: persons of a different race or ethnic group, women, children, older adults, rural residents, and those with limited or no health insurance, low health literacy, and/or low socioeconomic status. Nurses may unintentionally communicate lower expectations for persons who are disadvantaged, have a low literacy level, or have limited English proficiency.

Patients often hesitate asking for help with language skills. Some healthcare agencies include an assessment of a patient's ability to learn. However, the lack of assessment criteria may hinder nurses' efforts to institute appropriate teaching. Nurses can use the U.S. Census language screening questions. The person is asked if a language other than English is spoken at home, and if the answer is "yes," the person is asked to rate how well he or she speaks English: very well, well, not well, or not at all (Shin & Bruno, 2003). The National Standards for Culturally and Linguistically Appropriate Standards (CLAS) includes standards for cultural competence, language access, and organizational support (Office of Minority Health, 2001). The Joint Commission (2007) recommends that hospital leaders make a commitment to culturally and linguistically appropriate care highly visible to hospital staff and patients and that staff be provided with ongoing training to meet the unique needs of their patient population and to access language services for patients with limited English proficiency. A systematic review of research indicates that the use of professional interpreters raises the quality of clinical care for patients with limited English proficiency (Karliner, Jacobs, Chen, & Mutha, 2007).

Teaching can be simple or complex. In teaching elemental, task-oriented behaviors, the nurse uses basic materials, simple relationships, guides, sequencing of steps, and cause-and-effect relationships. Chronic disease self-management education programs can have a significant impact on health behavior and health focusing on a partnership between the patient and the healthcare provider. Nurses are involved in innovative program models that include Internet support, health coaching, and telemonitoring. Patients with chronic illnesses are often hospitalized for related complications. Therefore nurses need to be prepared to provide patient education. Education needs to consider various factors that might impede learning in a particular situation. The nurse manager role is to ensure that staff members have the resources to provide patient teaching, that it is done effectively, that it is appropriately documented, and that it is consistent with the patient's care plan.

In addition to being easy to read, written teaching materials need to reflect relevance, accuracy, and thoroughness and need to be updated regularly. They need to be appropriate for the patient's literacy level. Nurses have an ethical obligation to provide patients with education at a level that can be understood by their patients (Schaefer, 2008).

As a step-by-step process, teaching can be adapted to the problem-solving process model shown in Figure 22-1.

The following example uses the nursing process model in teaching a patient about diabetes:

Assess	Patient is a 16-year-old Hispanic boy with no previous knowledge of diabetes or skill in drug administration. English is a second language. He needs to administer insulin by the time he is discharged from the hospital.
Plan	Begin with a demonstration and return demonstration of basic subcutaneous injection. Progress step-by-step to basic understanding of diabetes, blood sugar, hypoglycemia, diet, and insulin dosage by the time of discharge. He is to return to a nurse-managed health center for follow-up care.
Implement	Set times to spend in instruction with patient. Begin with a demonstration, a return demonstration, and repeat instructions. Adjust learning materials to accommodate language barrier and age.
Evaluate	Patient has met minimal skill level of subcutaneous technique. He can administer insulin safely but has limited disease and cause-and-effect understanding. To be followed per nurse-managed health center with continued teaching.

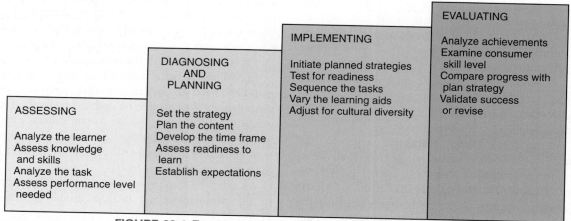

FIGURE 22-1 Teaching model adapted to the nursing process.

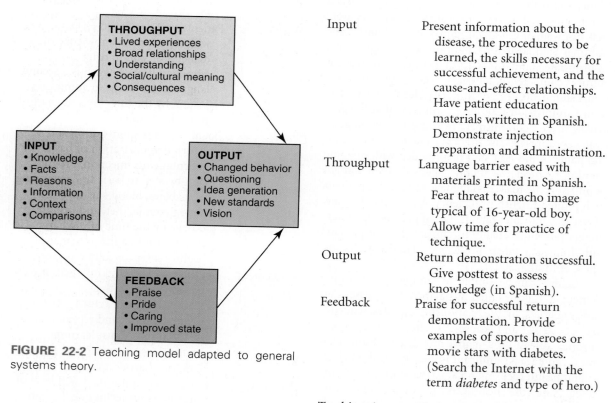

FIGURE 22-2 Teaching model adapted to general systems theory.

Conceptually, teaching also fits into the general systems theory model as shown in Figure 22-2. The following example uses the general systems theory model in teaching a patient with diabetes:

Input — Present information about the disease, the procedures to be learned, the skills necessary for successful achievement, and the cause-and-effect relationships. Have patient education materials written in Spanish. Demonstrate injection preparation and administration.

Throughput — Language barrier eased with materials printed in Spanish. Fear threat to macho image typical of 16-year-old boy. Allow time for practice of technique.

Output — Return demonstration successful. Give posttest to assess knowledge (in Spanish).

Feedback — Praise for successful return demonstration. Provide examples of sports heroes or movie stars with diabetes. (Search the Internet with the term *diabetes* and type of hero.)

Teaching is one of the most positive experiences nurses can have. Teaching can be fun and rewarding, but it is hard work.

Nurses need to be prepared and skilled to teach. They must be able to adapt to the learning styles of the consumer by using a variety of styles and flexible approaches in meeting the educational goals. For example, cancer detection and screening toolboxes were developed for migrant and seasonal farm workers with community input (Meade, Calvo, Rivera, & Baer, 2003). Examples of learning preferences include visual, auditory, kinesthetic, tactile, sequential, individual, and group. Having knowledge of the content, understanding consumer preferences, and being able to individualize the information to meet the consumer's ability to learn are critical to quality teaching.

EXERCISE 22-6
Use either the nursing process model or the general systems theory model as presented to prepare a teaching plan based on your actual nursing experience.

The family should also be included when providing patients with information. Numerous patient-satisfaction and family-satisfaction instruments are available to institutions, which can aid in understanding patient and family concerns. Furthermore, caregiver assessments should routinely be incorporated into practice improvement (Hannum Rose et al., 2007).

LEADERSHIP

Nurses are critically positioned to provide leadership for the twenty-first–century changes in health care. Understanding paradigm shifts in health care and the need to be responsive to change will prepare nurse managers to participate fully in shaping healthcare organizations of the future.

Nurse managers are well-positioned to influence the quality of care delivered by the staff. They set the tone for the unit's vision and mission and the focus for the staff. They must believe in and model a consumer-based service philosophy. One who believes in the need to provide service that is satisfying to the consumer knows that each consumer is different. What will satisfy one person will not satisfy another. Nurse managers, because they receive referrals when patients are dissatisfied with some aspect of their care, are in a unique position not only to find a solution but also to understand the types of problems being experienced by the patients on a unit and suggest

strategies for solving them. Being successful as leaders requires openness and flexibility; leaders are expected not only to do things right but also to do the right things and be effective role models for their followers. Leadership also involves the ability to relinquish control and a tolerance for ambiguity, as well as sudden and sometimes dramatic change.

Change is the modus operandi of the nursing environment in any healthcare setting. What works today may not work 6 months from now. Given the rapidly changing environment, the pressure to control costs, and advances in technology, science, and information, nurse managers need a whole new set of beliefs, behaviors, and skills.

Patient outcomes, standards of care, and evidence-based practice are attracting greater attention and receiving much more public scrutiny. Healthcare reform in the marketplace, the managed care movement, and consumer-directed health plans focus on the provision of quality care along with controlling costs. With this comes the realization that the evidence for certain nursing practices is limited and that nursing, as a profession, needs to be much stronger in making the case for value of the services provided by nurses.

In the area of consumer relations, patient satisfaction with care is a particularly relevant measure. A standardized survey of patients' perceptions of the quality of hospital care known as *Hospital Consumer Assessment of Healthcare Providers and Systems (HCAHPS)* was developed by the Centers for Medicare & Medicaid (CMS) and the Agency for Healthcare Research and Quality (AHRQ). Hospitals are now required to collect and publicly report HCAHPS results on the Hospital Compare website in order to receive their full CMS payment (Giordano, Elliott, Goldstein, Lehrman & Spencer, 2010). The first public reports comparing hospitals were released in 2008, allowing consumers to make meaningful comparisons among hospitals and creating incentives for hospitals to improve their quality. Nursing services researchers are particularly interested in responses to and satisfaction with nursing care. Valid measurement of patient satisfaction is an evolving science; nurses do not always accurately gauge what factors are most important to patients, and satisfaction measures are often skewed in a positive direction, with scores clustered at the top of the scale. These issues are

BOX 22-6	SAMPLE ITEMS FROM PATIENT'S ASSESSMENT OF QUALITY SCALE— ACUTE CARE VERSION (PAQS-ACV)

- The nurses treated me as if I am a special or important person.
- The nurses used touch to reassure or support me.
- The nurse knows who I am as a person.
- The nurses were calm when they were with me.
- The nurses were sensitive.
- The nurses were (im)patient.
- The nurses were caring people.
- I trusted the nurses.
- The hall was noisy.
- It was noisy in my room.
- The nurses were clear when teaching me about my care.
- The nurses were aware when I needed help from other health-care workers.
- The nurses were able to talk to me.

From Lynn, M.R., McMillen, B.J., & Sidani, S. (2007). Understanding and measuring patients' assessment of the quality of nursing care. *Nursing Research, 56*(3), 159-166.

addressed by Lynn, McMillen, and Sidani (2007), who developed an instrument to measure patient assessment of the quality of nursing care. Their instrument measures five dimensions: individualization, nurse characteristics, caring, environment, and responsiveness. Selected items appear in Box 22-6. Lynn et al. indicate that results from a traditional patient satisfaction tool should not be used to make statements about the nursing care or a nursing unit. More recently, Bacon, Hughes, and Mark (2009) tested structural contingency theory by examining the relationship between organizational influences and patient perceptions of symptom management, finding that better unit working conditions and collaboration with other disciplines significantly contributed to patient perceptions of better symptom management. Contingency theory, mentioned in Chapter 1, was developed by Lawrence and Lorsch (1967) and is a widely used organizational theory that emphasizes that design decisions are contingent on or depend on environmental conditions. The relationships among the contextual factors, structural factors, and organizational effectiveness are presented in the Theory Box

on p. 457. Thus it is incumbent upon nurses, both leaders and followers, to have a clear understanding of tools that are used to measure various aspects of patient satisfaction, the care delivered in an organization, and the relationships among them. Managers need to share the results of such surveys with their staff, examine what they are doing right so that they continue doing it, and determine how improvements could be made to address areas of concern.

Managers must be willing to give up direct control of every process. Staff must be supported in their use of power to be in control and to make decisions at the consumer-staff level of interaction. Some of our greatest successes derive from spontaneous actions. Giving up control involves being willing to take a risk and having a belief in the other person's ability to perform.

Leadership behaviors contributing to individual and personal excellence include the following:

- Allowing professionals more influence over their practice
- Giving staff opportunities to learn new and varied skills
- Giving recognition and reward for success and support and consolation for lack of success
- Fostering motivation and belief in the importance of each individual and the value of his or her contribution

The leader's role is to create within the worker a passion to do and contribute to the work effort successfully. This is supported by the seminal work of Aiken, Clarke, and Sloane (2002), who indicate that nurse staffing and organizational/managerial support for nursing are key to improving the quality of patient care.

Focusing on Consumers

We do best those things that we know how to do skillfully and those things about which we feel passionately. Fitting the right person to the right job is important. Maximum contribution is required from each staff member in today's healthcare agencies. Because the leader is the one who sets the standard for the success or failure of the staff's contributions, it is important to assess each staff member carefully—what is his or her skill level and commitment level, and what can be done to assist in making a maximum

THEORY BOX

Using Structural Contingency Theory to Test Patient Perceptions of Symptom Management

CONCEPT	KEY POINTS	COMPONENTS	VARIABLES (FACTORS)
Context	Includes external environment and the key tasks that an organization must perform	**External:** factors beyond the boundaries of the focal organization having the potential to influence the way the organization operates **Internal:** factors within the boundaries of the organization that affect its functioning **Factors influencing outcome measures**	**Hospital environment:** size, teaching status, Magnet™ status, illness severity, organizational life cycle **Nursing unit environment:** unit size, support services, patient acuity, work complexity **Patient characteristics:** age, gender, health status, education, previous hospitalizations
Structure	Administrative mechanisms used to balance coordination and control of work	**Staffing adequacy:** includes skills and knowledge of workers **Positive working conditions:** control over working conditions leads to positive outcomes	**Unit capacity:** RN staffing and education preparation of nurses **Work engagement:** personal involvement and commitment to work motivating an employee to invest more time, energy, and initiative **Autonomy** **Participation in decision making** **Relational coordination**
Organizational Effectiveness	Organizations are effective when structural features fit the demands of their internal and external environments	**Symptom management:** organizational characteristics may influence perceived effectiveness of symptom management	**Symptom distress:** extent to which nurses meet patients' expectations for management of troubling symptoms

Data from Bacon, C.T., Hughes, L.C., & Mark, B.A. (2009). Organizational influences on patient perceptions of symptom management. *Research in Nursing and Health, 32,* 321-334.

contribution? Figure 22-3 is an example of a completed staff assessment tool. Nurse managers can compile similar information for their staff members. Subsequently, the information can be used to form staff development plans.

When staff members know the leader is sincerely concerned about their welfare, they are better able to use their time, energy, and talents to serve the needs of the consumer. Staff members who are nurtured and cared for will be better able to nurture and care for the consumer.

EXERCISE 22-7

Form small groups and assess each member of the group using the headings shown in the staff assessment tool (see Figure 22-3).

Staff Member	Skill Level	Commitment Level	Suggested Action
(1) S. Baker, RN	High technical competence Able to teach others Learns quickly Needs improved people skills	Appears bored Does only what is assigned No enthusiasm Critical of any change	Assign challenges to use technical strengths Provide situations in which teaching others occurs Plan: Team assign with D. Carroll
(2) D. Carroll, RN	6-month postbasic program Learns quickly Slow with technical skills Needs technical supervision Excellent people skills	Excited about work Asks for new experiences Accepting of new ideas Volunteers to help others	Improve technical skills Provide safe and successful learning experiences Plan: Team assign with S. Baker
(3) J. Ratke, RN	Moderate technical competence Works best alone Not interested in teaching co-workers Good people skills	Restless, distracted Looking for a change Accepts new ideas Self-commitment—not group-oriented	Set up an independent project of her choosing (e.g., unit research idea) Provide some special technical training to increase skills
(4) C. Thomas, RN	High-level technical skills Enjoys helping others Excellent people skills Looks for challenges	Team player Interested in welfare of group Critical of poor performers Acts as cheerleader for change	Utilize willingness and group skills to plan and present a unit activity (e.g., in-service education production, unit open house)

FIGURE 22-3 Staff assessment tool.

THE SOLUTION

The vice president immediately met with the triage nurse and nurse manager. The nurse manager was surprised that her visit had not resolved the complaint. The vice president asked the triage nurse if she would have assessed a man with the same profile differently. Her immediate answer was "no." She stated that the staff was aware of the literary documents related to gender bias but that the protocol for assessing chest pain was well-designed and very objective, without bias to gender. With the approval of the nurse manager and triage nurse, the vice president invited the husband into the meeting. The husband and the nurse talked through the scenario of events and conversation that occurred during triage, especially the husband's perception that the triage nurse dismissed his request for immediate attention. They agreed that the husband might have said, "Does she really have to register herself?" The triage nurse had not interpreted his statement as a request for immediate action. Each realized that a miscommunication had occurred. Furthermore, the nurse responded to the husband's concern about gender bias. She explained that there had been information in the medical literature but that cardiologists, ethicists, and other healthcare experts had reviewed and approved the chest pain assessment protocol, ensuring no bias of gender. This situation was brought to resolution by an open line of communication. The result can often be "service recovery."

Several important points may be learned from this incident:
- Effective communication is critical for success. Clarification is always appropriate in situations of intense emotion. Active listening is an essential component of effective communication.
- Imagine yourself in the patient's situation and environment when analyzing communication.
- Engage the involved persons in the evaluation and solution related to a miscommunication.
- Healthcare practices, policies, and procedures should be updated to reflect new knowledge.
- Consumers are increasingly knowledgeable about health care; therefore expectations are more sophisticated and maintaining public trust is of great concern.
- Leadership must exude missionary zeal in educating personnel to the expectations for behavior in terms of consumer satisfaction.

—Suzanne Freeman

Would this be a suitable approach for you? Why?

THE EVIDENCE

1. Nurses are perceived as having great prestige, and nursing is perceived as the most trusted profession.
2. Nearly half of the adults in the United States have difficulty using and understanding health information.
3. Patients discharged from the emergency department are not prepared to manage their care at home.
4. Trust in healthcare providers is linked to their interpersonal skills.
5. Patients want to be treated fairly, with respect and attentiveness.
6. Sicker patients are less satisfied with the quality of their health care.
7. Patients' perceptions of care are affected by care focusing on individual needs and preferences.
8. Patients may be satisfied with care that is not of high quality.

NEED TO KNOW NOW

- Keep the consumer as the center of focus.
- Demonstrate commitment by serving as a patient advocate.
- Recognize that each staff member has a specific contribution to make to the unit's success.
- Understand the economic value of service.
- Evaluate patient outcomes and perceptions of care.

CHAPTER CHECKLIST

Times have changed, as has the role of the nurse manager. Healthcare's movement into the community, home, clinic, and outpatient setting has placed a whole new perspective on how to provide quality, cost-effective nursing care. Patients must participate in their care and need service-oriented nurses to be teachers, advocates, and leaders on their behalf. Managing care delivery in these diverse settings requires the use of flexible and creative skills. The key is to keep the patient as the center of focus and provide culturally and racially sensitive nursing care.

- Consumer relationships in health care typically involve interactions between the consumer and the following:

  The healthcare provider:
  - Healthcare provider–patient relationships are changing because of changes in the way health care is delivered.

  The nurse:
  - Nurses, as the healthcare providers who spend the most time with the consumer, set the tone for effective staff-patient interactions.

  The healthcare agency:
  - The agency's approach to care is determined by its mission and philosophy.

  The healthcare payers:
  - Insurance coverage and carriers usually dictate the services patients receive and where they receive them.

- Because of their favorable status with consumers, nurses are in a unique position to promote positive consumer relationships.
- Four major responsibilities of nurses in promoting successful consumer relationships are as follows:
  - Service
  - Advocacy
  - Teaching
  - Leadership
- A service orientation is consumer-driven and consumer-focused, emphasizing the quality of the nurse-patient relationship and the delivery of services in a caring atmosphere:

  Services differ from products:
  - Services are intangible, unpredictable, created and consumed simultaneously, and personal.
  - Products are tangible, predictable, produced and stored, and impersonal.

- The nurse can advocate by serving as a liaison between the consumer and the healthcare system:

- Nurses can interpret the agency's rules and customs for the consumer and negotiate if conflicts arise.
- Nurses also help secure culturally appropriate care and mediate cultural differences.
- Nurses are obligated legally and ethically to advocate for the recipients of care.
- Teaching is the sharing of information and education to help consumers become independent, self-responsible, and self-determining:
  - Nurses have an obligation to teach the consumer.
  - The three P's for successful consumer education are as follows:
    - Philosophy: Patient education is an investment with a significant positive return.
    - Priority: Education is important.
    - Performance: Clinical teaching excellence is a required skill for nurses.
  - Teaching can follow the five-step nursing process or a general systems model.

- Leadership fosters decision making at the consumer-staff level of interaction. Effective leadership strategies for the nurse manager include the following:
  - Keeping the central focus on the consumer and remembering that the consumer may be a whole population
  - Recognizing staff members' unique contributions and helping them maximize their personal excellence
  - Promoting staff members' sense of dignity, worth, caring, cultural diversity, and sensitivity
  - Understanding the economic value of service
  - Valuing interdisciplinary approaches to care
  - Evaluating patient outcomes, patients' perceptions of care, and patient satisfaction
  - Developing an effective service recovery plan

TIPS FOR PROMOTING A CONSUMER FOCUS

- Greet the patient by introducing yourself by full name and role.*
- Recap previous treatments or encounters.*
- Explain what to expect next.*
- Ask for questions.*
- Tell patients when they can expect you back.*
- Ask yourself if this service or approach is one you would wish to receive.

- Remember that in the pyramid of health services, it is the consumer who is the apex—the rest is there to support that person.
- Enter care relationships with the mindset of how to make care better from the recipient's perspective.
- Treat fellow employees, other healthcare professionals, families, and visitors with courtesy and respect.
- Ask staff members what they need to help them incorporate a customer service approach to care.
- Use the service, advocacy, teaching, leadership approach.

*From Baird, K. (2000). *Customer service in health care: A grassroots approach to creating a culture of service excellence.* San Francisco: Jossey-Bass.

REFERENCES

Agency for Healthcare Research and Quality (AHRQ). (January 2001). Health plans need culturally and linguistically appropriate materials for non-English speaking patients. *AHRQ Research Activities, 245*, 11. Retrieved April 11, 2010, from www.ahrq.gov/research/resact.htm.

Agency for Healthcare Research and Quality (AHRQ). (October 27, 2008). The CAHPS improvement guide: Practical strategies for improving the patient care experience. Retrieved April 11, 2010, from www.cahps.ahrq.gov.

Aiken, L. H., Clarke, S. P., & Sloane, D. M. (2002). Hospital staffing, organization, and quality of care: Cross-national findings. *Nursing Outlook, 50*, 187-194.

American Nurses Association (ANA). (2001). *Code of ethics for nurses with interpretive statements.* Washington, DC: Author.

American Nurses Association (ANA). (2009). *Gallup poll votes nurses most trusted profession.* Silver Spring, MD: Author. Retrieved April 9, 2010 from www.nursingworld.org.

American Nurses Association (ANA). (n.d.). NDNQI®: Transforming data into quality care. Silver Spring, MD: Author. Retrieved April 11, 2010, from www.nursingworld. org.

American Nurses Association (ANA). (2003a). *Nursing: Scope and standards of practice.* Washington, DC: Author.

American Nurses Association (ANA). (2003b). *Nursing's social policy statement* (2nd ed.). Washington, DC: Author.

Bacon, C. T., Hughes, L. C., & Mark, B. A. (2009). Organizational influences on patient perceptions of symptom management. *Research in Nursing and Health, 32,* 321-334.

Baird, K. (2000). *Customer service in health care: A grassroots approach to creating a culture of service excellence.* San Francisco: Jossey-Bass.

Bu, X., & Jezewksi, M. A. (2007). Developing a mid-range theory of patient advocacy through concept analysis. *Journal of Advanced Nursing, 57,* 101-110.

Bundorf, M. K., Wagner, T. H., Singer, S. J., & Baker, L. C. (2006). Who searches the Internet for health information? *Health Services Research, 41*(3 Pt 1), 819-836.

Calvin, A. O., Frazier, L., & Cohen, M. Z. (2007). Examining older adults' perceptions of health care providers: Identifying important aspects of older adults' relationships with physicians and nurses. *Journal of Gerontological Nursing, 33*(5), 6-12.

Cameron, J. I., & Gignac, M. A. (2008). "Timing it Right": A conceptual framework for addressing the support needs of family caregivers to stroke survivors from the hospital to the home. *Patient Education and Counseling, 70,* 305-314.

Dixon, A., Greene, J., & Hibbard, J. (2008). Do consumer-directed health plans drive change in enrollees' health care behavior? *Health Affairs, 27*(4), 1120-1131.

Donohue, J. M., Cevasco, M., & Rosenthal, M. B. (2007). A decade of direct-to-consumer advertising of prescription drugs. *New England Journal of Medicine, 357,* 673-681.

Doucette, J. N. (2003). Serving up uncommon service. *Nursing Management, 34*(11), 26, 28-30.

Engel, K. G., Heisler, M., Smith, D. M., Robinson, C. H., Forman, J. H., & Ubel, P. A. (2008). Patient comprehension of emergency department care and instructions: Are patients aware of when they do not understand? *Annals of Emergency Medicine, 53*(4), 454-461.

Ervin, N. (2006). Does patient satisfaction contribute to nursing care quality? *Journal of Nursing Administration, 36,* 126-130.

Flaskerud, J. (2007). Cultural competence: What is it? *Issues in Mental Health Nursing, 28,* 121-123.

Friele, R. D., & Sluijs, E. M. (2006). Patient expectations of fair complaint handling in hospitals: Empirical data. *BMC Health Services Research, 18,* 106.

Gardiner, R. (2008). The transition from 'informed patient care' to 'patient informed' care. *Studies in Health Technology Information, 137,* 241-256.

Giordano, L. A., Elliott, M. N., Goldstein, E., Lehrman, W. G., & Spencer, P. A. (2010). Development, implementation and public reporting of the HCAPHS survey. *Medical Care Research and Review, 67,* 27-37.

Hannum Rose, J., Bowman, K. F., O'Toole, E. E., Abbott, K., Love, T. E., Thomas, C., & Dawson, N. V. (2007). Caregiver objective burden and assessments of patient-centered, family-focused care for frail elderly veterans. *Gerontologist, 47,* 21-33.

Harris Interactive, Inc. (2008). Prestige paradox: High pay doesn't necessarily equal high prestige. Retrieved April 14, 2010, from www.harrisinteractive.com/harris_poll/.

Hobbs, J. L. (2009). A dimensional analysis of patient-centered care. *Nursing Research, 58,* 52-62.

Hupcey, J. E., & Miller, J. (2006). Community dwelling adults' perception of interpersonal trust vs. trust in health care providers. *Journal of Clinical Nursing, 15,* 1132-1139.

Jha, A. K., Orav, E. J., Zheng, J., & Epstein, A. M. (2008). Patients' perception of hospital care in the United States. *New England Journal of Medicine, 359,* 1921-1931.

Karliner, L. S., Jacobs, E. A., Chen, A. H., & Mutha, S. (2007). Do professional interpreters improve clinical care for patients with limited English proficiency? A systematic review of the literature. *Health Services Research, 42,* 727-754.

Kerfoot, K. (2007). Patient satisfaction and high reliability organizations: What's the connection? *Nursing Economic$, 25,* 119-120.

Kiger, P. J. (2004). The art of the apology. *Workforce Management, 81*(10), 57-58, 60-62.

Lawrence, P. R., & Lorsch, J. W. (1967). Differentiation and integration in complex organizations. *Administrative Science Quarterly, 12,* 1-47.

Leapfrog Group. (2009). The Leapfrog Group: Fact sheet. Retrieved October 2009, from www.leapfroggroup.org/media/file/FactSheet_LeapfrogGroup.pdf.

Lynn, M. R., McMillen, B. J., & Sidani, S. (2007). Understanding and measuring patients' assessment of the quality of nursing care. *Nursing Research, 56*(3), 159-166.

Meade, C. D., Calvo, A., Rivera, M. A., & Baer, R. D. (2003). Focus groups in the design of prostate cancer screening information for Hispanic farmworkers and African-American men. *Oncology Nursing Forum, 30,* 967-975.

Montalvo, I. (September 2007). The National Database of Nursing Quality Indicators® (NDNQI®). *Online Journal of Issues in Nursing, 12*(3). Retrieved October 2009, from www.nursingworld.org.

Naessens, J. M., Khan, M., Shah, N. D., Wagie, A., Pautz, R. A., & Campbell, C. R. (2008). Effect of premium, copayments, and health status on the choice of health plans. *Medical Care, 46,* 1033-1040.

National Alliance for Hispanic Health. (2000). *Quality health services for Hispanics: The cultural competency component.* Washington, DC: Department of Health and Human Services.

National Priorities Partnership. (2008). *National priorities and goals: Aligning our efforts to transform America's healthcare.* Washington, DC: National Quality Forum.

Nielson-Bohlman, L., Panzer, A. M., & Kindig, D. A. (Eds.). Committee on Health Literacy, Board on Neuroscience and Behavioral Health, Institute of Medicine. (2004). *Health literacy: A prescription to end confusion.* Washington, DC: National Academies Press.

Office of Minority Health. (2001). *National standards for culturally and linguistically appropriate services in health care (CLAS).* Washington, DC: U.S. Department of Health and Human Services. Retrieved April 11, 2010, from www.omhrc. gov.

Perlow, E. (2010). Accessibility: Global gateway to health literacy. *Health Promotion Practice, 11,* 123-131.

Pham, H. H., Grossman, J. M., Cohen, G., & Bodenheimer, T. (2008). Hospitalists and care transitions: The divorce of inpatient and outpatient care. *Health Affairs, 27,* 1315-1327.

Robert Graham Center. (2007). *The patient centered medical home: History, seven core features, evidence and transformational change.* Washington, DC: Author. Retrieved April 11, 2010, from www.graham-center.org.

Rosenthal, T. C. (2008). The medical home: Growing evidence to support a new approach to primary care. *Journal of the American Board of Family Medicine, 21,* 427-440.

Sahlsten, M. J., Larsson, I. E., Sjöström, B., & Plos, K. A. (2008). An analysis of the concept of patient participation. *Nursing Forum, 43,* 2-11.

Sarkar, U., Piette, J. D., Gonzales, R., Lessler, D., Chew, L. D., Reilly, B., Johnson, J., Brunt, M., Huang, J., Regenstein, M., & Schillinger, D. (2008). Preferences for self-management support: Findings from a survey of diabetes patients in safety-net health systems. *Patient Education and Counseling, 70,* 102-110.

Sauaia, A., Min, S. J., Leber, C., Erbacher, K., Abrams, F., & Fink, R. (2005). Postoperative pain management in elderly patients: Correlation between adherence to treatment guidelines and patient satisfaction. *Journal of the American Geriatrics Society, 53,* 274-282.

Schaefer, C. T. (2008). Integrated review of health literacy interventions. *Orthopaedic Nursing, 27,* 302-317.

Scott-Cawiezell, J., Vogelsmeier, A., McKenney, C., Rantz, M., Hicks, L., & Zellmer, D. (2006). Moving from a culture of blame to a culture of safety in the nursing home setting. *Nursing Forum, 41,* 133-140.

Shin, H. B., & Bruno, R. (October 2003). Language use and English speaking ability: 2000 (Census 2000 brief). U.S. Census Bureau, U.S. Department of Commerce, Economics and Statistics Administration. Retrieved April 11, 2010, from www.census.gov.

Smith, R. (May 20, 2008). Digital chasm: 18% of U.S. households are netless: 30% have never used PC to create a document. Retrieved April 11, 2010, from localtechwire.com/business/ local_tech_wire/opinion/blogpost/2911845/.

Tea, C., Ellison, M., & Feghali, F. (2008). Proactive patient rounding to increase customer service and satisfaction on an orthopaedic unit. *Orthopaedic Nursing, 27,* 233-240.

The Joint Commission. (2007). *What did the doctor say? Improving health literacy to protect patient safety.* Oakbrook Terrace, IL: Author. Retrieved April 11, 2010, from www. jointcommission.org/.

U.S. Department of Health and Human Services. (2008). Health communication activities: Health literacy. Office of Disease Prevention and Health Promotion. Retrieved April 11, 2010, from www.health.gov/communication/.

Wolf, D. M., Lehman, L., Quinlin, R., Zullo, T., & Hoffman, L. (2008). Effect of patient-centered care on patient satisfaction and quality of care. *Journal of Nursing Care Quality, 23,* 316-321.

Wolf, G., Triolo, P., & Ponte, P. R. (2008). Magnet Recognition Program: The next generation. *Journal of Nursing Administration, 38,* 200-204.

Wolff, J. L., & Roter, D. L. (2008). Hidden in plain sight: Medical visit companions as a resource for vulnerable older adults. *Archives of Internal Medicine, 168,* 1409-1415.

World Health Organization. (2008). 2008-2013 Action plan for the global strategy for the prevention and control of noncommunicable diseases. Retrieved April 11, 2010, from www.who.int/nmh/Actionplan-PC-NCD-2008.pdf.

Wylie, J. L., & Wagenfeld-Heintz, E. (2004). Development of relationship-centered care. *Journal of Healthcare Quality, 26*(1), 14-21, 45, 60.

Yoder-Wise, P. S. (2010). More serendipity: The Winkler County trial, *The Journal of Continuing Education in Nursing, 41,* 147.

SUGGESTED READINGS

Clark, P. A. (2006). *Patient satisfaction and the discharge process: Evidence-based best practices.* Marblehead, MA: Opus Communications.

Curley, M. A. (2007). *Synergy: The unique relationship between nurses and patients.* Indianapolis: Sigma Theta Tau International, Center for Nursing Press.

Laviest, T. (2005). *Minority populations and health: An introduction to health disparities in the United States.* Hoboken, NJ: Jossey-Bass.

Lipson, L. G., & Dibble, S. L. (Eds.). (2005). *Culture and clinical care.* San Francisco: UCSF Nursing Press.

Mol, A. (2008). *The logic of care: Health and the problem of choice.* New York: Routledge.

Osborne, L. (2004). *Resolving patient complaints: A step-by-step guide to service recovery* (2nd ed.). Boston: Jones & Bartlett.

Press, I. (2005). *Patient satisfaction: Understanding and managing the experience of care* (2nd ed.). Baltimore, MD: Health Administration Press.

Studer, Q. (2005). *Hardwiring excellence: Purpose, worthwhile work, making a difference.* Janesville, WI: Firestarter Publishing.

Studer, Q. (2008). *Results that last: Hardwiring behaviors that will take your company to the top.* Hoboken, NJ: Wiley.

WEBSITES

Agency on Healthcare Research and Quality Information for Consumers and Patients: www.ahrq.gov/consumer/

Cultural Diversity in Health Care: www.ggalanti.com/index.html

Cultural Diversity in Nursing: www.culturediversity.org/

EurasiaHealth Knowledge Network: www.eurasiahealth.org

Department of Health and Human Services: www.healthfinder.gov

Health Canada: www.hc-sc.gc.ca/index_e.html

Health on the Net Foundation: www.hon.ch

Healthsites: Your Portal to Medical Information on the Net: www.healthsites.co.uk/index.php

Hospital Compare: www.hospitalcompare.hhs.gov

Institute of Medicine: www.iom.edu

Medline Plus: Trusted Health Information for You: www.nlm.nih.gov/medlineplus/

National Health Information Center, U.S. Department of Health and Human Services: http://healthfinder.gov/

National Institutes of Health, Health Information: http://health.nih.gov/

Office of Minority Health: www.omhrc.gov

World Health Organization: www.who.int

Conflict: The Cutting Edge of Change

Victoria N. Folse

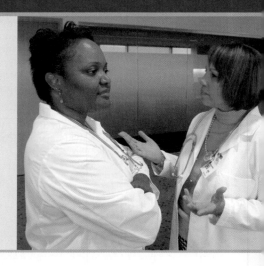

Appropriate conflict-handling strategies are essential in professional nursing practice because conflict cannot be eliminated from the workplace. To resolve conflicts, nurse leaders must be able to determine the nature of a particular issue, choose an appropriate approach for each situation, and implement a course of action. This chapter focuses on maximizing the nurse leader's ability to deal with conflict by providing effective strategies for conflict resolution.

OBJECTIVES

- Use a model of the conflict process to determine the nature and sources of perceived and actual conflict.
- Assess preferred approaches to conflict, and commit to be more effective in resolving future conflict.
- Determine which of the five approaches to conflict is the most appropriate in potential and actual situations.
- Identify conflict-management techniques that will prevent lateral violence from occurring.

TERMS TO KNOW

accommodating	compromising	lateral violence
avoiding	conflict	mediation
bullying	horizontal violence	negotiating
collaborating	interpersonal conflict	organizational conflict
competing	intrapersonal conflict	

THE CHALLENGE

Kimberly M. Wolski, RN, BSN
Staff Nurse, 4 Hope (Pediatric Hematology/Oncology and
Medical-Surgical Unit), Advocate Hope Children's Hospital,
Oak Lawn, Illinois

Over the past 6 months, I have gone through the exciting process of experiencing health care as a newly graduated registered nurse. I always dreamed of being a nurse who really could change the world one patient or family at a time and who could make some-one's stressful and sometimes scary hospital experience a little

brighter. The process of transitioning into the professiona[...] been an exhilarating and challenging one, but all of these hopes and dreams also created quite an intrapersonal conflict: how was I going to successfully transition into the independent professional nursing role when I have spent the past 4 years being supervised by highly educated, competent, and experienced nurses?

What do you think you would do if you were this nurse?

INTRODUCTION

Conflict is a disagreement in values or beliefs within oneself or between people that causes harm or has the potential to cause harm. Conflict is a catalyst for change and has the ability to stimulate either detrimental or beneficial effects. If properly understood and managed, conflict can lead to positive outcomes and practice environments, but if it is left unattended, it can have a negative impact on both the individual and the organization (Johansen, 2012; Kolb, 2013; Morrison, 2008). In professional practice environments, unresolved conflict among nurses is a significant issue resulting in job dissatisfaction, absenteeism, and turnover. Successful organizations are proactive in anticipating the need for conflict resolution and innovative in developing conflict resolution strategies that apply to all members (Trudel & Reio, 2011).

Conflict can be a strategic tool when addressed appropriately and can actually deepen and develop human relationships. Some of the first authors on organizational conflict (e.g., Blake & Mouton, 1964; Deutsch, 1973) claimed that a complete resolution of conflict might, in fact, be undesirable because conflict also stimulates growth, creativity, and change. Seminal work on the concept of organizational conflict management suggested conflict was necessary to achieve organizational goals and cohesiveness of employees, facilitate organizational change, and contribute to creative problem solving (Morrison, 2008). Moderate levels of conflict contribute to the quality of ideas generated and foster cohesiveness among team members, contributing to an organization's success (Greer et al., 2012). An organization without conflict is characterized by no change; and in contrast, an

optimal level of conflict will generate creativity, a problem-solving atmosphere, a strong team spirit, and motivation of its workers (Strack van Schijndel & Burchardi, 2007).

The complexity of the healthcare environment compounds the impact that caregiver stress and unresolved conflict has on patient safety. Conflict is inherent in clinical environments in which nursing responsibilities are driven by patient needs that are complex and frequently changing (Johansen, 2012). Healthcare providers are exposed to high stress levels from increased demands on an ever-limited and aging workforce, a decrease in available resources, a more acutely ill and underinsured patient population, and a profound period of change in the practice environment (Brinkert, 2011). Nurses employed in better care environments report more positive job experiences and fewer concerns about quality care. Positive practice environments and high core self-evaluations (self-esteem, self-efficacy, locus of control, and emotional stability) predicted nurses' constructive conflict management, and in turn, greater unit effectiveness (Siu et al., 2008). Favorable core self-evaluation was also a predictor of quality leader-staff relationships, empowerment, and job satisfaction for nurse managers (Laschinger, Purdy, & Almost, 2007). Moreover, hospitals with good nurse-physician relations are associated with better nurse and patient outcomes (Aiken et al., 2008).

An important factor in the successful management of stress and conflict is a better understanding of its context within the practice environment. The diversity of people involved in health care may stimulate conflict, yet the shared goal of meeting patient care needs provides a solid, ethical foundation for conflict resolution (Saltman, O'Dea, & Kidd, 2006). Because nursing remains a predominately female profession, this may contribute to the use of avoidance and accommodation as primary strategies. Emotions of empathy, compassion, and caring should not be suppressed, but neither should assertive communication and behavior. The stereotypical self-sacrificing behavior seen in avoidance and accommodation is strongly supported by the altruistic nature of nursing (Iglesias & Vallejo, 2012). Avoidance may be appropriate during times of high stress, but when overused, it threatens the well-being of nurses and retention within the discipline.

TYPES OF CONFLICT

The recognition that conflict is a part of everyday life suggests that mastering conflict-management strategies is essential for overall well-being and personal and professional growth. A need exists to determine the type of conflict present in a specific situation, because the more accurately conflict is defined, the more likely it will be resolved. Conflict occurs in three broad categories and can be intrapersonal, interpersonal, or organizational in nature; a combination of types can also be present in any given conflict.

Intrapersonal conflict occurs within a person when confronted with the need to think or act in a way that seems at odds with one's sense of self. Questions often arise that create a conflict over priorities, ethical standards, and values. When a nurse manager decides what to do about the future (e.g., "Do I want to pursue an advanced degree or start a family now?"), conflicts arise between personal and professional priorities. Some issues present a conflict over comfortably maintaining the status quo (e.g., "I know my newest charge nurse likes the autonomy of working nights. Do I really want to ask him to move to days to become a preceptor?"). Taking risks to confront people when needed (e.g., "Would recommending a change in practice that I learned about at a recent conference jeopardize the unit governance?") can produce intrapersonal conflict and, because it involves other people, may lead to interpersonal conflict.

Interpersonal conflict transpires between and among patients, family members, nurses, physicians, and members of other departments. Conflicts occur that focus on a difference of opinion, priority, or approach with others. A manager may be called upon to assist two nurses in resolving a scheduling conflict or issues surrounding patient assignments. Members of healthcare teams often have disputes over the best way to treat particular cases or disagreements in determining how much information is necessary for patients and families to have about their illness. Yet, interpersonal conflict can serve as the impetus for needed change and can accelerate innovation in approach.

Organizational conflict arises when discord exists about policies and procedures, personnel codes of conduct, or accepted norms of behavior and patterns of communication. Some organizational conflict is related to hierarchical structure and role differentiation among employees. Nurse managers, as well as their staff, often become embattled in institution-wide conflict concerning staffing patterns and how they affect the quality of care. Complex ethical and moral dilemmas often arise when profitable services are increased and unprofitable ones are downsized or even eliminated.

A major source of organizational conflict stems from strategies that promote more participation and autonomy of staff nurses. Increasingly, nurses are charged with balancing direct patient care with active involvement in the institutional initiatives surrounding quality patient care. Nurses who perceive themselves to work in a positive practice environment that creates a cooperative work context are more likely to report effective conflict-management approaches (Siu et al., 2008). The Magnet Recognition Program® of the American Nurses Credentialing Center (ANCC) (2008) identifies interdisciplinary relationships as one of the "Forces of Magnetism" necessary for Magnet™ designation. Specifically, collaborative working relationships within and among the disciplines are valued and must be demonstrated through mutual respect. Magnet™ hospitals must have conflict-management strategies in place and demonstrate effective use, when indicated. The following are other "forces" that are particularly germane to conflict in the practice environment:

- Organizational structure (nurses' involvement in shared decision making)
- Management style (nursing leaders create an environment supporting participation,

encourage and value feedback, and demonstrate effective communication with staff)

- Personnel policies and programs (efforts to promote nurse work/life balance)
- Image of nursing (nurses effectively influencing system-wide processes)
- Autonomy (nurses' inclusion in governance leading to job satisfaction, personal fulfillment, and organization success)

EXERCISE 23-1

Recall a situation in which conflict between or among two or more people was apparent. Describe verbal and nonverbal communication and how each person responded. What was the outcome? Was the conflict resolved? Was anything left unresolved?

STAGES OF CONFLICT

Conflict proceeds through four stages: frustration, conceptualization, action, and outcomes (Thomas, 1992). The ability to resolve conflicts productively depends on understanding this process (Figure 23-1) and successfully addressing thoughts, feelings, and behaviors that form barriers to resolution. As one navigates through the stages of conflict, moving into a subsequent stage may lead to a return to and change in a previous stage. To illustrate, the evening shift of a cardiac step-down unit has been asked to pilot a new hand-off protocol for the next 6 weeks, which stimulates intense emotions because the unit is already inadequately staffed (frustration). Two nurses on the unit interpret this conflict as a battle for control with the nurse educator, and a third nurse thinks it is all about professional standards (conceptualization). A nurse leader/manager facilitates a discussion with the three nurses (action); she listens to the concerns and presents evidence about the potential effectiveness of the new hand-off protocol. All agree that the real conflict comes from a difference in goals or priorities (new conceptualization), which leads to less negative emotion and ends with a much clearer understanding

of all the issues (diminished frustration). The nurses agree to pilot the hand-off protocol after their ideas have been incorporated into the plan (outcome).

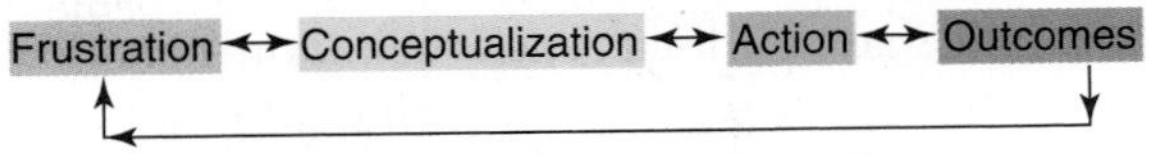

Frustration

When people or groups perceive that their goals may be blocked, frustration results. This frustration may escalate into stronger emotions, such as anger and deep resignation. For example, a nurse may perceive that a postoperative patient is noncompliant or uncooperative, when in reality the patient is afraid or has a different set of priorities at the start from those of the nurse. At the same time, the patient may view the nurse as controlling and uncaring, because the nurse repeatedly asks if the patient has used his incentive spirometer as instructed. When such frustrations occur, it is a cue to stop and clarify the nature and cause of the differences.

Conceptualization

Conflict arises when there are different interpretations of a situation, including a different emphasis on what is important and what is not, and different thoughts about what should occur next. Everyone involved develops an idea of what the conflict is about, and this view may or may not be accurate. This may be an instant conclusion, or it may develop over time. Everyone involved has an individual interpretation of what the conflict is and why it is occurring. Most often, these interpretations are dissimilar and involve the person's own perspective, which is based on personal values, beliefs, and culture.

Regardless of its accuracy, conceptualization forms the basis for everyone's reactions to the frustration. The way the individuals perceive and define the conflict has a great deal of influence on the approach to resolution and subsequent outcomes. For example, within the same conflict situation, some individuals may see a conflict between a nurse manager and a staff nurse as insubordination and become angry at the threat to the leader's role. Others may view it as trivial complaining, voice criticism (e.g., "We've been over this new protocol already; why can't you just adopt the change?"), and withdraw from the situation. Such differences in conceptualizing the issue block its resolution. Thus it is important for each person to clarify "the conflict as I see it" and "how it makes me respond" before all the people involved can define the

Frustration ↔ Conceptualization ↔ Action ↔ Outcomes

FIGURE 23-1 Stages of conflict.

conflict, develop a shared conceptualization, and resolve their differences. The following are questions to consider:

- What is the nature of our differences?
- What are the reasons for those differences?
- Does our leader endorse ideas or behaviors that add to or diminish the conflict?
- Do I need to be mentored by someone, even if that individual is outside my own department or work area, to successfully resolve this conflict?

Action

A behavioral response to a conflict follows the conceptualization. This may include seeking clarification about how another person views the conflict, collecting additional information that informs the issue, or engaging in dialog about the issue. As actions are taken to resolve the conflict, the way that some or all parties conceptualize the conflict may change. Successful resolution frequently stems from identifying a common goal that unites (e.g., quality patient care, good working relations). It is important to understand that people are always taking some action regarding the conflict, even if that action is avoiding dealing with it, deliberately delaying action, or choosing to do nothing. The longer ineffective actions continue, though, the more likely people will experience frustration, resistance, or even hostility. The more the actions appropriately match the nature of the conflict, the more likely the conflict will be resolved with desirable results.

Outcomes

Tangible and intangible consequences result from the actions taken and have significant implications for the work setting. Consequences include (1) the conflict being resolved with a revised approach, (2) stagnation of any current movement, or (3) no future movement. The outcome can be either constructive or destructive; effective strategies minimize destructive effects and maximize constructive outcomes (Saltman et al., 2006).

Constructive conflict results in successful resolution, leading to the following:

- Growth occurs.
- Problems are resolved.
- Groups are unified.

BOX 23-1   ASSESSING THE DEGREE OF CONFLICT RESOLUTION

I. Quality of decisions
   A. How creative are resulting plans?
   B. How practical and realistic are they?
   C. How well were intended goals achieved?
   D. What surprising results were achieved?
II. Quality of relationships
   A. How much understanding has been created?
   B. How willing are people to work together?
   C. How much mutual respect, empathy, concern, and cooperation has been generated?

Modified from Hurst, J., & Kinney, M. (1989). *Empowering self and others.* Toledo, OH: University of Toledo.

- Productivity is increased.
- Commitment is increased.

Unsatisfactory resolution is typically destructive and results in the following:

- Negativity, resistance, and increased frustration inhibit movement.
- Resolutions diminish or are absent.
- Groups divide, and relationships weaken.
- Productivity decreases.
- Satisfaction decreases.

Assessing the degree of conflict resolution is useful for improving individual and group skills in resolutions. Two general outcomes are considered when assessing the degree to which a conflict has been resolved: (1) the degree to which important goals were achieved and (2) the nature of the subsequent relationships among those involved (Box 23-1).

CATEGORIES OF CONFLICT

Categorizing a conflict can further define an appropriate course of action for resolution. Conflicts arise from discrepancies in four areas: facts, goals, approaches, and values. Sources of fact-based conflicts are external written sources and include job descriptions, hospital policies, standard of nursing practice, and The Joint Commission (TJC) mandates. Objective data can be provided to resolve a disagreement generated by discrepancies in information. Goal conflicts often arise from competing priorities (e.g., desire to empower employees vs. control through micromanagement); frequently, a common goal (e.g., quality patient care) can be identified and used to frame conflict resolution. Even when agreement exists on a common goal, different ideas about the best approach to achieve that goal may produce conflict. For example, if the unit goal is to reduce costs by 10 percent, one leader may target overtime hours and another may eliminate the budget for continuing education. Values, opinions, and beliefs are much more personal, thus generating disagreements that can be threatening and adversarial. Because values are subjective, value-based conflicts often remain unresolved. Therefore, a need to find a way for competing values to coexist is necessary for conflict management.

MODES OF CONFLICT RESOLUTION

Understanding the way healthcare providers respond to conflict is an essential first step in identifying effective strategies to help nurses constructively handle conflicts in the practice environment (Sportsman & Hamilton, 2007). Five distinct approaches can be used in conflict resolution: avoiding, accommodating, competing, compromising, and collaborating (Thomas & Kilmann, 1974, 2002). These approaches can be viewed within two dimensions: assertiveness (satisfying one's own concerns) and cooperativeness (satisfying the concerns of others). Most people tend to employ a combined set of actions that are appropriately assertive and cooperative, depending on the nature of the conflict situation (Thomas, 1992). See the conflict self-assessment in Box 23-2.

EXERCISE 23-2

Self-assessment of preferred conflict-handling modes is important. As you read and answer the 30-item conflict survey in Box 23-2, think of how you respond to conflict in professional situations. After completing the survey, tally, total, and reflect on your scores for each of the five approaches. Consider the following questions:
- Which approach do you prefer? Which do you use least?
- What determines if you respond in a particular manner?
- Considering the reoccurring types of conflicts you have, what are the strengths and weaknesses of your preferred conflict-handling styles?
- Have others offered you feedback about your approach to conflict?

As you read the rest of this section, use this pattern of scores and your reflections to examine the appropriate uses of each approach, assess your use of each approach more extensively, and commit to new behaviors to increase your future effectiveness.

Avoiding

Avoiding, or withdrawing, is very unassertive and uncooperative because people who avoid neither pursue their own needs, goals, or concerns immediately nor assist others to pursue theirs. Avoidance as a conflict-management style only ensures that conflict is postponed, and conflict has a tendency to escalate in intensity when ignored. That is not to say that all conflict must be addressed immediately; some issues require considerable reflection, and action should be delayed. The positive side of withdrawing may be postponing an issue until a better time or simply walking away from a "no-win" situation (Box 23-3). The self-assessment in Box 23-4 will help you recognize your own avoidance behaviors and use them more effectively.

Accommodating

When accommodating, people neglect their own needs, goals, and concerns (unassertive) while trying to satisfy those of others (cooperative). This approach has an element of being self-sacrificing and simply obeying orders or serving other people. For example, a co-worker requests you cover her weekends during her children's holiday break. You had hoped to visit friends from college, but you know how important it is for her to have more time with her family, so you agree. Box 23-5 lists some appropriate uses of accommodation.

Individuals who frequently use accommodating may feel disappointment and resentment because they "get nothing in return." This is a built-in by-product of the overuse of this approach. The self-assessment in Box 23-6 asks you to examine your current use of accommodation and challenges you to think of new ways to use it more effectively.

Competing

When competing, people pursue their own needs and goals at the expense of others. Sometimes people use whatever power, creativeness, or strategies that are available to "win." Competing may also take the form

BOX 23-2 CONFLICT SELF-ASSESSMENT

Directions: Read each of the following statements. Assess yourself in terms of how often you tend to act similarly during conflict at work. Place the number of the most appropriate response in the blank in front of each statement. Put *1* if the behavior is never typical of how you act during a conflict, *2* if it is seldom typical, *3* if it is occasionally typical, *4* if it is frequently typical, or *5* if it is very typical of how you act during conflict.

3 1. Create new possibilities to address all important concerns.
2 2. Persuade others to see it and/or do it my way.
4 3. Work out some sort of give-and-take agreement.
3 4. Let other people have their way.
3 5. Wait and let the conflict take care of itself.
5 6. Find ways that everyone can win.
2 7. Use whatever power I have to get what I want.
5 8. Find an agreeable compromise among people involved.
3 9. Give in so others get what they think is important.
3 10. Withdraw from the situation.
5 11. Cooperate assertively until everyone's needs are met.
3 12. Compete until I either win or lose.
3 13. Engage in "give a little and get a little" bargaining.
4 14. Let others' needs be met more than my own needs.
1 15. Avoid taking any action for as long as I can.
5 16. Partner with others to find the most inclusive solution.
4 17. Put my foot down assertively for a quick solution.
3 18. Negotiate for what all sides value and can live without.
3 19. Agree to what others want to create harmony.
1 20. Keep as far away from others involved as possible.
5 21. Stick with it to get everyone's highest priorities.
4 23. Argue and debate over the best way.
3 23. Create some middle position everyone agrees to.
2 24. Put my priorities below those of other people.
2 25. Hope the issue does not come up.
5 26. Collaborate with others to achieve our goals together.
3 27. Compete with others for scarce resources.
5 28. Emphasize compromise and trade-offs.
3 29. Cool things down by letting others do it their way.
3 30. Change the subject to avoid the fighting.

Conflict Self-Assessment Scoring

Look at the numbers you placed in the blanks on the conflict assessment. Write the number you placed in each blank on the appropriate line below. Add up your total for each column, and enter that total on the appropriate line. The greater your total is for each approach, the more often you tend to use that approach when conflict occurs at work. The lower the score is, the less often you tend to use that approach when conflict occurs at work.

Collaborating	Competing	Compromising	Accommodating	Avoiding
1. 3	2. 2	3. 4	4. 3	5. 3
6. 5	7. 2	8. 5	9. 3	10. 3
11. 5	12. 3	13. 3	14. 4	15. 1
16. 5	17. 4	18. 3	19. 3	20. 1
21. 5	22. 4	23. 3	24. 2	25. 2
26. 5	27. 3	28. 5	29. 3	30. 3
Total 28	Total 18	Total 23	Total 18	Total 13

Throughout the rest of this section, there are descriptions of each approach and related self-assessment and commitment-to-action activities. Use these totals to stimulate your thinking about how you do and could handle conflict at work. Most important, consider if your pattern of frequency tends to be consistent, or inconsistent, with the types of conflicts you face. That is, does your way of dealing with conflict tend to match the situations in which that approach is most useful?

From Hurst, J.B. (1993). *Conflict self-assessment.* Toledo, OH: Human Resource Development Center, University of Toledo.

BOX 23-3   APPROPRIATE USES FOR THE AVOIDING APPROACH

1. When facing trivial and/or temporary issues, or when other far more important issues are pressing
2. When there is no chance to obtain what one wants or needs, or when others could resolve the conflict more efficiently and effectively
3. When the potential negative results of initiating and acting on a conflict are much greater than the benefits of its resolution
4. When people need to "cool down," distance themselves, or gather more information

BOX 23-4   AVOIDANCE: SELF-ASSESSMENT AND COMMITMENT TO ACTION

If You Tend to Use Avoidance Often, Ask Yourself the Following Questions:

1. Do people have difficulty getting my input into and understanding my view?
2. Do I block cooperative efforts to resolve issues?
3. Am I distancing myself from significant others?
4. Are important issues being left unidentified and unresolved?

If You Seldom Use Avoidance, Ask Yourself the Following Questions:

1. Do I find myself overwhelmed by a large number of conflicts and a need to say "no"?
2. Do I assert myself even when things do not matter that much? Do others view me as an aggressor?
3. Do I lack a clear view of what my priorities are?
4. Do I stir up conflicts and fights?

Commitment to Action

What two new behaviors would increase your effective use of avoidance?
1.
2.

BOX 23-5   APPROPRIATE USES OF ACCOMMODATION

1. When other people's ideas and solutions appear to be better, or when you have made a mistake
2. When the issue is far more important to the other(s) person than it is to you
3. When you see that accommodating now "builds up some important credits" for later issues
4. When you are outmatched and/or losing anyway; when continued competition would only damage the relationships and productivity of the group and jeopardize accomplishing major purpose(s)
5. When preserving harmonious relationships and avoiding defensiveness and hostility are very important
6. When letting others learn from their mistakes and/or increased responsibility is possible without severe damage

BOX 23-6   ACCOMMODATION: SELF-ASSESSMENT AND COMMITMENT TO ACTION

If You Use Accommodation Often, Ask Yourself the Following Questions:

1. Do I feel that my needs, goals, concerns, and ideas are not being attended to by others?
2. Am I depriving myself of influence, recognition, and respect?
3. When I am in charge, is "discipline" lax?
4. Do I think people are using me?

If You Seldom Use Accommodation, Ask Yourself the Following Questions:

1. Am I building goodwill with others during conflict?
2. Do I admit when I have made a mistake?
3. Do I know when to give in, or do I assert myself at all costs?
4. Am I viewed as unreasonable or insensitive?

Commitment to Action

What two new behaviors would increase your effective use of accommodation?
1.
2.

of standing up for your rights or defending important principles, as when opposition to mandatory overtime is voiced (Box 23-7).

People whose primary mode of addressing conflict is through competition often react by feeling threatened, acting defensively or aggressively, or even resorting to cruelty in the form of cutting remarks, deliberate gossip, or hurtful innuendo. Competition within work groups can generate ill will, favor a win-lose stance, and commit people to a stalemate. Such behaviors force people into a corner from which there is no easy or graceful exit. Use Box 23-8 to help you learn to use competing more effectively.

BOX 23-7   APPROPRIATE USES OF COMPETING

1. When quick, decisive action is necessary
2. When important, unpopular action needs to be taken, or when trade-offs may result in long-range, continued conflict
3. When an individual or group is right about issues that are vital to group welfare
4. When others have taken advantage of an individual's or group's noncompetitive behavior and now are mobilized to compete about an important topic

BOX 23-9   APPROPRIATE USES OF COMPROMISE

1. When two powerful sides are committed strongly to perceived mutually exclusive goals
2. When temporary solutions to complex issues need to be implemented
3. When conflicting goals are "moderately important" and not worth a major confrontation
4. When time pressures people to expedite a workable solution
5. When collaborating and competing fail

BOX 23-8   COMPETING: SELF-ASSESSMENT AND COMMITMENT TO ACTION

If You Use Competing Often, Ask Yourself the Following Questions:
1. Am I surrounded by people who agree with me all the time and who avoid confronting me?
2. Are others afraid to share themselves and their needs for growth with me?
3. Am I out to win at all costs? If so, what are the costs and benefits of competing?
4. What are people saying about me when I am not around?

If You Seldom Compete, Ask Yourself the Following Questions:
1. How often do I avoid taking a strong stand and then feel a sense of powerlessness?
2. Do I avoid taking a stand so that I can escape risk?
3. Am I fearful and unassertive to the point that important decisions are delayed and people suffer?

Commitment to Action
What two new behaviors would increase your effective use of competition?
1.
2.

BOX 23-10   NEGOTIATION/COMPROMISE SELF-ASSESSMENT AND COMMITMENT TO ACTION

If You Tend to Use Negotiation Often, Ask Yourself the Following Questions:
1. Do I ignore large, important issues while trying to work out creative, practical compromises?
2. Is there a "gamesmanship" in my negotiations?
3. Am I sincerely committed to compromise or negotiated solutions?

If You Seldom Use Negotiation, Ask Yourself the Following Questions:
1. Do I find it difficult to make concessions?
2. Am I often engaged in strong disagreements, or do I withdraw when I see no way to get out?
3. Do I feel embarrassed, sensitive, self-conscious, or pressured to negotiate, compromise, and bargain?

Commitment to Action
What two new behaviors would increase your compromising effectiveness?
1.
2.

Compromising

Compromising involves both assertiveness and cooperation on the part of everyone and requires maturity and confidence. Negotiating is a learned skill that is developed over time. A give-and-take relationship results in conflict resolution, with the result that each person can meet his or her most important priorities as much of the time as possible. Compromise is very often the exchange of concessions as it creates a middle ground. This is the preferred means of conflict resolution during union negotiations, in which each side is appeased to some degree. In this mode, nobody gets everything he or she thinks he or she needs, but a sense of energy exists that is necessary to build important relationships and teams.

1. When seeking creative, integrative solutions in which both sides' goals and needs are important, thus developing group commitment and a consensual decision
2. When learning and growing through cooperative problem solving, resulting in greater understanding and empathy
3. When identifying, sharing, and merging vastly different viewpoints
4. When being honest about and working through difficult emotional issues that interfere with morale, productivity, and growth

| BOX 23-12 | COLLABORATION SELF-ASSESSMENT AND COMMITMENT TO ACTION |

If You Tend to Collaborate Often, Ask Yourself the Following Questions:
1. Do I spend valuable group time and energy on issues that do not warrant or deserve it?
2. Do I postpone needed action to get consensus and avoid making key decisions?
3. When I initiate collaboration, do others respond in a genuine way, or are there hidden agendas, unspoken hostility, and/or manipulation in the group?

If You Seldom Collaborate, Ask Yourself the Following Questions:
1. Do I ignore opportunities to cooperate, take risks, and creatively confront conflict?
2. Do I tend to be pessimistic, distrusting, withdrawing, and/or competitive?
3. Am I involving others in important decisions, eliciting commitment, and empowering them?

Commitment to Action
What two new behaviors would increase your collaboration effectiveness?
1.
2.

Negotiation and compromise are valued approaches. They are chosen when less accommodating or avoiding is appropriate (Box 23-9). Compromising is a blend of both assertive and cooperative behaviors, although it calls for less finely honed skills for each behavior than does collaborating. Negotiating is more like trading (e.g., "You can have this if I can have that" as in "I will chair the unit council taskforce on improving morale if you send me to the hospital's leadership training classes next week so I can have the skills I need to be effective."). Compromise is one of the most effective behaviors used by nurse leaders because it supports a balance of power between themselves and others in the work setting. The self-assessment in Box 23-10 will help you become more aware of your own use of negotiation and compromise and improve it.

Collaborating

Collaborating, although the most time-consuming approach, is the most creative stance. It is both assertive and cooperative because people work creatively and openly to find the solution that most fully satisfies all important concerns and goals to be achieved. Collaboration involves analyzing situations and defining the conflict at a higher level where shared goals are identified and commitment to working together is generated (Box 23-11). When nurses use cooperative conflict-management approaches, decision making becomes a collective process in which action plans are mutually understood and implemented. For example, when nurses and physicians work together, they can collaborate by asking, "What is the best thing we can do for the patient and family right now?" and "How does each of us fit into the plan of care to meet their needs?" This requires discussion about the plan, how it will be accomplished, and who will make what contributions toward its achievement and proposed outcomes. Use the self-assessment in Box 23-12 to determine your own use of collaboration.

At the onset of conflict, involved collaborating individuals can carefully analyze situations to identify the nature and reasons for conflict and choose an appropriate approach. For example, a conflict arises when a staff nurse and a charge nurse on a psychiatric unit disagree about how to handle a patient's complaints about the staff nurse's delay in responding to the patient's requests. At the point that they reach agreement that it is the staff nurse's responsibility and decision to make, collaboration has occurred. The charge nurse might say, "I didn't realize your plan of care was to respond to the patient at predetermined intervals or that you told the patient that you would check on her every 30 minutes. I can now inform the patient that I know about and support your approach." Or the staff nurse and the charge nurse might talk and subsequently agree that the staff nurse is too emotionally involved with the patient's problems and that it may be time for her to withdraw from providing the care and enlist the support of another nurse, even temporarily. Discussion can result in collaboration aimed at allowing the staff nurse to withdraw appropriately. Another, less-desirable choice could be to compete and let the winner's position stand (e.g., "I'm in charge; I'm going to assign another nurse to this patient to preserve our patient satisfaction scores" or "I know what is best for this patient; I took care of her during her past two admissions").

DIFFERENCES OF CONFLICT-HANDLING STYLES AMONG NURSES

The way in which conflict-management styles are used in health care has changed very little in the past 20 years. Previous studies suggest that avoidance and accommodation remain the predominant choices for staff nurses and that the prevalent style for nurse managers is compromise, despite the emphasis placed on collaboration as an effective strategy for conflict management (Sportsman & Hamilton, 2007). See the Research Perspective at right for a discussion about the correlation between emotional intelligence and the preferred conflict-handling styles among nurses. According to Iglesias and Vallejo (2012), the most common way nurses in clinical practice manage conflict is through accommodation. Nurses may use avoidance with physicians or managers because they may fear that engaging in conflict many jeopardize their career advancement. Further, nurses report they prefer to spend time with patients instead of solving a situation that requires excessive amounts of time and energy (Vivar, 2006). It is interesting to note that the prevalent conflict-management style for student nurses is compromise, followed by avoidance (Sportsman & Hamilton, 2007).

Research has found that nurses and physicians do not routinely collaborate with each other in conflict situations conducive to collaboration. Conflicts

RESEARCH PERSPECTIVE

Resource: Morrison, J. (2008). The relationship between emotional intelligence competencies and preferred conflict-handling styles. *Journal of Nursing Management*, 16(8), 974-983.

The purpose of this study was to determine if a relationship exists between emotional intelligence and the preferred conflict-handling styles of registered nurses in a healthcare setting. Emotional intelligence (EI) is the capacity to understand one's own feelings as well as the feelings of others and includes self-control, persistence, and motivation. It has been previously demonstrated that individuals who exhibit more emotional self-control can handle conflicting circumstances more effectively. A total of 92 nurses, over half of whom had graduated within the past 4 years, participated in the study. Nurses indicated they chose the accommodating style most frequently and used collaborating infrequently. Results showed that higher levels of EI positively correlated with collaborating and negatively with accommodating.

Implications for Practice
With the dynamic changes in health care today and the expanding role of the professional nurse, recognizing the issues affecting conflict in the practice environment is essential. Understanding how emotional intelligence levels and conflict skills correlate can be used to reduce conflict and improve interpersonal relationships in the practice environment. When conflict is approached with high levels of emotional intelligence, interpersonal skills are enhanced. Thus effective nurses and nursing leaders can enhance their EI competencies as a way of addressing conflict issues affecting the profession. EI development training can target the problems of conflict and stress in the practice environment.

between nurses and physicians may be intensified because of the overlapping nature of their domains and lack of clarification between roles. Also, when asked to describe relationships with physicians, nurses frequently reported power as a dominant theme. When nurse/physician interactions were examined, the compromising mode was found to be the significantly most common conflict-handling mode for both. A positive correlation existed between how long nurses had functioned in a leadership position and with what frequency they chose collaborating as a strategy for conflict management with physicians (Hendel, Fish, & Berger, 2007). The findings signal a need to strengthen a healthy professional alliance that relies on collaborative practice to ensure favorable patient outcomes.

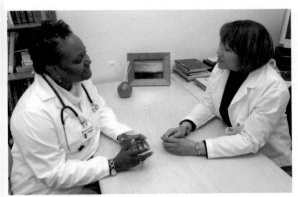

Compromise supports a balance of power between self and others in the workplace.

LITERATURE PERSPECTIVE

Resource: Almost, J. (2006). Conflict within nursing environments: Concept analysis. *Journal of Advanced Nursing*, 53(4), 444-453.

A concept analysis of conflict in nursing work environments was conducted using the evolutionary approach. Results following an exhaustive review of the literature published from 1980 to 2004 included a conceptual diagram of antecedents and consequences of conflict (Figure 23-2). Sources of conflict originate from individual characteristics, interpersonal factors, and organizational dynamics. Individual differences, typically generated by differing opinions and values, create potential conflict. Demographic dissimilarity (e.g., gender, educational levels, age, race, ethnicity) can stimulate conflict as well. Interpersonal factors such as distrust, perceptions of injustice or disrespect, and inadequate or poor communication style can lead to conflict. Organizational factors including the interdependence among team members and the changes that result from restructuring can set the stage for conflict within the practice environment.

Similarly, the effects of unresolved conflict are visible in individual characteristics, interpersonal factors, and organizational dynamics. Individual effects include job stress and dissatisfaction, absenteeism, and intent to leave, whereas interpersonal factors such as hostility and avoidance are dominant. The organizational impact of negative conflict management includes reduced productivity and ineffective teamwork.

Implications for Practice

Sources of conflict within the practice environment must be anticipated and addressed to enhance organizational effectiveness. Healthcare leaders must engage in conflict-management strategies to prevent or resolve conflict within nursing environments to ensure quality and safety.

THE ROLE OF THE LEADER

Encouraging positive working relations among healthcare providers requires effective conflict management as part of a healthy working environment (Johansen, 2012). The role of the nurse leader is to create a practice environment that fosters open communication and collaborative practices for achieving mutual goals that enable nurses to practice constructive approaches to conflict management (Johansen, 2012).

With the aging workforce and current nursing shortage, it is essential to create practice environments that will retain nurses and prevent premature departure from the discipline. Moreover, managers need to help challenge the stereotypical gender behavioral expectations and self-esteem issues frequently associated with a female-oriented profession and model effective management and leadership styles. One way to promote a positive work setting is to promote conflict prevention and ensure conflict resolution (Almost, 2006) (see the Literature Perspective at right). Nurse leaders must provide the best example of advocacy and empowerment to their staff by coaching newer nurses to think strategically about a mode of conflict handling that is appropriate for the situation. Poor communication often creates conflict (Kolb, 2013); most conflict can be resolved through careful listening and effective communication (Kolb, 2013). Nursing managers need to support their staff's use of effective conflict-management strategies by modeling open and honest communication, including staffing decision making, and securing resources that meet the staff's need in delivering quality care (Johansen, 2012).

Nurses in managerial positions spend inadequate time on conflict resolution. Many do not feel qualified or sufficiently experienced to deal with conflict (Brinkert, 2011). Moreover, some staff can be difficult to work with, so managers must remain focused on the problem and not the personalities of the team members. Nurse managers must also remain cognizant of other pitfalls of effective conflict resolution.

Conflict Concept Analysis

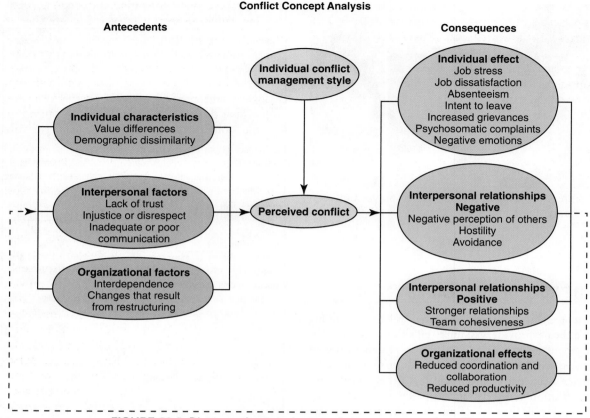

FIGURE 23-2 Diagram of antecedents and consequences of conflict.

For example, a common way for managers to avoid conflict in the workplace is to delay responding to colleagues' concerns voiced in staff meetings, to not reply to voice mails or e-mail messages, or to cancel or postpone important meetings. If this behavior is known and continues, the avoiding behavior is said to be endorsed or approved, leading to an unhealthy practice environment. Fostering collaboration requires a commitment of time and interpersonal energy to be effective, which many nurse leaders report as a barrier.

For example, a manager's need to give clear direction to a team automatically places less emphasis on the team deciding on the direction themselves. However, for the team to be successful, eventually that manager must recognize the need for the team to

work on its own even though the manager may at times need to intervene. Imagine a nurse manager was confronted by an angry team whose members felt like they were being treated like children, always being told what to do. Working together, they initiated team meetings and decision-making procedures (actions emphasizing participatory management, as in self-scheduling practices) that resulted in more ideas, a sense of ownership, and a noticeable self-direction from the team and its individual members. However, after a few months of continually emphasizing participation, the team began to lose its focus and cohesiveness and once again came to the manager for more direction. The manager listened and provided clarification, and the team regained its focus and efficiency.

The nature of the differences, underlying reasons, importance of the issue, strength of feelings, and commitment to shared goals all have to be considered when selecting an approach to resolving conflict. Preferred and previously effective approaches can be considered, but they need to match the situation. Sometimes, a third party may be introduced into a conflict so that mediation can occur. Mediation is a learned skill for which advanced training and/or certification is available. Principled negotiation can produce mutually acceptable agreements in every type of conflict. The method involves separating the people from the problem; focusing on interests, not positions; inventing options for mutual gain; and insisting on using objective criteria. The mediator is usually an impartial person who assists each party in the conflict to better hear and understand the other. In society, for example, there is much focus on who can control whom and on who is the "winner." The successful individual involved in conflict resolution and negotiation often moves beyond avoidance, accommodation, and compromise. In the nursing practice arena, there is often the added difficulty in negotiating conflicts when at least one of the parties is on an unequal or uneven playing field. This disadvantage is made even worse when the other party to the conflict does not even acknowledge the disparities involved.

MANAGING LATERAL VIOLENCE AND BULLYING

A significant source of interpersonal conflict in the workplace stems from lateral violence—aggressive and destructive behavior or psychological harassment of nurses against each other (Trudel & Reio, 2011). Nurses are particularly vulnerable because lateral or horizontal violence involves conflictual behaviors among individuals who consider themselves peers with equal power—but with little power within the system (Stanley et al., 2007). Nurses direct dissatisfaction toward one another in a variety of behavioral ways; Griffin (2004) was among the first to identify the 10 most common forms of lateral violence in the international literature as nonverbal innuendo, verbal confrontation, undermining activities, withholding information, sabotage, infighting, scapegoating, backstabbing, failure to respect privacy, and breaches of confidentiality. Bullying is closely related to lateral or horizontal violence, but a real or perceived power differential between the instigator and recipient must be present in bullying. Bullying is associated with psychological and physical stress, underperformance, professional disengagement, increased job turnover, and the potential for diminished quality of care (Vessey et al., 2009).

Understanding the sources of intraprofessional conflict in the practice environment is essential. Rowe and Sherlock (2005) report that nurses are the most frequent source of verbal abuse toward other nurses. Patients' families represent the second most frequent, followed by physicians, and then patients. Longo (2007) reported that over half of student nurses surveyed reported being put down by a staff nurse. In hostile work environments, the ability to provide quality patient care is compromised. The Joint Commission (TJC) (2008) acknowledges that unresolved conflict and disruptive behavior adversely affect safety and quality of care. Read and Laschinger (2013) also described the vulnerability of newly licensed nurses as they are socialized within the nursing workforce. New graduates reported feeling undervalued by other nurses and reported having learning opportunities blocked; many felt neglected and given too much responsibility without the appropriate support. New nurses experienced comments that were rude, abusive, humiliating, or unjustly critical. Lateral violence affects newly licensed nurses' job satisfaction and stress, as well as their perception of whether to remain in their current position and in the profession. This problem continues to be supported because students today have been exposed to bullying and may not be better prepared to handle it in school or in the workplace.

Lateral violence may be a response to the practice environment (Sheridan-Leos, 2008), in which ineffective leadership may exacerbate the problem (Stanley et al., 2007). TJC (2008) acknowledges that disruptive behavior that intimidates others and affects morale or staff turnover can be harmful to patient care. It mandates that organizations have a code of conduct that defines acceptable, disruptive, and inappropriate behaviors and that leaders create and implement a process for managing these conflictual situations. One-on-one conflict resolution must be encouraged, but a mechanism for confidential reporting is also necessary (Schaffner, Stanley, & Hough, 2006). Training on conflict management that includes how to recognize and defend against lateral violence is necessary to ensure a positive professional practice environment (Sheridan-Leos, 2008).

EXERCISE 23-3

Consider a conflict you would describe as "ongoing" in a clinical setting. Talk to some people who have been around for a while to get their historical perspective on this issue. Then consider the following questions:

- What are their positions and years of experience?
- How are resources, time, and personnel wasted on mismanaging this issue?
- What blocks the effective management of this issue?
- What currently aids in its management?
- What new things and actions would add to its management in the future?

THE SOLUTION

The solution to my conflict involved many components, including using my hospital's resources and looking inside of myself. Because a large part of my intrapersonal conflict involved apprehension about the ability to work as an independent nurse, I knew that I would have to maximize the education that I had received in nursing school and the educational opportunities, including orientation, offered by my employer. I had worked so hard during school and realized that critical thinking is one of the best assets that a health-care provider can use. I am also fortunate to work at an institution that values educating its new practitioners. I spent many hours in a classroom reviewing the principles of pediatric nursing and administering competent and safe nursing care. Many of the topics reinforced what I learned in school, but many of them were new to me, which was reassuring and rewarding.

During my orientation, I knew I wanted to be a sponge and experience as much as I could and learn as much as I could to prepare myself for the time that I would step into a patient's room without my preceptor next to me. As my days of orientation drew to a close, my apprehension was growing, but I realized I would not be left alone. Instead, I was left with wonderful support from my co-workers, mentors, and managers. The staff helped me grow and taught me that it is not only about helping your assigned patients but also about helping and supporting each other. We all have the goal of healing our patients and families, and if we use each other and work as a team, we can ensure the patients' needs are being met in the best possible way. I believe that, along with education, the realization of teamwork was the best solution to my conflict. Health care is a team effort with the ultimate goal of putting patients first and delivering quality and safe care.

I have been off orientation for a number of months and am still learning from my patients, my co-workers, and myself. I love the nursing profession and all of its challenges. Every day, I feel more confident in my independent professional nursing role and my ability to make a difference in the lives of patients and families.
—*Kimberly M. Wolski*

Would this be a suitable approach for you? Why or why not?

THE EVIDENCE

Conflict in the professional practice environment results in negative outcomes for nurses and other healthcare professionals, organizations, and patients. Lateral violence is toxic to the profession through its negative impact on the retention of staff and on detrimental outcomes for patients. It is essential for registered nurses to work in an effective and collaborative manner with other members of the healthcare team to eliminate lateral violence from the workplace (Center for American Nurses, 2008). The need for a culture change to abolish lateral violence has been endorsed by a number of professional organizations (e.g., American Nurses Association, The Joint Commission, International Council of Nurses, National Student Nurses Association). Nurses must enhance their knowledge and skill to eliminate hostile work environments, workplace intimidation, reality shock for new graduates, and the acceptance of "nurses eating their young."

NEED TO KNOW NOW

- Know how to assess preferred styles of conflict handling and to determine under what circumstances each mode is most effective.
- Identify appropriate behaviors to prevent or resolve conflict in your practice environment.

- Evaluate your practice environment for situations reflecting lateral violence. Know how to respond to a colleague who demonstrates lateral violence.

CHAPTER CHECKLIST

A more thorough understanding of conflict within the professional practice environment will enable the nurse to prevent or successfully manage nonproductive conflict. Navigating desirable conflict within the work environment will promote change resulting in organizational growth and personal and professional enrichment of nurses.

- The three types of conflict are as follows:
  - Intrapersonal
  - Interpersonal
  - Organizational
- The conflict process progresses through four stages:
  - Frustration:
    - Blocked goals lead to frustration.
    - Frustration is a cue to stop and clarify differences.
  - Conceptualization:
    - The way a person perceives a conflict determines how he or she reacts to the frustration.
    - Differences in conceptualizing an issue can block resolution.
- Action:
  - Intentions, strategies, plans, and behavior are formulated.
  - Outcome (may be both tangible and intangible).
- When assessing how well a conflict has been resolved, one must consider the following:
  - The degree to which important goals were achieved by assessing the outcomes
  - The nature of subsequent relationships among those involved in the conflict
- The five modes of conflict resolution are as follows:
  - Avoiding
  - Accommodating
  - Competing
  - Compromising
  - Collaborating
- Each mode of conflict resolution can be viewed within two dimensions:
  - From uncooperative to highly cooperative
  - From unassertive to highly assertive

TIPS FOR ADDRESSING CONFLICT

- Communicate to yourself and others that conflict is a necessary and beneficial process typically marked by frustration, different conceptualizations, a variety of approaches to resolving it, and ongoing outcomes.
- Assess the work environment to see what behaviors are endorsed and fostered by the leaders. Determine if these behaviors are worthy of imitation.

- Determine any similarities and differences in facts, goals, methods, and values in sorting out the different conceptualizations of a conflict situation.
- Assess the degree of conflict resolution by asking questions about the quality of the decisions (e.g., creativity, practicality, achievement of goals, breakthrough results) and the quality of the relationships (e.g., understanding, willingness to work together, mutual respect, cooperation).

REFERENCES

Aiken, L., Clarke, S. P., Sloane, D. M., Lake, E. T., & Cheney, T. (2008). Effects of hospital care environment on patient mortality and nurse outcomes. *Journal of Nursing Administration, 38*(5), 223-229.

Almost, J. (2006). Conflict within nursing environments: Concept analysis. *Journal of Advanced Nursing, 53*(4), 444-453.

American Nurses Credentialing Center (ANCC). (2008). Forces of Magnetism. Retrieved October 19, 2009, from www. nursecredentialing.org/Magnet.aspx.

Blake, R. R., & Mouton, J. S. (1964). *Solving costly organization conflict.* San Francisco: Jossey-Bass.

Brinkert, R. (2011). Conflict coaching training for nurse managers: A case study of a two-hospital health system. *Journal of Nursing Management, 19*, 80-91.

Center for American Nurses. (2008). *Lateral violence and bullying in the workplace.* Silver Spring, MD: Author.

Deutsch, M. (1973). *The resolution of conflict: Constructive and destructive processes.* New Haven, CT: Yale University Press.

Greer, L. l., Saygi, O., Aaldering, H., & de Dreu, C. (2012). Conflict in medical teams: Opportunity or danger? *Medical Education, 46*, 935-942.

Hendel, T., Fish, M., & Berger, O. (2007). Nurse/physician conflict management mode choices: Implications for improved collaborative practice. *Nursing Administration Quarterly, 31*(3), 244-253.

Iglesias, M. E. & Vallejo, R. B. (2012). Conflict resolution styles in the nursing profession. *Contemporary Nurse, 43*(1), 73-80.

Johansen, M. L. (2012). Keeping the peace: Conflict management strategies for nurse managers. *Nursing Management, 43*(2), 50-54.

Kolb, J. A. (2013). Conflict management principles for groups and teams. *Industrial and Commercial Training, 45*(2), 79-86.

Laschinger, H. K., Purdy, N., & Almost, J. (2007). The impact of leader-member exchange quality, empowerment, and core self-evaluation on nurse manager's job satisfaction. *Journal of Nursing Administration, 37*, 221-229.

Longo, J. (2007). Horizontal violence among nursing students. *Archives of Psychiatric Nursing, 21*, 177-178.

Morrison, J. (2008). The relationship between emotional intelligence competencies and preferred conflict-handling styles. *Journal of Nursing Management, 16*(8), 974-983.

Read, E. & Laschinger, H. K. (2013). Correlates of new graduate nurses' experiences of workplace mistreatment. *Journal of Nursing Administration, 43*(4), 221-228.

Rowe, M. M., & Sherlock, H. (2005). Stress and verbal abuse in nursing: Do burned out nurses eat their young? *Journal of Nursing Management, 13*(3), 242-248.

Saltman, D. C., O'Dea, N. A., & Kidd, M. R. (2006). Conflict management: A primer for doctors in training. *Postgraduate Medical Journal, 82*, 9-12.

Schaffner, M., Stanley, K., & Hough, C. (2006). No matter which way you look at it, it's violence. *Gastroenterology Nursing, 28*(6), 75-76.

Sheridan-Leos, N. (2008). Understanding lateral violence in nursing. *Clinical Journal of Oncology Nursing, 12*(3), 399-403.

Sportsman, S., & Hamilton, P. (2007). Conflict management styles in the health professions. *Journal of Professional Nursing, 23*(3), 157-166.

Stanley, K. M., Martin, M. M., Michel, Y., Welton, J. M., & Nemeth, L. S. (2007). Examining lateral violence in the nursing workforce. *Issues in Mental Health Nursing, 28*(11), 1247-1265.

Strack van Schijndel, R. J., & Burchardi, H. (2007). Bench-to-bedside review: Leadership and conflict management in the intensive care unit. *Critical Care, 11*(6), 234.

The Joint Commission (TJC). (2008). Accreditation participation requirements (pre-publication version). Retrieved February 4, 2009, from www.jointcommission.org/NR/rdonlyres/ B2AB8438-4BA7-4046-B96A-8834A90AA3C6/0/OME_ AllChapters.pdf.

Thomas, K. W. (1992). Conflict and conflict management: Reflections and update. *Journal of Organizational Behavior, 13*(3), 265-274.

Thomas, K. W., & Kilmann, R. H. (1974). *Thomas-Kilmann Conflict Mode Instrument,* Tuxedo, NY: Xicom.

Thomas, K. W., & Kilmann, R. H. (2002). *Thomas-Kilmann Conflict Mode Instrument* (revised edition), Mountain View, CA: CPP, Inc.

Trudel, J. & Reio, T. G. (2011). Managing workplace incivility: The role of conflict management styles—antecedent or antidote? *Human Resource Development Quarterly, 22*(4), 395-423.

Vessey, J. A., DeMarco, R. F., Gaffney, D. A., & Budin, W. C. (2009). Bullying of staff registered nurses in the workplace: A preliminary study for developing strategies for the transformation of hostile to healthy workplace environments. *Journal of Professional Nursing, 25*(5), 299-306.

Vivar, C. G. (2006). Putting conflict management into practice: A nursing case study. *Journal of Nursing Management, 14*(3), 201-206.

SUGGESTED READINGS

Autrey, P. S., Howard, J. L. & Wech, B. A. (2013). Sources, reactions, and tactics used by RNs to address aggression in an acute care hospital. *Journal of Nursing Administration, 43*(3), 155-159.

Brown, J., Lewis, L., Ellis, K., Stewart, M., Freeman, T. R. & Kasperski, M. J. (2011). Conflict on interprofessional primary health care teams—can it be resolved? *Journal of Interprofessional Care, 25*, 4-10.

Covey, S. R. (2004). *The 7 habits of highly effective people.* New York: The Free Press.

Goleman, D. (1996). Emotional intelligence. London: Bloomsbury.

Kudonoo, E., Schroeder, K., & Boysen-Rotelli, S. (2012). An Olympic transformation: Creating an organizational culture that promotes healthy conflict. *Organization Development Journal, 30*(2), 51-65.

O'Donnell, D. M., Livingston, P. M., & Bartram, T. (2012). Human resource management activities on the front line: A nursing perspective. *Contemporary Nurse, 41*(2), 198-205.

WEBSITES

Association for Conflict Resolution: http://acrnet.org

Center for Conflict Resolution: www.conflict-resolution.org/

Healthcare Conflict Management: Solutions to help you manage conflict to protect the quality and safety of care: www.healthcare-conflict-management.com/

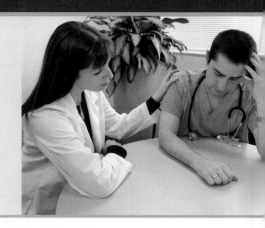

Managing Personal/
Personnel Problems

Karren Kowalski

The purpose of this chapter is to discuss various personal and personnel problems that a leader must face in all nursing settings. Some specific tips and tools are provided as ways to intervene, coach, correct, and document problem behaviors. Emphasis is placed on effective communication, both written and verbal.

OBJECTIVES

- Differentiate common personal/personnel problems.
- Relate role concepts to clarification of personnel problems.
- Examine strategies useful for approaching specific personnel problems.
- Prepare specific guidelines for documenting performance problems.
- Value the leadership aspects of the role of the novice nurse.

TERMS TO KNOW

absenteeism	nonpunitive discipline	role strain
chemically dependent	progressive discipline	role stress

THE CHALLENGE

Kathleen Bradley, RN, MSN, NE-BC
Director of Professional Resources, Porter Adventist Hospital,
Denver, Colorado

I work in a hospital that uses a float pool of well-prepared staff who are ready to be assigned to various areas so that the appropriate level of care can be provided. As you might expect, these nurses, especially when new to the hospital, are not always familiar with all of the aspects of every unit. One of the nurses employed at the hospital in the resource float pool was floated one day to the surgical unit. During her shift, she cared for a patient, who, while unattended, fell out of bed. The nurse manager of the float pool was asked to determine what happened.

What do you think you would do if you were this nurse?

INTRODUCTION

As a novice nurse, the question may be one of perception. "As a new staff nurse, I don't think of myself as a leader, so how is this information applicable?" In reality, even nurses with limited experiences (referred to here as *novice*) are responsible for and thus lead assistive and support personnel. They often lead a team consisting of licensed practical/vocational nurses (LPNs/LVNs) and nurse aides who are responsible for a group of patients. They are responsible for including other team members such as housekeeping personnel and allied health professionals (e.g., respiratory therapists, pharmacists, dietitians, and physical therapists) in providing excellent quality care for patients. The novice nurse must know how to handle difficult situations, including the decision to involve the unit leadership. It can be quite satisfying to work effectively with people. On the other hand, working with people presents some of the greatest challenges in the workplace. Problems such as absenteeism, uncooperative or unproductive employees, clinical incompetence, employees with emotional problems, and chemically dependent employees are only a few. If a nurse or a new leader wants to be successful, these problems must be dealt with in ways to minimize their effects on patient care and on staff morale. Just as documentation of patient care is critical, documentation of performance problems is critical. Overall goals are to assist the employee in the improvement of performance, to maintain the highest standards for the delivery of patient care, and to provide a supportive environment in which all staff members deliver the best care and attain work satisfaction. From this perspective, in this chapter we examine several specific employee problems and address the leader's role and options as well as the responsibilities of the novice nurse.

PERSONAL/PERSONNEL PROBLEMS

Absenteeism

One of the most vexing personnel problems is that of absenteeism. Inadequate staffing adversely affects patient care both directly and indirectly. When an absent caregiver is replaced by another who is unfamiliar with the routines, employee morale suffers and care may not meet established standards. Working with inadequate staffing or working overtime to cover for absent workers creates physical and mental stress. Replacement personnel usually need more supervision, which not only is costly but also may decrease productivity and the quality of patient care. Indirectly, co-workers may become resentful about being forced to assume heavier workloads and/or may be pressured to work extra hours. Chronic absenteeism may lead to increased staff conflicts, to decreased morale, and eventually to increased absenteeism among the entire staff. Given that nurses prefer to avoid conflict and negative behavior and to accommodate or make excuses for these situations (Sportsman, 2005), one way to confront persistent absenteeism is to discuss the situation directly with the employee (also see Chapter 18) by verbalizing:

- "I feel concerned when I see that you have been absent 3 days this month."
- "Can you see how excessive absences affect the smooth functioning of the unit, the work load of other team members, and the safety of patients?"

- "This rate of absences cannot continue. What is your plan for addressing this situation?"

Absenteeism also has a deleterious effect on the financial management of a nursing unit. Replacement of absent personnel by temporary personnel or overtime paid to other employees is very costly, and the cost of fringe benefits used by absent workers is very high. When employee costs are excessive, they compromise the ability to support other creative efforts of the unit such as staff education and new equipment and may affect staff-patient ratios. Also, as care delivery systems become more complex and technically oriented, successful nurse leaders realize that technology is not a replacement for human caregivers. Absent caregivers cannot be replaced with machines.

Absenteeism cannot be totally eliminated. There are always unplanned illnesses, accidents, bad weather, sick family members, a death in the family, and even jury duty, which are legitimate reasons for missing work and beyond the control of management. However, some portion of absenteeism is voluntary and preventable; thus the cause must be identified so that it may be addressed. Wallace (2009) identified issues leading to absenteeism including personal situations such as sick dependent family members, poor health, job stress or high work demands such as long hours, excessive workload, lack of control over work, and poor support from managers. These stressors lead to a poor work environment and lower the morale of fully engaged nurses.

Absenteeism may also indicate poor work satisfaction. Dissatisfied staff may in fact be completely disengaged, which can lead to increased absences. If the leader believes that the issue is attributable to work dissatisfaction, unit-based discussions may lead to insight about the sources. Such discussions provide an excellent opportunity for the novice nurse to listen, to learn, and to speak to issues. If the underlying cause can be identified, there may be a way to prevent the loss of the dissatisfied employee if retention is the goal. Some employees who convey that they are never happy with their jobs may continually disrupt the overall unit with their absenteeism and should be terminated. The Evidence section on p. 494 illustrates some of those factors to consider.

With role theory as a framework, absenteeism has been linked to role stress and role strain. Absence from work is a way of withdrawing from an undesirable situation short of actually leaving, and many employees increase their absenteeism just before submitting their resignation. If the healthcare worker is experiencing some form of role stress, it might be manifested through absenteeism. Role strain may be reflected by (1) withdrawal from interaction; (2) reduced involvement with colleagues and the organization; (3) decreased commitment to the mission and the team; and (4) job dissatisfaction. All of these could be manifested through absenteeism. With this framework, management of absenteeism is based on the belief that competent role performance requires interpersonal competence. "Role competence is the ability of a person in an interdependent position, which is ongoing in time, to carry out lines of action that are task and interpersonally effective" (Hardy & Conway, 1988, on p. 195). Role behavior occurs in a social context rather than in isolation. Therefore the nurse leader needs to understand the existing situation, when the situation changed to its current status, when it needs to change further, and how to accomplish such change. Because people who are more satisfied in their work usually commit to "be there" for their team, enhancing job satisfaction may be an effective strategy toward reducing absenteeism.

One model for nonpunitive discipline can be found in Figure 24-1. This model demonstrates how undesirable behaviors, such as absenteeism, can be successfully altered. Box 24-1 identifies specific steps that are involved in nonpunitive discipline.

This model of nonpunitive discipline allows employees to free themselves from some role stress by clarification of role expectations and assumptions. Employees can receive satisfaction from the realization that a problem may not be inadequate performance caused by personal faults but, rather, a lack of clarification of role expectations within the organization. Novice nurses may be called on to implement the process described in Box 24-1. For example, the novice nurse may be involved with the nurse manager or a support staff member or, in extenuating circumstances, the new nurse may be directly involved in the process. Remember, the focus is on the clear understanding of the situation, the growth of the individual, and the smooth and effective functioning of the team.

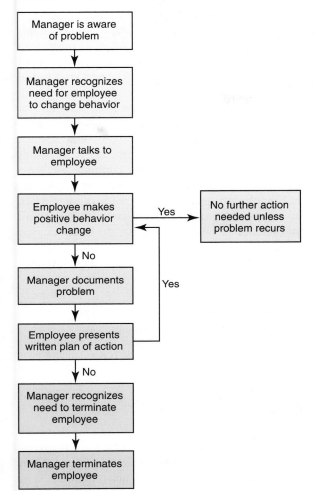

FIGURE 24-1 Model for behavioral change.

BOX 24-1   **STEPS TO CLARIFY ROLE EXPECTATIONS**

Step 1: Remind the employee of the employment policies and procedures of the agency. Sometimes an employee does not know or has forgotten the existing standards, and a reminder with no threats or discipline is all that is needed. The employee must remain ultimately accountable to the organization's policies and procedures.

Step 2: When the oral reminder does not result in a behavior change, put the reminder in writing for the employee. These oral and written reminders are simply statements of the problem and the goals to which both the manager and the employee agree. The employee must voluntarily agree with the manager that the behavior in question is not acceptable and must agree to change.

Step 3: If the written reminder fails, only then grant the employee a day of decision, which is a day off with pay to arrive at a decision about future action. Pay is given for this day so that it is not interpreted as punishment. The employee must return to work with a written decision as to whether or not to accept the standards for work attendance. Remember that this is a voluntary decision on the employee's part. Emphasize to the employee that it is the employee's decision to adhere to the standards.

Step 4: If the employee decides not to adhere to standards, termination results. However, if the employee agrees to adhere to the standards and in the future does not, he or she, in essence, has terminated employment. Keep a copy of the written agreements, and give the employee a copy. The manager should be clearly aware of the organization's policy for termination and request assistance from the human resources department as deemed necessary.

EXERCISE 24-1

Review the policy manual at a local healthcare organization. Determine what constitutes excessive absenteeism. What are the identified consequences?

Uncooperative or Unproductive Employees

The problem of uncooperative or unproductive employees is another area of frustration for the nurse leader. Hersey, Blanchard, and Johnson (2008) identified two major dimensions of job performance that relate to this problem: motivation and ability. The type and intensity of motivation vary among employees because of differing needs and goals that employees express. The leader can best handle employees with motivation problems by attempting to determine the cause of the problem and by working to provide an environment that is conducive to increased motivation for the employee. If the employee is uncooperative or unproductive because of a lack of ability, education and training are appropriate interventions.

The manager can determine lack of ability on the part of an employee in various ways. Frequent errors in judgment or techniques are often an indication of lack of knowledge, skill, or critical thinking. This illustrates the need for the nurse leader to document all variances or untoward events carefully after discussing them with the employee. When the nurse manager has thorough documentation, trends may be discovered that, in turn, suggest that a specific employee is having problems. The nurse manager can cite problem behaviors and perhaps even trends to the employee. Corrective action is easier to pursue and resolution is more effective with this strategy. When the problem is determined to result from a need for more education or training, the manager can work with the education department or the clinical specialist for the involved unit to help the employee improve his or her skills. Most employees are extremely cooperative in situations such as this because they want to do a good job but sometimes do not know how. Employees may deny they need help or may be too embarrassed to ask for help. When the manager can show an employee concrete evidence of a problem area, cooperation is enhanced.

Immature Employees

Sometimes an unproductive employee simply lacks maturity. This lack of maturity may be described as *emotional intelligence underdevelopment* that results in such problems as being socially inept or unable to control one's impulses (Strickland, 2000). The management tips column in *Health Care Manager* describes this situation in "Case in Health Care Management: Managing the Drama Queen" (2004). These employees are frequently defensive and emotional or tearful. They lack self-insight into their behavior. Sometimes immaturity in an employee may not be readily apparent to the leader but may be manifested in any of the following actions: defiance, testing of workplace guidelines, passivity or hostility, or little appreciation for any management decisions. The challenge for the nurse leader is not to react in kind but, rather, to relate to this employee in a positive and mature manner. A sense of humor and the ability to tease the employee into a more receptive, jovial mood are sometimes helpful. However, the leader needs to determine whether the undesirable behaviors are reflecting a state of being uncomfortable or incompetent (LaDuke, 2000). For example, if an employee states, "Administration is always making decisions to make our jobs harder," rather than making a hostile or defensive comment in reply, the manager could take the employee aside and say, "I notice that you seem to be angry about this new policy. Let's talk about it some more." Immature employees either act immaturely all of the time or regress to an immature level when stressed. The nurse leader must recognize

immaturity in an employee and react calmly and without anger. The leader must keep in mind that this employee may be displaying dynamics rooted in unresolved personal areas and that the behavior is not a personal attack on the leader. The best way to deal with this behavior is to confront the employee with the specific problem and define realistic limits of acceptable behavior with consequences for nonadherence. Generally, employees comply with specific limits but will test management in other areas. As this testing occurs, the leader must continue the same limit-setting technique. Remember that the immature employee usually has problems because of a lack of self-worth, power, and self-control. Praise and affirmation are valuable tools that the leader can use to help these employees feel better about themselves. Chapter 3 addresses generational issues if they are factors to consider.

EXERCISE 24-2

A nurse comes to you, the nurse leader, and states that one of the other nurses is tying a knot in the air vent (pigtail) of nasogastric tubes. This nurse does not know how to approach the employee to discuss the problem. What would you do?

Clinical Incompetence

Clinical incompetence is possibly one of the most frustrating problems that the nurse leader faces, although it may be entirely correctable. The problem may surface immediately in a new employee. It is possible that despite an effective interview process, a lack of fit exists between the new nurse's strengths or skill set and the needs of the unit. Such a nurse can be coached and supported to find a different position, one that fully utilizes his or her strengths and skills. At other times, clinical incompetence comes as a surprise if co-workers "cover" for another employee. Some nurses are unwilling to report instances of clinical incompetence because they do not want to feel responsible for getting one of their peers in trouble. When other employees are engaged in enabling behavior by covering for the mistakes of one of their peers, the nurse leader may be surprised to discover that the employee does not know or cannot do what is expected of him or her at work. Sadly, the employee in question has been able to cover incompetence by hiding behind the performance of another employee.

The nurse leader must remind employees that part of professional responsibility is to maintain quality care and thus they are obligated to report instances of clinical incompetence, even when it means reporting a co-worker. Ignoring violations of a safety rule or poor practice is unprofessional and cannot be tolerated.

Most healthcare agencies use skills checklists or a competency evaluation program to ascertain that their employees have and maintain essential skills for the job they are expected to do. A skills checklist is one way to determine basic clinical competency (Table 24-1). This checklist typically contains a number of basic skills along with ones that are essential for safe functioning in the specific area of employment. Any type of skills review should be directly linked to quality-improvement indicators. The employee may be asked to do a self-assessment of the listed skills or competencies and then have performance of the skills validated by a peer or co-worker. This is a very effective method for the leader to assess the skill level of employees and to determine where additional education and training may be necessary. In addition, if the leader discovers that an employee cannot perform a skill adequately, the skills list can easily be checked and directly observed behaviors can be assessed to determine at what level the employee is functioning. At the completion of the assessment, a specific plan for remediation can be developed. Sometimes, an employee may be able to perform all of the tasks on a skills checklist but still cannot manage overall patient care effectively. If, in questioning the employee or in evaluating the employee's performance, the manager/leader determines that there is a lack of knowledge or that there are problems with time management, formal education may be the proper course of action. In either event, the leader must establish a written contract containing a plan of action that sets time limits within which certain expectations must be achieved. This ensures compliance on the part of the employee. A more comprehensive program for competency evaluation might include not only the skills checklist but also unit-specific objectives, an overall framework for evaluation, and critical-thinking exercises that are interactive in nature (Johnson, Opfer, VanCura, & Williams, 2000). The role of the novice nurse leader, particularly with ancillary personnel, is to support the nurse

manager as well as be helpful and supportive of the team members who are striving to improve.

Emotional Problems

Emotional problems among nursing personnel may affect not only the involved individual but also co-workers and ultimately the delivery of patient care. The nurse leader must be aware that certain behaviors, such as poor judgment, increased errors, increased absenteeism, decreased productivity, and a negative attitude, may be manifestations of emotional problems in employees.

A nurse manager began hearing complaints from patients about a nurse named Nancy. Patients were saying that Nancy was abrupt and uncaring with them. The manager had not received any complaints about Nancy before this time, so she questioned Nancy about why this was occurring. Nancy reported that her mother was very ill and she was so worried about her and so upset that she could not sleep and was tired all of the time. She went on to say that she was having trouble being sympathetic with complaining patients when they did not seem to be as sick as her mother.

When an employee's behavior changes significantly, personal problems with which the person cannot cope may be the cause. The nurse leader is not and should not be a therapist but must intercede, not only to help the individual with the problems but also to maintain proper functioning of the unit. In dealing with the employee who exhibits behaviors that indicate emotional problems, the manager assists the individual to obtain professional help to cope with the problem. The individual's work setting and schedule may need to be adjusted. This may require support from other staff members so there is no negative effect on patient care. The manager acknowledges that an employee is experiencing emotional difficulties and yet the standards of patient care cannot be compromised. It is reassuring for staff to witness the care and concern shown a fellow staff member who is in great difficulty. They can interpret that similar support would be given to them if they were in a difficult situation.

The most important approach that the manager can take with an emotionally troubled employee is to provide support and encouragement and to assist the individual to obtain appropriate help. Many agencies have some kind of employee assistance program

TABLE 24-1   EXAMPLE OF A SKILLS CHECKLIST

Purpose

1. The clinical skills inventory is a three-phase tool to enable the newly hired RN and the nurse manager to determine individual learning needs, verify competency, and plan performance goals.
2. The RN will complete the self-assessment of clinical skills during the first week of employment. The RN will use the appropriate scale to document current knowledge of clinical skills.
3. The nurse manager will document observed competency of the orientee or delegate this to a peer. All columns must be completed on the inventory level.
4. At the end of orientation, the new RN and the manager will use the inventory to identify performance goals on the plan sheet. The skills inventory will be in a specified place on the nursing unit so that it is available to the manager and other RNs. It should be updated at appropriate intervals as specified by the manager.

Scale for Self-Assessment

1 = Unfamiliar/never done
2 = Able to perform with assistance
3 = Can perform with minimal supervision
4 = Independent performance/proficient

Score for Validation of Competency

1 = Unable to perform at present
2 = Able to perform with assistance
3 = Progressing/repeat performance necessary
4 = Able to perform independently

CLINICAL SKILLS (EXAMPLES)	SELF-ASSESSMENT		COMMENT	VALIDATION			COMMENT
	SCALE	DATE		SCORE	DATE	INITIALS	
Epidural catheter care							
NG/Dobbhoff							
Insertion							
Management							
Preoperative care/ teaching							
Postoperative care/ teaching							

Plan Sheet for Skills Inventory

Name _____
Date _____

Goals   **Date to Be Completed**

_____
_____
_____
_____
_____
_____
_____

Orientee's signature _____
Manager's signature _____
Date _____

(EAP) to which the manager should refer any troubled employee. (The Literature Perspective below describes a counseling service and how it helps retain nurses.) During this process, the manager must remember to check with the human resources department about any implications that may occur because of the Americans with Disabilities Act (ADA). If an employee has a documented mental illness, the employing agency may be under certain legal constraints as specified in the ADA. The nurse manager should always remember that many resources are available to assist with personnel problems. The manager should never feel required to know all of the legal implications regarding employment policies. Rather, the manager must know that help is available and how to access it.

EXERCISE 24-3

As a nurse manager in a community health agency, you have just had a meeting that was called by several of your staff nurses. They expressed concern regarding another nurse colleague who has come to work tearful several times during the past week. They state she often goes into the break room when she is in the agency and appears as if she has been crying when she comes out. She has refused to discuss her distress with her colleagues. These nurses express concern and want you to help her. What is your response? What would you do?

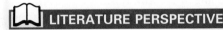 **LITERATURE PERSPECTIVE**

Resource: Luquette, J. S. (2005). The role of on-site counseling in nurse retention. *Oncology Nursing Forum, 32,* 234-236.

This article describes various aspects of an on-site counseling service and how it demonstrates value to nurses. The key cornerstone beliefs of the service are confidentiality, minimal financial cost, professionalism of the provider, and convenient appointment times and office locations. Services can be both group and individually based. To be effective, the services must be available when nurses work and also be available by phone. The offices need to be in less trafficked areas to help maintain confidentiality. Numerous professional and personal issues are cited. In addition, the service should include crisis intervention and services devoted to team-building.

Implications for Practice

The availability of on-site counseling during any work schedule helps charge nurses and nurse managers refer individuals for help and allows individual nurses to seek the support they may need during challenging times.

Chemical Dependency

Chemical dependency among nursing personnel places patients and the organization at risk. Such an employee adversely affects staff morale by increasing stress on other staff members when they have to assume heavier workloads to cover for the chemically dependent employee who is not performing at full capacity or who is often absent. As a result, patient care may be jeopardized because staff is focusing more on the problems of a co-worker than on those of the patients. For the novice nurse, it is critical to be aware of the professional responsibilities of reporting incidents in which peers or team members exhibit signs of chemical dependency.

The manager is responsible for early recognition of chemical dependency and referral for treatment when appropriate (McAndrew & McAndrew, 2000). State laws vary as to the reportability of chemical dependency. As is true of all nurses, a nurse manager is responsible for upholding the nurse practice act and should be familiar with the legal aspects of chemical dependency in the state in which he or she is employed. As with the employee with emotional problems, the nurse manager should be aware of ADA issues and check with the human resource department for help with how to handle the employment of a chemically dependent employee. Most states and agencies have reporting requirements regarding substance abuse. The state board of nursing is a key place to determine specific details required by a given state. All nurse managers should familiarize themselves with the nurse practice act in the state in which they are employed and with the personnel policies relating to substance abuse in their employing agency. Furthermore, nurse managers should ensure that staff is familiar with legal requirements.

In the present social climate, there is more interest in helping affected individuals than in punishing them and there is also more empathy and understanding toward them than in the past. Identification of an employee with a chemical dependency is usually difficult, especially because one of the primary symptoms is denial. The primary clue to which a manager should be alert when chemical dependency is suspected is any behavioral change in an employee. This change could be any deviation from the behaviors the employee normally exhibits. Some specific behaviors to note might be mood swings, a change from a tidy appearance to an untidy one, an unusual interest in patients' pain control, frequent changes in jobs and shifts, or an increase in absenteeism and tardiness.

When a manager suspects that an employee may be chemically dependent, the manager must intervene because patient care may be jeopardized. A manager facing a problem with an impaired nurse must be compassionate yet therapeutic. Knowing that denial may be one of the primary signs of substance abuse, the manager must focus on performance problems that the nurse is exhibiting and urge the nurse to seek counseling or treatment voluntarily. EAPs always protect the employee's privacy and are usually available free or at a minimal charge to the employee. The manager should strive to refer any troubled employee to the EAP. This removes the manager from the counseling role and helps employees get the professional help they need without fear of a breach in confidentiality. If a nurse refuses to seek help voluntarily for a substance abuse problem, the manager is responsible for following the established policy for such employees. The manager must remember that if the substance-abusing employee is terminated and not reported to the State Board of Nursing, the manager not only may be violating a law but also may be enabling this employee to obtain employment in another agency and potentially be in a position to harm patients and co-workers.

Many states have rehabilitation programs for chemically impaired nurses so that they may return to nursing if rehabilitated. Nurse managers are sometimes asked to assist with monitoring the progress of a chemically impaired nurse. Specific guidelines are established through the rehabilitation program with the cooperation of the employee, the agency, and the manager. The manager is typically asked to provide feedback about the employee's progress to the employee and to the state or rehabilitation program involved. These programs vary, but, for example, a nurse who has been an admitted abuser of meperidine may be allowed to work in a setting in which this drug is never used, or the nurse may not be permitted to administer any controlled substances to patients. This, of course, puts an added burden on other staff members, but it can be a positive experience for all because nurses face some of their professional responsibility by helping another nurse while upholding patient care. Often, as a part of their therapy, these nurses are required to share openly with other staff members what their problem is and what they are doing to control it. When handled in a positive, professional way, the nurse manager can turn a potentially destructive situation into a positive, constructive one.

Regardless of the type of personnel issue, the manager needs to have a plan in place for ongoing monitoring and follow-up of issues/problems.

EXERCISE 24-4

Review your state's nurse practice act and rules and regulations. What are you required to do if you believe a nurse has a problem with chemical dependency?

Incivility

Incivility or lateral violence in the workplace is disruptive behavior or communication that creates a negative work environment, thus interfering with quality patient care and safety (Simpson, 2008). Such behavior is often nurse to nurse or provider to provider. These behaviors include nonverbal innuendo such as eye-rolling or eyebrow raising, verbal affronts, undermining activities, withholding information, sabotage, infighting, scapegoating, backstabbing, failure to respect privacy, and broken confidences (Bigony et al., 2009; Griffin, 2004) (see the Literature Perspective on p. 491). Uncivil behavior must be addressed. The first step by the manager when he or she has observed the unwanted behavior may be a discussion with the nurse; the next step is written documentation in the personnel file if the behaviors do not abate, followed by a stepwise disciplinary action in association with the human resources department (Clark, Farnsworth, & Springer, 2008). It is important for the new nurse to be cognizant and aware of behaviors of incivility and to understand the guidelines/rules relevant to such behavior in the facility. Also, it is important for the new nurse to support increased teamwork by behaving in a positive, upbeat manner and to not become enmeshed in negative behavior on the unit.

LITERATURE PERSPECTIVE

Resource: Bigony, L., Lipke, T. G., Lundberg, A., McGraw, C. A., Pagac, G. L., & Rogers, A. (2009). Lateral violence in the perioperative setting. *AORN Journal, 89* (4), 688-696.

Lateral violence is counterproductive to quality health care and has negative repercussions not only on staff but also on the safety of patients. The effects of such behavior on the victims (other staff members) include increased job stress, frustration, disenchantment, disengagement, and "burnout." Victims will exhibit increased absenteeism and provide substandard care because of anxiety from anticipating the next episode of violence. Violent behavior toward peers is a deterrent to strongly developed and functioning teams and nurse collegiality and contributes to nurse vacancy rates.

Implications for Practice
Recommendations for combating lateral violence among nurses include nursing self-governance models, multidisciplinary task forces, employee assistance programs, effective orientation for new employees including increased consciousness about lateral violence, and protection from reprisal for reporting incidents of lateral violence.

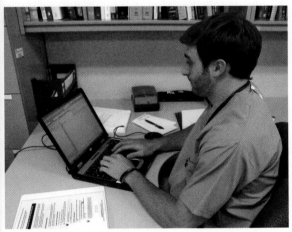

Documentation of personnel problems is an important aspect of the nurse manager's job.

DOCUMENTATION

Documentation of personnel problems is unquestionably one of the most important but also one of the most onerous aspects of the nurse manager's job.

As much as some managers may wish they would, personnel problems probably will not "disappear" and therefore will eventually have to be resolved. Through careful, ongoing documentation of problems, the manager makes the task of identifying and correcting problems much less burdensome.

Documentation cannot be left to memory! At the time that an employee is involved in a problem situation or receives a compliment or does something extremely well, a brief notation to this effect must be placed in the personnel file. This entry includes the date, time, and a brief description of the incident. Adding a small notation as to what was done about a problem when it occurred is also helpful. Along with this, the nurse manager should keep a log or summary sheet of all reported errors, unusual incidents, and accidents. These extremely important data should include the date, time, and names of involved individuals and should be tallied monthly for analysis by the manager. The few extra minutes each day that the manager spends tracking these data provide invaluable information to him or her about organizational and individual functioning. This tracking can then be used to pinpoint an individual's problem areas, areas of excellence in individual performance, and overall organizational problem areas. The manager who keeps careful records about organizational functioning has greater control in the management of personal and personnel problems. Box 24-2 describes content and format for such documentation and provides an example as an illustration.

PROGRESSIVE DISCIPLINE

When an employee's performance falls below the acceptable standard despite corrective measures that have been taken, some form of discipline must be enacted. Most organizations use some form of **progressive discipline** to correct problem behaviors. When the nurse leader suspects that specific behaviors may lead to progressive discipline, it is critical that all interactions be documented and that the human resources department is involved in the process to ensure accurate adherence to all policies. Progressive discipline consists of evaluating performance and providing feedback within a specified structure of increasing sanctions. These sanctions,

BOX 24-2 DOCUMENTATION OF PROBLEMS

- Description of incident—an objective statement of the facts related to the incident
- Actions—statements describing the plan to correct and/or prevent future problems
- Follow-up—dates and times that the plan is to be carried out, including required meeting with the employee

Example

Several patients reported that Becky, one of the night-shift registered nurses, was "curt" and "gruff" and seemed uncaring with them. I called Becky into my office and reiterated the complaints that I had received, including the specifics of times and incidents. I reminded Becky about what my expectations were relating to patient care, emphasizing the importance of a caring attitude with all patients. We discussed what the possible cause of Becky's behavior might be, such as problems at home or lack of sleep. Becky denied being curt or gruff but agreed that some of her mannerisms might be misinterpreted. I suggested to Becky that perhaps she needed to be particularly aware of her body language and to soften her tone of voice. After discussing this incident and reminding Becky of the importance of caring in nursing, I cited the policy regarding behavior and told Becky that this behavior would not be tolerated. I told Becky we needed to meet every Friday morning at the end of Becky's shift to discuss how the week had gone and to determine how she was interacting with the patients assigned to her. I also told Becky I would be checking with patients to see what they had thought of Becky, pointing out that I do this routinely.

These weekly meetings are to be conducted for 6 weeks, followed by monthly meetings for a 3-month period. If problems do not recur, the meetings will be discontinued after this time.

Joseph P. Riley, RN, MSN
Nurse Manager
Hanson Way Hospital

BOX 24-3 STEPS IN PROGRESSIVE DISCIPLINE

1. Counsel the employee regarding the problem.
2. Reprimand the employee. A verbal reprimand usually precedes a written one, but some organizations issue both a verbal and a written reprimand simultaneously. When the documentation is written, the employee must sign to verify that the problem was discussed. This does not mean that the employee agrees with the reprimand. It means only that he or she is aware of a written reprimand that is to be placed in the employee's personnel file. The employee always receives a copy of a written reprimand.
3. Suspend the employee if the problem persists. He or she will be suspended without pay for a specified period, usually several days or longer according to the agency policy. During this time, the employee may realize the seriousness of the problem based on the resulting discipline.
4. Allow the employee to return to work with written stipulations regarding problem behavior.
5. Terminate the employee if the problem recurs.

progressing from least severe to most severe, are described in Box 24-3. Examples of the kind of workplace behavior that usually involves progressive discipline and could even result in immediate termination are harassment and chemical abuse.

TERMINATION

At times, even though the manager has done everything possible to gain the cooperation of a problem employee, the problems may persist. In such cases, there is no choice but to terminate the employee.

Because termination is one of the most difficult things a manager does, the following guidelines should be followed:

1. The manager must be confident that everything possible has been done to help the employee correct the problem behaviors.
2. The manager must recognize that if employment continues, this employee will have a deleterious effect on overall organizational functioning and, more important, on nursing care.
3. The employee must have been made fully aware of the problem performance and of the fact that all of the correct disciplinary steps have been followed.
4. The nurse manager should check with the human resources and legal departments before proceeding to ensure that termination is justifiable legally and that proper steps have been followed.

The nurse manager needs to be confident in the knowledge that all policies regarding termination have been followed before having an actual termination meeting with the employee. It is always preferable to err on the side of caution when proceeding with termination of an employee. Remember that termination is something that the employee has caused as a result of persistent problem behaviors or certain behaviors for which the organization has zero tolerance. Termination is not done at the whim of management; it results from failure on the part of the employee to change a problem behavior.

Situations that may warrant immediate dismissal include theft, violence in the workplace, and willful abuse of the patient, to name a few. Again, the manager should use the assistance of the human resource department to ensure that all of the organization's policies are being upheld correctly. The following example illustrates that a manager needs to anticipate a termination to ensure ongoing standards:

Linda has gone through all of the steps in the progressive discipline process as a result of her abusive behavior toward her co-workers. She returned to work and seemed to be doing well until about 6 weeks later, when she slammed down her clipboard during report and angrily accused the charge nurse of always giving her the worst assignments. The nurse manager was present and asked Linda to come into her office. At this point, she told Linda she was relieving her of her assignment that day and asked her to go home to cool off. The manager told her that she would call her the following day about what would be done. Linda went home, and the manager reviewed the incident with her nurse administrator. They both agreed that Linda's behavior not only was intolerable but also violated the terms of her probation and therefore she should be terminated. The manager

called Linda the following day as she had agreed to do and asked her to come and meet with her. The manager and administrator met with Linda and reviewed the incidents and the disciplinary measures leading up to this incident. The nurse manager asked the administrator to be present at the scheduled meeting because it is a good practice to have a witness in a confrontational situation such as termination. The manager stated to Linda that she regretted it had come to this but pointed out to her that her behavior had violated all of the agreed-upon stipulations and, as a result, she would be terminated immediately. Linda was tearful and had numerous excuses, but the manager remained firm and merely repeated that Linda, in not fulfilling the agreement, had chosen to end her employment.

EXERCISE 24-5
Review a healthcare organization's policies regarding termination. What are the conditions, such as stealing or violence, that are described as cause for immediate dismissal? Is abusing substances at work one of those conditions?

CONCLUSION

All employees share a role with managers to prevent and control personal/personnel problems in their work setting. Everyone must be willing to refuse to allow unethical behavior from co-workers and to speak out and act appropriately when problems occur.

THE SOLUTION

The nurse manager in charge of the resource float pool wanted to assess the float pool nurses' critical-thinking skills and did this through weekly rounding. The charge nurses of each unit also completed a peer assessment form whenever a nurse floated to the unit so that the nurse who floated there could receive feedback. In this manner, if a pattern emerged from either the rounding assessment or the peer reviews, the float nurse could receive immediate coach-

ing. Finally, the nurse manager decided to have the staff review published information about hourly rounding and review the patient fall protocols from the various units where the float nurse worked.
—*Kathleen Bradley*

Would this be a suitable approach for you? Why?

THE EVIDENCE

Davey, Cummings, Newburn-Cook, and Lo (2009) sought to identify predictors of short-term absenteeism in staff nurses. Such absenteeism contributes to lack of continuity in patient care and decreases staff morale, which is costly to the facility. A systematic review of studies conducted between 1986 and 2006 led to the inclusion of 16 peer-reviewed research studies. Findings were that the individual "nurse's history of prior absences," "work attitudes" (e.g., job satisfaction, organizational commitment, and work involvement), and other "retention factors" such as shared governance reduced absenteeism, whereas poor leadership, "burnout," and "job stress" increased absenteeism. It became clear that the reasons underlying absenteeism are still poorly understood and that a robust theory for nurse absenteeism is lacking. Further theory development and research are needed.

NEED TO KNOW NOW

- The human resources department is my friend. It is there to help both new staff and leaders.
- Successful nurses:
  - Have a positive attitude about patients and families.
  - Demonstrate respect for all co-workers from housekeeping to the CEO.
- Participate in open discussion and decision making that is fair and reflects the organizational mission.
- Recognize and celebrate the contributions of co-workers.

CHAPTER CHECKLIST

To obtain satisfaction from working with people, a nurse manager must be knowledgeable about personal and personnel issues that are likely to occur in the work setting. The nurse manager must be able to detect, prevent, and correct problems that affect nursing care and staff morale in a nursing agency. Proper documentation and follow-up are key elements in the successful management of all personnel issues.

- Absenteeism's detrimental effects are as follows:
  - Patient care may be below standard.
  - Replacement personnel require additional supervision.
  - Absenteeism may increase among the entire staff.
  - Financial management of the unit suffers adverse effects.
- Effective strategies to reduce absenteeism include the following:
  - Enhance nurses' job satisfaction.
  - Use Haddock's model (1989) of nonpunitive discipline:
    - Remind the employee of the problem orally.
      - Follow up with a written reminder if the oral one fails.
      - Grant the employee a day of decision if the written reminder fails.
      - Terminate if the employee decides not to adhere to standards.
- Uncooperative or unproductive employees may lack motivation, ability, or maturity:
  - The nurse manager can try to provide an environment that is more conducive to motivation.
  - Education and training are appropriate interventions for lack of ability.
  - Praise and affirmation are often the most effective strategies for an employee who lacks maturity.
- Clinical incompetence is a highly correctable problem for nurse managers:
  - Clinical incompetence may be masked by co-workers' enabling behavior.
  - A skills checklist helps determine basic clinical competency and pinpoint the need for additional training and education.

- A comprehensive competency program may include not only a skills checklist but also a means for evaluating critical-thinking ability of the employee.
- When emotional problems are evident, the nurse manager must assist the employee in getting professional help. The nurse manager is responsible for early recognition of chemical dependency and referral for treatment when appropriate:
  - The manager must do the following:
    - Uphold the state's nurse practice act.
    - Be familiar with state laws on chemical dependency.
    - Know the healthcare organization's personnel policy on chemical dependency.
  - Some warning signs of possible chemical dependency are as follows:
    - Behavioral changes such as mood swings
    - Sudden and unusual neglect of personal appearance
    - Unusual interest in patients' pain control
    - Increased absenteeism and tardiness
- Documentation of problems must include the following:
  - A description of the incident
  - A description of the manager's actions
  - A plan to correct/prevent future occurrences
  - Dates and times of follow-up measures
- Progressive discipline may be used when other corrective measures have failed. Steps in progressive discipline are as follows:
  - Counsel the employee regarding the problem.
  - Reprimand the employee (first verbally, then in writing).
  - Suspend the employee if the problem persists.
  - Allow the employee to return to work, with written stipulations regarding problem behavior.
  - Terminate the employee if the problem recurs.

■ TIPS IN THE DOCUMENTATION OF PROBLEMS

- Identify the incident and related facts.
- Describe actions taken by the manager when the problem was identified.
- Develop an action plan for everyone involved.
- Schedule a follow-up meeting to evaluate progress of the action plan.
- Remember to document everything objectively and completely!

REFERENCES

Bigony, L., Lipke, T. G., Lundberg, A., McGraw, C. A., Pagac, G. L., & Rogers, A. (2009). Lateral violence in the perioperative setting. *AORN Journal, 89*(4), 688-696.

Case in health care management: Managing the drama queen. (2004). *The Health Care Manager, 23*(4), 318-320.

Clark, C. M., Farnsworth, F., & Springer, P. J. (2008). Policy development for disruptive student behaviors. *Nurse Educator, 33*(6), 259-262.

Davey, M. M., Cummings, G., Newburn-Cook, C. V., & Lo, E. A. (2009). Predictors of nurse absenteeism in hospitals: A systematic review. *Journal of Nursing Management, 17*(3), 312-330.

Griffin, M. (2004). Teaching cognitive rehearsal as a shield for lateral violence: An intervention for newly licensed nurses. *Journal of Continuing Education in Nursing, 35*(6), 257-263.

Haddock, C. (1989). Transformation leadership and the employee discipline process. *Hospital Health Service Administration, 34*(2), 185-194.

Hardy, M. E., & Conway, M. E. (1988). *Role theory: Perspectives for health professionals* (2nd ed.). Norwalk, CT: Appleton & Lange.

Hersey, P., Blanchard, K., & Johnson, D. E. (2008). *Management of organizational behavior: Utilizing human resources* (9th ed.). Englewood Cliffs, NJ: Prentice Hall.

Johnson, T., Opfer, K., VanCura, B., & Williams, L. (2000). A comprehensive interactive competency program. Part I: Development and framework. *MedSurg Nursing, 9*(5), 265-268.

LaDuke, S. (2000). Nurses' perceptions: Is your nurse uncomfortable or incompetent? *Journal of Nursing Administration, 30*(4), 163-165.

Luquette, J. S. (2005). The role of on-site counseling in nurse retention. *Oncology Nursing Forum, 32*, 234-236.

McAndrew, K. G., & McAndrew, S. J. (2000). Workplace substance abuse impairment: The occupational health care provider's role. *AAOHN Journal, 48*(1), 32-47.

Simpson, K. R. (2008). Horizontal hostility. *MCN. The American Journal of Maternal Child Nursing, 33*(5), 328.

Sportsman, S. (2005). Build a framework for conflict assessment. *Nursing Management, 36*(4), 32-40.

Strickland, D. (2000). Emotional intelligence: The most potent factor in the success equation. *Journal of Nursing Administration, 30*(3), 112-117.

Wallace, M. (2009). Occupational health nurses: The solution to absence management. *AAOHN Journal, 57*(3), 122-127.

SUGGESTED READINGS

Barnes, B., Leis, S., Brammer, I. M., Gustin, T. J., & Lupo, T. C. (1999). A developmental evaluation process for nurses: Enhancing professional excellence. *Journal of Nursing Administration, 29*(4), 25-32.

DeCampti, P., Kirby, K. K., & Baldwin, C. (2010). Beyond the classroom to coaching: Preparing new nurse managers. *Critical Care Nursing Quarterly, 33*(2), 132-137.

Hojat, M. (2009). Ten approaches for enhancing empathy in health and human services cultures. *Journal of Health and Human Services Administration, 31*(4), 412-450.

Huseman, R. C. (2009). The importance of positive culture in hospitals. *Journal of Nursing Administration, 39*(2), 60-63.

Lewis, R., Yarker, J., Donaldson-Feilder, E., Flaxman, P., & Munic, F. (2010). Using a competency-based approach to identify the management behaviours required to manage workplace stress in nursing: An incident study. *International Journal of Nursing Studies, 47*(3), 307-313.

Osborne, J., Blais, K., & Hayes, J. S. (1999). Nurses' perceptions: When is it a medication error? *Journal of Nursing Administration, 29*(4), 33-38.

Quinn, C., & Barton, A. (1999). The implications of drug treatment and testing orders. *Nursing Standard, 14*(27), 38-41.

Wildman, S. & Hewison, A. (2009). Rediscovering a history of nursing management: From Nightingale to the modern matron. *International Journal of Nursing Studies, 46*(12), 1650-1661.

Wilson, S. (2009). Developing interpersonal skills. *Nursing New Zealand, 15*(11), 3-4.

Wright, D. (1998). *The ultimate guide to competency assessment in health care.* Eau Claire, WI: PESI HealthCare.

Yoder, L. H. (1995). Staff nurses' career development relationships and self-reports of professionalism, job satisfaction, and intent to stay. *Nursing Research, 44*(5), 290-297.

Workplace Violence and Incivility

Crystal J. Wilkinson

Nurses working in hospitals and other healthcare facilities are at disproportionally high risk for physical violence because of the very nature of their job. We screen patients and their visitors to the best of our ability, but we never know who will walk through the door and in what mental status. To maintain personal safety and an environment free from the potential of physical violence, nurses must be alert to signs of trouble. Not all healthcare workplace violence is of a physical nature or from patients or their families; like any other business, it is subject to horizontal violence and interdisciplinary incivility. Horizontal violence comes in the form of intimidating or derisive behavior between and among staff, managers, or physicians; it interferes with optimal job performance and has negative effects on the delivery of high-quality patient care. Research suggests that workplace violence/incivility can be prevented if people are aware of warning signs and have training on how to effectively deal with potentially violent situations. No organization can completely prevent or eliminate workplace violence, but with proper planning and effective programs, the chances of such violent occurrences can be dramatically reduced.

OBJECTIVES

- Categorize the types of violence/incivility that may occur in the workplace.
- Analyze risk factors for potential violence or disruption.
- Describe guidelines for preventing workplace violence and incivility.
- Evaluate your organization's plan for preventing workplace violence and incivility.
- Evaluate interventions that help prevent horizontal violence and incivility.

TERMS TO KNOW

bullying	incivility	lateral aggression
horizontal violence	interpersonal conflict	toxic workplace

THE CHALLENGE

Lori Jeffries, RN
University Medical Center Brackenridge, Austin, Texas

I had recently come to work in the emergency department (ED) from a general medical-surgical unit in a different hospital. I had been working in the ED only a few months when the incident occurred. My patient was an older man with mental illness who had not been taking his medication. He appeared to have been living on the streets and presented to the ED confused and mumbling. He did not have a shirt, and he was having difficulty keeping his pants on because the zipper was broken. Our ED keeps donated clean clothing for just such occasions. The clothes were in a long narrow closet where we also kept a gurney used to transport expired patients.

You had to squeeze by the gurney to get to where the clothes were. I wanted to make my patient more comfortable by getting him some clean clothes to wear. At the time, I did not think that he was the type of person who might be dangerous. I had him come with me to the closet to make sure the items I picked would fit him because he was tall and solidly built. I went into the closet first, with him following a few feet behind me. I picked up a pair of pants and turned around to hold them up to see if they were about the right size. That is when he backed up and closed the door. I knew then I was in trouble.

What do you think you would do if you were this nurse?

INTRODUCTION

Workplace violence and incivility in health care have emerged as an important safety issue over the past decade. It is seen on a continuum from threats or intimidation to its most extreme form, homicide. Violence, whether from persons outside or within an organization, has been shown to have negative effects including increased job stress, reduced productive work time, decreased morale, increased staff turnover, and loss of trust in the organization and its management. The purpose of this chapter is to increase awareness of the risk factors for violence and incivility in healthcare facilities and to provide strategies for decreasing or preventing those events in the workplace.

Defining Workplace Violence/Incivility

As part of the Centers for Disease Control and Prevention (CDC), the National Institute for Occupational Safety and Health (NIOSH) conducts research and makes recommendations to prevent work-related illness and injury. NIOSH works with industry and labor organizations to understand and improve worker safety and health. NIOSH (2002) defines workplace violence as "violent acts (including physical assaults and threats of assaults) directed toward persons at work or on duty." The definition of violence includes overt and covert behaviors ranging from offensive or threatening language to homicide. In recent years, additional descriptions of other forms of workplace violence have been added. Horizontal violence or lateral aggression has been used to describe aggressive and destructive behavior of co-workers against each other. Other terms associated with this type of violence include bullying and interpersonal conflict. These behaviors exist in what has been termed toxic workplaces. Incivility includes a wide range of behaviors from ignoring, to rolling one's eyes, to yelling, and eventually to personal attacks, both physical and psychological. Both types of workplace violence are addressed in this chapter and are referred to as violence.

Scope of the Problem

The true scope of workplace violence in health care is difficult to determine. The main source of data for workplace violence and injuries is the Bureau of Labor Statistics (BLS). Fatal and nonfatal occupational injury statistics are collected by the BLS in two major categories: goods-producing and service-providing industries. In a 2006 BLS report of service-providing organizations, healthcare and social assistance organizations had the highest percentage of reported nonfatal injuries (Figure 25-1).

Because the reporting category includes both healthcare and social assistance organizations, accurate data for health care alone are hard to determine. In another BLS summary report released in 2007 (Figure 25-2), more specific analysis indicated employees working in general medical and surgical hospitals had the highest number of nonfatal occupational injuries in private-sector industries. Ambulatory health services and nursing care facilities

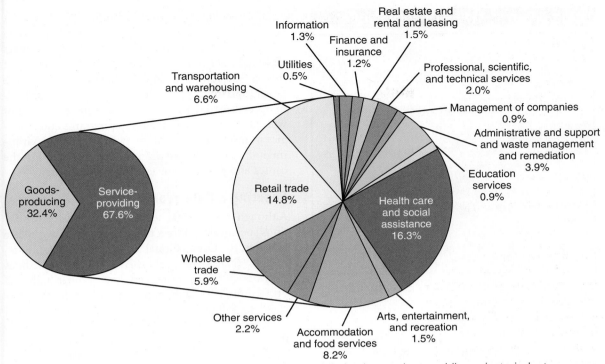

FIGURE 25-1 Distribution of nonfatal occupational injuries by service-providing private industry sector, 2006.

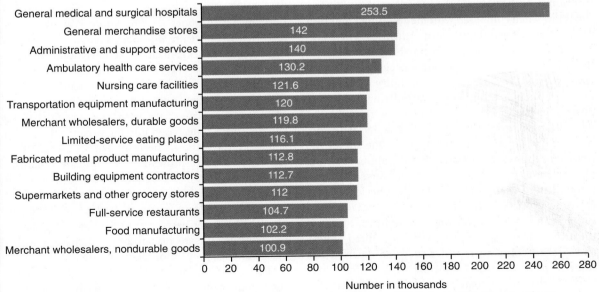

FIGURE 25-2 Industries with at least 100,000 nonfatal occupational injuries and illnesses, private industry, 2007.

BOX 25-1	TYPES OF VIOLENCE	
Intimidation		75.9%
Angry outbursts		71.9%
Hypersensitivity to criticism		71.5%
Belligerence		66.9%
Threatening/disruptive behavior		64.6%
Bullying		59.8%
Harassment		51.6%
Threats of physical violence		38.9%
Obsession with a supervisor		28.5%
Ominous or specific threats		27.9%
Physical violence		25.8%
Intentional property damage		17.0%
Preoccupation with recently publicized violent events		8.3%
Carrying or storing weapons		7.5%
Preoccupation with violent themes		5.9%
Recent acquisition of or fascination with weapons		5.6%

From Hader, R. (2008). Workplace violence survey 2008. *Nursing Management, 39*(7), 13-19.

appeared fourth and fifth in frequencies. When combined, the disproportional incidence in these three healthcare settings is cause for concern.

In addition, 114 fatal injuries were reported in preliminary BLS data for health care in 2007. Although this number is a concern, the incidence of fatal injuries is low when compared with the combined number of fatalities or for other types of industries. There are concerns that the true rate is much higher because many incidents are not reported, especially when violence does not result in a physical injury or is verbal in nature such as intimidation or bullying. Underreporting in health care is thought to be related to a perception within nursing that assaults with or without injuries are "part of the job." One survey of nurses in Minnesota reported that the annual rate of physical and non-physical assaults on nurses per 100 respondents was 13.2 (Nachreiner, Gerberich, Ryan, & McGovern, 2007). According to Hader (2008) in a survey conducted by *Nursing Management,* 80% of the 1377 nurse respondents from the United States and 17 other countries reported they had experienced some form of violence within the work setting (Box 25-1). Verbal rather than physical forms of violence were reported most often. According to the survey, the perpetrator was a patient 53.2% of the time, with

nurse colleagues a close second at 51.9% of the time. Next in the ranking were physicians (49%), visitors (47%), and other healthcare workers (37.7%). Nurses observed their colleagues being the primary target of this violence (79.7%) and had personally been the target (56.1%). Many earlier studies with similar findings demonstrate the need to examine the causes of workplace violence and develop programs and strategies to improve personal safety in the work environment. In particular, attention needs to be paid to the causes and remedies for lateral violence issues.

Ensuring a Safe Workplace

Although no national legislation or federal regulations specifically address the prevention of workplace violence, the Occupational Safety & Health Administration (OSHA) has published voluntary guidelines for workers in healthcare and several other high-risk professions. Although employers are not legally obligated to follow these guidelines, the Occupational Safety and Health Act (OSH Act) (1970) mandates that, in addition to complying with hazard-specific standards, all employers have a general duty to provide their employees with a workplace free from recognized hazards likely to cause death or serious physical harm. An organization can be cited if its leaders fail to address such hazards. Because healthcare workers are at increased risk, OSHA (2004) developed *Guidelines for Preventing Workplace Violence for Health Care and Social Service Workers* to assist healthcare organizations in developing violence prevention plans. Several states are also enacting or developing laws, standards, or recommendations that address healthcare workplace security and safety. Many of these laws have been created with strong support from state-based nursing organizations with support from the American Nurses Association (ANA) and other professional healthcare organizations (ANA, 2009). A few states have passed laws that enhance criminal penalties on crimes committed against licensed or certified health professionals. Many other states have or are working on legislation requiring healthcare organizations to have a workplace violence prevention plan (Figure 25-3).

The Joint Commission (TJC) (2008) has strengthened requirements in their Leadership standards for dealing with disruptive behavior. Citing studies that suggest intimidating and disruptive behaviors

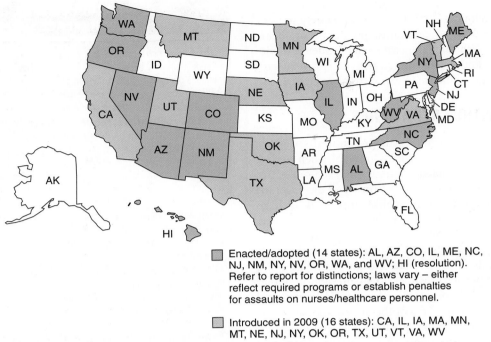

Enacted/adopted (14 states): AL, AZ, CO, IL, ME, NC, NJ, NM, NY, NV, OR, WA, and WV; HI (resolution). Refer to report for distinctions; laws vary – either reflect required programs or establish penalties for assaults on nurses/healthcare personnel.

Introduced in 2009 (16 states): CA, IL, IA, MA, MN, MT, NE, NJ, NY, OK, OR, TX, UT, VT, VA, WV

FIGURE 25-3 The American Nurse Association's Nationwide State Legislative Agenda for workplace violence, June 2009.

contribute to poor patient satisfaction and preventable adverse outcomes, the standards calls for codes of conduct and processes for managing such behaviors. These standards became effective in January 2009.

The Cost of Workplace Violence

Our knowledge of the scale of workplace violence remains incomplete because no consistent system of data collection exists. Data regarding the less severe forms of workplace violence are particularly sparse. Even less clear is the financial toll workplace aggression exacts on businesses. A Workplace Violence Research Institute (1995) study estimated the aggregate cost of workplace violence to U.S. employers to be more than $36 billion as a result of expenses associated with lost business and productivity, litigation, medical care, psychiatric care, higher insurance rates, increased security measures, negative publicity, and loss of employees. Pearson and Porath (2009) suggest that estimates of cost should consider how many times people report they are sick when they are really

avoiding bad behavior and decreases in productivity because employees no longer feel comfortable in the environment. These costs mount rapidly.

Researchers (Hartley, Biddle, & Jenkins, 2005) from the National Institute for Occupational Safety and Health (NIOSH) have attempted to determine the cost of the most extreme workplace violence using a model that calculates direct and indirect costs of workplace fatalities, including medical expenses and lost earnings. NIOSH estimated the average mean cost of a workplace homicide incident, from 1992 to 2001, to be $800,000. The total cost of workplace homicides during this same period totaled nearly $6.5 billion. Studies have yet to capture the full cost of workplace violence in its many forms. More measurement is also needed to assess the cost and effectiveness of known intervention strategies.

Making a Difference

So what is the nurse in a leader, manager, or follower role to do given the serious and complex issue of violence in the workplace? Making a difference includes promotion of an organizational culture of safety, developing and implementing a safety strategy, providing training programs, predicting problems, and using technology to reduce the incidence of violence. In addition, personal strategies to prevent being victimized by violence in any setting are critical.

PREVENTION STRATEGIES

The old adage "an ounce of prevention is worth a pound of cure" is particularly relevant when dealing with workplace violence. Preventing even one act of violence can save money and time and diminish the possible negative psychological impact of such an event. The costs from lost work time and wages, reduced productivity, medical costs, workers' compensation payments, and legal and security expenses may be difficult to estimate but are clearly excessive when compared with the cost of prevention. Other future costs of workplace violence include increased staff turnover rates. Loss of the organizational investment required to train qualified staff and departure of experienced existing staff can increase operating expenses and reduce the quality of care. By taking a proactive approach that includes preventing violence, organizations can also avoid being victimized. To address the issue of violence, it is necessary to have a broad understanding of types of violence that may be encountered and the signs that portend a potentially violent situation. In short, prevention is the right thing to do for people and for the organization.

Types of Violence

Since 1990, the University of Iowa Injury Prevention Research Center (IPRC) has been one of 11 injury "Centers of Excellence" funded by the National Center for Injury Prevention and Control, a branch of the CDC. Workplace violence has been one of their research focus areas (2001). The University collects and uses epidemiologic data on groups at high risk in order to develop prevention strategies and training to control and prevent injuries. In their investigations, they categorize workplace violence into four types (Box 25-2).

These categories can be very helpful in the design of strategies to prevent workplace violence, because each type of violence requires a different approach for prevention, acknowledging the fact that some work-

---

BOX 25-2	CATEGORIES OF WORKPLACE VIOLENCE

Criminal Intent (Type I): The perpetrator has no legitimate relationship to the business or its employees and is usually committing a crime in conjunction with the violence. These crimes can include robbery, shoplifting, and trespassing. The vast majority of workplace homicides (85%) fall into this category.

Customer/Client (Type II): The perpetrator has a legitimate relationship with the business and becomes violent while being served by the business. This category includes customers, clients, patients, students, inmates, and any other group for which the business provides services. A large proportion of customer/client incidents are believed to occur in the healthcare industry, in settings such as nursing homes or psychiatric facilities; the victims are often patient caregivers. Police officers, prison staff, flight attendants, and teachers are some other examples of workers who may be exposed to this kind of workplace violence.

Worker-on-Worker (Type III): The perpetrator is an employee or past employee of the business who attacks or threatens another employee(s) or past employee(s) in the workplace. Worker-on-worker fatalities account for approximately 7% of all workplace violence homicides.

Personal Relationship (Type IV): The perpetrator usually does not have a relationship with the business but has a personal relationship with the intended victim. This category includes victims of domestic violence assaulted or threatened while at work.

From Iowa Injury Prevention Research Center. (February 2001). *Workplace violence: A report to the nation.* University of Iowa—Iowa City. Retrieved October 28, 2009, from www.public-health.uiowa.edu/iprc/resources/workplace-violence-report.pdf.

---

places may be at higher risk for certain types of violence. Understanding the types of violence allows leaders to conduct a more focused risk assessment based on what types of crimes may occur.

Risk Assessment

Although anyone working in health care is at risk for becoming a victim of violence, those with direct patient contact are at higher risk. NIOSH (2002) reports that healthcare workers in hospitals, specifically those in the emergency department, are at particular risk. Violence is also a frequent occurrence in psychiatric and geriatric settings. Unlike in other settings, hospital violence differs in that it is usually the result of patients or their family members feeling frustration or anger. This is usually related to feelings of vulnerability, stress, and loss of control that accom-

BOX 25-3   **RISK FACTORS FOR VIOLENCE IN HEALTHCARE FACILITIES**

- Working when understaffed, especially during visiting hours and meal times
- Transporting patients between areas in a facility
- Long waits for patient care
- Overcrowded, uncomfortable waiting areas
- Working alone or in an area isolated from other staff
- Solo work with patients in areas with no back-up or way to get assistance, such as communication devices or alarm systems
- Poor environmental design
- Inadequate security
- Lack of staff training in handling potentially violent situations
- Lack of policies for preventing and managing crises with potentially violent individuals
- Unrestricted movement of patients or visitors
- Poorly lit corridors, rooms, parking lots, or other areas
- Prevalence of handguns or other weapons among patients, their families, or friends
- Increasing presence of gang members, drug or alcohol abusers, trauma patients, or distraught family members
- Use of hospitals or healthcare facilities for holding criminals, violent individuals, and the acutely mentally disturbed
- Serving chronically mentally ill patients being released without adequate resources for follow-up care
- Availability of money or drugs within the facility

Adapted from Occupational Safety & Health Administration (OSHA). (2004). *Guidelines for preventing workplace violence for health care and social service workers.* Retrieved October 28, 2009, from www.osha.gov/Publications/osha3148.pdf.

BOX 25-4   **WORKPLACE VIOLENCE PROGRAM CHECKLISTS**

OSHA and ANA have provided comprehensive checklist documents that can assist leaders and managers in conducting an organizational workplace violence assessment. The checklist titles are provided here. The checklists provide detailed step-by-step instructions to conduct an in-depth assessment and establish a monitoring program. To see the complete document, go to *www.osha.gov* (OSHA Publication No. 3148-01R 2004).

Checklist 1: Organizational Assessment Questions Regarding Management Commitment and Employee Involvement

Checklist 2: Analyze Workplace Violence Records

Checklist 3: Identifying Environmental Risk Factors for Violence

Checklist 4: Assessing the Influence of Day-to-Day Work Practices on Occurrences of Violence

Checklist 5: Post-Incident Response

Checklist 6: Assessing Employee and Supervisor Training

Checklist 7: Recordkeeping and Evaluation

Adapted from American Nurses Association: *Promoting Safe Work Environments for Nurses, 2002.* (From Occupational Safety and Health Administration (OSHA). (2004). *Guidelines for preventing workplace violence for health care and social service workers* (OSHA Publication No. 3148-01R). Washington, DC: U.S. Department of Labor. [www.osha.gov])

pany illness. Many factors have been identified that can increase the risk for violence erupting in healthcare facilities. Risk factors identified in OSHA's *Guidelines* (2004) are listed in Box 25-3.

Other risk factors for violence include the location of the facility, its size, and the type of care provided. Facilities located in inner-city areas that serve a wide variety of the disadvantaged, especially those with mental illness or a history of violent behavior or those who are under the influence of drugs or alcohol, are at increased risk for violence to occur. Review of reports of violent incidents reveals they often take place during times of high activity and interaction with patients, such as at meal times and during visiting hours and patient transportation. Assaults may occur when service is denied, when a patient is involuntarily admitted, or when a healthcare worker attempts to set limits on eating, drinking, or use of tobacco or alcohol.

Similar to the nursing process, prevention of workplace violence begins with a systematic assessment. Assessing risk and planning for prevention of workplace violence call for input and expertise from a variety of staff. A risk assessment based on a multidisciplinary team approach to workplace violence prevention is often the most effective. A team with representation from administration, staff, security, facilities engineering, human resources, legal counsel, and risk management is needed to address risks from all perspectives. A worksite assessment involves a step-by-step, common-sense look at the facility and the surrounding areas for existing problems and potential hazards. OSHA's *Guidelines* (2004) provide a comprehensive assessment with checklists and forms developed by the ANA to assist with the process. These are helpful to managers and leaders who are not familiar with this type of assessment (Box 25-4).

When looking at possible threats or hazards, those from within an organization also must be considered. Determining if current employees pose a danger in the workplace is a critical factor that is often overlooked. In addition to personal and psychological factors, behaviors can be observed in employees that may be related to violence or aggression in the workplace (Paludi, Nydegger, & Paludi, 2006). The most obvious of these is a previous history of aggression and substance abuse. Screening potential employees through drug testing, background checks, and references can help reduce these risks. Paludi et al. (2006) also advise of warning signs that can alert employers of problems with current employees that warrant intervention to prevent a violent incident.

Firing Right

Organizational conditions or outcomes may magnify the potential for violence to erupt. This includes prolonged high levels of stress or factors that create what is known as a *toxic workplace environment*. Rapid change, layoffs, changes in schedules and workloads, or wage freezes could have this effect. The employment situation with the highest potential to create this kind of stress is the firing or layoff process. Most organizations have specific protocols that deal with the process of terminating employees, because firing is cause for strong emotions that can increase the potential for violence. As a manager, you may be responsible for staff terminations. The goal always is to conduct the process in the most professional manner possible, although organizational rules may specify a detailed procedure. A few tips on how to prepare for this potentially problematic situation are provided in Box 25-5.

BOX 25-5	FIRING RIGHT

Firings should be planned with forethought for any potential problems. Steps should be taken to avoid potential violence during employee separation. A key step is protecting the employee's dignity and avoiding humiliation. The reasons for termination should be clear and leave no room for debate. All details should be arranged, including timing, the room used, and who is present. The room should provide privacy but not contain any objects that could be used as a weapon. The person being terminated should not be blocked from accessing the exit door. Termination notices and severance checks along with any other documentation should be on hand. Arrangements should be made to clean out the person's desk or locker. There should be no reason for the person to return to the worksite. This saves everyone from embarrassment and any potential scenes. It is important to try to determine how the person will react to make appropriate arrangements. If there is a perceived need, a security officer or off-duty police officer can be called to stand by.

Adapted from Winfeld, L. (2001). *Training tough topics*. New York: American Management Association.

There is no profile or litmus test to identify whether a current employee might become violent. It is important for employers and employees alike to remain alert to problematic behavior that, in combination, could point to possible violence. Because no one behavior in and of itself suggests a greater potential for violence, behaviors must be looked at in totality. Problem situations, circumstances that may heighten the risk of violence, can involve a particular event or employee or the workplace as a whole.

HORIZONTAL VIOLENCE: THE THREAT FROM WITHIN

Horizontal or lateral violence describes a wide variety of behaviors, from verbal abuse to physical aggression between co-workers. This term, though commonly used, may be limiting because it suggests the violence is perpetrated between those at the same level of authority. It may be better termed *relational aggression* (Dellasega, 2009), which can occur between people at different levels. This includes bullying behavior and intimidation. *Horizontal violence* or *bullying* is used in this section because these are terms common in the literature. Horizontal violence and its effects have been reported in nursing literature for more than 20 years. In a review of five research studies

---

EXERCISE 25-1

Assess several clinical settings for workplace violence risks. Can you identify any based on what you have read? What security measures are currently in place? Can any of them be improved? How safe would you feel in the different geographical areas?

Once the risk assessment is completed, the next step is to analyze the data and prioritize the problems that need to be addressed. Priorities can be established by asking a few basic questions: What are the risks? Who might be harmed and how? What is the level of risk? What measures need to be taken to reduce or eliminate risk? Do we need to implement changes now or later? Once the priorities are set, the business of designing or improving prevention programs can begin. (See the "Developing a Safety Plan" section on p. 508.)

on horizontal violence, researchers (Woelfle & McCaffrey, 2007) found that horizontal violence is experienced by not only student nurses but also the novice and veteran nurses. Many of the research reports found infighting and a general lack of support of nurses for each other to be common occurrences. The studies also indicate that new graduates were likely to experience horizontal violence, which resulted in high absentee rates and thoughts of leaving nursing after their first year. This caused the researchers to ask this question: How can nurses treat patients kindly and give them the respect they need when they treat each other so poorly? In light of the looming nursing shortage, these consistent findings among nurses were cause for concern.

Many theories exist as to why horizontal violence exists in nursing, ranging from nursing's traditional hierarchical structure, to oppression of nursing as a profession, to feminism (Farrell, 2001). However, it is also noted that workplace aggression is common in other professions and is most likely the result of a complex myriad of individual, social, and organizational characteristics (Farrell, 2001, Hutchinson, Vickers, Jackson, & Wilkes, 2006). Regardless of the reasons why it happens, the concerns are that impaired intrapersonal relationships between nurses at work can cause errors, accidents, and poor work performance (Farrell, 1997) and may play a significant role in attrition (Johnson, 2009). In a survey on workplace intimidation published by the Institute for Safe Medication Practices (2003), almost half of the 2095 respondents recalled being verbally abused when questioning or clarifying medication prescriptions. This intimidation played a role in not questioning an order as a way of not directly confronting the prescriber. The results of the survey had professional healthcare and nursing organizations issue calls to action to address all types of workplace violence in the interest of promoting a safe and respectful work environment that promotes the delivery of high-quality care instead of threatening it. Shortly after the publication of the release of the Institute's report, the International Council of Nurses (ICN) (2006) published a position statement on healthcare workplace violence. The ICN also asserted the following:

> Violence in the workplace threatens the delivery of effective patient services and, therefore, patient safety. If quality care is to be provided, nursing

personnel must be ensured a safe work environment and respectful treatment. Excessive workloads, unsafe working conditions, and inadequate support can be considered forms of violence and incompatible with good practice.

In 2008, the Center for American Nurses published a position paper stating there is no place in a professional practice environment for lateral violence and bullying among nurses or between healthcare professionals. These disruptive behaviors are toxic to the nursing profession and have a negative impact on retention of quality staff. Horizontal violence and bullying should never be considered normally related to socialization in nursing nor be accepted in professional relationships. The statement goes on to assert that all healthcare organizations should implement a zero tolerance policy related to disruptive behavior, including a professional code of conduct and educational and behavioral interventions to assist nurses in addressing disruptive behavior. See the Literature Perspective on p. 506. A number of other state and national nursing organizations also have issued statements regarding the detrimental effect of disruptive behavior on both patients and nurses and have called for solutions to address the problem. TJC (2008) proposed a revision in its standards for disruptive behavior, identifying manifestations of abuse and violence in the workplace and providing avenues for ending this phenomenon. With professional groups calling for change from within nursing and accreditation groups calling on administration to fix problems, we must examine how to implement a change.

Increasing Awareness of Horizontal Violence

The causes of horizontal violence within nursing are many, and it has been found to be pervasive and long-standing. No definitive actions have been shown to significantly decrease its occurrence. One thing is certain—recognizing the tendency toward bullying, harassment, or intimidation in the workplace is a prerequisite to preventing it. The true depth of the problem is difficult to determine. Commonly, horizontal violence is significantly underreported for any number of reasons, and organizational leaders often are not aware of its extent. To get an accurate picture of employee satisfaction and concerns about bullying and other forms of violence, anonymous surveys

Resource: Nachreiner, N., Gerberich, S., McGovern, P., Church, T., Hansen, H., Geisser, M., & Ryan, A. (2005). Impact of training on work-related assault. *Research in Nursing & Health, 28* (1), 67-78.

This article is based on data collected from the Minnesota Nurses' Study on perceptions of violence and the work environment. The same researchers who conducted the Minnesota study turned their focus to the relationship between violence prevention policies and workplace violence. Little literature is available on the topic, and there is a growing need to understand what interventions can reduce physical assaults and other violent behavior in healthcare settings. One of the primary recommendations from governmental and professional organizations is to establish policies that address workplace violence, but there is no clear evidence that this is effective. From the study results, it appears that certain types of policies, specifically zero tolerance and defining the specific behaviors that are prohibited, are the most protective for the nurse population. Another revealing finding was the lack of surety about the existence of policy among the nursing staff. Organizational culture, effective communication, and dissemination of policy were all factors identified as variables for reducing the effectiveness of policy.

Implications for Practice

The presence of policy alone will not protect workers from violence, although emerging research indicates policy can have an impact on reducing it. Beyond policy, there must be an organizational commitment to enforcement of policy and an obvious dedication to ensuring safety. Communication about policy, particularly how to identify, prevent, and report violence, is crucial. If staff is unsure what to do, the policy may not be worth the paper it is written on.

should be conducted. Surveying staff can help identify problems and provide a basis for developing appropriate interventions. To understand if violence or intimidation is a reason for leaving, organizations should conduct exit interviews with the assurance that the information will remain confidential if an employee fears retaliation. This is an important step in gauging if the problem is bullying or intimidation by managers. In a recent survey study (Johnson, 2009), 50% of the respondents indicated that they were bullied by their manager or director. The researcher suggests that when management is part of the problem, victims have a harder time feeling they have adequate support to end the negative cycle of violence. This may serve to perpetuate the existence of a toxic environment within an organization.

Nursing leaders can set the stage for addressing workplace bullying by examining and addressing their own behaviors and by fostering an environment that encourages open communication and collaboration. With personal insight in hand, they can lead their nurses to examine their own behavior and work together to create a work environment in which bullying is not tolerated. An atmosphere of openness can encourage dialog and brainstorming to find solutions. The importance of this type of mutual support was a major theme in a study by Woelfle & McCaffrey (2007). Lack of support leads many victims of bullying to decide that the best alternative was to leave the organization and to give this advice to others who found themselves in similar situations (Johnson, 2009). Employees who are supported in reporting workplace aggression may feel they have options other than leaving. The worst outcome would be for the nurse to feel that using formal and informal organizational channels to bring about an end to bullying was emotionally draining, time-consuming, and futile.

Organizational culture and working conditions also can contribute to bullying and horizontal violence. High stress levels, inadequate staffing, organizational change, and unrealistic expectations can contribute to a toxic environment and foster increased incivility among staff. A culture of zero tolerance for horizontal violence is an effective leadership strategy to prevent its occurrence. For organizations that have tolerated horizontal violence, developing a new shared set of values and goals that promote empowerment, communication, and collaboration is a positive step (Longo, 2007). Leaders need to set the tone for establishing a civil workplace in which all members are treated with respect and in which conflicts are dealt with in a healthy and open manner. TJC suggests 11 actions for organizations to address disruptive behavior that can be used as a blueprint for developing a program (Box 25-6). No violence prevention program will work if management does not endorse it.

Encouragement to report violence in all its forms is crucial to understanding the root of the problem and implementing plans to eradicate it. Acts of good faith by organizational management in supporting

BOX 25-6   THE JOINT COMMISSION SUGGESTED ACTIONS

1. Educate all team members—both physicians and non-physician staff—on appropriate professional behavior defined by the organization's code of conduct.
2. Hold all team members accountable for modeling desirable behaviors, and enforce the code consistently and equitably among all staff, regardless of seniority or clinical discipline, in a positive fashion through reinforcement as well as punishment.
3. Develop and implement policies and procedures/processes appropriate for the organization that address the following:
   - "Zero tolerance" for intimidating and/or disruptive behaviors
   - Medical staff policies regarding intimidating and/or disruptive behaviors
   - Reducing fear of intimidation or retribution and protecting those who report or cooperate in the investigation of intimidating, disruptive, and other unprofessional behavior
   - Responding to patients and/or their families who are involved in or witness intimidating and/or disruptive behaviors
   - How and when to begin disciplinary actions (e.g., suspension, termination, loss of clinical privileges, reports to professional licensure bodies)
4. Develop an organizational process for addressing intimidating and disruptive behaviors that solicits and integrates substantial input from an interdisciplinary team including representation of medical and nursing staff, administrators, and other employees.
5. Provide skills-based training and coaching for all leaders and managers in relationship-building and collaborative practice, including skills for giving feedback on unprofessional behavior, and conflict resolution.
6. Develop and implement a system for assessing staff perceptions of the seriousness and extent of instances of unprofessional behaviors and the risk of harm to patients.
7. Develop and implement a reporting/surveillance system (possibly anonymous) for detecting unprofessional behavior.
8. Support surveillance with tiered, non-confrontational interventional strategies, starting with informal "cup of coffee" conversations directly addressing the problem and moving toward detailed action plans and progressive discipline, if patterns persist.
9. Conduct all interventions within the context of an organizational commitment to the health and well-being of all staff, with adequate resources to support individuals whose behavior is caused or influenced by physical or mental health pathologies.
10. Encourage interdisciplinary dialogs across a variety of forums as a proactive way of addressing ongoing conflicts, overcoming them, and moving forward through improved collaboration and communication.
11. Document all attempts to address intimidating and disruptive behaviors.

staff include a policy of non-retaliation for reporting. Making sure that reporting is easier and doing an impartial investigation are critical. Ensuring appropriate discipline for identified problems that is proportional to the seriousness of the event goes a long way in building employee trust. People are the greatest resource in an organization, and wise management invests time and effort in addressing culture, safety, and satisfaction of nursing staff. Finally, organizations that implement interventions aimed at addressing workplace bullying need to collect data to determine whether these interventions are successful.

Nurses themselves must work to actively develop a culture in which violence is not tolerated. This involves a critical self-assessment of personal behaviors and looking for patterns or situations that could trigger subtle types of lateral aggression. Awareness and understanding of the types of horizontal violence can help them to actively not participate in the behaviors. This is a powerful tool in eradicating a toxic environment. Many subtle forms of horizontal violence are listed in Box 25-7 that may not be readily recognized as violent behavior but are psychologically and emotionally harmful. Recognizing these behaviors and efforts to eliminate them can create a healthier working environment that is based on mutual respect.

EXERCISE 25-2

Think about your behavior in the workplace. Have you ever acted in a way that might be described as lateral aggression or horizontal violence? How might you guard against such behaviors? Do you think you could confront a co-worker participating in an act of lateral aggression? What would you say?

BOX 25-7 COMMON SUBTLE BEHAVIORS IN NURSE-NURSE BULLYING

- Giving a nurse "the silent treatment"
- Spreading rumors
- Using humiliation and put-downs, usually regarding a nurse's skills and abilities
- Failing to support a nurse because you do not like him or her
- Excluding a nurse from on-the-job or off-the-job socializing
- Repeating information shared by one nurse out of context so that it reflects badly on him or her
- Sharing confidences you were asked to keep private
- Making fun of another nurse's appearance, demeanor, or another trait
- Refusing to share information with another nurse or otherwise setting him or her up to fail
- Manipulating or intimidating another nurse into doing something for you
- Using body language (e.g., eye rolling or head tossing) to convey an unfavorable opinion of someone
- Saying something unfavorable and then pretending you were joking
- Calling names
- Teasing another nurse about his or her lack of skill or knowledge
- Running a smear campaign or otherwise trying to get others to turn against a nurse

Modified from Dellasega, C. (2009). Bullying among nurses. *American Journal of Nursing, 109*(1), 52-58.

Education

Education on workplace violence should be provided to all employees but initially to supervisors, whose support is crucial to the success of the program (Gallant-Roman, 2008). Interventions aimed at nurse leaders regarding ways to change organizational climates that perpetuate bullying have proved to be a better option than directing education at individual nurses (Johnson, 2009). Education should focus on identifying the potential for violence, managing violent situations, and behavioral and de-escalation techniques. In some settings, more focused training on applying restraints and take-down techniques would be appropriate. This type of training should start in nursing school to prepare those going into the workforce for the realities of their day-to-day work. Training needs to be annual and ongoing, addressing topics that have been identified through survey, reporting, and data analysis.

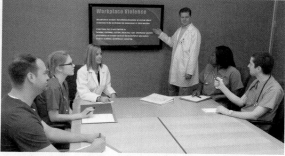

Participating in violence prevention education can prepare staff to deal with situations that contribute to bullying or intimidation.

Participating in violence prevention education can prepare staff to deal with situations that contribute to bullying or intimidation. In her study, Griffin (2004) used a cognitive behavior technique called *cognitive rehearsal* as an intervention for lateral violence. Cognitive rehearsal involves listening and then holding the information provided in the mind to allow time to process a response in a way the staff have been taught. This change in the way they responded allowed opportunities to change negative perceptions and confront laterally violent nurses. This opens the door to better communication and has been shown to help nurses better cope with potentially violent situations (Oostrom & van Mierlo, 2008).

DEVELOPING A SAFETY PLAN

No "one-size-fits-all" strategy exists for an effective safety and violence prevention program or plan. Effective plans may share a number of features, but a good plan must be tailored to the needs, resources, and circumstances of a particular employer and a particular work force. Activities related to developing a good prevention program fall into three domains: administrative, environmental, and interpersonal.

Administrative

To develop an effective workplace violence strategy, there must be support from the top. If an organization's senior executives are not truly committed to a prevention program, it is unlikely to be effectively implemented. Part of the organization's responsibility is to provide a written program for job safety and security. Developing and maintaining a program requires time and resources. Allocations need to be made to allow for a multidisciplinary safety committee, regular worksite analysis, prevention activities, safety and health training, documentation, and evaluation of the overall program. The program should outline the organization's commitment to a safe work environment and the staff's involvement in the plan. The program should be proactive, not reactive, and have clear goals and objectives to prevent workplace violence that is specific to the organization and its characteristics. Personnel, work environments, business conditions, and society all change and evolve. A successful prevention program must change and evolve with them. Policies and practices should not be set in concrete and should be regularly evaluated to determine if they are keeping current with a changing environment. The administration needs to communicate the safety plan effectively and consistently enforce policy to ensure that the staff feels its safety is of paramount importance.

A written workplace violence policy sets the standard for acceptable workplace behavior *and* should be available to all employees. The statement should affirm the company's commitment to a safe workplace, employees' obligation to behave appropriately on the job, and the employer's commitment to take action on any employee's complaint regarding harassing, threatening, and violent behavior. The statement should be in writing and distributed to all employees. In defining acts that will not be tolerated, the statement should make clear that not only physical violence but also threats, bullying, harassment, and weapons possession are against company policy and are prohibited.

Plans should consider the workplace culture: work atmosphere, relationships, and management styles. Policies on workplace conduct should be written to clearly state the employer's standards and expectations. Attention should be paid to elements in an organization's culture that foster a toxic work environment, such as the following:

- Tolerance of bullying or intimidation
- Lack of trust among workers
- Lack of trust between workers and management
- High levels of stress, frustration, and anger

The organization should be actively addressing root causes of problems to reduce the potential for frustration to lead to violence. If significant problems are identified, disciplinary actions for violent behavior of any kind must be proportionate, consistent, reasonable, and fair. Erratic or arbitrary discipline, favoritism, and a lack of respect for employees' dignity and rights are likely to undermine an employer's violence prevention efforts. Workers who perceive an employer's practices as unfair or unreasonable will be more unlikely to report problems. Lack of reporting allows unfavorable situations to continue with many negative impacts. If there is a complaint or incident, an incident response team should conduct or ensure a thorough investigation of the facts and, based on the results, determine appropriate disciplinary measures. Likewise with patients or visitors to a healthcare facility, expectations about acceptable behavior and the consequences of violent behavior should be clearly communicated. Strong administrative commitment to a safety plan serves to reaffirm the employer's commitment to a workplace free from threats and violence.

Environmental

Engineering controls and other environmental adaptations to remove safety hazards can be very effective. Deciding what interventions are needed is the "intelligence" work of organizations. The counter-measures applied can reduce potential risks. The selection of measures to be used is based on the hazards identified in the security risk analysis. Some environmental interventions, such as providing better lighting or restricting access to care areas, can have a significant impact on safety at very low cost. The types of interventions that may be identified by security risk assessment are listed in Box 25-8.

Administrative and work practice controls can also be evaluated to determine the effect on how staff members perform their jobs and how changes in procedures can help reduce the potential for violent incidents. Any process changes that reduce waiting times or improve customer service can help reduce frustration that may lead to violent outburst. Staff training on handling aggressive behavior and how to respond in violent events is discussed in the next section.

BOX 25-8   ENVIRONMENTAL SAFETY CONTROLS

- Assess any plans for new construction or physical changes to the facility or workplace to eliminate or reduce security hazards.
- Install and regularly maintain alarm systems and other security devices, panic buttons, handheld alarms or noise devices, cellular phones, and private channel radios where risk is apparent or may be anticipated. Arrange for a reliable response system when an alarm is triggered.
- Provide metal detectors—installed or handheld, where appropriate—to detect guns, knives, or other weapons, according to the recommendations of security consultants.
- Use a closed-circuit video recording for high-risk areas on a 24-hour basis. Public safety is a greater concern than privacy in these situations.
- Create security alert overhead paging protocols and response teams.
- Place curved mirrors at hallway intersections and concealed areas.
- Enclose nurses' stations and install deep service counters or bullet-resistant, shatterproof glass in reception, triage, and admitting areas or patient service rooms.
- Provide employee "safe rooms" for use during emergencies.
- Establish "time-out" or seclusion areas with high ceilings without grids for patients who "act out," and establish separate rooms for criminal patients.

- Provide comfortable client or patient waiting rooms designed to minimize stress.
- Ensure that counseling or patient care rooms have two exits.
- Lock doors to staff counseling rooms and treatment rooms to limit access.
- Arrange furniture to prevent entrapment of staff.
- Use minimal furniture in interview rooms or crisis treatment areas, and ensure that it is lightweight, without sharp corners or edges, and affixed to the floor, if possible. Limit the number of pictures, vases, ashtrays, or other items that can be used as weapons.
- Provide lockable and secure bathrooms for staff members separate from patient/client and visitor facilities.
- Lock all unused doors to limit access, in accordance with local fire codes.
- Install bright, effective lighting, both indoors and outdoors.
- Replace burned-out lights and broken windows and locks.
- Keep automobiles well maintained if they are used in the field.
- Lock automobiles at all times.
- Provide administrative controls such as codes for door access in staff or restricted areas.
- Improve processes to decrease wait times or other activities that create frustration for patients and family members.

Adapted from American Nurses Association: Promoting Safe Work Environments for Nurses, 2002. (From Occupational Safety and Health Administration (OSHA). (2004). *Guidelines for preventing workplace violence for health care and social service workers* (OSHA Publication No. 3148-01R). Washington, DC: U.S. Department of Labor. [www.osha.gov]).

Interpersonal

Little research has been done on the effectiveness of training staff to anticipate, recognize, and respond to conflict and potential violence in the workplace (see the Research Perspective on p. 511). A recent study of nurses suggests that training is an important factor to help protect their employees. Helping staff to be alert to warning signs of violence and to know how to respond when there are indications of a problem seems to be beneficial. Training about workplace violence prevention will vary according to different employee groups and issues specific to their work environment. Training should be provided to new and current employees, supervisors, and managers. All training should be conducted on a regular basis and cover a variety of topics, including the following:

- The workplace violence prevention policy, including reporting requirements

- Risk factors that can cause or contribute to threats and violence
- Early recognition of warning signs of problematic behavior
- Where appropriate, ways of preventing or defusing volatile situations or aggressive behavior
- Information on cultural diversity to develop sensitivity to racial and ethnic issues and differences
- A standard response action plan for violent situations, including availability of assistance, response to alarm systems, and communication procedures
- The location and operation of safety devices such as alarm systems, along with the required maintenance schedules and procedures
- Ways to protect oneself and co-workers, including use of a buddy system

RESEARCH PERSPECTIVE

Resource: Nachreiner, N., Gerberich, S., Ryan, A., & McGovern, P. (2007). Minnesota Nurses' Study: Perceptions of violence and the work environment. *Industrial Health, 45* (5), 672-678.

In this study, a sample of 6300 randomly selected Minnesota nurses (RN and LPN) working in hospitals, nursing homes, and long-term care facilities were surveyed and asked to describe their experience with work-related violence in the previous year. From the survey data, rates of both physical and non-physical violence were calculated. The annual physical assault rate was 13.2 per 100 nurses. The non-physical violence rate was 38.8. Non-physical violence included threats, sexual harassment, and verbal abuse. Additional findings from the study included a high level of perceived work-related stress but an overall feeling of respect and trust from co-workers and reports of good supervisor support. In contrast, many reported that morale among personnel was poor or fair. As identified in other research studies, when stress and violence interact, the negative effects on staff accumulate. Another finding that was consistent with other research was that nurses tend to perceive violence as just a part of their job. They may rationalize that if they were harmed by a patient, it was caused somehow by poor performance on their part. This perception of violence being part of the job and a lack of awareness or resistance to thinking that nurses are at risk for violence may diminish corrective actions or prevention of such occurrences.

Implication for Practice
Workplace violence is a complex problem for health care. We know that healthcare providers are at high risk because of the nature of their work and their close dealings with patients and their families. We know that nurses may tend to minimize violent behavior because they consider it part of the job. We tolerate some non-physical abuses from patients and from each other for many varied reasons. All of these things contribute to high levels of stress and potential burn out. We must not only look at the stressors on nurses but also consider the ability of organizations to respond to these reports of stressors. This is an important issue to address because violence and stress have been cited as significant reasons that nurses leave the workforce. Understanding the role of workplace violence, interventions tailored to the needs of nurses to prevent it have a more urgent importance as we face a significant nursing shortage in the very near future. Helping nurses feel less stressed and feel safe and supported in their work environment is a key issue for leaders and managers.

- Policies and procedures for reporting and record-keeping
- Policies and procedures for obtaining medical care, counseling, workers' compensation, or legal assistance after a violent episode or injury

Training employees in nonviolent response and conflict resolution has been suggested to reduce the risk that volatile situations will escalate to physical violence. Training that addresses hazards associated with specific tasks or worksites and relevant prevention strategies is also critical. Training should not be regarded as the sole prevention strategy but, instead, as a component in a comprehensive approach to reducing workplace violence. To increase vigilance and compliance with stated violence prevention policies, training should emphasize the appropriate use and maintenance of protective equipment, adherence to administrative controls, and increased knowledge and awareness of the risk of workplace violence.

No matter how thorough or well-conceived, preparation will not be effective in an emergency if no one remembers or implements the plan. Training exercises should be a regular part of the process. Training must include managers and senior executives who will be making decisions in a real incident. Exercises must be followed by careful evaluation with rapid responses that fix whatever weaknesses have been revealed.

EXERCISE 25-3
Look at your organization's workplace safety plan. Does it have a statement about zero tolerance for violent behaviors? Does it include instructions on how to report violent behavior? Has it been updated recently? Based on what you have read, do you think the plan is comprehensive?

Understanding the Potential for Violence

Though violent incidents can occur seemingly without warning, some theories allow us to assess and predict potential occurrences. Research by John Monahan (1981), a psychologist at the University of Virginia Law School, describes basic mental and behavioral cycles and circumstances that can escalate over time into violence. The cycle or spiral has four parts:

1. An individual encounters a stressful event.
2. The individual reactions to the event with certain types of thoughts that are predisposed based on personality.

3. The thoughts lead to emotional responses.
4. These responses in turn determine the behavior used to respond to the situation.

Extreme stress may lead to a belief that violence is the only viable way to cope with the situation or to relieve the stress. The responses of the individuals involved can either de-escalate or escalate the situation, influencing the ultimate outcome. Awareness of this basic pattern can help manage the potential for violent situations. Understand that the individual's perception of the stress is what precipitates the spiral. What seems like a minor issue to you may be a huge event for someone else depending on his or her subjective experience. Things as minor as a change in routine or seemingly small annoyances can be a trigger. The stressful event can become magnified when a person is not sure whether he or she has the resources to successfully respond to the stress. It then becomes important to appraise how a person responds to stressors, how he or she views the situation, and what he or she expects to happen.

If the individual is contemplating an assault, anything that can be done to improve communication and decrease frustration can have a significant impact. At this point, the perpetrator may be struggling to overcome internal barriers to lashing out. Taking advantage of this internal struggle and allowing the person a way to back down without embarrassment can de-escalate the situation. This takes good communications skills that can be taught and rehearsed. Another strategy is to not allow an environment that is conducive to a physical assault. In many cases, an assault will not take place in the presence of other staff, in a public area, or where there are surveillance cameras. If an attack is initiated, the goal is minimization of harm and control of the situation or escape.

Physical attacks often occur after several indicators have pointed toward the potential of violence. Case studies of violent behavior are filled with information that show that people felt threatened, intimidated, or unsafe in the presence of the person who later committed an act of violence. In his book *The Gift of Fear: Survival Signals That Protect Us From Violence*, DeBecker (1997) asserts that fear is an internal warning system, alerting us to potentially threatening situations. In interviews with survivors of violent attacks, they frequently related that they "had a bad

feeling" about the situation or that they knew that something was not right. DeBecker postulates that the "gut feeling" or "intuition" is the result of rapid cognitive processing of a complex web of cues or patterns of behavior that the subconscious brain alerts to before the logical part of the brain has the chance to catch up. Learning to use this awareness has formed the basis for many self-defense and workplace violence trainings. Training on subtle clues as well as day-to-day experience in dealing with a variety of people can add to adeptness in reading situations and recognizing danger. Validating that this fear response is useful may help in situations in which that moment of trying to rationalize the fear can give a perpetrator the edge needed to carry out an attack. The trick is not only to listen to your intuition but also to look for behaviors that predict violence or to provide an opportunity for escape. Many overt cues may predict violence. Body language is the most significant of these cues. These are usually easy to identify and may include standing too close, threatening gestures, tense posture, furtive glances, and rapid or repetitive movements. Being aware of your body language can be a critical factor in keeping a situation from escalating. We are generally aware of the body language of others but may not recognize our own body language.

Assessing behaviors that may precede violence and any other clues about a person's history such as mental illness and drug or alcohol abuse may also help predict violent behavior. Luck, Jackson, and Usher (2007) devised a system that helps identify observable behaviors that indicate the potential for violence. Through their research with emergency department personnel, they created five distinctive elements that portend violent behavior. They use the easily remembered acronym *STAMP* to outline cues for an assessment of the behaviors (Box 25-9).

Often a violent act is preceded by a threat. A threat may be explicit or veiled, spoken or unspoken, specific or vague. It may be an offhanded remark or comments made to people close to the patient or family that may suggest problematic behavior. Detecting threats and/or threatening behavior, evaluating them, and finding a way to address them are important keys to preventing violence. All staff members need to be educated on how to detect threatening behavior and how to report it. All threats should be evaluated to determine when someone is making a

BOX 25-9	STAMP ASSESSMENT COMPONENTS AND CUES

Assessment Component	Assessment Cue
Staring	Prolonged glaring at the nurse while she/he is engaged in nursing practice
Tone and volume of voice	Sharp or caustic retorts Sarcasm Demeaning inflection Increase in volume
Anxiety	Flushed appearance Hyperventilation Rapid speech Dilated pupils Physical indicators of pain: grimacing, writhing, clutching body Confusion and disorientation Expressed lack of understanding about emergency department processes
Mumbling	Talking "under their breath" Criticizing staff or the institution just loudly enough to be heard Repetition of same or similar questions or requests Slurring or incoherent speech
Pacing	Walking around confined areas such as a waiting room or bed space Walking back and forth to the nurses' area Flailing around in bed "Resisting" health care

Adapted from Luck, L., Jackson, D., & Usher, K. (March 2007). STAMP: Components of observable behavior that indicate potential for patient violence in emergency departments. *Journal of Advanced Nursing, 59*(1), 11-19, Blackwell Publishing Ltd.

threat versus posing a threat. In most cases, a threat will not lead to a violent act, but it still requires a response. The goal of threat assessment is to place a threat somewhere on a hierarchy of dangerousness and, on that basis, determine an appropriate intervention (Office of Workforce Relations [OWR], 1998).

Personal Safety Training

You are more likely to survive any life-threatening situation if you confront reality and develop a plan.

This requires preparation and keeping your wits. Frequent training and rehearsal of what to do in a particular situation can help remain clearheaded when fear kicks in. Knowing whom to call, what escape routes are available, and how to defuse violent situations provides readily accessible skills when violent events occur.

Most training on workplace violence prevention is based on basic self-defense techniques that are important for everyone to know. This type of training consists primarily of using common sense and awareness to avoid potentially dangerous situations. Key points are (1) being constantly aware of your surroundings and (2) planning ahead or thinking about potential problems and how you would respond. Knowing how to call for help or memorizing code names for emergency situations is part of this preparation. Assessing work areas for potential security problems and how you might escape if trapped in particular areas is key. Running different scenarios in your head will help you respond more quickly. Assessing how you respond in tense situations can be helpful and provide insight into whether your behavior would escalate a situation. Learning how to project confidence and not being afraid to yell if you need help are also simple self-defense techniques that everyone can use.

Other conflict-management techniques that can be taught include defusing the aggressive individual. This technique is grounded in basic therapeutic communication theory. The goal is to manage situations in which people experience an escalation of emotion that may lead to violence. De-escalation can reduce the level of tension to the point at which the person under stress can regain control and avoid violence. To defuse situations, you must remain rational in the face of the irrational. If the affected person senses you are losing control, it will increase his or her anxiety and loss of control. Understanding how you handle your own stress can influence your ability to effectively de-escalate others. By practicing therapeutic communication techniques, it is possible to more readily access the behaviors so that, in a crisis, you can use your skills without freezing. Most important to remember is that you must look and act calm even if you are not. Helping someone stay calm is often easier if you appear warm and approachable. The person you are de-escalating will notice and take cues from your behaviors, even if he or she is too irrational to hear your words.

People exhibit some identifiable elements of escalation when they become upset. Challenging authority or asking questions that may not seem related to the situation is one common behavior. Another is to refuse or balk when given directions. A person may also temporarily lose some control and use words he or she may not normally use. The agitated person may even become threatening or intimidating. This agitation can rapidly turn life-threatening, so it is important to gain control of the situation quickly. As the situation escalates, you must retain your professionalism. If you become defensive or irrational, the situation only gets worse. It is often easier to react in a professional manner if you are not alone. Using the buddy system can be an easy way to help you retain your professionalism and reduce the chance of injury. Caution must be used when additional people come into an aggressive situation. The aggressor may become more agitated if he or she feels that people are ganging up on him or her. On the other hand, a witness may cause the aggressor to reconsider his or her behavior and regain control. One way to help those who are out of control is to validate or empathize with them. When we empathize with others, we are considering their needs and feelings. Expressing empathy helps the other person feel understood. Often, repeating the *feelings* you hear rather than the *content of what was said* is a good strategy. This can highlight the speaker's concerns and fears and may help him or her begin to mentally process what is happening. This validation is powerful in de-escalating a situation. Keeping a calm tone of voice and a relaxed posture can help an agitated person hear the content of your message. Another way to demonstrate we are in control and responsive is to make sure our words and actions match (are congruent). This means that our words and actions communicate the same thing and form a clear message. For example, nodding and paying attention to the person talking to you is congruent with both sending the message that you would like to hear more and that you are listening. Being incongruent or acting in a way that does not match your words may be interpreted as being untrustworthy or inauthentic. For example, saying "I want to help you" while looking repeatedly at your watch sends a mixed message to the person you are trying to help.

Body language can be used to de-escalate situations. Most communication is nonverbal and involves body language. A basic awareness of body language of people under stress is useful. For example, when someone is upset, his or her personal space tends to increase. The best way to ensure that you are not invading the personal space of others is to stand at an angle to the person rather than face to face, slightly outside his or her personal space (usually about 3 feet or so). Your shoulders should be at about a 90-degree angle to the person to whom you are talking. Keep your arms relaxed and at your sides, and stand with your feet slightly parted. Again, if your body language is aggressive, it may further escalate a situation. You should also be aware of your relationship to an exit. An agitated person may become more aggressive if he or she feels his or her escape from an area is being blocked. You do not want to be the person blocking an exit route if the person does decide to attack. Gender and culture may play into a situation and can influence how you may potentially use eye contact, touching, or head movements. It is also important to assess the body language of potentially violent persons, looking for clues as to what they may do next or when they may become violent. Pounding or clenching fists or pointing fingers may indicate the person is about to physically lash out. If these warning signs are present, it may be time to disengage and find help. If you are the one being threatened, any one of these techniques may buy the time needed to get out. The key is to recognize the signs and take action to de-escalate the situation.

EXERCISE 25-4

Have you ever received training from your employer on workplace violence? Would you feel comfortable asking for training from your manager? What type of training would you want?

After a Violent Event

Violence can and will occur despite best efforts at prevention. Like all violent crime, workplace violence creates ripples that go beyond what is done to a particular victim. It damages trust and the sense of security every worker has a right to feel while on the job. In that sense, everyone loses when a violent act takes place. When it does occur, leaders must be prepared to deal with the consequences by providing an environment that fosters honest communication and support. Lack of commitment in addressing violence can lead to economic loss in the form of high turnover rates, lost work time, damaged employee morale, and reduced productivity. In addition, the organization could face possible legal action from state and federal agencies, increased workers' compensation payments, medical expenses, and possible lawsuits and liability costs. Employees who have been harmed at work in an act of violence should receive assistance with any documentation needed to receive necessary medical care. Psychological and other supportive therapies should be offered, and the victims should avail themselves of these services.

When a violent event occurs, the organization should take immediate action to prevent recurrence. An investigation should always follow any violent event to determine if new emergency procedures need to be implemented and if any existing policies or procedures need to be changed to protect staff. Any staff member involved in a violent incident should be supported and offered counseling. Care should be taken to determine if the problem may be related to underreporting of warning signs. Staff of the affected areas should be involved with the investigation and should be given as much information as possible to ensure that they know that the safety issue is being addressed. Additional training should be offered. Existing training should be evaluated to determine if it addresses current situations. Advice from safety experts should be sought to ensure that interventions are addressing any problem areas. This will help the organization keep abreast of new strategies for dealing with workplace violence as they develop.

EXERCISE 25-5

You have been asked to help an inner-city hospital. The administration staff has advised you that the current safety plan may not be adequate because several incidents have occurred in the hospital in the past year involving violent attacks on staff members. How would you go about conducting an assessment of the facility? What types of things would you look for? What tools would you use to guide your assessment?

Finally, the success of safety interventions should be regularly evaluated. An evaluation program should examine the reporting system for incidents to determine whether problems exist with not identifying situations because of underreporting. Data related to the frequency and severity of workplace violence and the subsequent interventions should be examined along with the outcomes to determine if changes need to be made. Staff surveys before and after implementing safety interventions should be assessed. The question is, Do they believe the intervention made a difference?

Employees have the right to expect a safe work environment, but they are also expected to participate in active prevention through gaining knowledge of safety policies, participating in training, and reporting potential problems. Through communication and attention to problems, organizations can foster a climate of trust and respect among workers and between employees and management. This helps reduce the potential for toxic work environments that can allow horizontal violence to flourish.

SUMMARY

Workplace violence affects us all. Its burden is borne not only by victims of violence but also by their co-workers, their families, their employers, and every worker at risk of violent assault. Although we know that, each year, workplace violence results nationwide in hundreds of deaths, more than 2 million injuries, and billions of dollars in costs, our understanding of workplace violence in health care is still in its infancy. Much remains to be done in the area of research, particularly in data collection and interventions for horizontal violence. Without basic information on who is most affected and which prevention measures are effective in what settings, we can expect only limited success in addressing this problem. The first steps have been taken, but a number of key issues have been identified that require future research. All nurses and healthcare leaders need a broader understanding of the scope and impact of workplace violence to reduce the human and financial burden of this significant public health problem.

THE SOLUTION

It was dark, and I started to panic. I knew he was physically much bigger and stronger than I. At that point, all kinds of things were running through my mind. You always hear people say that if they were in that situation, they would fight, but I froze and felt like I would faint. I never thought a patient would attack me. I had come from a work environment in which no incidents like this occurred. I had a perception that just being a nurse was a shield from anything bad happening. As all these thoughts were racing through my mind, he grabbed me and started trying to put his hands down my pants. I heard a far-away voice calling for help and then realized the voice was mine. Luckily, someone in the office next to the closet heard me call. He opened the door and grabbed the patient by his shoulders and dragged him out of the closet. He started asking the patient what he was doing. At that point, the patient became very frightened. In a whirlwind, I recall security coming to control the patient, and before I knew it, the social worker was taking me to the charge nurse's office. They made sure I was not injured and asked what had happened. I did not have any physical injuries but I was pretty shaken. The police were called, and a report was filed. I had to go to the police station to give a statement. After that, I went home. I asked for a few days off because I had to think about whether I could return to that job. I struggled with my thoughts and emotions, and I did go back to work. Most of the staff were supportive when I returned, but I was surprised to find out that some of my co-workers were rather cavalier about the event, saying that I should have known better than to let the patient go with me and that I wasn't physically hurt, so it was no big deal. That was hurtful, but

it made me realize that I may have been naïve about things that were apparent to them based on their years of experience. That incident changed the way I look at all things in my day-to-day work. I know not to be blocked from an exit. I know the kinds of patients who may turn violent. When I get that "hair raised on the back of my neck" feeling, I pay attention to it. I am not afraid to ask for help if I feel there is any risk of violence. I wanted to share this story, I hope, to spare someone else the same experience. The main thing is never assume a patient won't hurt you. I would have benefitted from safety training during my orientation to the ED because that was something I had never experienced in my previous work. After the incident, a large window was installed in that closet so it was not dark and people passing by could see in. Ultimately, charges were filed against the patient. When the case came up and the police talked to me about testifying, I was not sure if I wanted to pursue the issue. The patient had been mentally ill and was not in control. I felt that I was supposed to be taking care of him, not prosecuting him. They told me he did have previous charges for aggressive incidents and a charge of rape. Ultimately, I did testify and the patient was sentenced to 7 years in prison. I reconcile the conflict I felt with the understanding that his incarceration would prevent someone else being harmed.

—*Lori Jeffries*

Would this be a suitable approach for you? Why?

THE EVIDENCE

Workplace violence is recognized as a significant problem within health care. Reviews of nursing literature indicate that violence in the workplace is a significant reason why many nurses leave their jobs and, in some cases, the profession of nursing. With growing concern about a nursing shortage, nurse leaders need to implement effective intervention programs that can foster a healthier workplace. Education and training have been the main interventions used in the past, but little research has been done to evaluate their effectiveness. In a study by Oostrom and van Mierlo (2008), the aim was to evaluate the effectiveness of an aggression management training program. A three-part training program was offered to voluntary participants. The program consisted of a variety of

teaching methods. The participants were asked to complete a questionnaire developed to evaluate the training. Based on a principal component analysis, two separate scales were constructed: insight into assertiveness and aggression and ability to cope with adverse working situations. The results of the study showed considerable and significant improvement on both scales. The improvements persisted after the training and indicated an enduring change in knowledge and behavior. The participants' scores on ability to cope showed further increase after the training. From the finding, the researchers concluded that aggression management training may be an effective instrument in the fight against workplace violence.

- Know how to access the workplace safety plan in your area of practice.
- Be aware of your surroundings at all times, keeping in mind that you are at increased risk for violence.

- Use the STAMP assessment tool to help you identify behaviors that predict violence.
- Practice what to say to stop workplace bullying.

CHAPTER CHECKLIST

This chapter focused on two kinds of workplace violence: physical attacks and bullying. Nursing research indicates violence in any form can drain nurses of their enthusiasm for their work and undermines efforts to create a satisfied workforce. At a time when we are facing a nursing shortage, it is imperative to prevent or eliminate violence from health care. All nurses—leaders, managers, and followers—must be aware of the potential for all forms of violence and strive to not participate in horizontal violence, which weakens us as a profession. The key to preventing violence is understanding the potential for it and implementing interventions to minimize that potential.

Key organizations calling for action to reduce workplace violence include the following:
- OSHA
- NIOSH
- American Nurses Association
- International Council of Nurses
- Institute for Safe Medication Practices
- The Joint Commission
- International Nurses

Organizations need to allocate time and resources to develop and maintain a workplace safety and violence prevention program. The basic steps in accomplishing this goal are as follows:
- Conducting a comprehensive safety risk assessment
- Prioritizing problems and interventions
- Writing a plan that includes a zero tolerance policy for violence

- Developing a reporting plan
- Instituting a multidisciplinary committee to update and maintain the plan, as well as document and analyze problems and develop solutions
- Implementing administrative, environmental, and interpersonal measures and strategies to prevent violence
- Planning and delivering training related to safety based on the individual needs of different departments
- Providing support for victims of violence including appropriate investigation and corrective measures
- Evaluating the effectiveness of the safety plan

Organizational leaders can implement strategies to reduce workplace violence to promote a positive workplace culture. This includes the following:
- Surveying staff to identify problems
- Implementing innovative interventions to rid the workplace of bullying
- Ensuring non-retaliation for reporting of horizontal violence
- Enforcing zero tolerance policies
- Providing training on violence prevention
- Promoting honest, open communication and an atmosphere of trust

Nurses, nurse leaders, and administrators must invest time and resources to prevent nurses from leaving the profession because of workplace violence.

More research is needed to identify effective interventions to prevent violence in health care.

TIPS FOR PREVENTING WORKPLACE VIOLENCE

- Take a self-defense course to help you develop other skills to keep you safe at work and elsewhere.
- Take advantage of training offered on workplace violence. If training is not offered, ask your employer to consider providing it.

- Make a personal commitment to not participate in any behaviors that perpetuate horizontal violence.
- Practice precautionary strategies such as the STAMP assessment.
- Analyze workplaces for safety risk factors using the checklists provided by OSHA.

REFERENCES

American Nurses Association (ANA). (November 23, 2009). *Workplace violence.* Retrieved April 14, 2010, from www.nursingworld.org/MainMenuCategories/ANAPoliticalPower/State/StateLegislativeAgenda/WorkplaceViolence.aspx.

Bureau of Labor Statistics, U.S. Department of Labor. (2006). *Workplace injuries and illnesses in 2006.* USDL 07-1562. Retrieved October 28, 2009, from www.bls.gov/iif/home.htm.

Bureau of Labor Statistics, U.S. Department of Labor. (2007). *Workplace injuries and illnesses in 2007.* USDL 08-1498. Retrieved March 22, 2009, from www.bls.gov/news.release/pdf/osh.pdf.

Center for American Nurses. (2008). *Policy statement on lateral violence and bullying in the workplace.* Author. Approved February 2008. Retrieved July 2010 from http://centerforamericannurses.com/associations/9102/files/Position%20StatementLateral%20/Violence%20and%20Bullying.pdf.

DeBecker, G. (1997). *The gift of fear: survival signals that protect us from violence.* New York: Little, Brown and Co.

Dellasega, C. (2009). Bullying among nurses. *American Journal of Nursing, 109*(1), 52-58.

Farrell, G. (1997). Aggression in clinical settings: Nurses' views. *Journal of Advanced Nursing, 25*(3), 501-508.

Farrell, G. (2001). From tall poppies to squashed weeds: Why don't nurses pull together more? *Journal of Advanced Nursing, 35*(1), 26-33.

Gallant-Roman, M. (2008). Strategies and tools to reduce workplace violence. *AAOHN: official journal of the American Association of Occupational Health Nurses, 56*(11), 449-454.

Griffin, M. (2004). Teaching cognitive rehearsal as a shield for lateral violence: An intervention for newly licensed nurses. *Journal of Continuing Education in Nursing, 35*(6), 257-263.

Hader, R. (2008). Workplace violence survey 2008. *Nursing Management, 39*(7), 13-19.

Hartley, D., Biddle, E., & Jenkins, E. (2005). *Societal costs of workplace homicides in the United States, 1992-2001.* Morgantown, WV: National Institute for Occupational Safety and Health, Division of Safety Research.

Hutchinson, M., Vickers, M., Jackson D., & Wilkes, L. (2006). Workplace bullying in nursing: Towards a more critical organizational perspective. *Nursing Inquiry, 15*, 118-126.

Institute for Safe Medication Practices. (2003). *Survey on workplace intimidation.* Retrieved October 28, 2009, from www.ismp.org/Survey/surveyresults/Survey0311.asp.

International Council of Nurses (ICN). (2006). *Abuse and violence against nursing personnel.* ICN Position Statement. Retrieved October 28, 2009, from www.icn.ch/psviolence00.htm.

Johnson, S. (2009). Workplace bullying: Concerns for nurse leaders. *Journal of Nursing Administration, 39*(2), 84-90.

Longo, J. (2007). Leveling horizontal violence. *Nursing Management, 38*(3), 34-37, 50-51.

Luck, L., Jackson, D., & Usher, K. (March 2007). STAMP: Components of observable behavior that indicate potential for patient violence in emergency departments. *Journal of Advanced Nursing, 59*(1), 11-19.

Monahan, J. (1981). *Predicting violent behavior: An assessment of clinical techniques.* Beverly Hills, CA: Sage.

Nachreiner, N., Gerberich, S., McGovern, P., Church, T., Hansen, H., Geisser, M., & Ryan, A. (2005). Impact of training on work-related assault. *Research in Nursing & Health, 28*(1), 67-78.

Nachreiner, N., Gerberich, S., Ryan, A., & McGovern, P. (2007). Minnesota Nurses' Study: Perceptions of violence and the work environment. *Industrial Health, 45*(5), 672-678.

National Institute for Occupational Safety and Health (NIOSH). (2002). *Violence: Occupational hazards in hospitals (NIOSH Publication No. 2002-2101).* Washington, DC: U.S. Department of Health and Human Services, Public Health Service, Centers for Disease Control and Prevention. Retrieved October 28, 2009, from www.cdc.gov/niosh/docs/2002-101/.

Occupational Safety and Health Administration (OSHA). (2004). *Guidelines for preventing workplace violence for health care and social service workers* (OSHA Publication No. 3148-01R). Washington, DC: U.S. Department of Labor.

Occupational Safety & Health Act (OSH Act). (1970). Public Law 91-596, 84 STAT. 1590, Section 5. 91st Congress, S.2193, December 29, 1970, as amended through January 1, 2004.

Office of Workforce Relations (OWR), OWR-09. (February 1998). *Dealing with workplace violence: A guide for agency planners.* Washington, DC: U.S. Office of Personnel Management.

Oostrom, J., & van Mierlo, H. (2008). An evaluation of an aggression management training program to cope with workplace violence in the healthcare sector. *Research in Nursing & Health, 31*, 320-328.

Paludi, M., Nydegger, R., & Paludi, C. (2006). *Understanding workplace violence: A guide for managers and employees.* Westport, Connecticut: Praeger Publishers.

Pearson, C., & Porath, C. (2009). *The cost of bad behavior: How incivility is damaging your business and what to do about it.* London: Portfolio.

The Joint Commission. (July 9, 2008). Behaviors that undermine a culture of safety. *Sentinel Event Alert, 40.* Retrieved October 28, 2009, from www.jointcommission.org/SentinelEvents/SentinelEventAlert/sea_40.htm.

Woelfle, C., & McCaffrey, R. (2007). Nurse on nurse. *Nursing Forum, 42*(3), 123-131.

Workplace Violence Research Institute. (1995). The cost of workplace violence to American businesses. Retrieved October 28, 2009, from www.workviolence.com/articles/cost_of_workplace_violence.htm.

SUGGESTED READINGS

American Nurses Association (ANA). (2004). *Occupational safety and health.* Retrieved April 14, 2010, from http://www.nursingworld.org/MainMenuCategories/ANAMarketplace/ANAPeriodicals/OJIN/TableofContents/Volume92004/No3Sept04/ViolenceinHealthCare.aspx.

American Nurses Association (ANA). (2002). *Preventing workplace violence.* Retrieved October 28, 2009, from www.nursingworld.org/MainMenuCategories/OccupationalandEnvironmental/occupationalhealth/workplaceviolence/ANAResources/PreventingWorkplaceViolence.aspx.

Corporate Alliance to End Partner Violence. Retrieved October 28, 2009, from www.caepv.org.getinfo/facts_stats.php

Occupational Safety and Health Administration (OSHA). (2002). *Fact sheet: Workplace violence.* Retrieved October 28, 2009, from www.osha.gov/OshDoc/data_General_Facts/factsheet-workplace-violence.pdf.

Family Violence Prevention Fund (FVPF). *Domestic violence in the workplace.* Retrieved October 28, 2009, from http://endabuse.org/programs/workplace/.

Federal Bureau of Investigation. (2004). *Workplace violence: Issues in response.* Retrieved October 28, 2009, from www.fbi.gov/publications/violence.pdf.

National Institute for Occupational Safety and Health (NIOSH), CDC. *Occupational violence.* Retrieved October 28, 2009, from www.cdc.gov/niosh/topics/violence/.

National Institute for Occupational Safety and Health (NIOSH). (1995). *Preventing homicide in the workplace.* Retrieved October 28, 2009, from www.cdc.gov/niosh/homicide.html.

National Institute of Occupational Safety and Health (NIOSH). (1996). *Violence in the workplace: Risk factors and prevention strategies.* Retrieved October 28, 2009, from www.cdc.gov/niosh/violcont.html.

National Institute for Occupational Safety and Health (NIOSH). (2002). *Violence: Occupational hazards in hospitals.*

Retrieved October 28, 2009, from www.cdc.gov/niosh/docs/2002-101/.

National Institute for Occupational Safety and Health (NIOSH). (2004). *Violence on the job.* Retrieved October 28, 2009, from www.cdc.gov/niosh/docs/video/violence.html.

National Institute of Occupational Safety and Health (NIOSH). (2004). *Worker health chartbook, 2004.* Retrieved October 28, 2009, from www.cdc.gov/niosh/docs/2004-146/.

Occupational Safety & Health Administration (OSHA), U.S. Department of Labor. *Workplace violence.* Retrieved October 28, 2009, from www.osha.gov/SLTC/workplaceviolence.

Occupational Safety & Health Administration (OSHA). (2002). *Hospital eTool.* Retrieved October 28, 2009, from www.osha.gov/SLTC/etools/hospital/index.html.

Occupational Safety & Health Administration (OSHA). (2004). *Guidelines for preventing workplace violence for health care and social service workers.* Retrieved October 28, 2009, from www.osha.gov/Publications/osha3148.pdf.

Safe@Work Coalition. Domestic violence in the workplace. Retrieved April 14, 2010, from http://www.safeatworkcoalition.org/dv/whatisdv.htm.

U.S. Department of Justice, Bureau of Justice Statistics. (2001). *Violence in the workplace: 1993-1999.* Retrieved October 28, 2009, from www.ojp.usdoj.gov/bjs/pub/pdf/vw99.pdf.

U.S. Office of Personnel Management (USOPM). (1998). *Dealing with workplace violence: A guide for agency planners.* Retrieved October 28, 2009, from www.opm.gov/Employment_and_Benefits/WorkLife/OfficialDocuments/handbooksguides/WorkplaceViolence/index.asp.

U.S. Office of Personnel Management (USOPM). (2003). *A manager's handbook: Handling traumatic events.* Retrieved October 28, 2009, from www.opm.gov/Employment_and_Benefits/WorkLife/OfficialDocuments/handbooksguides/Trauma/index.asp.

Delegation: An Art of Professional Practice

Patricia S. Yoder-Wise

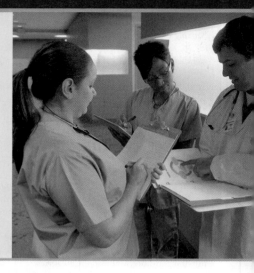

Delegation is a complex process that can be quite effective in accomplishing work. Registered nurses who work in settings where there are other members of the nursing staff are likely to face this task daily. This chapter defines various aspects of delegation, including legal perspectives and how to make delegation decisions. The emphasis is on the role of the nurse as delegator, irrespective of the formal position an individual may hold.

OBJECTIVES

- Define *delegation* and its component parts.
- Evaluate how tasks and relationships influence delegation to a specific individual.
- Comprehend the legal authority for a registered nurse to delegate.
- Value the complexity of decision making related to delegation.

TERMS TO KNOW

accountability	delegation	responsibility
delegatee	delegator	unlicensed nursing personnel

Cindy Joy-McCoy, BSN, RN
Director of Emergency Nursing Services, University Medical Center Brackenridge, Austin, Texas

All emergency departments (EDs) receive trauma patients at one level or another. Outlying EDs often receive trauma patients who are critical and are brought there as the first place for treatment. They are brought by emergency medical services (EMS) and by family members. Many level 3 and level 4 trauma centers have limited resources, so their challenge is to stabilize and transfer these patients to the closest level 1 trauma center. They also get "walk-ins" who have a laceration or broken bone that needs attention and can be more serious than it appears. Level 1 and level 2 trauma centers have their challenges also, because they need to use their resources to the maximum to provide the best care to those patients.

All of our hospitals use ED technicians. Recently we created a new classification for trauma technicians to provide a promotional opportunity for the ED technicians, who are not licensed and are more skilled than the traditional nursing assistants. To work in trauma situations, these technicians need specific skills. This mix of licensed staff (predominantly registered nurses) and unlicensed staff (the two levels of technicians) can be confusing in emergency situations in which everyone is supposed to respond to any event. Everyone has to be clear about what can be delegated to someone else and what cannot. We had to be sure the unlicensed staff members were trained sufficiently to participate at high levels without exceeding their designated role.

What do you think you would do if you were this nurse?

INTRODUCTION

Delegation is a complex, convoluted, work-enhancing strategy. It can make the difference between caring for a group of patients and experiencing great anxiety and caring for that same group with a controlled expectation of what can be achieved. Used properly, delegation can enlarge the effect you have on patient care; used improperly, it can be frustrating and scary. Delegation is an art and a skill that can be developed and honed into one of the most effective professional management strategies any registered nurse can use. Each of the following sections is designed to foster the best of delegation.

HISTORICAL PERSPECTIVE

Until the early 1970s, registered nurses (RNs) were quite familiar with the art of delegation. Most care occurred in acute care hospitals, which were staffed by RNs (mostly diploma graduates, frequently prepared in the hospital in which they worked), licensed practical/vocational nurses (LPNs/LVNs), and nurse aides (commonly called *unlicensed assistive personnel* or unlicensed nursing personnel, or *UAPs* or *UNPs*, today). Note that the term *unlicensed nursing personnel* is used to distinguish those for whom nurses are accountable as opposed to the numerous unlicensed

assistive personnel providing aid in other clinical disciplines. Team nursing was used, and staffing ratios were such that it was not uncommon for relatively few RNs to be present on a nursing unit. Much of the direct care was provided by LPNs/LVNs and aides. Of course, because there were few complex procedures, the direct care provided was related primarily to physical comfort and to what today would be called *simple treatments.*

As care became far more intricate and monitoring demands and expectations placed on nursing increased, moving to a higher ratio of RNs was logical. Thus, during the 1970s and 1980s, many nurses entered the profession with relatively limited experience or knowledge about the details of delegation—no one was in the clinical area to whom one could delegate anything related to patient care except the basic physical care. Sometimes the professional staff even dealt with that.

In the mid-1990s, a dramatic shift from primary nursing (an all-professional staff concept) to a multi-level nursing staff occurred. As a result, addressing the topic of delegation in some detail became critical to safe care. This return, however, was not to delegation as it was known earlier. In part, the difference today is based on the sophisticated demand for cost containment and reduction and the new complexities that are present in health care. As the healthcare industry emphasizes community-based care, the challenge of delegation and the resultant supervision become even more difficult. The increase, especially in UNPs, related in the past to a shortage of nurses. An even more dramatic one is predicted over the next several years, rising to a predicted need of 500,000 more RNs by 2025 (Buerhaus, 2009). Therefore, in addition to the supply of nurses and healthcare cost-control measures, the role of the RN will change to meet the increasing demands for care. Nursing's flexibility to alter how we function based on the changes we find has allowed nursing to survive and sometimes thrive. The consistent element, irrespective of how we function, is care.

During the early part of the twenty-first century, both the National Council of State Boards of Nursing (NCSBN) and the American Nurses Association (ANA) became increasingly concerned about the quality of delegation decisions. The NCSBN stated it believes that "state boards of nursing should regulate nursing assistive personnel" (NCSBN, 2005, p. 160). This means that it believes the current approach in many states of having certified nursing assistants regulated through the health or hospital division of the state no longer meets the needs of nursing. In addition, the NCSBN has added an expectation that basic training for nursing assistive personnel includes an emphasis on the concepts related to how to receive delegation. The ANA (2005) focused on the principles of delegation that an RN must use. Together they created a joint statement on delegation to guide nurses in their practice (Joint Statement, 2009). Basically, the statement acknowledges that the authority for delegation resides within the nursing practice act of each state, acknowledges the value of unlicensed personnel in meeting patient needs, and acknowledges that decisions should be made based on protection of the health, safety, and welfare of the public. In addition, the statement identifies that the decision to delegate tasks is based on a variety of complex factors such as the patient's condition, the complexity of the task, and the predictability of outcomes.

Although it is apparent that nursing's need to delegate work will likely increase across the spectrum of care, content related to how to perform this task remains limited in schools of nursing, especially related to community settings. According to a report from the Nursing Executive Center of The Advisory Board Company (2008) of 36 competencies surveyed, nursing school leaders reported that they spent 1.8% of their instruction time teaching delegation. Of the six items with scores that tied this percentage or represented a lesser time, several related to delegation. For example, conflict resolution also represented 1.8% of the time, and conducting appropriate follow-up and ability to accept constructive criticism represented 1.7% and 1.6%, respectively. Although registered nurses do not supervise all unlicensed assistive personnel (e.g., physical therapy technicians), they often have exchanges with unlicensed nursing personnel and LPNs/LVNs. Further, only 10% of frontline leaders identified new graduates as proficient in delegation of tasks. Gaining experience and confidence in this important skill can enhance success early in the profession.

Delegation can be further complicated by multiple cultural factors such as ethnicity, age, and gender. Although it might be possible to speak in generalities about each of those factors (e.g., saying men are better leaders than women), various studies have shown commonalities across these cultural differences. For example, Deal (2007) identified that there are differences among employees based on age. Younger generations, for instance, tend to morph rules to fit their logic, whereas the traditional generation follows the details of the rules. Although these generational differences exist, the differences tend to be in demonstrated behavior. The values tend to be comparable across generations.

DEFINITION

Delegate, or *delegation,* is defined in multiple ways. However, consistent elements can be found in each definition. Each definition calls for at least two people (a delegator and a delegatee), work, and some kind of transfer of authority and responsibility to perform the work. No definition suggests it is an abdication of accountability for the overall outcomes or performance or the abdication of the need to be involved. This is an important point because remaining in touch with others who are completing work on behalf of a delegator is sometimes difficult. Figure 26-1 shows that accountability remains fixed and that some portion of work is transferred along with the authority and responsibility for that delegated work.

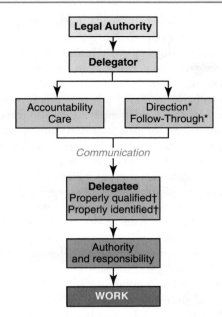

```
        ┌─────────────────┐
        │  Legal Authority │
        └────────┬────────┘
                 ▼
        ┌─────────────────┐
        │    Delegator     │
        └────────┬────────┘
         ┌───────┴────────┐
         ▼                ▼
┌──────────────┐  ┌──────────────────┐
│ Accountability│  │    Direction*    │
│     Care      │  │ Follow-Through*  │
└──────────────┘  └──────────────────┘

          Communication

        ┌─────────────────────┐
        │     Delegatee        │
        │ Properly qualified†  │
        │ Properly identified† │
        └──────────┬──────────┘
                   ▼
        ┌─────────────────────┐
        │     Authority        │
        │  and responsibility  │
        └──────────┬──────────┘
                   ▼
        ┌─────────────────────┐
        │        WORK          │
        └─────────────────────┘
```

*Two common failures identified by Standing, Anthony, and
Hertz (2001).
†Two key recommendations by Fagin (2001).

FIGURE 26-1 A delegation framework: delegation to achieve care outcomes.

The importance of communication suggests that it must be constant to ensure basic, safe care. In fact, as tragic as Hurricane Katrina was when it struck in August 2005, critical healthcare lessons emerged. "Communication was the most critical factor in the determination to evacuate and the ease with which that process was completed" (McGlown, O'Connor, & Shewchuk, 2009, p. 277). Communication must be timely, often redundant, and reliable.

A definition of *delegation,* therefore, might be as follows: achieving performance of care outcomes for which you are accountable and responsible by sharing activities with other individuals who have the appropriate authority to accomplish the work. Acceptance of the delegated work must occur, either passively (i.e., no protest occurs) or actively (i.e., communication indicates acceptance). Therefore delegation can occur only when two people are involved in a mutual work situation and one of the persons has accountability and the other has some authority for perform-

ing specific tasks. When two RNs work together sharing activities, delegation does not occur. However, if one RN has specific accountability for an outcome and that nurse asks another RN to perform a specific component of the overall function, that is delegation (see the "Assignment versus Delegation" section on p. 527 for further information).

The terms *delegators* and *delegatees* represent the two key roles enacted in a delegation situation. *Delegators* are registered nurses who convey a portion of a patient's care to another person. *Delegatees* comprise licensed practical/vocational nurses and unlicensed personnel, which may be referred to as aides, assistants or technicians.

Delegation occurs when an RN assigns an LPN/LVN or UNP to perform a specific function or aspect of care. The term *UNP* incorporates a variety of workers, such as nursing assistants, orderlies, nurse associates, and patient care assistants. This role, as the word *assistive* conveys, provides help to the registered nurse who is accountable for care. Most UNPs today are prepared in some formal program, but that program may range from less than a week to several weeks. Consistency in preparation and job descriptions for UNPs is lacking! The NCSBN *(www.ncsbn. org)* has expressed concern about preparation inconsistency and suggests that programs and UNPs both need greater public accountability.

The RN needs to be aware of the qualifications needed by a delegatee to perform safely. Authority is a critical component. It may be designated by law, such as the nursing practice act, or it may be designated by educational preparation/certification. Typically, a position description further defines what the nature of the authority is for a specific position. Knowing someone's abilities is critical to successful delegation—that is true for both the delegator and the delegatee.

Although the study is fairly old, Standing, Anthony, and Hertz (2001) found the two most common errors associated with poor patient outcomes related to (1) giving improper directions and (2) providing improper follow-through of agency protocol. These findings suggest that communication and agency protocols are crucial to achieving positive performance outcomes. Examples of improper directions could include not indicating when to report important findings or not alerting the delegatee to what the important findings might be. Examples of improper follow-through of agency protocol might be found when the delegator fails to validate findings that are not anticipated or when the delegator encourages the individual to perform functions beyond the stated position description for the delegatee. In addition, failure of the delegatee to report findings is an example of failure to follow through.

Achieving Outcomes

Achieving performance outcomes is the driving force of all health care. If what someone does has little or no benefit in improving the delivery of care, it is, of course, ineffective. Therefore all care is based on attaining expected outcomes, whether that care is provided directly by an individual or group of professionals or whether that care was shared between professionals and assistants. Performance of care outcomes relates to the profession's keeping its trust with the public, that is, to perform safely and competently. Standing et al. (2001) suggest that negative outcomes seem more related to delegation situations in which the nurse is less experienced in practice and the UNP is less experienced in a specific setting. In ever-changing healthcare settings, it is critical to know that you must delegate to achieve all that is expected of you. In essence, this means that if you cannot trust others or if you are frustrated because you cannot do it all yourself, you will be very frustrated with the way in which health care is delivered and your career opportunities will be fairly limited.

Learning about another and developing trust are critical to success. Lencioni, in what is now an established, classic publication (2002), cites lack of trust as the number-one dysfunction of a team. Comfortable, confident delegation requires considerable trust to function as a smooth pairing. Hansten (2008) pointed out that few nurses planned specific times to check with assistive personnel and thus much time was spent looking for each other. She recommends a minimum number of checks being done before and after breaks and meals.

Accountability and Responsibility

The terms *accountability* and *responsibility* refer to the legal expectation the state has vested in persons with the designation of RN. *Accountability* means that someone must be able to explain actions and results.

Legally, the RN is accountable for nursing care. *Responsibility* refers to reliability, dependability, and obligation to accomplish work. It also refers to each person's obligation to perform at an acceptable level. Thus assistants, whether UNPs or LPNs/LVNs, are obligated to perform that which they can at acceptable quality levels. Those individuals are also responsible for informing the delegator what limitations, if any, would prevent the accomplishment of expected outcomes. The *Code of Ethics for Nurses*, Provision 4 (ANA, 2008), identifies the expectation of accountability and responsibility and makes specific reference to delegation. For example, even when some portion of care is delegated to someone else, each individual nurse is accountable and responsible for his or her practice, including the decision to delegate and the outcome of the delegated tasks.

Organizational accountability is another aspect. Making solid decisions depends on how well the organization provides adequate resources, including appropriate staffing and mix. Organizations that function in positive ways, such as Magnet™ organizations, typically have supportive environments that help teams function effectively. The NCSBN concurs with the ANA that the driving principle in decision making is patient (public) safety.

Sharing Activities

Sharing activities may sound simplistic; however, when someone with the legal accountability for a role shares tasks, that individual is not giving away those tasks. In essence, sharing does not negate the nurse's accountability for the total care. So, when delegating, the nurse is merely sharing activities or functions to ensure total outcomes. The delegation definition emphasizes that care itself is not delegated—only tasks (activities) are. Thus accountability rests with the delegator. Sharing may consist of many strategies ranging from asking an assistant to perform a specific task to expecting the same performance as the day before. For delegation to be effective, the RN must accept that sharing activities is important and benefits patient care. Professional aspects of care may never be delegated—only basic skills (frequently thought of as daily living/personal hygiene activities). In addition, some monitoring/technical skills may be delegated. Some organizations provide a two-level or three-level approach to UNP positions, with each level allowing more skills to be performed. In the future, we might anticipate that more, rather than fewer, skills might be delegated to others as the stability and predictability of those skills increase and the need to assist nurses in more ways increases.

Span of Control

The registered nurse may have responsibility for a group of people who work as part of the team he or she leads. Those people may include persons with no formal preparation or recognition (e.g., unit secretary), those with dependent status (e.g., LPNs/LVNs who function under the direction of a physician or RN), or others who are designated as being accountable to the delegator (e.g., other RNs or healthcare providers who report to a designated delegator, such as a nurse manager).

Span of control is an important concept to keep in mind when interacting with others to achieve care. This term refers to how many people for whom you have responsibility. For example, if a nurse has responsibility for 5 staff members, each of whom cares for 10 patients, the nurse, in effect, has responsibility for 5 staff members *and* 50 patients. This may not be as overwhelming as it may seem at first if the patients are in stable condition and their needs are predictable; if the staff are well-prepared, experienced providers of routine care; and if the geographic area is restricted. On the other hand, if any of these factors is lacking, this responsibility may be overwhelming, even if each staff member provides care for only 5 patients. Thus, if others render elements of care, multiple factors must be assessed to determine how manageable the situation is.

Appropriate Authority

Appropriate authority to perform certain functions stems from various sources. For example, the practice of LPNs/LVNs is defined by state titling or practice acts, as well as by institutional policies. UNPs, such as certified nursing assistants, are prepared to meet a specific set of functions. As mentioned, the preparation of UNPs varies considerably. That preparation, coupled with institutional policies, defines what UNPs may do. Position descriptions may provide more specific insight about the authority designated in certain positions. These elements—the titling or practice acts, position descriptions, and policies—form the expectations for what individuals in certain categories are expected to be able to do.

All organizations have descriptors of what tasks may be performed by someone in a particular position. When a position description contains functions that are normally performed or are believed to be an essential part of the practice of a licensed person (e.g., physician, nurse, pharmacist), the person performing in that role is doing so through a passive delegation act. There is, in essence, no active decision being made by the RN in determining what to delegate or to whom. When active delegation occurs, the RN assesses the situation, determines what is best for patient care, directs a UNP to perform certain tasks, and holds the person accountable. Even when organizational protocols indicate that someone else may perform a task on behalf of the RN, the employee must be competent to perform the tasks. This expectation suggests that the delegator will make initial and ongoing assessments related to the delegatee's performance in addition to assessment of patients and their needs. Furthermore, state laws governing the practice of professional nursing typically define what the RN must do when someone else assumes certain tasks.

A FRAMEWORK FOR DELEGATION

In addition to the framework laid out in Figure 26-1, another way to consider the concept of delegation can be found in Hersey and Blanchard's (1988) original work about leadership style (see the Theory Box on p. 526). Although the terms have changed in subsequent revisions, the key concepts have not. These researchers explained followership behavior in the context of two factors: ability and willingness. Both factors relate to specific situations. *Ability* relates to knowledge and skills; *willingness* relates to attitude. Thus, if a delegatee indicates reluctance to perform some work, the delegator assumes more control of the situation to determine whether knowledge is lacking; whether there is some psychomotor interference with performing the work; or whether the delegatee is bored, anxious, or upset and thus unwilling to meet the expectations of the situation. The less able or willing the delegatee is in a situation, the more involvement is needed from the delegator. This theory was not designed for application to delegation, but

THEORY BOX

Situational Theory

THEORY/CONTRIBUTOR	KEY IDEAS	APPLICATION TO PRACTICE
Hersey and Blanchard (1988) created this theory to explain how leaders/managers need to behave differently.	A wise leader analyzes how an individual interacts in a specific situation. The analysis consists of the sophistication of the employee and the task itself and the need for interaction. A leader then responds accordingly based on this analysis.	Treating people equally is unfair. Before delegating, an RN must know what a specific employee needs in a specific situation.

TABLE 26-1 COMMUNICATING WITH A DELEGATEE

CONDITION FOR THE DELEGATEE	RELEVANCE TO DELEGATOR	TERMINOLOGY	CLINICAL EXAMPLE
Has limited knowledge and ability to perform the task	Requires more guidance	Tell (if the relationship is not going to be ongoing)	"Take his blood pressure every 15 minutes."
Has ongoing relationship, new task	Requires explanation	Sell	"Here is what you need to do; in fact, let me show you what is necessary."
Has willingness and ability, but the relationship is new	Requires that both create mutual expectations and conditions of performance	Participate	"Tell me how you go about performing this procedure, and I will share with you my expectations about how frequently and under what conditions we need to report to each other."
Has established relationship and expertise	Little guidance is needed	Delegate	"I know you know what you are doing and when to report, and just remember that I am available to you at any time an issue or concern arises. Thanks for being part of my team."

many nurses find it helpful as they make delegation decisions.

The original research about the follower's relationship with the leader focused on how the two interacted. To simplify how nurses use the model in clinical settings, Table 26-1 presents the conditions for the delegatee, the meaning for the delegator, the original terminology, and a clinical example related to how communication might be structured.

EXERCISE 26-1

Ask three staff nurses what their top three assessment factors for delegatees are. Compare these cited factors to determine any commonalities among the lists.

So, what strategy does the delegator use to interact with a delegatee? In essence, the greater the ability and willingness of the delegatee is, the more likely it is that the delegator could use the strategy of delegation as the strategy for interacting with that person in a specific situation. In other words, both the amount of guidance (task behavior) and the amount of support (relationship behavior) would be relatively low. This seems logical for established work relationships. However, not all situations are established.

Delegation can be viewed as a spectrum of behaviors based on the context and needs in a specific situation. Knowing how to interact with a given delegatee is one of the key challenges of a delegator if effective outcomes are desired.

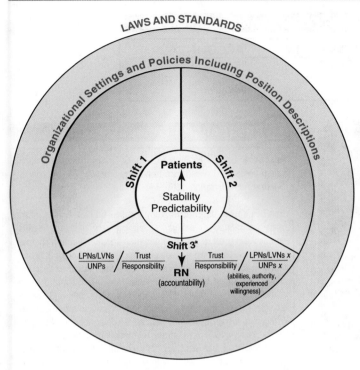

FIGURE 26-2 Delegation framework.

x = Number of LPN/LVNs and UNPs working with a specific RN.
*Repeated for other shifts.

Figure 26-2 integrates the various considerations for delegation. Each registered nurse has assistants available during a designated shift. Mutual trust and shared responsibility must exist between the registered nurse and the assistants, and their focus is on the patients at the center of the model. The registered nurse retains accountability for the patient and considers each assistant's abilities, authority, experiences, and willingness in relation to various patient care tasks to meet the needs of the patient. This decision process occurs in light of organizational settings and policies and the broader legal and standard perspective.

ASSIGNMENT VERSUS DELEGATION

Two meanings are attributed to the term *assignment.* The most common meaning refers to the work each person is to accomplish in a designated work period. This assignment consists of patient care expectations and unit-related activities, which may include such aspects as learning activities, regulation activities, and unit-management activities. The second meaning relates to assignment as the transference of both responsibility and accountability. This strategy is most common when one RN assigns a patient to another RN. Although nurses typically refer to the way work is distributed as an assignment, in reality, some portions of the work distribution are delegated care, not assigned. Thus UNPs receive delegated activities, whereas RNs receive assigned care/assignments. When an RN assigns care to another RN, both accountability and responsibility are transferred. When an RN delegates care to someone such as a

TABLE 26-2	DELEGATION VERSUS ASSIGNMENT	
ASPECT	**RESPONSIBILITY**	**ACCOUNTABILITY**
Delegation	Yes	No
Assignment	Yes	Yes

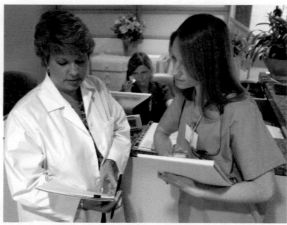

Nursing managers face complex decisions with delegation involving patients and staff.

UNP, responsibility is transferred; accountability is not. Table 26-2 depicts the differences.

IMPORTANCE OF DELEGATING

Delegation is a critical skill for accomplishing care in a timely manner. It usually saves time in the long run and, when effective, is cost-effective. At its worst, however, it is exceedingly costly. Therefore making the best decisions about care is imperative. One of the burdensome misconceptions about the profession of nursing is nursing care being defined in terms of psychomotor tasks. Therefore professional nurses must convey the consistent message that doing a task is one component of care. Although the performance of a psychomotor task is critical, the critical analyses "behind the scenes" are clearly the precipitators of the actions. Research indicates that it is truly the careful decision making of nurses and their ability to synthesize information from various sources that matter in terms of effective nursing care. It is logical to consider the importance of the professional role in safe patient care, whether that care is performed by an individual

 RESEARCH PERSPECTIVE

Resource: Bittner, N. P., & Gravlin, G. (2009). Critical thinking, delegations, and missed care in nursing practice. *The Journal of Nursing Administration, 39*(3), 142-146.

This qualitative, descriptive study focused on how nurses make decisions related to delegating nursing care elements. Focus groups were used to gather information about delegation competence. Participants were medical-surgical nurses from a 300-bed teaching hospital. The participants were then asked to describe clinical situations in which delegation was needed and then to relate examples in which delegation was successful and unsuccessful. Finally, they were asked about care omissions. Seven categories were determined related to delegation: tasks delegated, knowledge expectation, relationships, role uncertainty, communication barriers, system support, and omitted care. Nurses often did not say how they ensured that the UAP understood the task or accepted the delegation. In addition, the lack of follow-up often resulted in learning important information at the end of the shift. Often UAPs had little or no information about the patients for whom they were providing care. Further, the lack of clerical support and missing equipment and supplies deterred the smooth provision of nursing care.

Implications for Practice
The authors identified that some care was missed or omitted, which could result in negative patient outcomes.

RN or by others through delegation. The Research Perspective above cites the relevance of delegation and missed care. In seminal research, Kalisch and Williams (2009) identified the creation of a tool to measure missed nursing care—one of the major concerns when delegation fails (see The Evidence section on p. 534).

Delegation has direct patient and professional benefits. One of these is the availability of the professional staff to patients to teach the basics of safe activities of daily living (ADL). Seldom should a decision to delegate be based on time-saving considerations alone; however, in an effective team, delegation *can* conserve time.

LEGAL AUTHORITY TO DELEGATE

Most state nursing practice acts address the concept of delegation; some explicate rules and regulations governing what may be delegated and when. State boards of nursing are vested with protecting the public; therefore they regulate practice and the educational preparation required to practice nursing. The expectation that specific knowledge about nursing and delegation is needed to perform safely makes the nurse legally accountable and thus liable. Because nursing roles evolve over time, thinking about the scope of liability for the RN is valuable. Many acute care hospitals have decreased their use of LPNs/LVNs, leaving only UNP-type personnel available to assist with care.

Legally, the concept of delegation is complex. First, the individual doing the delegation is personally responsible for prudent action. If delegation is not performed within acceptable standards, malpractice may be the outcome. In addition, according to Guido (2007), failure to delegate and supervise within acceptable standards may extend to direct corporate liability for the institution. Furthermore, whenever care is provided by other than a registered nurse, the accountability for care remains with the manager (of care)/delegator even though others provide various aspects of care. This view of professional liability is consistent with the idea that licensure conveys both privilege and expectations.

SELECTING THE DELEGATEE

In many settings, you are one of a group of professional staff members who have the authority to delegate; therefore you probably will not be able to select the person with whom you will work. On the other hand, opportunities may occur in your career when you have a chance to select your own assistant. Several aspects of selecting an assistant are important. For example, knowing that you can communicate readily is important. If an LPN/LVN who has functioned in a physician's office for some time and is not familiar with working under the directions of an RN or having nursing care supervised is concerned about your supervision, talking about it can eliminate or diminish feelings of concern.

Appreciating and valuing each other's cultural perspectives can help with communication and with care itself. For example, an assistant who does not concur with you about the goals of hospice might actually work at counter-purposes to the organizational philosophy. In addition, if the assistant is like you in terms of strengths, you will both want to do the same things, possibly leaving gaps in care. So, selecting someone with strengths that are different from yours enhances the work the two of you can accomplish together. This approach is consistent with the classic strengths theory (Buckingham & Clifton, 2001), which suggests that we all should focus on building our strengths rather than "fixing" our weaknesses to be most effective at what we do. Realistically, however, it is often impossible to balance your strengths through the deliberate selection of a delegatee. In such cases, it is even more important to consider the whole aspect of patient care to ensure that the full spectrum of needs is addressed. An experienced UNP is likely to be able to adapt to changing situations, including changing delegators.

SUPERVISING THE DELEGATEE

Because the RN is always accountable for assessment, diagnosis, planning, and evaluation, it is important that UNPs understand what elements of implementation they may carry out and why the RN is responsible for analyzing data gathered. Thus RNs are accountable for an initial assessment and then intermittent evaluations. Both elements must be present to ensure effectiveness in entrusting an element of care to someone else.

Delegators may have lessened the amount of direct care work they will do. However, this practice has simultaneously increased their supervisory work.

📖 LITERATURE PERSPECTIVE

Resource: Hansten, R. I. (2008). Why nurses still must learn to delegate. *Nurse Leader, 6*(5), 19-25.

This article addresses a three-level professional practice certification program that was implemented across 14 organizations with 217 experienced nurses participating. The participants rated themselves on skills deficits related to delegation before and after an education program. Twelve skill areas were assessed and included initial direction, practice feedback, assign tasks, checkpoints, ask and use feedback, accountability, and evaluate care. Ratings improved in all areas in the post-course assessment. "RN-to-nursing assistant hand-offs are as vital as any in our vigilance to save lives" (p. 21).

Implications for Practice
Better delegation skills can help nurses be more effective in capitalizing on the availability of quality nursing care.

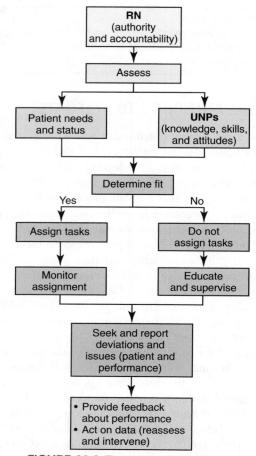

FIGURE 26-3 The delegation process.

Creating a plan to evaluate how both patients and delegatees are doing throughout the work period is critical and is influenced by factors such as knowledge of and experience with the delegatee, the number of delegatees and patients for whom the delegator is accountable, the geographic design of the unit, the stability of the patients, and other resources available to staff. The Literature Perspective above identifies some important skills in delegation.

DELEGATION DECISION MAKING

Figure 26-3 illustrates the delegation process, which begins with assessing the patient and the UNP. Four key factors must be considered before the UNP's abilities are assessed. They are safety, critical thinking, stability, and time. If the patient is unsafe for any reason, delegation may be inappropriate. Exceptions tend to focus around monitoring behaviors (e.g., when patients are placed on suicide precautions). *Critical thinking* refers to the intensity and complexity of decisions that are needed. For example, simple teaching, such as washing hands, can be performed by a UNP; complex teaching, such as diabetic care, cannot. *Stability* suggests that the more stable a patient is, the more likely a UNP could provide care. Finally, *time* refers to the length and intensity of interaction. Thus relatively few UNPs are found in emer-

gency departments; many are found in extended-care facilities.

Assuming the patient-assessment outcomes suggest someone could assist with care, the RN next assesses the abilities of the UNP. When a "fit" (elements of work and performance abilities) occurs, tasks can be assigned. If a fit does not occur, tasks can still be assigned but the delegator will need to educate, monitor, or evaluate more closely to ensure adequate care. Although the UNP is performing tasks (their responsibility), the RN is monitoring (accountability) care and outcomes. The RN should seek information, and the UNP should report information. This two-way follow-through allows care to be altered in a timely manner. At times, especially as new skills are acquired or new relationships are forged, the

TABLE 26-3	GETTING TO THE RIGHT ANSWERS

CHECK THESE QUESTIONS	QUESTIONS YOU MIGHT ASK YOURSELF
The right task	_____ Is it appropriate to delegate (based on legal and institutional factors)? _____ Is the person able and willing to do this specific task?
The right circumstances	_____ Would the delegation process suggest that the circumstances are right? _____ Is staffing such that the circumstances demand delegation strategies?
The right person	_____ Is the prospective delegatee a willing and able employee? _____ Are the patient needs a "fit" with the delegatee?
The right direction/communication	_____ Do you and the delegatee have "common language"? (Do words, such as *time frames, needs,* and *critical,* mean the same to both of you?) _____ Does the delegatee know what and when to report? Is your communication based on a "fit" with the situation and culture?
The right supervision	_____ Do you know how and when you will interact about patient care with the delegatee? _____ How often will you need to provide direct observation?

Based on work by the National Council of State Boards of Nursing. (2005).

RN will want to provide feedback during the care process. In all situations, the RN needs to provide feedback about performance at the end of such activity. In addition to making it known that the UNP was monitored and supported, the UNP knows how to perform better next time because feedback should be directed toward quality.

Sometimes we fail to delegate to others. We may think it is too time-consuming or energy-consuming. Sometimes we frankly believe we can do a better job ourselves or we seek the recognition for specific care. But, when we delegate, we leverage our contributions to care.

> **EXERCISE 26-5**
> Select three patient records from a clinical setting in which delegation occurs. On the basis of the documentation only, evaluate if there are indications/assumptions about safety, critical thinking, stability, and time. If you are familiar with any UNPs in the setting, use Figure 26-3 to identify how you would work with prospective delegatees to accomplish the care. Finally, in one or two sentences, state the rationale for your conclusions about delegation.

Integrating Factors

Combining these factors into an integrated whole for making decisions is valuable. One factor may be the overriding element. For example, when critical-thinking needs are great, the other factors may be relatively less influential. Thus reaching decisions about to whom to delegate, what to delegate, and when to delegate is a complex process.

Providing specific feedback about performance is the best strategy for shaping future behavior. Therefore statements such as "You performed that procedure with ease" are more effective than saying "Nice job." Equally important is the feedback from the person performing the tasks. Was the work completed? How did the patient respond? What changes were noted? These are examples of what the RN must know from the person who performed the delegated portion of care. The wise RN also listens for clues about the UNP's perception of the delegation interaction and uses that information to continue building trust.

When possible, provide positive feedback; however, it undermines your credibility to convey satisfaction when the performance is less than desirable. Therefore being honest about feedback is the best strategy. Being honest about the circumstances and performance and what we can do to change them helps the delegatee develop for the future. Attacking the person or personal characteristics not only has little or no positive effect on care but also has the potential to undermine a long-term relationship. Table 26-3 poses some appropriate questions for reaching decisions about delegation.

Finally, keep in mind that some individuals occupy positions for which they are not qualified. One strategy for dealing with this is to lower your expectations so that the individual can be successful. *Before doing that, however, think about the effect on others.* For example, why is one employee held to a standard and another is not? Who becomes responsible for accomplishing the work the one person cannot achieve? Is it fair to compensate for someone who cannot meet performance expectations? What are the potential liabilities of altering the standards of performance? Reaching decisions about delegating elements of care is a complex process. When the professional nurse knows the individual is incapable of appropriate performance and does not intervene, the potential for liability increases. Even eliminating the legal questions, ethical considerations should influence the nurse.

DELEGATION-PROCESS CHALLENGES

Delegation clearly is complex, but there are some ways to simplify the process. For example, when possible, selecting the delegatee whose talents match the task is better than merely selecting a competent individual. In large organizations, having a choice about who the delegatee is is more likely to occur than in smaller facilities. In rural settings, the delegatees tend to be more predictable, long-term employees; thus delegation is made easier because more is known about them and their abilities.

Delegation may be difficult early in careers and in specific circumstances. In those situations, it may be helpful to initiate working together with an oral acknowledgment that the delegatee's abilities are unknown but that, together, this team is committed to providing the best care for its patients. Stating up front that offense or insult is not intended and then seeking feedback later make the delegatee more receptive to hearing messages. The key is to seek specific feedback so that messages that are offensive can be changed. The goal, however, remains the same: to focus on the outcomes of patient care.

Letting the delegatee implement the task in his or her own way can be a challenge. Someone else will be unlikely to do a task just as the delegator would. However, assuming that no safety or ethical discrepancies are likely, delegation really is a matter of trust.

BOX 26-1	DELEGATION COMMUNICATION TEMPLATE

- State exactly what is being delegated and what the expected outcome is.
- Convey recognition of the authority to perform what is expected.
- Identify priorities.
- Acknowledge monitoring activities you may perform.
- Specify any performance limitations, such as time limits on performing a procedure.
- Specify deadlines, including exact timing if that is important.
- Specify report time lines and data expected.
- Specify parameter deviations, including when immediate action must be taken.
- Identify appropriate resources, including people who may be consulted.
- Be clear about what may not be delegated.

If the delegator intervenes, the delegatee loses confidence or becomes frustrated and the delegator has lost the benefits of delegating.

In delegating, the delegator must be sure that the two most critical elements of managing are considered. Assess or recall, first, that the individual knows what is expected and, second, that the necessary resources to accomplish the work are available (Wagner & Harter, 2006). Having deadlines helps keep the delegatee on target without oversupervising. Being clear about the need to check quality and effectiveness ensures that monitoring will be ongoing.

In settings other than those of confined geography, such as hospitals, long-term care facilities, and clinics, one of the greatest challenges of delegation relates to supervision. In such situations, it is especially important to be clear about what is expected of the delegatee. Box 26-1 presents a communication template to use when delegating. The more that is understood between the delegator and the delegatee about a particular delegation situation, the greater the chances are of being effective in patient care.

EXERCISE 26-6

Think about what you could delegate, and then use the delegation communication template found in Box 26-1 to practice with a classmate the transfer of specific responsibilities for care.

BOX 26-2 **CRITICAL COMMUNICATION**

1. State the facts (this care is substandard). If that does not correct the situation,
2. Challenge (use his or her first name and a qualifier [e.g., Susan, isn't this a sterile procedure?]), and if that does not correct the situation,
3. TAKE ACTION (INTERVENE).

Finally, situations may occur in which you see issues associated with delegation but you have no authority. Assuming no negative patient outcomes or safety issues are involved, you can help other delegators achieve positive outcomes by doing three things: asking, offering, and doing. Begin by asking questions related to the problem/issue/mission. This in itself may help the delegator see a situation differently. Making an offer such as an idea to move the process ahead toward a favorable outcome may be necessary or desirable. Finally, whatever you advocate is best valued if you can demonstrate the behavior you propose (doing). Brafman and Brafman (2008) cited a situation in which communication is critical—the pilots in an airborne plane. Through crew resource management training, the cabin crew learned to communicate in a manner to prevent disasters. Briefly, the approach is described in Box 26-2.

EXERCISE 26-7

Using the assignments made by a nurse manager or charge nurse where you have a clinical experience, answer the following questions: Was it clear what was delegated? Why or why not? Were delegation decisions logical? Why or why not? From what you know about your nursing practice act and professional standards, did the assignments make sense legally and ethically? What is your rationale?

CHARGE NURSES

If no other RN delegates (usually because of the limited numbers of LPNs/LVNs or UNPs), the charge nurse always does. Charge nurses frequently emerge as such within the first year of practice or within a few months when they are experienced and working in a new situation. Connelly, Yoder, and Miner-Williams (2003) studied this group of people and found that the group needs to have four areas of competencies—clinical/technical, critical thinking, organizational, and human relation skills. Because these are skills characteristic of a "good nurse," taking on a larger role is possible.

INTEGRATED CARE

In the late 1990s, care moved from multidisciplinary, coordinated care to an integrated approach. Again, this move provides an impetus for a multiskilled worker. Having someone who performs "what is needed now" for the patient or the professional staff is the focus rather than the "me and my assistants" approach. This is consistent with the Institute of Medicine (IOM) (2003) report, *Health Professions Education: A Bridge to Quality*. Patient-centered care is a key factor in redirecting health care to what patients need as opposed to what we offer. However, as McCloskey, Bulechek, Moorhead, and Daly (1996) suggested with a classic term, the nurse will continue to provide the important "glue role" so that care achieves positive outcomes. In other words, in many settings, nursing's presence on a regular basis predisposes nurses to the "glue" role (holding patient care together) for logical reasons. Integrating care enhances the potential of both for *safe* patient care *and* for *quality* patient care.

CONCLUSION

Delegation is a complex and yet critical process that is needed to provide sufficient care to people requiring nursing services. A structured process helps nurses and their assistants increase the probability of providing safe care.

THE SOLUTION

Seton is a network system with eight EDs at all levels. The solution was to create an educational program that would be pertinent to the needs of trauma centers across the network. The directors developed the program that would be applicable to their care needs.

The position descriptions for the two types of technicians were the same throughout the network. In addition, even though the needs of a trauma technician in a rural environment would be different from those of the trauma technician in a level 1 facility, we decided to use the same educational curriculum and meet the same competency requirements across the network. The difference in the curriculum would be the clinical hours that they spent in training. All of the trauma technician competencies had to be validated by an RN III or IV, one who is nationally certified in trauma nursing and has had experience with these skills.

In addition, the registered nurses wore navy scrubs and the technicians wore burgundy so that others could identify their posi-

tion visually and thus know what role in delegation each could assume. This was exceptionally helpful for the trauma surgeons, who would know immediately who was who.

Finally, we required everyone at one of the hospitals to engage in mock trauma situations. This included the EMS, the RNs, the technicians, the ED and trauma physicians, the respiratory therapists, and the x-ray and laboratory personnel. Irrespective of where trauma technicians are employed in the network, they are required to participate in a mock trauma simulation. Thus every ED was prepared for a system of delegation at a level appropriate to the organization's needs.

—*Cindy Joy-McCoy*

Would this be a suitable approach for you? Why?

THE EVIDENCE

A sample of staff nurses ($n = 459$ and $n = 639$ in two separate studies) from 35 acute care hospital units participated in a study designed by Kalisch and Williams (2009) to create a quantitative tool to measure missed nursing care.

The model is a middle-range theory with three antecedents: labor resources, material resources, and communication. To determine missed care in a systematic way, a tool that quantifies what was previously described in qualitative terms provides evidence about the nature of care that is missed and the reasons attributed to that missed care. The content validity index was 0.89.

The tool was self-administered and anonymous. The final tool contained 22 questions related to the type of care missed and 16 questions related to the reasons attributed to missing the care.

Implications for Practice

This tool creates a way to measure an important aspect of care, that which was not provided. The tool provides a way to measure individual nurse capabilities including delegation.

NEED TO KNOW NOW

- Analyze tasks that may be delegated.
- Practice how to use the delegation aids that are available to you.
- Be familiar with your nursing practice act and the corresponding rules and regulations.

- Assess your patients with the perspective that some of their care will be provided by others.

CHAPTER CHECKLIST

Delegation obviously is a complex issue. It has many facets, each of which by itself is complex. One of the critical roles of RNs is that of the "glue factor," by which the RN coordinates care across the spectrum of providers and affects the quality of care. Current

research suggests that many indirect care interventions are not delegated by RNs because of the complexities and quality implications.

- Delegation involves achieving outcomes and sharing activities with other individuals who have

the authority to accomplish work for which the delegator is accountable and responsible.
- The ways in which delegation can actually be enacted can be based on a situational leadership model.
- Nursing practice acts, rules, and regulations provide the legal structure for delegation; the *Code of Ethics for Nurses* provides the ethical structure.

- Knowing the skills and abilities of the delegatees is critical to feeling comfortable and confident in delegation.
- The delegation process provides a comprehensive approach to a productive interaction.
- Building a trusting relationship takes time and has tremendous value in working effectively.

TIPS FOR DELEGATING

- Ascertain the skills of unlicensed nursing personnel to whom you may delegate tasks.
- Use the communication template to enhance successful delegating.
- Use a decision-making framework to screen what can be delegated to unlicensed nursing personnel.
- Evaluate on a regular basis your effectiveness in delegating to others.

- Know the nursing practice act, standards for the area of clinical practice, organizational policies, and position description.
- Know the skills, knowledge, and attitudes of the people working with you.
- Monitor, monitor, monitor.

REFERENCES

American Nurses Association (ANA). (2005). *Principles for delegation.* Silver Spring, MD: Author.

American Nurses Association (ANA). (2008). *Code of ethics for nurses with interpretive statements.* Washington, DC: Author.

Bittner, N. P., & Gravlin, G. (2009). Critical thinking, delegations, and missed care in nursing practice. *The Journal of Nursing Administration, 39*(3), 142-146.

Brafman, O., & Brafman, R. (2008). *Sway: The irresistible pull of irrational behavior.* New York: Doubleday.

Buckingham, M., & Clifton, D. O. (2001). *Now, discover your strengths.* New York: The Free Press.

Buerhaus, P. I. (2009). *The future of the nursing workforce in the United States.* Sudbury, MA: Jones & Bartlett.

Connelly, L. M., Yoder, L. H., & Miner-Williams, D. (2003). A qualitative study of charge nurse competencies. *Med Surg Nursing, 12*, 298-305.

Deal, J. J. (2007). *Retiring the generation gap: How employees young and old can find common ground.* San Francisco: Wiley.

Fagin, C. M. (2001). *When care becomes a burden: Diminishing access to adequate nursing.* New York: Milbank Memorial Fund.

Guido, G. W. (2007). Legal and ethical issues. In P. S. Yoder-Wise (Ed.), *Leading and managing in nursing* (2nd ed.). St. Louis: Mosby.

Hansten, R. I. (2008). Why nurses still must learn to delegate. *Nurse Leader, 6*(5), 19-25.

Hersey, P., & Blanchard, K. H. (1988). *Management organizational behavior* (5th ed.). Englewood Cliffs, NJ: Prentice Hall.

Institute of Medicine (IOM). (2003). *Health professions education: A bridge to quality.* Washington, DC: National Academies Press.

Joint Statement on Delegation. (2009). Retrieved October 20, 2009, from www.ncsbn.org.

Kalisch, B. J., & Williams, R. A. (2009). Development and psychometric testing of a tool to measure missed nursing care. *The Journal of Nursing Administration, 39*(5), 211-219.

Lencioni, P. (2002). *The five dysfunctions of a team.* San Francisco: Jossey-Bass.

McCloskey, J. C., Bulechek, G. M., Moorhead, S., & Daly, J. (1996). Nurses' use and delegation of indirect care interventions. *Nursing Economic$, 14*, 22-33.

McGlown, K. J., O'Connor, S. J., & Shewchuk, R. M. (2009). Evidence-based criteria for hospital evacuation: The case of Hurricane Katrina. In A. R. Kovner, D. J. Fine, & R. D'Aquila (Eds), *Evidence-based management in healthcare.* Chicago: AUPHA.

National Council of State Boards of Nursing. (2005). *Business Book, Annual Meeting.* Chicago, IL: Author.

Nursing Executive Center. (2008). *Bridging the preparation-practice gap: Volume I—Quantifying new graduate nurse improvement needs.* Washington, DC: The Advisory Board Company.

Standing, T., Anthony, M. K., & Hertz, J. E. (2001). Nurses' narratives of outcomes after delegation to unlicensed assistive personnel. *Outcomes Management for Nursing Practice, 5*(1), 18-23.

Wagner, R., & Harter, J. K. (2006). *The 12 elements of great managing.* New York: Gallup Press.

SUGGESTED READINGS

Anthony, M. K., Standing, T., & Hertz, J. E. (2000). Factors influencing outcomes after delegation to unlicensed assistive personnel. *The Journal of Nursing Administration, 30,* 474-481.

Moll, J. A., & Tripp, E. (2002). Nursing delegation: Implications for home care. *Caring, 21*(9), 24-28, 30, 32.

Munroe, D. J. (2003). Assisted living issues for nursing practice. *Geriatric Nursing, 24*(2), 99-105.

Rodwell, J., Noblet, A., Demir, D., & Steane, P. (2009). Supervisors are central to work characteristics affecting nurse outcomes. *Journal of Nursing Scholarship, 41,* 310-319.

Role Transition

Diane M. Twedell

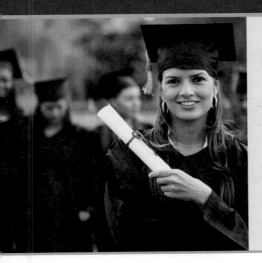

This chapter provides information about role transition—the process of moving from a clinically focused position to a supervisory position with increased responsibility. The basic overview of management roles illustrates the complexity of managing work done by others and provides a foundation for understanding role transition. The exercises offer opportunities to recognize one's own expectations, resources, and management potential.

OBJECTIVES

- Construct the full scope of a manager role by outlining Responsibilities, Opportunities, Lines of communication, Expectations, and Support (ROLES).
- Analyze specific examples of role transitions as a staff nurse and a nurse manager.
- Describe the phases of role transition by using a life experience.
- Construct a response to an unexpected role transition.
- Compare strategies to facilitate a successful role transition.

TERMS TO KNOW

mentor	role internalization	role transition
role development	role negotiation	ROLES
role discrepancy	role strain	
role expectations	role stress	

Lindsey M. Worden, RN, BSN
Medical Nephrology Nurse Manager, Mayo Clinic, Rochester,
Minnesota

I started my career in nursing on the same medical/nephrology unit that I currently manage. In my previous 4 years as a staff nurse on the unit, I was actively involved with committee work and I wore many hats on the unit as a charge nurse and preceptor. I became interested in management because I enjoyed working with others and the challenges of looking at how to improve current processes on the patient care unit.

I was aware that the nurse manager role was complex and pivotal for a quality work environment for nurses and patients. I was not aware of just how difficult the role was to carry out. I was not prepared for all the personnel issues, paperwork, and problems that popped up unexpectedly. I felt lost and unsure when working with budgeting and finances. I wondered if I would ever understand everything I needed to. I also noticed how I missed the intense patient contact and missed the day-to-day patient interaction.

I was engulfed in a whirlwind of change and found that not being able to lean on friends from the unit was one of the biggest changes I encountered. I had accepted this opportunity to develop myself as a leader and manager and did not realize how it would affect me personally. The relationships I had with my friends from the unit had changed, and the people I called my peers were now my employees. This concept was tough to handle, and often I felt alone. I could feel how employees looked at me differently. I think it is difficult to transition to a new role with staff with whom you have already formed relationships. I was challenged to adapt to this new role with caution and ensure I treated everyone equally and fairly.

What do you think you would do if you were this nurse?

INTRODUCTION

Role transition involves transforming one's professional identity. A new graduate makes a transition from the student role to the nurse role. Expectations of students are clearly specified in course and clinical objectives. Expectations for a new nurse as an employee may not be so clear. The new graduate nurse faces the first of several professional transitions. The Literature Perspective and Research Perspectives on p. 539 provide further information on role transitions for new graduate nurses, which are helpful for new graduates, their co-workers, and their managers.

Consider the staff nurse who becomes a nurse manager. The staff nurse performs tasks related to the care of patients. As a follower, the staff nurse has accountability and responsibility for the work that is accomplished. A staff nurse who becomes a nurse manager must transition into the new role as a generalist, orchestrating diverse tasks and getting work done through others.

A staff nurse who moves from an acute care setting to a home health agency must also undergo a role transition. Instead of balancing the needs of multiple patients, the home health nurse can focus on one patient at a time. Yet, when a collegial opinion is needed during a visit, peers with whom to consult are not readily available. Registered nurses who transition to nurse practitioner roles and other advanced practice roles experience this same type of role transition.

Organizations play a key role in assisting employees through role transitions. Changes in roles can be either painful or exciting and depend largely on the work culture and support provided. According to Sewell (2008), "role transition is a hurdle encountered by every nurse entering the workforce. A host of new experiences await the neophyte beyond the clinical experiences of nursing school" (p. 49).

Knowing what to expect during the transformation can reduce the stress of accepting and transitioning into a new role and result in quality outcomes. After an overview of the roles of leader, manager, and follower, this chapter describes the process of role transition, with an emphasis on strategies that can be used to ease the transition.

TYPES OF ROLES

Accepting a management position dictates accepting three roles that involve complex processes. The roles of leader, manager, and follower are complex because they involve working through and with unique individuals in a rapidly changing environment. Examples of the people with whom you interact and the pro-

LITERATURE PERSPECTIVE

Resource: Salera-Vierira, J. (2009). The collegial clinical model for orientation of new graduate nurses: A strategy to improve the transition from student nurse to professional nurse. *Journal for Nurses in Staff Development, 25* (4), 174-181.

The collegial clinical model is used in nursing schools in which one nursing clinical instructor oversees several students on a patient care unit. This manuscript focuses on utilization of the model in an acute care setting using a nurse educator with new graduate nurses rather than the traditional preceptor orientee model alone. This model was based on Lev Vygotsky's sociocultural development theory utilizing a concept defined as the *zone of proximal development (ZPD).* Learning takes place in the zone of proximal development as the learner moves from various types of learning—from classroom, to precepted clinical environment, to independent work.

The model was found to support preceptors and assist with the transition of new graduate nurses and did not present an increased economic burden on the employer. The conclusion noted that this model can help graduate nurses make the transition into their position.

Implications for Practice
Using a model to create a plan for intensified orientation provides a strategy for comparison across organizations. Intense orientation is an expensive endeavor and one that leads to the potential for new nurse satisfaction and thus the potential for retaining that new employee.

 RESEARCH PERSPECTIVE

Resource: Sewell, E. (2008). Journaling as a mechanism to facilitate graduate nurses' role transition. *Journal for Nurses in Staff Development, 24* (2), 49-52.

Academia has a rich background with journaling occurring on both the faculty and student side of nursing education programs. Sewell describes the journaling experience to assist new nurses in transitioning to the clinical setting. Journaling styles used included freestyle, thinking-in-action, and reflective. Journaling gives new nurses the opportunity to use introspection, reflection, and dialog as they transition into their new role. Journaling can assist new nurses in understanding their new role. This is another tool that staff educators can use in orientation and staff development of the graduate nurse.

Implications for Practice
Journaling is a long tradition and expectation in many countries and roles. Having new graduates (and others) journal is a powerful strategy for identifying growth and emotions related to particular experiences. Documenting experiences shortly after experiencing them helps staff identify issues, patterns of response, and potentials for changing behaviors.

 RESEARCH PERSPECTIVE

Resource: Young, M., Stuenkel, D., & Bawel-Brinkley, K. (2008). Strategies for easing the role transformation of graduate nurses. *Journal for Nurses in Staff Development, 24* (3), 105-110.

This study describes the effects of a 6-week newly graduated nurse hospital orientation on role conceptions and role discrepancy of newly graduated nurses. The three role conceptions focused on in the study were bureaucratic, professional, and service roles. The difference between ideal and actual role conception was calculated. The findings indicated that formal structured orientation programs for the new graduate nurse ease the transition from student to practicing RN.

Implications for Practice
Because registered nurses fulfill the three types of roles described above, role conflict can easily ensue. Being aware of which role one is performing at any given time helps new nurses, and others, identify where role strengthening can help. New graduates arrive with concepts of what a role should be, only to find that the ideal may not be in place. Knowing the discrepancies between real and ideal can help new graduates make the transition to the new role and can help form the basis for discussions that may help the organization improve roles.

cesses involved in each role are shown in Table 27-1. In nursing, each of these roles relates to patients and clients.

The transition from a staff nurse role to a nurse manager/leader role can occur overnight. The nurse moves from the clinical work of patient care to lead a group of employees. Clark (2008) notes that "leadership is not simply granted to individuals and is not about responding passively to events. It is about creating possibilities that were absent before" (p. 30). McConnell (2008) says that a healthcare professional who takes on a manager position is taking on a second occupation. "The professional who enters management must wear two hats" (p. 278). One role is as the professional on technical and clinical matters, and one is as a generalist manager.

The role of follower involves respecting the authority of others and working within the system to contribute to the organizational outcomes. Managers as

TABLE 27-1	LEADER, MANAGER, AND FOLLOWER ROLES: PEOPLE WITH WHOM YOU INTERACT AND PROCESSES INVOLVED IN EACH ROLE	

ROLE	PEOPLE WITH WHOM INTERACTIONS OCCUR	PROCESSES INVOLVED IN THE ROLE
Leader	Persons being led Peers	Listening Encouraging Motivating Organizing Problem solving Developing Supporting
Manager	Persons being supervised Administrators Supervisors Regulating agencies	Organizing Budgeting Hiring Evaluating Reporting Disseminating
Follower	Supervisor Peers	Conforming Implementing Contributing Completing assignments Alerting

BOX 27-1	"ROLES" ACRONYM

Responsibilities
Opportunities
Lines of communication
Expectations
Support

followers recognize their accountability to the persons above them on the organizational chart. Within a team, the manager recognizes the leadership being provided by others and supports decisions made by the group.

In the evolving healthcare environment, the nurse providing direct patient care also must function as a leader, manager, and follower. As *leader,* the nurse recognizes the uniqueness of each patient and provides feedback on clinical progress. As *manager,* the nurse links the patient to the resources to achieve clinical outcomes. Medical information is translated into a format that the patient can use to make informed decisions about treatment and self-care. Through referrals, the nurse facilitates continuity of care within the larger system. As *follower,* the nurse is accountable to the team and the supervisor for completing the work that is assigned. The nurse as a follower practices within the policies and procedures of the organization and the standards of the profession.

Learning the leader, manager, and follower aspects of any new role can be overwhelming. Another approach to the complexity of role transition is the acronym *ROLES,* in which each letter represents a component common to all roles.

ROLES: THE ABCs OF UNDERSTANDING ROLES

Acronyms help us retain and organize information. "ROLES" (Box 27-1) is an acronym that is useful in role transition.

R **stands for responsibilities.** What are the specified duties in the position description for the new position? What tasks are to be completed? What decisions must the person in this position make? For example, the job for a nurse manager might include 24-hour accountability, whereas a job description for a nurse practitioner may involve direct care in a primary care setting. Every position has specific tasks for which the position holder is responsible.

O **stands for opportunities,** which are untapped aspects of the position. In the employment interview, the nurse executive may have said that the previous manager did not encourage the staff nurses to participate in continuing education. Or, while touring the unit, a manager observes that the report room lacks amenities. Maybe there is a new method of delivering patient care that is appropriate for the unit. These possibilities represent opportunities for a manager to influence organizational and unit goals.

L **represents lines of communication,** which are at the heart of every leadership role. No matter what

THEORY BOX

Hardy's Role Theory

THEORY/CONTRIBUTOR	KEY IDEAS	APPLICATION TO PRACTICE
Hardy (1978) is credited with applying role theory to healthcare professionals. Role is the expected and actual behaviors associated with a position. Role expectations are the attitudes and behaviors others anticipate that a person in the role will possess or demonstrate. Role stress is a social condition in which role demands are conflicting, irritating, difficult, or impossible to fulfill. Role strain is the subjective feeling of discomfort experienced as the result of role stress.	Role stress is a precursor to role strain. Role stress is associated with low productivity and performance. Role stress and role strain can lead a person to withdraw psychologically from the role. Clear, realistic role expectations can decrease the role stress for a new nurse manager.	Clear, realistic role expectations can increase productivity.

Data from Hardy, M.E. (1978). Role stress and role strain. In M.E. Hardy & M.E. Conway (Eds.), *Role theory: Perspectives for health professionals*. New York: Appleton-Century-Crofts.

role an individual is in, there are relationships with multiple individuals including supervisors and peers. Roles incorporate patterns of structured interactions between the manager and people in these groups. The nurse manager receives and sends messages. Being a skillful listener can be more important than being skillful in sending messages. Skill is required to communicate both the content and the intent of the message effectively. Only through practice can one develop skill. In Chapter 18, techniques of effective communication are described that are extremely important to a new manager in building the team.

E **stands for expectations.** Expectations vary depending on your goals. Colleagues may expect a new nurse anesthetist to be on call every weekend. Staff nurses have specific expectations of their managers and particularly want the manager to be a facilitator and a leader. The nursing executive or administrator will likely have expectations about how managers spend their time on the job—even about how much time they spend at work. Nurse executives' expectations evolve from their perspectives of the manager's accountability and duties.

Finding out in advance what the explicit and implicit expectations are of the people involved can facilitate a smoother role transition by decreasing role ambiguity (Hardy, 1978). Hardy's work with role theory suggests a strong relationship between role ambiguity (one type of role stress) and role strain.

The major concepts of role theory are presented in the Theory Box above.

There are also personal expectations related to performance as a manager. You have a mental image of the role of a manager or person in this position. The process of role transition unfolds as a new manager identifies expectations, recognizes the similarities and differences, and develops the roles of leader, manager, and follower.

S **stands for support,** which is closely tied to expectations about performance. All roles are shaped to some degree by the support and services others provide. The acute care nurse has peers readily available when a second opinion is needed. The same nurse may feel lost when confronted with questionable findings during a home visit. The nurse manager who must develop the unit's budget in a skilled care facility may have no accounting department to provide services, such as a detailed analysis of the facility's expenditures. Each role has some support available. When a new position is being considered, it is important to evaluate whether support is available in areas in which a manager may lack knowledge or skill. When implementing changes in roles, the organization needs to develop support services to facilitate role transition. The *Research Perspectives* and the *Literature Perspective* describe the support needed by new graduate nurses during role transition to the practice environment.

BOX 27-2   ROLE TRANSITION PROCESS

Unlearning old roles while learning new roles requires an identity adjustment over time. The persons involved must invest themselves in the process. In this way, role transition can be compared to developing a relationship. The process of developing an intimate relationship with another person provides a familiar framework for considering role transition. Relationships typically move through the phases of dating, commitment, honeymoon, disillusionment, resolution, and maturity.

Role Preview

During the dating phase, the interested persons spend structured time together. Both parties present their best characteristics and dedicate much energy to developing the relationship. Although both parties present their best characteristics, both also are alert to clues that the other party cannot meet their expectations. For example, one may consider the financial and emotional resources that the other person would bring to the relationship. The individuals might spend time with each other's families to get a feel for the emotional climate in which the other person grew up.

Interviewing for a management position is similar to dating. An interview involves touring the unit, visiting with people, and attempting to make a good impression. The potential employer is also attempting to make a favorable impression. The interviewee wants to find out whether this is an organization that will support his or her growth as he or she supports the growth of the organization. Questions are asked about the role of the manager, and the potential manager mentally evaluates whether the described role matches personal expectations about management. Both of these examples represent the phase "role preview."

Role Acceptance

Through the dating process, two people may decide that they want to spend the rest of their lives together and commit to the relationship. Sometimes, one or both of the people decide that they do not want to establish a long-term relationship. In a similar way, following the role preview of the interview process, both parties may agree to establish a relationship as employee and employer. Or one or both of the parties may decide not to establish the relationship. In dating, the public decision to leave other similar relationships and establish this new relationship represents a formal commitment. In role transition, the formal commitment of the employment contract implies acceptance of the management role, or "role acceptance."

Role Exploration

In new relationships, a time of dating and commitment is usually followed by a honeymoon. More than a trip to a vacation spot, the honeymoon has become synonymous with excitement, happiness, and confidence. In a new work role, people also experience a honeymoon phase. The new graduate may be relieved that the educational program was successfully completed and now a salary can be earned. When a new manager is hired, the employer is excited that the search is over. The staff is happy to have a leader, especially if staff members had input into the hiring decision. The new manager is happy, excited, and, most of all, confident in exploring the new roles involved in the management position.

Role Discrepancy

Whether by a gradual process or as the result of a particular event that serves as the turning point, eventually the honeymoon is over and disillusionment about the relationship occurs. For example, one person may make an expensive purchase without consulting the partner. An argument is followed by a period of painful silence. Similarly, the honeymoon phase in a new employment position can be followed by a period of disillusionment.

Role discrepancy, a gap between role expectations and role performance, causes discomfort and frustration. Role discrepancy can be resolved by either dissolving the relationship or by changing expectations and performance. The importance of the relationship and the perceived differences between performance and expectations, the basis of role discrepancy, must be considered in light of personal values. When the relationship is valued and the differences are seen as correctable, the decision is made to stay in the relationship. This decision requires the couple or the manager to develop the role.

Role Development

Choosing to change either role expectations or role performance or to change both is the process of role development. In an intimate relationship, open communication can clarify expectations. Negotiation may result in reasonable expectations. Certain behaviors may be changed to improve role performance. For example, one person in the relationship learns to call home to let the other know about the possibility of being late.

To reduce role discrepancy in a new management position, the same open communication and negotiation must occur.

ROLE TRANSITION PROCESS

One way to think about the way in which someone transitions to a new role is illustrated in Box 27-2 and Table 27-2. Thinking about transitions in terms of a common social perspective may be helpful for some.

STRATEGIES TO PROMOTE ROLE TRANSITION

Becoming a manager or assuming a new role requires a transformation—a profound change in identity. Such a transformation invokes stress as the person unlearns old roles and learns the management role.

BOX 27-2   **ROLE TRANSITION PROCESS—cont'd**

Expectations need to be clarified and stipulated by both parties. New managers evaluate management styles and techniques to determine which ones best fit them and the situation. The personal management style evolves as the individuals develop the management roles in their own unique ways. If role discrepancy can be reduced and the role developed to be satisfactory to both parties, the new manager can focus on developing the roles of the position and proceed to the phase of role internalization.

Role Internalization

Role internalization occurs in relationships as they mature. No longer do the persons in the relationship consciously consider their roles. They have learned the behaviors that maintain and nurture the relationship. The behaviors become second nature. The energy spent on establishing and developing the relationship can be redirected toward achieving mutual goals. In the same way, managers who have been in management positions for several years have internalized their roles. Usually they do not consciously consider their roles. Managers know they have reached the stage of role internalization when they focus on accomplishing mutual goals instead of contemplating whether their role performance matches their role expectations. Managers who have internalized their roles have developed their own unique personal style of management. Table 27-2 summarizes the comparison between the phases of developing an intimate relationship and the phases of role transition to a nurse manager.

Unexpected Role Transition

Not every relationship is successful. Some relationships end in an argument, divorce, or death. When a relationship ends unexpectedly, a person goes through a grieving process. In a similar way, when a person is fired, a position is eliminated, or a job description changes dramatically, the person may have to grieve before being able to engage in role transition. Health care is in a tumultuous state. Mergers, acquisitions, and reductions in force are commonplace. To be successful, workplace restructuring must be undertaken with the same sensitivity afforded a person who has lost a relationship through death or divorce. Role transition takes time, even in reverse.

The initial response to a change in role can be shock and disbelief. The person may feel numb and unable to function. As the numbness wears off, the person may become angry. The anger fuels resistance to the change and may be directed toward those who initiated the role change. The anger may be directed internally, leading to depression. If the person is unable to acknowledge and talk about the loss, the period of grief may be extended or emotional baggage may be created that is carried into the next role. Grieving can eventually resolve in acceptance. Lessons learned from the experience are identified and internalized. A new role is sought, and the "dating" begins again.

When a relationship is dissolved in the case of death or divorce, a legal document is prepared to formally dissolve the financial and social obligations between the persons involved. The loss of a position as a result of restructuring or a buyout should involve a similar process. The employer may offer the nurse a severance package that includes financial compensation and outplacement services. If the employer does not offer a written agreement, the nurse should formally request and negotiate reasonable compensation and assistance. Similar to signing a prenuptial agreement, a nurse may have signed a contract with the employer when hired. The terms of that agreement may require the employer to buy out (pay the salary and benefits) for the time remaining on the contract.

Written by Jennifer Jackson Gray.

Several strategies can be helpful in easing the strain and speeding the process of role transition (Box 27-3).

Internal Resources

A key strategy in promoting role transition is to recognize, use, and strengthen one's values and beliefs. Behavior is influenced by values and beliefs. Clark (2008) notes that values and beliefs "shape how individuals think, and see the world, and the meanings they attribute to their experiences, actions and relationships with others" (p. 30). It is important that new leaders do not lose sight of their own values and beliefs. The role of manager is not for everyone. One must consider whether personal goals and profes-

BOX 27-3   **STRATEGIES TO PROMOTE ROLE TRANSITION**

- Strengthen internal resources
- Assess the organization's resources, culture, and group dynamics
- Negotiate the role
- Grow with a mentor
- Develop management knowledge and skills

TABLE 27-2	COMPARISON OF PHASES IN DEVELOPING AN INTIMATE RELATIONSHIP AND IN UNDERGOING ROLE TRANSITION AS A NURSE MANAGER	
PHASE IN DEVELOPING AN INTIMATE RELATIONSHIP	**PHASE IN ROLE TRANSITION AS A NURSE MANAGER**	**CHARACTERISTICS OF PHASE**
Dating	Role preview	Presentation of best characteristics to make favorable impression; both parties evaluate each other to determine likelihood of the other being able to fulfill one's expectations
Commitment to relationship	Role acceptance	Public announcement of mutual decision to initiate contract
Honeymoon	Role exploration	Experience of excitement, confidence, and mutual appreciation
Disillusionment	Role discrepancy	Awareness of difference between role expectations and role performance; reconsideration of whether to continue with contract
Resolution	Role development	Negotiation of role expectations; adjustment of role performance to approximate expectations and to find own unique style
Maturation of relationship	Role internalization	Performance of role congruent with own beliefs and individual style; achievement of mutual goals

sional fulfillment can best be achieved through management. One's commitment to the challenges of managing can provide the desire to persevere during the process of role transition.

Clark (2008) notes that "nurses typically work according to two sets of values; professional values, which are determined by their code of professional conduct, and personal values" (p. 31). If an individual in transition understands his or her own personal values, these will help the person respond to situations and relationships. A person's value does not depend on the quality or quickness of the adjustment to the management role. An exercise such as writing down short statements of belief or self-affirmations and posting this information may be helpful as a visual reminder.

Changing circumstances in health care raise the need for flexibility. The effective leader must be able to learn and master new skills, translate information for staff, and adapt behavior to the situation. It is also important for the new leader to not expect too much of oneself all at once; understanding that this transition takes time will help with flexibility.

Organizational Assessment

A new manager is much like an immigrant in a new country. An immigrant learns how to access the available resources to acclimate to the new environment. Cultural practices of the new country may seem strange or odd. Such differences can be analyzed and decisions made about which aspects to incorporate into one's own culture. More subtle differences in communication patterns or group dynamics can also be identified. Understanding the nuances of social interactions is often the most difficult aspect of acclimating to a new country. The transition is smoother for the immigrant who understands himself or herself, assesses the new environment, and learns how to communicate within groups.

The new manager must also learn how to access resources in the organization. Approaching the organization as a foreign culture, the new manager can keenly observe the rituals, accepted practices, and patterns of communication within the organization. This ongoing assessment promotes a speedier transition into the role of manager. The immigrant who spends energy bemoaning the difficulties of the new

---

EXERCISE 27-1

ROLES Assessment

Answer these questions for a position in management that you would consider.

Responsibilities

1. From the position description, what are the responsibilities?
2. For what decisions are you responsible?
3. Consider information about the management position that you learned during the interview (this may be role-played). Also consider the responsibilities of managers you have observed. Are there other responsibilities to add to your list?

Opportunities

4. What would you like to do differently from the previous manager?
5. How could your strengths or expertise benefit the people or nursing unit you would manage?
6. Dream a little (or a lot). If a person who had been a patient on the unit were describing the nursing care to another potential patient, what would you want the first patient to say? Describe the unit as you want it to be known.

Lines of Communication

7. Draw yourself in the middle of a separate piece of paper. Now fill in the people above you and below you with whom you would communicate. Draw lines from you to each person or group. On the line, identify the form of communication. For example, if you communicate with the director of nursing through a weekly report, write on the line, "Written report."

Expectations

8. This may be the most difficult part to assess. List in short sentences or phrases the expectations each person or group may have for you in relation to your management position.

SELF	FAMILY
ADMINISTRATION	IMMEDIATE SUPERVISOR
PEOPLE YOU WILL MANAGE	

Support

9. What people do you know in the organization who could provide information that you will need to do your job?
10. What departments provide services that you could access for assistance?

Next Steps

Now compare the lists.

Place a star next to those expectations that are held by more than one person or group. For example, you want to handle the budget of the unit efficiently, an expectation shared with nursing administration.

Circle those items that could cause conflicts.

Refer to the Strategies to promote role transition section in this chapter on how to resolve these conflicts.

Save your responses to these questions to review in 3 months. You may be surprised how your own perception of your ROLES may change over time.

---

country may fail to enjoy the advantages that drew him or her to the country in the first place. In the same way, the manager who focuses on the weaknesses of the organization may lack the energy to internalize the new role, a step that is critical to being an effective leader.

Role Negotiation

A strategy that is helpful during conflicting role expectations is role negotiation. The ROLES assessment (see Exercise 27-1) may have identified areas of significant conflict. Writing down the expectations is the first step in resolving areas of conflict. It is important to review the expectations listed to determine whether they are realistic. Unrealistic expectations strongly held by others may require diplomatic reeducation so that their expectations can become more realistic.

The priority of different role expectations may also require role negotiation with the person above you in the line of command. Ask for input as to which expectations have the highest priorities. Explain personal and family expectations, and clearly state the priority that meeting those expectations has. The process may have to be repeated several times before agreement on the expectations related to roles and the priority of each expectation is found. Rewriting the unrealistic expectations to be achievable can reduce three common sources of role stress—ambiguity, overload, and conflict. Each person's role contributes to the end result. All individuals must understand their roles, or the team may fail.

Mentors

The process of mentoring is not a new concept. This concept has been alive since Homer's *Odyssey*. Odysseus leaves Ithaca to fight in the Trojan War. Before leaving, he entrusts his son to Mentor. Mentor was to develop and prepare him for his life and duties. Stewart (2006) states that "mentor has become the

BOX 27-4	BENEFITS OF MENTORING

Mentor	Mentee
Stimulation of new ideas	One-to-one relationship
Development	Advice about career development
Self-awareness	Enlarged network
Enlarging colleague pool	Self-confidence
New relationships	Insight into organization
	Professional development

Modified from Funderburk, A. (2008). Mentoring: The retention factor in the acute care setting. *Journal for Nurses in Staff Development, 24*(3), E1-E5.

term used to describe a person who takes on the responsibility for guiding the development of another person" (p. 114). Mentors are an important component of a nurturing environment that promotes staff retention. Dyer (2008) notes that "mentoring is hoped for by most new nurses and is most commonly requested during the beginning phase of a nursing career" (p. 87).

Mentors can be a tremendous source of guidance and support for staff nurses and managers, serving both career functions and psychosocial functions. Career functions are possible because the mentor has sufficient professional experience and organizational authority to facilitate the career of the "mentee." Box 27-4 highlights some key functions of mentors. The Robert Wood Johnson Nurse Executive Fellows program has identified five competencies of leaders and mentors (Center for the Health Professions, 2009). These comprise interpersonal and communication effectiveness, risk taking and creativity, self-knowledge, inspiring and leading change, and strategic vision *(www.rwjf.org)*.

Sponsorship involves volunteering or nominating the mentee for additional responsibilities. A mentor can be a sponsor by creating opportunities for individual achievement and providing encouragement. The mentor may suggest the mentee be appointed to a key nursing committee or volunteer for a special assignment. Sponsorship leads to exposure or opportunities for the mentee to build a reputation of competence. With exposure, the mentor provides protection by absorbing negative feedback, sharing responsibility for controversial decisions, and teaching the unwritten rules about "how things are done

around here." These unwritten rules may be more important to job success than the written rules.

Coaches provide information about how to improve performance, including feedback on current performance. *Coaching* requires frequent contact and willingness on the part of the mentee to accept feedback. Challenging assignments are given to the mentee that will stretch the limits of knowledge and skill. The mentor helps the mentee learn the technical and management skills necessary to accomplish the task, such as which numbers on the budget printout are added to achieve the total expenditures.

The interpersonal relationship between the mentor and the mentee involves mutual positive regard. Because the mentee respects the career accomplishments of the mentor, the mentee identifies with the mentor's example. This role modeling is both conscious and unconscious. The mentee with character and self-respect will evaluate the behaviors of the mentor and select those behaviors worthy of being emulated.

Counseling, as another psychosocial function of the mentor, allows the mentee to explore personal concerns. Confidentiality is a prerequisite to sharing personal information. Because the opinion of the mentor is respected, the mentor may provide guidance to the mentee. The best mentors can provide guidance while recognizing that the mentee may choose to disregard the advice.

Being mentored is a learning process. Admiration for a mentor and recognition of the mentor's commitment to self-success can provide an environment of trust in which a mentor-mentee relationship begins. Both persons develop positive expectations of the relationship, and both take the initiative to nurture the new relationship. As more of the mentor functions are experienced, the bond between the mentor and mentee grows stronger.

Relationships between mentors and mentees vary because of individual characteristics and the career phase of each. During the early phases of a career, a nurse manager is concerned about competence and a mentor can provide valuable coaching. As the nurse manager develops, sponsorship by a mentor can prepare the manager for a promotion. A mentor nearing the end of the work career can find fulfillment in sharing knowledge with new managers and at the same time benefit from the counsel of a recently retired colleague.

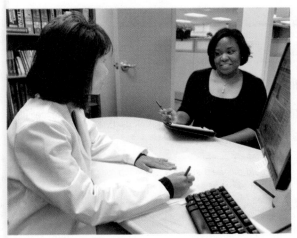

Keeping up with current research is an effective management and education strategy.

Management Education

Management performance can be hindered by a specific knowledge deficit. For example, the manager may lack business skills or knowledge about legal aspects of supervision. Weston et al. (2008) note that "leadership education is needed to develop competencies in nurses transitioning from clinical to front-line supervisory positions" (p. 472). The Arizona Nurse Leadership Model is based on the work of Longest (1998), which describes six critical leadership competencies: conceptual, technical, interpersonal or collaborative, political, commercial, and governance.

Experience and education provide a firm basis for seeking additional credentials. A nurse holding an administrative position at the nurse executive level with a baccalaureate preparation and 24 months of experience can take an examination to become a certified nursing executive. Nursing administrators with master's degrees and experience at the executive level can take an examination to become a certified nurse executive, advanced. The website of the American Nurses Credentialing Center (ANCC, 2009) has more detailed information about certification examinations (*www.nursecredentialing.org*). A certification credential also was developed by the American Organization of Nurse Executives (AONE) in 2008 exclusively for the nurse executive—the Certification in Executive Nursing Practice (CENP). (*www.aone.org/certification*).

FROM ROLE TRANSITION TO ROLE TRIUMPH

Developing an intimate relationship can be a difficult process, but most people still value relationships enough to make the effort. Making the transition and transformation into a management role is also worth the effort. Leading lives of integrity and commitment, nurse managers set examples, bringing out the best in staff nurses and thereby multiplying their influence on quality patient care.

SUMMARY

Transitions from staff nurse to charge nurse or nurse manager pose new challenges. Nurses who make these transitions with minimal discomfort are reflective of role theory in action. Although nurses today are better prepared to take on more formal leadership roles, the roles themselves are more challenging. Charge nurses and managers are responsible for mentoring and coaching new staff as they transition to the new roles they are assuming. These transition activities take time and effort to achieve the best results possible.

THE SOLUTION

It has taken me a number of months to feel comfortable with my new routine, and I know that it will be around 2 years before I feel completely comfortable in my new role. I continue to learn day by day, and I set achievable goals for myself and the patient care unit. I am currently pursuing my master's in nursing with a leadership/administration emphasis. I am learning so much about the type of leader I want to be. I continue to use my resources on a daily basis including my patient care unit collaborative practice framework team consisting of a nursing education specialist and clinical nurse specialist. I have a nurse manager preceptor who has done a great job of supporting me and illustrating how to juggle the new responsibilities and accountability. I feel less stressed and more proficient.

I have also developed a new group of friends within the medical specialty leadership group who have helped me achieve balance in my life.

Role transition is a challenge, and I look at it as a learning opportunity in which I can grow as an individual. This has been a life-changing experience for me. I'm proud to say that I'm extremely glad I took this leap.

—*Lindsey M. Worden*

Would this be a suitable approach for you? Why?

THE EVIDENCE

Etheridge's descriptive, longitudinal, phenomenological study (2007) examined the perceptions of recent nursing graduates about learning to make clinical judgments. Semi-structured interviews were conducted to determine the meaning of making clinical nursing judgments. These interviews were conducted on three different dates: within a month after the end of a preceptor experience, 2 to 3 months later, and 8 to 9 months after the first interview.

Major components of learning to think like a nurse included building confidence, accepting responsibility, adapting to changing relationships with others, and thinking more clinically. Discussions with peers were a powerful experience for the individual nurses transitioning to their new role.

NEED TO KNOW NOW

- Obtain a complete and detailed position description for the new role.
- Identify critical resources available in the organization to assist with role transition: nurse managers, nurse educators, clinical nurse specialists, preceptors, charge nurses, peers, employee assistance program, healthy living center.
- Be open to feedback, and ask for it on a regular basis.

- Be prepared to identify a mentor in the first 6 to 9 months of a new role.
- Plan to attend educational programs that expand knowledge base and enhance self-confidence.
- Identify stress points during role transition, and seek help accordingly

CHAPTER CHECKLIST

Role transition is a process that takes time and energy—two scarce resources for nurse managers. Knowing what to expect and how to facilitate the process can speed role transition and minimize the expenditure of energy as the nurse manager negotiates new roles.

- Responsibilities, opportunities, lines of communication, expectations, and support are aspects common to all roles. When considering a management role, gather information about each of these aspects.
- Managers are also leaders and followers.

- Role transition is a process of unlearning old roles and learning new roles.
- The phases of role transition are as follows:
  - Role preview
  - Role acceptance
  - Role exploration
  - Role discrepancy
  - Role development
  - Role internalization
- Unexpected role transitions involve a grieving process. Financial and social obligations of the manager and the employer may need to be formally dissolved with appropriate compensation and outplacement services.
- The phase of role preview is similar to dating in that both parties present their best characteristics to make a favorable impression.
- Commitment to a relationship is analogous to role acceptance—a public announcement of a mutual decision to initiate a contract.
- Role exploration is similar to the honeymoon phase of an intimate relationship.
- Role discrepancy has its roots in the disillusionment experienced when role expectations do not match role performance.
- Role development is a time of resolution, when role expectations are negotiated and performance is adjusted to approximate expectations.
- A maturing relationship is similar to role internalization; during role internalization, the performance of the role is congruent with one's own beliefs.
- Commitment, character, self-respect, and flexibility are internal resources that can facilitate the process of role transition.
- Role negotiation involves communicating with your supervisor to come to an agreement as to role expectations.
- Mentors can provide career and psychosocial functions, enhancing the career development of the manager.
- Educational programs provide information needed by nurses to fulfill management roles.

TIPS FOR ROLE TRANSITIONING

- Role transition is a normal process. Anticipate and prepare for role changes.
- Identify the responsibilities, opportunities, lines of communication, expectations, and support for the role.
- Use your internal resources to negotiate a role that is consistent with your values and life commitments.

REFERENCES

American Nurses Credentialing Center (ANCC). (2009). *Nurse executive certification eligibility criteria.* Retrieved October 21, 2009, from www.nursecredentialing.org.

American Organization of Nurse Executives (AONE). (2008). *AONE launches new nurse executive certification credential.* Retrieved October 21, 2009, from www.aone.org.

Center for the Health Professions. (2009). *RWJ program eligibility.* Retrieved October 21, 2009, from www.futurehealth.ucsf.edu.

Clark, L. (2008). Clinical leadership: Values, beliefs and vision. *Nursing Management, 15,* 30-35.

Dyer, L. (2008). The continuing need for mentors in nursing. *Journal for Nurses in Staff Development, 24,* 86-90.

Etheridge, S. A. (2007). Learning to think like a nurse: Stories from new nurse graduates. *Journal of Continuing Education in Nursing, 38*(1), 24-30.

Hardy, M. E. (1978). Role stress and role strain. In M. E. Hardy & M. E. Conway (Eds.), *Role theory: Perspectives for health professionals.* New York: Appleton-Century-Crofts.

Longest, B. (1998). Managerial competence at senior levels of integrated delivery systems. *Journal of Healthcare Management, 43*(2).

McConnell, C. (2008). The health care professional as a manager: Balancing two important roles. *The Health Care Manager, 27,* 277-284.

Salera-Vierira, J. (2009). The collegial clinical model for orientation of new graduate nurses: A strategy to improve the transition from student nurse to professional nurse. *Journal for Nurses in Staff Development, 25*(4), 174-181.

Sewell, E. (2008). Journaling as a mechanism to facilitate graduate nurses' role transition. *Journal for Nurses in Staff Development, 24,* 49-52.

Stewart, D. (2006). Generational mentoring. *Journal of Continuing Education in Nursing, 37*, 113-120.

Weston, M., Falter, B., Lamb, G., Mahon, G., Mallock, K., Provan, K., Roe, S., & Webylo, L. (2008). HealthCare Leadership Academy: A statewide collaboration to enhance nursing leadership competencies. *Journal of Continuing Education in Nursing, 37*, 468-472.

Young, M., Stuenkel, D., & Bawel-Brinkley, K. (2008). Strategies for easing the role transformation of graduate nurses. *Journal for Nurses in Staff Development, 24*(3), 105-110.

SUGGESTED READINGS

Fleming, M., & Kayser-Jones, J. (2008). Assuming the mantle of leadership: Issues and challenges for directors of nursing. *Journal of Gerontological Nursing, 34*(11), 18-25.

Scott, E., & Smith, S. (2008). Group mentoring: A transition to work strategy. *Journal for Nurses in Staff Development, 24*(5), 232-238.

Steiner, S., McLaughlin, D., Hyde, R., Brown, R., & Burman, M. (2008). Role transition during RN-to-FNP education. *The Journal of Nursing Education, 47*(10), 441-447.

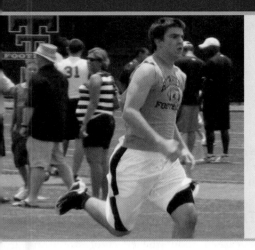

Self-Management: Stress and Time

Catherine A. Hill

This chapter examines the concept of self-management—developing self-expression and behaviors that match organizational cultures, social contexts, and the occupational expectations as a professional nurse so you can effectively re-order your day, engage in powerful persistence, and enjoy daily renewal. Three components of self-management are explored: stress management, time management, and meeting management. Methods for managing stress and organizing your time are introduced. Practical exercises and suggestions for stress management and time management are presented that can be used for personal and professional situations to reduce stress and enhance efficiency.

OBJECTIVES

- Define self-management.
- Explore personal and professional stressors.
- Analyze selected strategies to decrease stress.
- Assess the manager's role in helping staff manage stress.
- Evaluate common barriers to effective time management.
- Critique the strengths and weaknesses of selected time-management strategies.
- Evaluate selected strategies to manage time more effectively.

TERMS TO KNOW

agenda	employee assistance program	perfectionism
burnout	general adaptation syndrome	procrastination
coping	(GAS)	role stress
delegation	information overload	self-management
depersonalization	overwork	time management

THE CHALLENGE

William John Gonzolez, MSN, RN
DNP Student, Texas Woman's University College of Nursing,
Dallas, Texas

Stress seems to come at me from different directions and never disappears! This is a high-stress time for me. I am a full-time graduate student in nursing, and I have a full-time job at Parkland Hospi- tal. I have a wife and children who deserve my time and attention too. It seems I always have to be somewhere and I still have to try to get homework done!

What do you think you would do if you were this nurse?

INTRODUCTION

What should you do when you have tried your best, but things are not going well? What needs changing? Where do you begin? Self-management involves self-directed change to achieve important goals (Stuart & Laraia, 2008). As a nurse leader, your goals will require balancing personal and professional objectives and organizing your time and activities to reach them. The literature suggests that stress hardiness of nurse leaders is essential to safe, high-quality patient care (Halm et al., 2005), as well as staff recruitment and retention (Bailey, 2009). In the past, nursing research on stress focused on individual acceptance of demanding work environments, complex role requirements, and staff shortages instead of proactive problem solving (Shirey, 2006). Several thought leaders, reflected in the meta-analysis of Zangaro and Soeken (2007), suggest that cultivating stress hardiness produces nurse managers with a leadership style and resilience that improves working conditions. However, using both internally and externally available psychosocial resources did not compensate for the stress experienced by nurse managers and physicians (Lindholm, 2006). Luckily, stress hardiness can be taught (Judkins, Reid, & Furlow, 2006).

To develop stress hardiness, we must actively improve our skills related to stress management, adaptive coping, healthy communication, and problem solving. The three key strategies introduced in this chapter—stress management, time management, and meeting management—are important ways to do more with fewer resources. Time and stress are somewhat of a "chicken and egg" phenomenon—not enough time contributes to stress, and stress can erode efficiency and thus decrease time on task. The key lies in our ability to manage both time and stress, not only personally but also profes- sionally. The outcome of effective self-management is hardiness and the ability to accomplish professional and personal goals.

UNDERSTANDING STRESS

Nurses have learned about the effect of stress on patients and how to teach them to manage its conse- quences. However, only one third of nurse managers have any sort of formal leadership or managerial training (Bailey, 2009) that would prepare them for dealing with multiple sources of stress at the same time. Nurses need to recognize the unique stressors in their professional and personal lives. Everyone experiences stress—the exhilaration of a joyous event, as well as the negative feelings and unpleasant physi- cal symptoms that may be associated with a difficult life situation or even the anticipation of difficulty. Stress is the uncomfortable gap between how we would like our life to be and how it actually is. Nurses are not immune to the effects of stress. Learning what stress is, its dynamics, and some strategies to manage distress is a part of the personal and professional maturation of nurses.

Definition

In this chapter, *stress* and *distress* (Selye, 1965) are used interchangeably, although some writers regard stress as neutral and refer to the positive and negative attributes of eustress and distress, respectively. Stress is a consequence or response to an event or stimulus. Stress is not inherently bad. It is each individual's interpretation that determines whether the event is viewed as positive or threatening. In addition, stress management does not necessarily mean stress reduc- tion. Rather, stress management is characterized by emotional and behavioral control, perseverance, and challenge in the face of stressful events (Kobasa,

Maddi, & Kahn, 1982). Stress management is a nurse manager competency (Jennings, Scalzi, & Rodgers, 2007). Stress management has important implications for the workplace because of its link to low absenteeism rates, improved quality, and increased productivity (Judkins, Reid, & Furlow, 2006).

SOURCES OF JOB STRESS

Job stress can be defined as the physical and emotional responses that arise when the job requirements do not match the abilities, resources, or needs of the worker. Work-related stress can lead to poor physical and emotional health and injury. There is a difference between job-related challenges (eustress), which motivate us to learn new skills and master our jobs, and distress, which can lead to exhaustion, feelings of inadequacy, and failure. If you are involved in an oral interview for a job, you will benefit from a certain amount of stress (eustress). It is stress that provides you with determination and gives you your "edge" that will help you think quickly and clearly and express your thoughts in ways that will benefit your interview process. Having your car break down on the way to the interview creates stress (distress) as you realize that you will be late for the appointment. As more is learned about the relationship of stress to physiologic changes, stressors will become even easier to identify. When one looks at job-related stressors, the stressors fall into one of two categories: external (working conditions) and internal (worker characteristics).

External Sources

Occupational stress in nursing has been well-defined and documented. Work-related stressors, such as workload, rotating shifts, high patient acuity, inadequate staffing, ethical conflicts, dealing with death and acute illness, role ambiguity, the intensity of complexity compression, and job insecurity have all been associated with increased stress and burnout. Nurses spend more time at work, and nurse managers report 12- to 14-hour days with 24-hour accountability (Rudan, 2002).

Change

Although the distress that results from change takes many forms, two underlying patterns appear to be constant. Often, nurses feel trapped by conflicting expectations. They expect to furnish care, to meet patients' needs, and to be nurturing. However, organizations require nurses to be managers of patient care and of systems and value their contribution to efficiency and cost-effectiveness while simultaneously preserving quality of care. Because nurses cannot comply with both expectations, they experience considerable role conflict, frustration, and distress.

Social

Interpersonal relations can buffer stressors or can in themselves become stressors. Outside the work setting, home can be a refuge for harried nurses; however, stresses at home, when severe, can impair work performance and relationships among staff or even result in violence that may invade the workplace.

Changes in healthcare delivery systems, as well as the current nursing shortage, have reduced the number of professional nurses, often creating situations of minimally safe staffing levels. Consequently, some nurses lose supportive, collegial relationships that may have been established over many years. Many institutions now depend on supplemental staffing with agency or "traveling" nurses, thus creating a very transient nursing staff. In other situations, nurses are reassigned or they "float" to various patient-care units, which requires that they work with unfamiliar staff. Thus they may feel isolated or become unwillingly involved in dysfunctional politics on the unit. Such situations may also necessitate that nurses work with patients whose requirements for care may be unfamiliar, resulting in further stress related to patient safety concerns.

Persons in management-level positions may also become stressors. Communication may come from the top down, with little opportunity for nurses to participate in decisions that affect them directly or that they may need to implement without proper training or support. Nurses may experience distress from feelings of frustration and helplessness with this lack of opportunity for input to decisions.

In addition, disruptive behavior poses considerable work stress. Although healthy workplaces include freedom from such behavior, too many instances occur in healthcare settings. In addition to being stressful for nurses, such behavior can disrupt

RESEARCH PERSPECTIVE

Resource: Rosenstein, A. H., & O'Daniel, M. (2008). A survey of the impact of disruptive behaviors and communication defects on patient safety. *Joint Commission Journal on Quality and Patient Safety, 34,* 464-471.

This study involved a survey related to nurses and physicians and the effect of disruptive behavior on patient care. Although the sample was a convenience sample, over 4500 responses were analyzed. Nurses (88%) observed disruptive behaviors in physicians. Physicians (51%) acknowledged observing disruptive physician behaviors. In addition, 67% identified that disruptive behaviors contributed to adverse events.

Implications for Practice
Although it may be difficult to confront situations in which a physician is disruptive, nurses now know that this behavior does not affect only them. Disruptions affect patient care.

patient safety efforts (see the Research Perspective above).

The Position

Upon entering nursing school, most students expect that caring for patients who are chronically or critically ill and for families who have experienced tragedy will be stressful. The current environment in many healthcare agencies, however, is more complex and is often characterized by overwork, as well as by the stresses inherent in nursing practice. In some settings, direct care nurses have been expected to stay beyond the designated assignment period, often with little or no notice. Some managers experience stress in those situations and resort to threatening behaviors and statements, such as the potential for dismissal. These situations often escalate when direct care nurses do not believe they can deliver safe care and nurse managers exhaust creative ways to provide adequate coverage.

Role stress is an additional stressor for nurses. Viewed as the incongruence between perceived role expectations and achievement (Chang & Hancock, 2003), role stress for new graduates is related to role ambiguity and role overload. Role stress is particularly acute for new graduates, whose lack of clinical experience and organizational skills, combined with new situations and procedures, may increase feelings of overwhelming stress. Conflict between what was learned in the classroom and actual practice may add additional stress.

Gender Roles

Approximately 94% of the nation's 2.9 million nurses are women (Health Resources and Services Administration, 2005), and many go home to traditionally gender-related responsibilities that may include household management, children, and aging parents. When added to the already stressful workday of the nurse, the additional responsibilities often contribute to the level of distress felt by the nurse. Thanks to generation Y's entry into the workforce, greater emphasis on work-life balance has become increasingly important.

Evans and Steptoe (2002) examined the associations of work stress and gender-role orientation to psychological well-being and sickness-related work absences in male-dominated (accounting) and female-dominated (nursing) occupations in England. They concluded that when men and women are occupationally engaged in gender-dominated occupations in which they are in the gender minority, the men and women perceived more work-related hassles and exhibited gender-specific health effects.

Internal Sources

Personal stress "triggers" are events or situations that have an effect on specific individuals. A personal trigger might be a specific event such as the death of a loved one, an automobile accident, losing a job, or getting married. These events are in addition to daily personal stressors such as working in a noisy environment, job dissatisfaction, or a difficult commute to work. Negative self-talk, pessimistic thinking, self-criticism, and overanalyzing can be significant ongoing stressors. These internal sources of stress usually stem from unrealistic self-beliefs (unrealistic expectations, taking things personally, all-or-nothing thinking, exaggerating, or rigid thinking), perfectionism, or the type A personality.

An individual's ability to deal with stress may be moderated by psychological hardiness. According to Lambert, Lambert, and Yamase (2003), psychological hardiness is a composite of commitment, control, and challenge. These form a constellation that (1) dampers the effects of stress by challenging the perception of the situation and (2) decreases the negative impact of a situation by moderating both cognitive appraisal and coping. Maddi (2002), in a 12-year longitudinal study, found that individuals thriving in a stressful work environment displayed the same psychological hardiness. The commitment attitude led the individuals to be actively involved in the changes that decreased isolation. The control attitude led them to try to influence outcomes rather than sink into powerlessness and passivity. The challenge attitude led them to believe that the stressful events were opportunities for new learning.

Lifestyle choices, such as the use of caffeine, lack of exercise, poor diet, inadequate sleep and leisure time, and cigarette smoking, have a direct effect on the amount of one's stress. Most of the stress an individual has is self-generated. Recognizing that we create most of our own stress is the first step to dealing with it.

Dynamics of Stress

Stress may result from unrealistic or conflicting expectations, the pace and magnitude of change, human behavior, individual personality characteristics, the characteristics of the position itself, or the culture of the organization. Other stressors may be unique to certain environments, situations, and persons or groups. Initially, increased stress produces increased performance. However, when stress continues to increase or remains intense, performance decreases. Hans Selye's mid-century investigations of the nature of and reactions to stress (Selye, 1956) have been very influential. In his classic theory, Selye (1991) described the concept of stress, identified the general adaptation syndrome (GAS), and detailed a predictable pattern of response (see the Theory Box on p. 556 and Figure 28-1).

More recent investigations of the relationship among the brain, the immune system, and health (psychoneuroimmunology) have generated models that challenge Selye's general adaptation syndrome. Although Selye states that all people respond with a similar set of hormonal and immune responses to any stress, Kemeny (2003) proposes that there are two stress responses: (1) the classic GAS and (2) a withdrawing reaction, in which the person pulls back to conserve energy. Kemeny hypothesizes that people respond to the same psychological event in different ways, depending on their independent appraisal of the situation (DeAngelis, 2002).

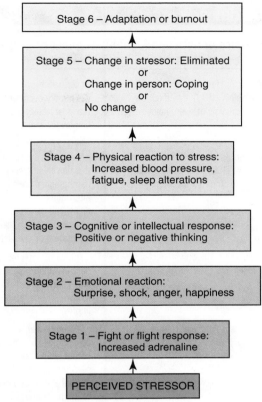

FIGURE 28-1 The stress diagram.

Critical of stress research using predominately (87%) male subjects, Taylor et al. (2000) proposed a model of the female stress response, the "tend and befriend," as opposed to the male's "fight or flight" model. The "tend and befriend" response is an estrogen and oxytocin–mediated stress response that is characterized by caring for offspring and befriending those around in times of stress to increase chances of survival.

Most nurses can easily recognize the origins of stress and its symptoms. For example, a healthcare agency may make demands on nurses, such as excessive work, that the nurses regard as beyond their capacity to perform. When they are unable to resolve the problem through overwork, with more staff, or by looking at the situation in another way, the nurses may feel threatened or depressed. They may also experience headache, fatigue, or other physical symptoms. If the stress persists, such symptoms may

THEORY BOX

Theories Applicable to Self-Management

KEY CONTRIBUTORS	KEY IDEAS	APPLICATION TO PRACTICE
Maslow's Hierarchy of Needs: Maslow (1943) identified five need levels of every human.	Although recent research shows the five levels are not always present or in order, it is reasonable that unmet needs motivate most employees most of the time.	Nurse wages should be sufficient to provide shelter and food. Job security and a social environment that rewards and recognizes nurse performance are important.
General Adaptation Syndrome: Selye (1956) is credited with developing this theory.	The "stress response" is an adrenocortical reaction to stressors that is accompanied by psychological changes and physiologic alterations that follow a pattern of fight or flight. The general adaptation syndrome includes an alarm, resistance, and adaptation or exhaustion.	Change, lack of control, and excessive workload are common stressors that evoke psychological and physiologic distress among nurses.
Complex Adaptive Systems: Plsek and Greenhalgh (2001).	This theory of unpredictable interactions between interdependent people and activities emphasizes the importance of innovation and rapid information sharing to improve performance.	Nurse engagement in self-managed groups and teams allows organizations to shape their environment through controlled "experimentation" using the rapid-cycle plan-do-study-act improvement method.
The Pareto Principle: Hafner (2001).	The "Pareto Principle" refers to a universal observation of "vital few, trivial many." Pareto (1848-1923) studied distribution of personal incomes in Italy and observed that 80% of the wealth was controlled by 20% of the population. This concept of disproportion often holds in many areas. Although the exact values of 20 and 80 are not significant, the observation of considerable disproportion is important to remember.	The 80-20 rule can be applied to many aspects of health care today. For example, 80% of healthcare expenditures are on 20% of the population, and 80% of personnel problems come from 20% of the staff. In quality improvement, 80% of improvement can be expected by removing 20% of the causes of unacceptable quality or performance. A nurse can also expect that 80% of patient-care time will be spent working with 20% of his or her patient assignment.

increase; nurses may attempt to cope by becoming apathetic or by resigning their positions. Table 28-1 gives physical, mental, and spiritual/emotional signs of overstress in individuals.

In 2004, Segerstrom and Miller published a meta-analysis of research on the relationship between stress and the human immune system. They found that acute stressors (very short-term) "revved up" the immune system, preparing for infection or injury. Short-term stressors, such as tests, tended to suppress cellular immunity while preserving humoral immu-nity. The immune systems of those who are older or already sick are more prone to stress-related immune system changes.

Physical illnesses linked to stress include visceral adiposity, type II diabetes, cardiovascular disease (hypertension, heart attack, stroke), musculoskeletal disorders, psychological disorders (anxiety, depres-sion), workplace injury, neuromuscular disorders (multiple sclerosis), suicide, cancer, ulcers, asthma, and rheumatoid arthritis. Stress can even cause life-threatening sympathetic stimulation.

TABLE 28-1	SIGNS OF OVERSTRESS IN INDIVIDUALS	
PHYSICAL	**MENTAL**	**SPIRITUAL/EMOTIONAL**
Physical signs of ill health: • Increase in flu, colds, accidents • Change in sleeping habits • Fatigue **Chronic signs of decreased ability to manage stress:** • Headaches • Hypertension • Backaches • Gastrointestinal problems **Unhealthy coping activities:** • Increased use of drugs and alcohol • Increased weight • Smoking • Crying, yelling, blaming	• Dread going to work every day • Rigid thinking and a desire to go by all the rules in all cases; inability to tolerate any changes • Forgetfulness and anxiety about work to be done; more frequent errors and incidents • Returning home exhausted and unable to participate in enjoyable activities • Confusion about duties and roles • Generalized anxiety • Decrease in concentration • Depression • Anger, irritability, impatience	• Sense of being a failure; disappointed in work performance • Anger and resentment toward patients, colleagues, and managers; overall irritable attitude • Lack of positive feelings toward others • Cynicism toward patients, blaming them for their problems • Excessive worry, insecurity, lowered self-esteem • Increased family and friend conflict

MANAGEMENT OF STRESS

Individuals respond to stress by eliciting coping strategies that are a means of dealing with stress to maintain or achieve well-being. These strategies may be ineffective because of their reliance on methods such as withdrawal or substance abuse, or they may be effective in helping restore a greater sense of well-being and effectiveness. Some of these effective strategies are discussed here.

Stress Prevention

One effective way to deal with stress is to determine and manage its source. Discovering the origin of stress in patient care may be difficult because some environments have changed so rapidly that the nursing staff is overwhelmed trying to balance bureaucratic rules and limited resources with the demands of vulnerable human beings. *Complexity compression* is the name given to conditions in which change occurs with great intensity (Krichbaum et al., 2007). When in distress, nurses may need to step back and look at the "big picture." By identifying daily stressors, the nurse can then develop a plan of action for management of the stress. This plan may include elimination of the stressor, modification of the stressor, or changing the perception of the stressor (e.g., viewing mistakes as opportunities for new learning) using a reframing technique.

Many of the day-to-day activities of nursing can create workplace stress. Consider the critical nature of nursing work and the potential for serious injury to others. Staffing shortages create situations of caring for more patients with less help. Nurses may have inadequate rest because of rotating shifts or irregular schedules. Nurses are subject to significant musculoskeletal stress caused by lifting, pulling, and turning patients. Nurses give physical care to those who are physically unclean or verbally abusive. Nurses watch patients and families suffer with pain and grief. These stressors are often counterbalanced by the rewards of patient appreciation, the joy of seeing a healthy baby born, or seeing the relief brought by a medication or repositioning. However, given the stressful nature of nursing, it is wise for the nurse to be alert to his or her own signs of stress and to develop lifestyle habits that help reduce stress. Adequate sleep, a balanced diet, regular exercise, and frequent interactions with friends are excellent stress-buffering habits to develop.

According to Stöppler (2005), the top five stress-management mistakes are poor calendar habits, clutter, perfectionism, self-treatment, and following others' expectations. These may be high on your list of stress experiences. Analyze your stress experiences by completing Exercise 28-1.

Symptom Management

Unpredictable and uncontrollable change, coupled with immense responsibility and little control over the work environment, produces stress for nurses and other healthcare professionals. Consequently, nurses may develop emotional symptoms such as anxiety, depression, or anger; physical alterations such as fatigue, headache, and insomnia; mental changes such as a decrease in concentration and memory; and behavioral changes such as smoking, drinking, crying, and swearing. The important factor is not the stressor but, rather, how the individual perceives the stressor and what coping mechanisms are available to mediate the hormonal response to the stressor.

Multiple "stress-buffering" behaviors can be elicited to reduce the detrimental effects of stress. The stressor-induced changes in the hormonal and immune systems can be modulated by an individual's behavioral coping responses. These coping responses include leisure activities and taking time for self, decreasing or discontinuing the use of caffeine, positive social support, a strong belief system, a sense of humor, developing realistic expectations, reframing events, regular aerobic exercise, meditation, and use of the relaxation response.

Everyone needs to balance work and leisure in his or her life. Leisure time and stress are inversely proportional. If time for work is more than 60% of awake time or if self-time is less than 10% of awake time, stress levels will increase. Changes should be made to relieve stress, such as decreasing the number of work hours or finding more time for leisure activities. Caffeine is a strong stimulant and, in itself, a stressor. Slowly weaning off caffeine should result in better sleep and more energy. Positive social support can offer validation, encouragement, or advice. By discussing situations with others, one can reduce stress. A great deal of stress comes from our belief systems, which cause stress in two ways. First, behaviors result from them, such as placing work before pleasure. Second, beliefs may also conflict with those of other people, as may happen with patients from different cultures. Articulating beliefs and finding common ground will help reduce anger and stress. Humor is a great stress reducer and laughter a great tension reducer. A common source of stress is unrealistic expectations. Realistic expectations can make life feel more predictable and more manageable. *Reframing* is changing the way you look at things to make you feel better about them or to obtain a different perspective. Recognizing that there are many ways to interpret the same situation, taking the positive view is less stressful. Regular aerobic exercise is a logical method of dissipating the excess energy generated by the stress response.

Meditation to elicit the relaxation response can be beneficial. The benefits of practicing relaxation techniques for 20 minutes daily include a feeling of well-being, the ability to learn how tension makes the body feel, and the sense that tension can be controlled. In cases of some stress-related disorders (e.g., hypertension), biofeedback may be used to monitor physiologic relaxation processes. Exercise 28-2 outlines one systematic relaxation technique.

Social support in the form of positive work relationships, as well as nurturing family and friends, may be an important way to buffer the negative effects of a stressful work environment (Erdwins, Buffardi, Casper, & O'Brien, 2001). Although friendships may be formed with colleagues, the workload and the shifting of staff from one unit to another often make it difficult to establish and maintain close relationships with peers. However, managers and co-workers who are supportive may improve morale in the workplace (Zangaro & Soeken, 2007) (see the Research Perspective at right). Nurses in a new position or in an unfamiliar geographic area must anticipate that they will benefit from the security of being part of a group that can furnish emotional support. Without easily accessible family and friends, nurses need to be intentional about seeking new, supportive personal relationships. Such efforts may help nurses cope with workplace demands that seem to exceed their capabilities. Positive coping strategies may also make nurses less likely to adopt such potentially negative coping strategies as withdrawing, lowering their standards of care, and abusing alcohol or other substances.

EXERCISE 28-2
This exercise can be used in the middle of a working day, the last thing at night, or at any time you feel tense or anxious. Review the information and strategies at the Mayo website: *www.mayoclinic.com/health/meditation/HQ01070*. Make a short list of steps to take, and put it in your smart phone, personal digital assistant (PDA), or notepad.

Burnout

Sometimes individuals cannot manage stress successfully through their own efforts and require assistance. Examples of behavior related to stress that feels overwhelming are found in Table 28-1 on p. 557. Coping strategies, such as those described previously, may furnish temporary relief or none at all. With this level of distress, one can feel overwhelmed or helpless and may be at greater risk for mental or physical illness. This constellation of emotions is commonly called *burnout*.

A classic definition of burnout is a "prolonged response to chronic emotional and interpersonal stressors on the job" (Maslach, Schaufeli, & Leiter, 2000, p. 398). The sources of the stressors may exist in the environment, in the individual, or in the interaction between the individual and the environment. Some stressors, such as employment termination, appear to be universal, whereas other stressors, such

 RESEARCH PERSPECTIVE

Resource: Zangaro, G. A., & Soeken, K. L. (2007). A meta-analysis of studies of nurses' job satisfaction, *Research in Nursing & Health, 30,* 445-458.

This study looked at the strength of the relationship between job satisfaction, autonomy, stress, and collaboration in 31 studies that included 14, 567 subjects. Although the findings varied, job satisfaction correlated most strongly with job stress, followed by collaboration and autonomy. These findings have important implications for improving nurses' work environment.

Implications for Practice
Given the current nursing shortage, nurse job satisfaction and employee retention are very important to current healthcare industry demands for safe, effective, patient-centered, timely, efficient, and equitable care. Nurses and nurse managers in all settings are faced with resource constraints. Identifying and validating nurse perceptions about stress, collaboration, and autonomy facilitate accurate assessment and effective management of staff, turnover rates, and performance.

---

as meeting deadlines, are more personal. For example, some nurses thrive on goals and timetables, whereas others feel constrained and frustrated and thereby experience distress. Burnout is not an objective phenomenon as if it were the accumulation of a certain number and type of stressors. How the stressors are perceived and how they are mediated by an individual's ability to adapt are important variables in determining levels of distress.

Nurses who are burned out feel as though their resources are depleted to the point that their well-being is at risk. A self-analysis usually uncovers the characteristics of burnout. First, a feeling of physical, mental, and emotional exhaustion can be recognized. Greenglass, Burke, and Fiksenbaum (2001) found that emotional exhaustion was directly related to workload. For example, recent graduates may value total, detailed care for individuals and may have little experience in caring for more than two patients simultaneously. When confronted with the responsibility of caring for a group of six to eight acutely ill patients, they may have difficulty adapting to the realities of the workplace and emotional exhaustion ensues. Emotional exhaustion in turn has a direct effect on levels of cynicism and somatization. A second characteristic of burnout is

TABLE 28-2	STRESS-MANAGEMENT STRATEGIES	
PHYSICAL	**MENTAL**	**EMOTIONAL/SPIRITUAL**
• Accept physical limitations • Modify nutrition: moderate carbohydrate, moderate protein, high in fruits and vegetables, low caffeine, low sugar • Exercise: participate in an enjoyable activity five times a week for 30 minutes • Make your physical health a priority • Nurture yourself by taking time for breaks and lunch • Sleep: get enough in quantity and quality • Relax: use meditation, massage, yoga, or biofeedback	• Learn to say "no"! • Use cognitive restructuring and self-talk • Use imagery • Develop hobbies or activities • Plan vacations • Learn about the system and how problems are handled • Learn communication, conflict resolution, and time-management skills • Take continuing education courses	• Use meditation • Seek solace in prayer • Seek professional counseling • Participate in support groups • Participate in networking • Communicate feelings • Identify and acquire a mentor • Ask for feedback and clarification

depersonalization, a state characterized by distancing oneself from the work itself and developing negative attitudes toward work in general (Greenglass et al., 2001). Depersonalization is commonly described as a feeling of being outside one's body, feeling as if one is a machine or robot, an "unreal" feeling that one is in a dream or that one "is on automatic pilot." Generally, subjective symptoms of unreality make the nurse uneasy and anxious. Others may view this as callousness. Nurses pushed to do too much in too little time may distance themselves from patients as a means of dealing with emotional exhaustion.

A decreased sense of professional accomplishment and competence is the third hallmark of burnout. Low professional efficacy has been found to be a function of higher levels of cynicism (Greenglass et al., 2001). *Efficacy* is one's belief in his or her capabilities to organize and execute goal-oriented activities. Nurses are more inclined to take on a task if they believe they can succeed. Low efficacy can lead nurses to believe tasks are harder than they actually are. This can lead to a sense of failure, perceived helplessness, and finally crisis. Coping skills are no longer effective. At this point, help from others is needed.

RESOLUTION OF STRESS

Resolution of stress in its early stages can be accomplished through a variety of techniques. Nurses must be able to reach a balance of caring for others and caring for self. Table 28-2 summarizes physical, mental, and emotional/spiritual strategies.

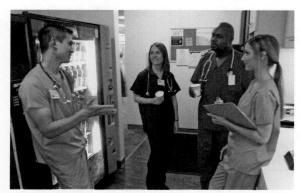

Peers and followers can be supportive and help reduce stress.

Social Support

Peers and followers can be supportive and help reduce stress by assisting with problem solving and by developing new perspectives. Family and friends can provide a safe haven and a vacation from stress. Social isolation increases stress. Social support allows one to be playful, have fun, laugh, and vent emotions.

Counseling

Persistent, unpleasant feelings, problem behavior, and helplessness during prolonged stress may suggest the need for assistance from a mental health professional. Examples of problem behaviors include tearfulness or angry outbursts over seemingly minor incidents, major changes in eating and/or sleeping patterns, frequent unwillingness to go to work, and substance abuse. In such cases, the aforementioned coping strategies afford only temporary relief; nurses with this level of distress feel overwhelmed and believe that their well-being cannot be maintained. In these stressful situations, nurses may feel helpless and require professional assistance from an advanced practice psychiatric nurse, clinical psychologist, psychiatrist, or other mental health worker.

In some organizations, employee assistance programs (EAPs) provide free, voluntary, confidential, short-term professional counseling and other services for employees either via in-house staff or by contract with a mental health agency. This type of counseling can be effective because the counselors may already be aware of organizational stressors. Some nurses may have confidentiality concerns when using employer-recommended or employer-provided counseling services. Mental health professionals are bound by their professional standards of confidentiality. Nonetheless, there may be times when it is in the nurse's best interest to sign a release of information, such as when seeking employer accommodation for a certain physical or emotional problem.

Those who seek counseling outside of the workplace may be guided in their selection of mental health professionals by a personal physician, a knowledgeable colleague, or such publications as the most recent edition of the *Official American Board of Medical Specialties (AMBS) Directory of Board Certified Medical Specialists* (American Board of Medical Specialties [ABMS], 2008), which is available on the Internet and in many hospital libraries. When the problem underlying the distress is ethical or moral, a trained pastoral counselor may be helpful. Some clergy are certified in pastoral care or have earned a degree in another discipline such as psychology. Referrals can be obtained from hospital pastoral-care departments or churches that sponsor regional centers where certified counselors are available. When private counseling is being arranged, the health insurance contract should be checked to determine mental health benefits and the payment limitations and types of providers eligible for reimbursement.

Leadership and Management

Although social support and counseling can alter how stressors are perceived, time management and effective leadership can modify or remove stressors. Nurse managers have limited formal authority as individuals in most organizations, although managerial groups may be able to influence policy and resource allocation. Nurse managers can, however, control some environmental stressors on their units. First, managers can examine their own behavior as a source of subordinates' stress.

In some cases, a controlling or autocratic style of management is appropriate, such as in emergency situations and when working with a large percentage of new and inexperienced employees. For the most part, however, professional nurses need and want the latitude to direct their activities within their sphere of competence. "Letting go," or delegating, means that the nurse leader trusts the personal integrity and professional competence of the team. It does not mean abdicating accountability for achieving accepted standards of patient care and agreed-upon outcomes.

Assistance with problem solving is another way to reduce environmental stressors. Nurse leaders may provide technical advice, refer staff to appropriate resources, or mediate conflicts. Often, nurse leaders enable staff to meet the demands of their work more independently by providing time for continuing education and professional meetings to enhance competence.

Another way in which nurse leaders can reduce stress is to be supportive of staff. Support is not equated with being a friend but, rather, with helping one's peers accomplish good care, develop professionally, and feel valued personally. Leaders can ensure that the expected workload is in line with the nurses' capabilities and resources. They can work to ensure meaningfulness, stimulation, and opportunities for nurses to use their skills. Nurses' roles and responsibilities need to be clearly and publicly defined. Work schedules should be posted as far in advance as possible and should be compatible with what is known about patient safety. Encouraging innovation and experimentation, for example, can motivate staff and give them a sense of greater control over their environment. Affirming a good idea or finding resources to study or implement a promising new procedure or proposal by a staff nurse is supportive. In contrast, when staff members struggle with overwork and other stressors, support is recognizing the condition and helping the nurses avoid such passive coping strategies as feeling helpless or lowering standards of care in favor of active problem solving. Nurse leaders must be sensitive to the distress of the nursing staff and recognize it verbally without becoming counselors, which is in conflict with their role. Support may involve making nursing staff aware of resources that furnish counseling while being careful to avoid diagnostic labels and to maintain strict confidentiality. When distress relates to the personal life of subordinates, managers should focus on the effect of such situations on workplace performance—not on the events that have produced the stress.

In addition, leaders can enhance the workplace by dealing effectively with their own stressors. Maintaining a sense of perspective as well as a sense of humor is important. Some stressors, in fact, can be ignored or minimized by posing three questions:

1. "Is this event or situation important?" Stressors are not all equally significant. Do not waste energy on little stressors.
2. "Does this stressor affect me or my unit?" Although some situations that produce distress are institution-wide and need group action, others target specific units or activities. Do not borrow stressors.
3. "Can I change this situation?" If not, then find a way to cope with it or, if the situation is intolerable, make plans to change positions or employers. This decision may require gaining added credentials that may produce long-term career benefits.

Keeping stressful situations in perspective can enable nurses to conserve their energies to cope with stressful situations that are important, that are within their domain, or that can be changed or modified.

MANAGEMENT OF TIME

A very close relationship exists between stress management and time management. Time management is one method of stress prevention or reduction. Stress can decrease productivity and lead to poor use of time. Time management can be considered a preventive action to help reduce the elements of stress in a nurse's life.

Everyone has two choices when managing time: organize or "go with the flow." There are only 24 hours in every day, and it is clear that some people make better use of time than others do. *How* people use time makes some people more successful than others. The effective use of time-management skills thus becomes an even more important tool to achieve personal and professional goals. Time management is the appropriate use of tools, techniques, and principles to control time spent on low-priority needs and to ensure that time is invested in activities leading toward achieving desired, high-priority goals. More simply, time management is the ability to spend your time on the things that matter to you and your organization. However, it does take time to plan daily time-management strategies! By setting goals and eliminating time stealers, you will have the extra time to accomplish them.

Where Does Your Time Go?

Have you ever wasted time? Time, although a cheap commodity, is our most valuable resource. There are some commonly identified time stealers, and individuals must recognize them to guard against them. At the heart of time management is an important shift in focus. Concentrate on results, not on being busy.

Doing Too Much

Do you try to do too much at once? At work, do you have three or four major projects going simultaneously? Are you a member of more than one organizational committee? Do you have to worry about what will be on the table for dinner while you are hanging an IV and planning a staff meeting? Have you ever completed a nursing intervention and realized that your mind was really somewhere else and you had ignored the patient? If you *think* you have too much to do, you probably do! Learn to have fewer projects running simultaneously and to concentrate your efforts on one thing at a time. The first step is to be realistic and limit major commitments, and then give each activity your full and undivided attention. Sometimes completing one task before starting another is the most efficient method for getting everything done. Prioritization of goals and activities each day is very helpful.

In the nursing profession, however, limiting commitments is not always possible. When you are feeling overwhelmed by the sheer volume of tasks to be completed, take the time to establish priorities for the day.

Decide what must be done versus what would be nice to do. Do not let yourself get distracted from your priority tasks. Nursing is a balancing act; priorities are always changing.

Inability to Say "No"

Sometimes the smallest and simplest words are the most difficult to learn. If you are suffering from overload, you probably have gotten there by not being able to say "no." Learning to say "no" to requests is difficult, and in the process, others may be displeased. If you do not say "no," however, you may end up spending much time on projects that are uninteresting or have no relationship to your personal goals and priorities. When someone asks you to do something, you need to stop and consider the request. Do you want to do the task now or sometime in the future? If not, then say so. If you wish to do the task but simply do not have the time, consider delegation. However, be honest with the requester—if you simply do not have the time, say so as politely as possible. If you wish to take on the task but at a later date, negotiate. Remember, accepting an assignment you will never be able to complete sheds an unfavorable light on you.

Procrastination

Do you put off important tasks because they are not enjoyable or because they may be difficult? Do you find excuses for not starting or completing tasks? Are you a procrastinator? By engaging in procrastination, or doing one thing when you should be doing something else, you give up time to complete your task and therefore limit the quality of the work you produce. There are techniques to help deal with procrastination. First, identify the reason for procrastinating. Then make that task your highest priority the next day. Reward yourself after you finish the task. Another technique is to select the least attractive element of the task to do first, and the rest will seem easy.

Some people find that they procrastinate when the task ahead is very large. The solution is to break the task down into manageable pieces and plan rewards for accomplishing each of the smaller tasks. Developing a **p**rogram **e**valuation and **r**eview **t**echnique (PERT) chart or a Gantt chart may help in this process. PERT charts were originally developed as tools to assist in complex projects that require a series of activities, some of which must be performed sequentially and others that can be performed in parallel with other activities. Envisioned as a network diagram, a PERT chart indicates dependent activities that must be completed before a new activity is undertaken. A Gantt chart (Table 28-3) consists of a table of project task information and a bar chart that graphically displays the project schedule. This method of tracking project activities in relation to time is often used in planning and project management. Both chart techniques can be used to outline how you will approach a large project.

Complaining

Complaining is the act of expressing dissatisfaction or annoyance with persons, places, things, and situations (Merriam-Webster Online, 2009). Often, the time people spend complaining about a task or a particular

TABLE 28-3	SAMPLE GANTT CHART							
TASK	**ACCOUNTABILITY**	**JAN**	**FEB**	**MAR**	**APR**	**MAY**	**JUNE**
1. Conduct literature search	Unit clinical nurse specialist	————	→→				
2. Hold nursing practice committee meeting to review material	Chair, nursing practice committee		X				
3. Create a report for the medical staff	Chair, nursing practice committee			————	→→		
4. Disseminate findings to nursing and medical staff	Chair, nursing practice committee					————	→→

situation is greater than the time needed to complete the task or to deal with the issue. If you find yourself complaining repeatedly about something, stop and ask yourself what would be the ideal solution and then take the risk to act on it. If the complaint is related to another person, either take the time to talk with the person and get the problem out in the open or write a letter to the person discussing your point of view (even if you do not mail it). If you find yourself complaining about something within the workplace, rethink the problem, generate some possible solutions, and then talk to your manager. Look for solutions that are very simple or "outside the box." Talk to your manager and be prepared to discuss solutions—not just your dissatisfaction or annoyance. In this way, your manager will see you as interested in contributing to the goals of the organization.

Perfectionism

Perfectionism is the tendency to never finish anything because it is not yet perfect. This approach tends to consume much time when your expected outcome is not attainable. Overcoming perfectionism takes considerable effort. However, this does not mean that you should do less than your best. Being aware of perfectionism means that you occasionally need to give yourself permission to do slightly less than a perfect job, such as buying a carryout dinner rather than preparing a four-course meal after a day at work.

Interruptions

One common distraction from priority activities is interruptions. Some interruptions are integral to the positions that you hold, but others can be controlled. A home care nurse with a large caseload can expect to be paged at any time. More commonly, however, are the numerous small interruptions by individuals who want just a "minute of your time" and take 2 minutes getting to the point! Box 28-1 identifies some specific strategies to prevent and control interruptions. The two keys to dealing with interruptions are to resume "doing it now" so that an interruption does not destroy your schedule and to maintain the attitude that whatever the interruption, it is a part of your responsibility. When you make a conscious decision not to worry about the things you cannot control, you

have more energy to maintain a positive perspective and to move projects forward.

Disorganization

One of the most serious time wasters of all is disorganization. How many times have you had to spend 5 minutes trying to find something you have misplaced or misfiled? Organization can be a great time saver. Remember that the guiding principle is that organization is a process rather than the product. You can spend so much time organizing that you will never get to the task at hand (procrastination). Simple organizing guidelines include eliminating clutter, keeping everything in its place, and doing similar tasks together. In contrast, Abrahamson and Freedman (2006) make the case that there are benefits to disorder because disorder often is more efficient and may produce better outcomes.

BOX 28-1   TIPS TO AVOID INTERRUPTIONS AND WORK MORE EFFECTIVELY

- Ask people to put their comments in writing—do not let them catch you "on the run."
- Let the office/unit secretary know what information you need immediately.
- Conduct a conversation in the hall to help keep it short or in a separate room to keep from being interrupted.
- Be comfortable saying "no."
- When involved in a long procedure or home visit, ask someone else to cover your other responsibilities.
- Break projects into small, manageable pieces.
- Get yourself organized.
- Minimize interruptions—for example, allow voice mail to pick up the phone; shut the door.
- Keep your work surface clear. Have available only those documents needed for the task at hand.
- Keep your manager informed of your goals.
- Plan to accomplish high-priority or difficult tasks early in the day.
- Develop a plan for the day and stick to it. Remember to schedule in some time for interruptions.
- Schedule time to meet regularly throughout the shift with staff members for whom you are responsible.
- Recognize that crises and interruptions are part of the position.
- Be cognizant of your personal time-waster habits, and try to avoid them.

Too Much Information

The newest time waster to evolve is data proliferation. The technology within our workplace forces us to receive huge amounts of data and to transform these data into useful information. The computer workstation, once touted as a time-saving device, has become the driving force behind care delivery. Nurses can view the computer either as a stress-producing slave driver or as a simple tool to assist them in their daily activities.

Information overload, or "data smog," occurs when you are overwhelmed by too much information, too fast, and too often and do not have the skills to interpret the data into useful information. Developing data and information gathering, receiving and sending skills (known as *information literacy*) can greatly reduce stress and improve efficiency and productivity (Englebardt & Nelson, 2002). Gaining a new appreciation for information is important. Information is simply a tool to use to plan action or make decisions. By learning what information is important, you can learn to use it to your advantage.

Time-Management Concepts

Table 28-4 presents a classification scheme for time-management techniques. The unifying theme is that each activity undertaken should lead to goal attainment and that goal should be the number-one priority at that time.

Goal-Setting

The first steps in time management are goal-setting and developing a plan to reach the goals. Set goals that are reasonable and achievable. Do not expect to reach long-term goals overnight—*long-term* means just that. Give yourself time to meet the goals. Determine many short-term goals to reach the long-term goal, giving you a frequent sense of goal achievement. Give yourself flexibility. If the path you chose last year is no longer appropriate, change it. Write your goals, date the entry, keep it handy, and refer to it often to give yourself a progress report.

Setting Priorities

Once goals are known, priorities are set. They may, however, shift throughout a given period in terms of goal attainment. For example, working on a budget may take precedence at certain times of the year, whereas new staff orientation is high priority at other times. Knowing what your goals and priorities are helps shape the "to do" list. On a nursing unit or as you work in a community setting, you must know your personal goals and current priorities. How you organize work may depend on geographic considerations, patient acuity, or some other schema.

A particular strategy to assist in prioritization suggests that people generally focus on those things that are important and urgent. By placing the elements of importance and urgency in a grid (Figure 28-2), all

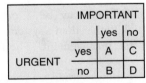

FIGURE 28-2 Classification of priorities.

TABLE 28-4	CLASSIFICATION OF TIME-MANAGEMENT TECHNIQUES	
TECHNIQUE	**PURPOSE**	**ACTIONS**
Organization	Designed to promote efficiency and productivity	Organize and systematize things, tasks, and people. Use basic time-management skills.
Keep focused on goals	Focuses on goal achievement	Assemble a prioritized "to do" list based on goals daily.
Tool usage	Uses the right tool for planning and preparation	Use tools such as a smart phone.
Time-management plan	Helps to refocus, to gain control, and to use information	Develop a personal time-management plan appropriately.

activities can be classified as shown (Covey, Merrill, & Merrill, 1994).

Typically, we tend to focus on those items in cell A because they are both important and urgent and therefore command our attention. Making shift assignments is an A task because it is both important to the work to be accomplished and commonly urgent because there is a time frame during which data about patients and qualifications of staff can be matched. Conversely, if something is neither important nor urgent (cell D), it may be considered a waste of time, at least in terms of personal goals. An example of a D activity might be reading "junk" e-mail. Even if something is urgent but not important (cell C), it contributes minimally to productivity and goal achievement. An example of a C activity might be responding to a memo that has a specific time line but is not important to goal attainment. The real key to setting priorities is to attend to the B tasks, those that are important but not urgent. Examples of B activities are reviewing the organization's strategic plan or participating on organizational committees.

Organization

A number of simple routines for organization can save many minutes over a day and enhance your efficiency. Keeping a workspace neat or arranging things in an orderly fashion may be a powerful time-management tool. Rather than a system of "pile management," use "file management." The following are a few hints:

- Plan where things should go: your desk or your disk
- Keep a clean workspace
- Create a "to do" folder
- Create a "to be filed" folder for any papers
- Schedule time to work your way through the folders

Determine your priority goals for the next day, and have the materials ready to work on when you start the next morning.

Time Tools

Sometimes, the real problem is that the events of the day become the driving force, rather than a planned schedule. Days may become so tightly scheduled that any little interruption can become a crisis. If you do not plan the day, you may be responding to events rather than prioritized goals. If you think you are a reactor rather than a proactive time user, use a time log to list work-related activities for several days. You may not be able to plan well because you really do not have a good estimate of how long a particular activity actually takes or you do not know how many activities can be accomplished in a given time frame.

As the nurse's role in care management becomes more complex, the need for organizational tools increases. Tracking the care of groups of patients, either as the member of a care team or in a leadership capacity, can be overwhelming. Each nurse must devise a method for tracking care and organizing time, as well as delegating and monitoring care provided by others. Although some nurses depend on a shift flowsheet or a Kardex system, others have the benefit of computerized information tracking systems. Handheld computer devices such as PDAs or bar-code scanners for medication administration are other methods to track information and increase safety and efficiency. However, the issue of patient confidentiality cannot be ignored when entering data into a PDA that you take home at the end of your shift.

Managing Information

The first step in managing information is to assess the source. Once you have identified the sources of your data, you have a better idea of how to deal with the information. Track incoming information for a few days. Patterns will begin to emerge and will give clues as to how to deal with it. You can generally predict that, using the Pareto principle, 80% of your incoming data comes from approximately 20% of your sources and that 80% of useful information comes from 20% of information received (see the Theory Box on p. 556).

By developing information-receiving skills, you can quickly interpret the data and convert them to useful information, discarding unneeded data. Initially, you should reduce or eliminate that which is useless. Delete the e-mail, or toss the memo in the trash. Next, monitor the information flow and decide what to do with incoming data. Find and focus on the most important pieces, and then quickly narrow down the specific details you need. Identify resources that are most helpful, and have them readily available. Be able to build the "big picture" from the masses of data you receive. Finally, recognize when you have enough information to act.

Once you have mastered the receiving end of information, concentrate on information-sending skills. Remember, your information is simply another person's data! Try to keep your outflow short; make it a synthesis of the information. Finally, select the most appropriate mode of communication for your message from the technology available. You may be sending your information in written (memo or report) or verbal (face-to-face or presentation) form or via telephone, voice mail, e-mail, text, twitter, or fax. Remember, the most important skill is to know when you have said enough. Exercise 28-3 will help you consider how you have dealt with information.

EXERCISE 28-3

Think of the last time you were in the clinical area. How often did you record the same piece of data (e.g., a finding in your assessment of the patient)? Remember to include all steps, from your jotting down notes on a piece of paper or entering data into the computer to the final report of the day. What information processing tools could decrease the number of steps?

MEETING MANAGEMENT

Two key time-management strategies that are critical to success are managing meetings and delegation, which are discussed in the next two sections of this chapter. Even nurses who may not have extensive management responsibilities usually are in the position of delegating tasks to less-skilled workers and can benefit from learning to make the most of meetings, either as the leader or as a group member.

Managing Meetings

Meetings serve various purposes, ranging from creating social networks to setting formal policy. Lencioni (2004) defines four types of meetings, as follows:

- The first meeting type is the daily check-in, which takes about 5 minutes and is the opportunity to check schedules and activities. This might be analogous to a "touch base" or huddle meeting to ensure that everyone is progressing as planned and that no patient-care issues are unattended.

- The second meeting type is the weekly tactical meeting, which is used to resolve issues. This type would be reflective of what the unit staff needs to address to ensure that it has the resources to achieve what it needs to do for patients.

- The monthly strategic meeting type is used to address big issues that have longer-term implications. These meetings are frequently standing committees of the organization on which staff serve.

- The fourth meeting type is the quarterly off-site review, which is designed to analyze progress and to develop the team. It is uncommon to find that many organizations provide this frequency and intensity (Lencioni suggests this type of meeting should be 1 to 2 days) except at higher levels in the organization.

Meetings may be designed to solve problems, disseminate information, seek input, inspire the group, delegate work or authority, or create/maintain a formal power base. Unless the purpose of a meeting is to socialize, the meeting is unlikely to be effective if it is poorly managed.

Tips for Managing Meetings Effectively

Consider if this meeting is necessary. For example, a phone call, posted notice, e-mail, or brief "huddle" (a short, check-in meeting) might suffice. If the right people are not available, rescheduling may be a good option.

Schedule meetings right before lunch or at the end of the day. Participants will have an incentive to stick to the schedule. Set a start time and a stop time, and reward prompt members by starting on schedule. Avoid meetings lasting longer than $1\frac{1}{2}$ to 2 hours. Select an appropriate setting in which the participants are not readily accessible to interruptions. If necessary, plan the seating arrangement to prevent inappropriate behaviors such as whispering or other interruptions. If the group meets over a period of time, have group members set rules for conduct and behavior.

Distribute an agenda. Whenever possible, provide a written agenda to each member in advance of the meeting. Establish and make known the goal of the meeting. Attach all needed preparation reading to the agenda. The more advanced the reading or preparation that is required, the earlier members should receive agendas. Different types of agendas can be used for different purposes:

- *Structured agendas:* If a topic is particularly controversial, consider setting a rule that requires any negative comment to be preceded by a positive one.
- *Timed agendas:* Consider setting a specific amount of time to be dedicated to each item on the agenda. If you stick to the schedule, discussion will stay focused and you will be more likely to make it through the agenda. However, setting realistic times is critical to the success of this strategy.
- *Action agendas:* Consider submitting an agenda with a description of the needed/desired action, such as review proposals, approve minutes, or establish outcomes.

Keep the group on task. Use rules of order to facilitate meetings. Robert's Rules of Order (Robert, Evans, Honemann, & Balch, 2000) may seem overly structured; however, this structure is particularly helpful when diversity of opinion is likely or important. Specifically, these rules help the person chairing the meeting by setting limits on discussion and using a specific order of priorities to deal with concerns.

Keep minutes, and distribute them to participants. The minutes provide a record for reference if needed and convey contents to persons unable to attend.

Planning for the meeting is a group leader's best strategy for a satisfactory experience. Participants must also prepare for meetings. Reviewing the agenda (or requesting one in advance if not provided), reviewing preparatory materials, and thinking through agenda items are ways that group members may assist in accomplishing the meeting goals. Meeting participants should be on time for all meetings or communicate that they will be late or unable to attend. Participants should be prepared to leave on time as well. When a meeting is poorly chaired, a committee member could volunteer to ensure that the meeting agendas and minutes are distributed. It is important to recognize that some people deliberately avoid preparing agendas and distributing minutes in an attempt to control the meeting. Exercise 28-4 will help you understand the importance of well-run meetings.

> **EXERCISE 28-4**
> Have you ever sat in a meeting and wondered why you were there? Perhaps the purpose of the meeting, where the meeting was heading, or even who was in charge was unclear to you! Write down the three things about the meeting that were most annoying, and then analyze how the situation could have been handled better.

Delegating

Delegation is a critical component of self-management for nurse managers and care managers. Appropriate delegation not only increases time efficiency but also serves as a means of reducing stress. Delegation is discussed in depth in Chapter 26, but it is also appropriate to discuss briefly as a time-management strategy. Delegation works only when the delegator trusts the delegatee to accomplish the task and to report findings back to the delegator. The delegator wastes time if he or she checks and redoes everything someone else has done. Delegation requires empowerment of the delegatee to accomplish the task. If the nurse does not delegate appropriately, with clear expectations, the delegatee will constantly be asking for assistance or direction. Delegation can also be a means of reducing stress if used appropriately. If the nurse does not understand delegation and does not use it appropriately, it can be a major source of stress as the nurse assumes accountability and responsibility for care administered by others.

SUMMARY

Self-management is a means to achieve a balance between work and personal life, as well as a way of life to achieve personal goals within self-imposed priorities and deadlines. Time management is clock-oriented, and stress management is the control of external and internal stressors.

To achieve a balance in life and minimize stressors, nurses must learn to sit back and see their own personal "big picture" and examine their personal and professional goals. Personal priorities also must be established. Stressors and coping strategies need to be identified and used. By developing these techniques, nurses can gain a sense of control and become far better nurses in the process.

THE SOLUTION

I do feel I handle the stress better than I used to. Considering the increased load, I guess I must! I definitely take better care of myself than I used to: I get enough sleep; I try to eat a balanced diet; I take a vitamin daily; I exercise at least 15 to 30 minutes everyday; and I try not to procrastinate too much, as that just increases the stress because I am thinking about the project the whole time I am putting off doing it.

My wife is really supportive, and I have a good friend who takes some classes with me. I often take myself out for lunch when it's getting really bad. I also pray each day, and I find that helps tremendously. Probably the most important thing I have learned to do is really be in the present moment. For example, when I am playing with the kids, I don't fixate on how long until I can go work on whatever project, or when I'm out on Friday night, I really don't think about all the stuff that just happened that week or that is coming up the next week. That helps because the effect stress has is really what we do with it. So if I don't focus on all that stuff all the time, my stress level is much more manageable! I think having many options to manage stress is important ... not every method works for me every time, so I pick and choose what I can do at the time to get some benefit.

—*William John Gonzolez*

Would this be a suitable approach for you? Why?

THE EVIDENCE

Melchior et al. (2007) studied increased work stress and its effect on depression and anxiety. This study is based on a birth cohort that was most recently assessed in 2004-2005. These men and women, age 32 years, were interviewed regarding their work stress. Those individuals with highly intense, demanding work had an increased risk for a depressive disorder or an anxiety disorder. Other factors that were analyzed and eliminated as affecting depression and anxiety included history of psychiatric disorders, socioeconomic status, and general negativity.

NEED TO KNOW NOW

- Create an organization system that works for you.
- Be alert to personal stress levels.
- Use a healthy intervention strategy.
- Eliminate unnecessary information from your personal and professional life.

CHAPTER CHECKLIST

Stress management and time management are two strategies for self-management. Balancing stress means caring for your emotional, physical, and mental needs. Delegating effectively, using schedules and calendars and other planners, using time-management principles, and managing meetings are key strategies to be integrated into the nurse leader role. By accomplishing self-management, managers, leaders, and followers will find themselves in control of work time and stressors, as well as more confident in achieving both personal and work-related goals.

Stress and overwork are inherent in the nursing profession, and nurses can adapt and cope with stress and time pressures by learning effective ways to care for themselves and to manage time. By assessing and reducing specific stressors and time wasters, nurses can thrive within the healthcare challenges before them. Increasing skills in coping, organization, delegation, and effective time management is vital for effective leadership. A nurse manager who can be a role model and support his or her staff in turbulent times is a true leader.

- Stress management includes using cognitive and psychosocial activities to decrease the stress or enhance the ability to handle stress.
- Time management includes using tools and strategies to ensure that priority goals are achieved.

- Signs of excess stress must be heeded to prevent burnout or chronic health problems.
- Strategies to reduce stress include physical, mental, and emotional.
- Strategies to improve time management include identification of potential time wasters, use of time-management strategies, and appropriate delegation.
- Strategies to improve meeting management include effective organization and use of a process to facilitate the meeting.

TIPS FOR SELF-MANAGEMENT

- Know what your high-priority goals are, and use them to filter decisions.
- Know your personal response to stress, and self-evaluate frequently.
- Make your health a priority, and use strategies that keep yourself in control.
- Use organizational systems that meet your needs; the simpler, the better.
- Simplify.
- Refocus on your priorities whenever you begin to feel overwhelmed.

REFERENCES

Abrahamson, E., & Freedman, D. H. (2006). *A perfect mess: The hidden benefits of disorder*. New York: Little, Brown and Co.

American Board of Medical Specialties (ABMS). (2008). *Official American Board of Medical Specialties (ABMS) directory of board certified medical specialists*. Retrieved October 21, 2009, from www.abms.org/Who_We_Help/Consumers/.

Bailey, J. (2009). The challenge for today's nurse managers: How to be fiscally competent & efficient while nurturing the workforce and sustaining self. *Spinal Cord Injury, 29*(1), 25-28.

Chang, E., & Hancock, K. (2003). Role stress and role ambiguity in new nursing graduates in Australia. *Nursing and Health Sciences, 5*, 155-163.

Covey, S. R., Merrill, A. R., & Merrill, R. R. (1994). *First things first: To love, to learn, to leave a legacy*. New York: Simon & Schuster.

DeAngelis, T. (2002). A bright future for PNI. *Monitor on Psychology, 33*(6). Retrieved September 1, 2006, from www.apa.org/monitor/jun02/brightfuture.html.

Englebardt, S. P., & Nelson, R. (2002). *Health care informatics: An interdisciplinary approach*. St. Louis: Mosby.

Erdwins, C. J., Buffardi, L. C., Casper, W. J., & O'Brien, A. S. (2001). The relationship of women's role strain to social support, role satisfaction, and self-efficacy. *Family Relations, 50*(3), 230-238.

Evans, O., & Steptoe, A. (2002). The contribution of gender-role orientation, work factors, and home stressors to psychological well-being and sickness absence in male- and female-dominated occupational groups. *Social Science and Medicine, 54*(4), 481-492.

Greenglass, E., Burke, R., & Fiksenbaum, L. (2001). Workload and burnout in nurses. *Journal of Community and Applied Social Psychology, 11*, 211-215.

Hafner, A. W. (2001). Pareto's Principle: The 80-20 rule. Retrieved May 25, 2010, from http://www.bsu.edu/libraries/ahafner/awh-th-math-pareto.html.

Halm, M., Peterson, M., Kandels, M., Sabo, J., Blalock, M., Branden, R., et al. (2005). Hospital nurse staffing and patient mortality, emotional exhaustion, and job dissatisfaction. *Clinical Nurse Specialist, 19*(5), 241-251.

Health Resources and Services Administration. (2005). *National sample survey of registered nurses*. Retrieved October 21, 2009, from http://bhpr.hrsa.gov/healthworkforce/rnsurvey04/default.htm.

Jennings, J. M., Scalzi, C. C., & Rodgers, J. D. (2007). Differentiating nursing leadership and management compencies. *Nursing Outlook, 55*(4), 169-175.

Judkins, S., Reid, B., & Furlow, L. (2006). Hardiness training among nurse managers: Building a healthy workplace. *Journal of Continuing Education in Nursing, 37*(5), 202-207.

Kemeny, M. (August, 2003). The psychobiology of stress. *Current Directions in Psychobiological Science, 12*, 124-129.

Kobasa, S. C., Maddi, S. R., & Kahn, S. (1982). Hardiness and health: A perspective study. *Journal of Personality and Social Psychology, 42*(1), 168-177.

Krichbaum, K., Diemert, C., Jacox, L., Jones, A., Koenig P., Mueller, C., et al. (2007). Complexity compression: Nurses under fire. *Nursing Forum, 42*(2), 86-94.

Lambert, V., Lambert, C., & Yamase, H. (2003). Psychological hardiness, workplace stress and related stress reduction strategies. *Nursing and Health Sciences, 5*, 181-184.

Lencioni, P. (2004). *Death by meeting*. San Francisco: Jossey-Bass.

Lindholm, M. (2006). Working conditions, psychosocial resources and work stress in nurses and physicians in chief managers' positions. *Journal of Nursing Management, 14*, 300-309.

Maddi, S. R. (2002). The story of hardiness: Twenty years of theorizing, research and practice. *Consulting Psychology Journal, 54*, 173-185.

Maslach, C., Schaufeli, W., & Leiter, M. (2000). Job burnout. *Annual Review of Psychology, 52*, 397-422.

Maslow, A. H. (1943). A theory of human motivation. *Psychological Review, 50*, 370-396.

Melchior, M., Caspi, A., Milne, B. J., Danese, A., Poulton, R., & Moffitt, T. E. (2007). Work stress precipitates depression and anxiety in young, working women and men. *Psychological Medicine, 37*, 1119-1129.

Merriam-Webster Online. (2009). *Complain.* Retrieved October 21, 2009, from www.merriam-webster.com/dictionary/complain.

Plsek, P. E., & Greenhalgh, T. (2001). The challenge of complexity in health care. *British Medical Journal, 323*(7313), 625-628.

Robert, H., Evans, W., Honemann, D. H., & Balch, J. (Eds.). (2000). *Robert's rules of order newly revised.* Cambridge, MA: Perseus Book Group.

Rosenstein, A. H., & O'Daniel, M. (2008). A survey of the impact of disruptive behaviors and communication defects on patient safety. *Joint Commission Journal on Quality and Patient Safety, 34*, 464-471.

Rudan, V. T. (2002). Where have all the nursing administration students gone? *Journal of Nursing Administration, 32*, 185-188.

Segerstrom, S., & Miller, G. (2004). Psychological stress and the human immune system: A meta-analytic study of 30 years of inquiry. *Psychological Bulletin, 130*(4), 601-630.

Selye, H. (1956). *The stress of life.* New York: McGraw-Hill.

Selye, H. (1965). The stress syndrome. *American Journal of Nursing, 65*, 97-99.

Selye, H. (1991). History and present status of the stress concept. In A. Monat & R. Lazarus (Eds.), *Stress and coping: An anthology* (pp. 21-36). New York: Columbia University Press.

Shirey, M. (2006). Stress and coping in nurse managers: Two decades of research. *Nursing Economic$, 24*(4), 193-211.

Stöppler, M. (2005). *Top five stress management mistakes. Your guide to stress management.* Retrieved October 21, 2009, from http://stress.about.com/cs/copingskills/a/mistakes_p.htm.

Stuart, G. W., & Laraia, M. T. (2008). Self modification assistance. In G. M. Bulechek, H. K. Butcher, & J. M. Dochterman (Eds.), *Nursing interventions classifications* (5th ed., pp. 644-645), St. Louis: Mosby.

Taylor, S. E., Klein, L. C., Lewis, B. P., Gruenewald, T. L., Gurung, R. A., & Updegraff, J. A. (2000). Biobehavioral responses to stress in females: Tend-and-befriend, not fight-or-flight. *Psychological Review, 107*, 411-429.

Zangaro, G. A., & Soeken, K. L. (2007). A meta-analysis of studies of nurse's job satisfaction. *Research in Nursing & Health, 30*, 445-458.

SUGGESTED READINGS

Drucker, P. (1999). *Management challenges for the 21st century.* New York: HarperCollins.

Field, T., Quintino, O., Henteleff, T., Wells-Keife, L., & Delvecchio-Feinberg, G. (1997). Job stress reduction therapies. *Alternative Therapies in Health & Medicine, 3*(4), 54-56.

Lenson, B. (2002). *Good stress, bad stress.* Cambridge, MA: De Capo Press.

Lyon, B. (2000). Conquering stress. *Reflections on Nursing Leadership, 26*(1), 22-23, 43.

Oncken, W., & Wass, D. (November/December, 1999). Management time: Who's got the monkey? *Harvard Business Review*, reprint 99609.

Skovholt, T. (2001). *The resilient practitioner: Burnout strategies for counselors, therapists, teachers and health professionals.* Upper Saddle River, NJ: Allyn & Bacon (Pearson).

Tracy, B. (2004). *Time power.* New York: AMACOM.

29

Managing Your Career

Debra Hagler

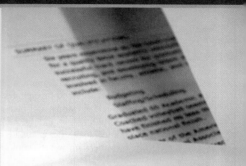

Curriculum Vit

Successful people actively manage their careers rather than wait for "lucky breaks." Although trusted others may guide or influence career development, every individual must manage his or her own career. Tools to document accomplishments and ways to extend career development beyond the work setting are considered in this chapter. Continuous lifelong learning and the ability to demonstrate and document competency are critical elements in effective career management.

OBJECTIVES

- Differentiate among career styles and how they influence career options.
- Analyze person-position fit.
- Develop a cover letter and résumé targeted for a specific position.
- Analyze critical elements of an interview.
- Describe a variety of professional development activities, including academic and continuing education programs.
- Identify contributions you could make and benefits you could derive from active involvement in professional organizations.

TERMS TO KNOW

career	curriculum vitae	professional association
certification	licensure	(organization)
continuing education	portfolio	résumé

Daniel Weberg, RN, BSN, MHI, CEN
Director, Academy of Continuing Education, Arizona State
*   University College of Nursing and Health Innovation,*
*   Phoenix, Arizona*

When I graduated from nursing school 5 years ago, I knew that I wanted to work in the emergency department right away. I was surprised at the opposition from most faculty and friends who told me, "You have to get at least a year of experience in med-surg first." Another challenge for me early on was the drive I felt to expand my

skills in different directions, not only in direct bedside care. During my undergraduate nursing courses, I had taught myself how to run the human patient simulators used in the learning laboratory, and I thought there might be a market for those skills. My struggle during this time was finding the direction to get to an objective that I could not clearly express and find a unique type of job that had not been created yet.

What do you think you would do if you were this nurse?

INTRODUCTION

The number of career options and paths within nursing is staggering. Some of these options are the "traditional" and highly valued roles nurses have performed for centuries—providing direct care to patients, leading teams or organizations, teaching, providing public health or school health services, or working in an occupational field. Other options have emerged over the past decade, and new options continue to emerge. Serving all patients and healthcare consumers as a legislative aide, for example, is not a common role, but it is one that helps shape the state's or nation's view of health care. Screening patients for insurance benefits and working in the clinic at a local grocery or chain store are other examples of the less traditional roles nurses fill. However, these numerous options provide a challenge: how to build a career, which education best serves the role, which experiences best prepare nurses for a specific field or role, and what new activities and roles need to be developed? Because a career extends over a lifetime and because nursing is defined by law, not by employing organizations, making choices can redirect a nurse's future. Some options build primarily on experience and others on education and experience; all, however, require that a nurse engage in professional development and continue to advanced expertise to meet the evolving challenges in health care. How nurses reach their career goals depends on the goals they set and how they manage their career development.

A FRAMEWORK

A career can be defined as progress throughout an individual's professional life. It can be developed in

numerous ways, but it begins with selecting positions that contribute to career goals. Because so many roles can be performed in the name of nursing, the driving force for a career option should be the same as the force that drives a decision about a particular position. That force is the fit between a person and the position or career path. There is a relationship between an individual and a position, and that same relational fit is exhibited in a career path (Figure 29-1). A good fit is built on strong, similar goals and tolerable (or growth-producing) differences. The whole of any work situation is composed of the two elements—person and position—interacting in an environment in which other elements influence both. The whole is symbolized by blending a person's talents with a position's expectations to create the productive whole. Analyzing positions and the required skills in light of individual talents can help

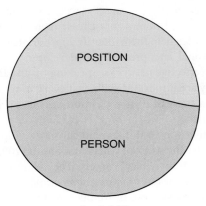

Goal: A Fit
FIGURE 29-1 Person-position fit.

applicants determine positions that fit with their strengths and define gaps to be addressed. When gaps occur, skills development might be needed to form a fit or the position may not be a good fit.

The person/position fit and how that fit evolves throughout a career are critical considerations in appreciating positions held throughout a career. Thus, when considering a career path, such as practitioner or administrator or educator, the person needs to recall prior positions held and the aspects of those positions that were most rewarding. As an example, if a nurse held multiple positions and then he determined that the teaching and learning opportunities were the most rewarding aspects, the career plan of educator might emerge. Whatever career is pursued, one key strategy is planning to obtain the right education and experience.

Generations may view work, positions, and careers differently, yet many similarities exist across generations. For example, Deal (2007) reported that all generations prefer face-to-face coaching. Younger generations, however, sought more frequent feedback than did older generations. In addition, Deal reported that almost everyone surveyed wanted to learn and thought learning was important. The learning related to the work he or she needed to do, not to the generational group in which he or she was categorized. An important finding was related to the stereotype of younger generations wanting to learn everything via a computer; that was a wrong assumption. The key to applying these points about coaching and learning is that leaders and managers must listen to others to learn what others want and need. This strategy can apply to career development as well. Listening to what individuals tell others about their own interests and strengths can help them identify appropriate resources for personal and professional development and for creating effective networks. Speaking up and listening carefully are important skills that every nurse can use in being successful in a position and in pursuing a career path.

Another way to think about career development is to consider the work of Citrin and Smith (2003), who studied "extraordinary" careers. They identified three broad categories of *promise, momentum,* and *harvest.* These terms suggest movement from early to late career. Thus, early in one's career, the focus is on developing skills, establishing credentials, and socializing into the role. Mid-career, the focus often shifts

to honing specific areas of expertise (the things by which we will be known) and being more aware of the fit of positions within the broad array of opportunities that will enhance some goal. Finally, in a later career stage, many individuals focus on the profession (the broad view of the work) and how to leave it better off as a result of being a member of the profession. This movement through nursing life is predicated on having a vision of a career as opposed to a series of jobs.

Finally, the classic work of Friss (1989) provides another way to look at careers through considering styles (Table 29-1). Her view of four possible career styles describes one being no better than another; rather, each is different. *Steady state* (positional plateau) careers describe those individuals who select a role and stay in that role throughout the career. This type of career style is common in rural settings and for those individuals who commit their working life to a positional category such as staff nurse, clinic nurse, or nurse practitioner. The focus of this career style is to become increasingly competent in the role and clinical area. *Linear* careers are those that represent vertical movement in the organizational hierarchy. This movement often creates more organizational knowledge and a more diversified view of what comprises nursing. This movement is characterized by changes in title; for example, moving from staff nurse to nurse manager to director represents this kind of career style. *Entrepreneurial and transient* style is appealing to nurses who wish to "see the world" or have a creative bent. The final style, *spiral,* focuses on the movement in and out and up and down. For example, nurses who move from within an organization as a staff nurse to nurse manager at another organization, then move in that organization to a nursing director role, and later leave for another opportunity exemplify this style.

It would be easy to label nurses' careers if they could each be described by a single style; however, the fluidity of the profession allows nurses to switch foci along a career path to gain a specific experience or meet a personal need. This dynamic suggests that it is difficult at best to label a nurse's style, career category, or generational attributes. The same dynamic makes leading and managing a group of nurses a challenge and provides for great diversity to meet organizational needs and nurses' career goals. The best opportunity for nurses to manage their careers and for a

TABLE 29-1   CAREER STYLES

	EXAMPLE	DESCRIPTION	MOTIVATION AND CHARACTERISTICS	MANAGERIAL CONSIDERATIONS
Steady State	Staff nurses	Constancy in position with increasing professional skill	Increasing expertise High professional identity Obligation to serve Maintenance of standards Autonomy in performance of care Preference for action Personal accountability The work itself Stability	Hold work in high esteem Decentralize Use and recognize abilities Provide feedback about patient outcomes Reward competence and tenure Provide continuing education Provide permanent assignment
Linear	Nursing service administrator	Hierarchical orientation with steady climb	Requisite authority and power Had a challenging first job Guided by internalized norms Money Recognition Opportunities for self-development	Provide management development Reward and value both education and competence Modify management selection and development systems Provide decreasing supervision
Entrepreneurial and Transient	Nurses in private practice; temporary assignments	Desire to create new service; meeting own priorities	Limited organizational commitment Opportunists Novelty/creativity Other people Achievement	Use flexibility to organization's benefit Avoid burdening them with organizational and practice decisions Provide immediate feedback
Spiral	Nurse who returns after raising a family	Rational, independent responsibility for shaping career	Novelty Prestige Intense period of employment followed by non-employment or a different employment Care for others Opportunities for self-development Typically well paid, service-oriented Recognition	Configure specific job that needs doing Be flexible about terms and length of commitment Find challenging initial assignment Negotiate Encourage creativity

Data from Friss, L. (1989). *Strategic management of nurses: A policy oriented approach.* Owings Mills, MD: AUPHA Press.

manager to help nurses gain important experiences is for the individuals to know themselves.

Knowing Yourself

Being a professional holds both privileges and obligations. The legal privileges and expectations are codified in the state nursing practice acts, rules, and regulations. Because licensure is designed to provide the baseline (i.e., the minimum expectation), it does not identify or obligate any practitioner to function in a professional manner as defined by the profession itself. For example, no practice act identifies membership in a professional association or providing community/professional service as an expectation.

Yet the profession, through various professional organizations, embraces the expectation that nurses will belong to professional associations and provide leadership in improving communities. For example, the Forces of Magnetism *(www.nursecredentialing.org/Magnet/ProgramOverview/ForcesofMagnetism.aspx)* identifies the expectation that nurses are involved in their community. The challenge, of course, is how to incorporate these activities into a busy, committed life! It often is those "additional" activities and interests that enrich a career and provide for invaluable insight into clinical and professional issues. Knowing what is important, what is valued, and the commitment needed forms the basis for understanding one's self.

Whether positions are plentiful or scare, knowing one's self can focus the available work or selection process toward capitalizing on one's strengths. Even assessing one's strengths through a formal avenue (e.g., Strengths Finder 2.0 at *www.strengthsfinder.com/113647/Homepage.aspx* or Buckingham's [2008] *The Truth about You: Your Secret to Success*) can provide insight. Therefore the beginning of creating a person/position fit is understanding the person involved. Throughout school and initial experiences in nursing, insight begins to evolve that helps each of us determine our preferences for our life work. It is not that some positions are valueless; rather, it is that some positions add more to what we want to be able to achieve in the long term than other positions. As an example, any position that offers educational compensation or flexible scheduling might work well for the short term if the goal is to return to school and complete advanced education for a specialized role.

Being able to describe yourself from various perspectives is useful. First, knowing your strengths tells you what you bring to a position and what you can rely on. When you know your strengths, you can say what they are in a succinct manner and use them as a filter in reading position descriptions to find your fit and to learn the organizational language. An analysis of your competencies allows you to see what work needs to be done to meet required or desired standards and competencies. Finally, entering into such analyses can help you see the bigger picture of your career and how what you can learn from a particular position might contribute to your overall goals. The career styles described in Table 29-1 include the motivation and characteristics of each style. Seeing how your self-analysis fits with the descriptors in the third column may suggest how you see yourself approaching your career. The goal of all this work is to know yourself well so that your pursuit of a position or career path fits you and your strengths.

Knowing the Position

Few people, including nurses, assume a position and remain in that position forever. Exceptions occur in rural areas and in highly specialized positions. Thus most nurses hold more than one position throughout their work life. Those positions can be selected by chance or by plan. Chance positions should not be ignored, but they should be evaluated in light of career goals and an assessment of the position and the organization. Managing a career actively allows for these chance opportunities to enrich the career rather than detract from it. Rapid changes in health care require an evaluation of each employment opportunity. Can a position contribute to increased skills and competencies? Does a position have the potential to recast one's professional profile so that others see the potential for greater contributions? Are the benefits of the position so enticing that they offset limitations of the position itself? These are the kinds of questions to ask yourself when considering a particular position.

Position assessment begins with understanding the basics of the organization and its vision and mission. Assessment also requires finding out specifics of the position, which may be available only through an interview. Bolles (2009) points out that most managers look first within the organization to promote

---

EXERCISE 29-1

Using an established description of a registered nurse—for example, the one created by the Texas Board of Nursing to describe beginning competencies of new graduates describes personal interests, skills, and abilities in the following areas. Consider your talents and values from the multidimensional view of nursing: communication, physical and psychological care, management, learning, teaching, scholarship, and involvement in the profession.

someone rather than looking broadly at the talent available. This is in contrast to how many people seek jobs; they look broadly first. So, one key strategy to use is selecting an organization where you want to work, even if the position is not exactly the right one. The potential for inside connections and networking, in addition to knowledge about management styles in the organization and future position openings, can lead you to the position that is the right fit for you.

CAREER DEVELOPMENT

A career extends beyond employment positions. A career includes the various ways in which an individual engages in activities that provide care to patients, support that care, educate for that care, support the providers of that care, study the ways in which to deliver the care, and engage in the broader perspective of professional and community service. Thinking broadly about a career in a rapidly changing field such as health care is critical to remaining competent and relevant. Licensure carries certain expectations about maintaining competence and reflecting professional standards. Legislators enact legislation based on the needs of the citizens and in response to political pressures. When a profession is protected by legislation, others, such as consumers, insurers, regulatory agencies, and employers, expect that professional standards have been and will continue to be met. Continuing competence is a focal issue for every professional.

In today's rapidly changing society, a position that was once "a fit" may no longer work. The position may have evolved as much as the person did. If the movement was in harmony, the fit remains, but if the position changes one way and the person another, the fit devolves.

Bolles (2009) also suggests that there are life-changing positions. These can best be described as changing positions and fields simultaneously (such as may occur with a spiral career style). For example, when a charge nurse in a critical care unit assumes the role of a chief nursing officer in a rural community hospital, a major shift has occurred. Nurses who follow a spiral career path, especially if they are second-degree students (meaning they have a degree in another field and then enter nursing), may also

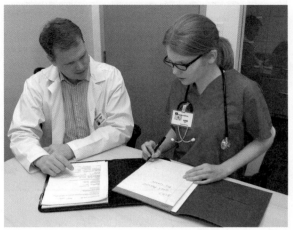

A mentor can inspire new thinking and new opportunities and steer you toward various roles and clinical areas.

experience this phenomenon. These individuals may have worked in another field and now are pursuing their hearts. They may have become bored with a career that had few interactions with people, or they may have studied in fields such as science and realized that the best application of knowledge could occur in patient care. Because of prior career successes, these individuals may craft career patterns that appear very different from the majority of the profession: they are using talents from two fields and are trying to capitalize on both.

Core career development strategies are important to success. Selecting professional peers and mentors to share in your development is crucial to gaining good, ongoing advice. Having a few well-chosen peers, mentors, and role models who respond openly from various perspectives can enrich career planning and development.

EXERCISE 29-2

Think about an experienced nurse who serves as a role model to you. Would you want that person as a mentor? If so, consider how you would enlist that person's assistance in molding your career.

Table 29-2 defines six key aspects of creating and managing a career. Although each aspect is important, one aspect that can be most useful to consider is

TABLE 29-2	KEY ASPECTS OF CREATING AND MANAGING A CAREER
Who	Mentor
What	Role and clinical options
When	"Timing is everything"; always open to opportunities; don't leave in the middle of a critical project
Where	Local or not; inpatient or outpatient
How	Proactive; your search is your job
Why	Seeking challenge/testing out ideas

the "who"—the mentor you choose. That person can inspire new thinking and new opportunities and steer you to various roles and clinical areas. That person can also create connections for you and help guide decisions related to timing and context. Mentors might even be able to create opportunities for you to test new approaches to clinical care or to new aspects of a position you thought of as boring.

CAREER MARKETING STRATEGIES

Even the steady-state or experienced nurse who is not seeking a new position needs to have a curriculum vitae (CV) or résumé that can document continued development of expertise. Interviewing, which is a two-way process, also contributes to successful position choices and career development.

Although professional data can be recorded in numerous ways, most people do not do so in a systematic manner. Therefore, when information about one's career is needed quickly, it is difficult to recall and then to hone the most pertinent information for a position. A goal of this chapter is to develop a systematic strategy for creating marketing documents that you can use throughout your professional career. Some organizations use an electronic form of professional records so that an individual can readily access and convert the information into various documents. The National Student Nurses Association; the American Nurses Credentialing Center; and the Honor Society of Nursing, Sigma Theta Tau International, provide access to such an electronic approach. Portability of information is an important consideration so

that information moves with an individual throughout a career.

Many position searches, even those internal to an organization, begin with a résumé. The key is to make information distinctive in telling your professional story and in establishing the appearance of a competent professional.

Data Collection

Depending on your unique background, the extent of data collection varies considerably. The first step is to collect all your professional career information. If you are fairly new in the profession, analyze anything special you did in school, such as electives, offices held, and special assignments, honors, and recognitions. If you are a second-career nurse, consider your previous work and how it relates to your profession now. If you have an employment history, start with your nursing positions. Include relevant information from volunteer roles, which can illustrate skills such as in leadership, ability to balance budgets, communication, and political astuteness, as well as indicate professional commitment.

To begin data collection, especially if you have not kept records before, begin with where you are and think back. If you have short experience or no difficulty recalling details, you are in great shape to start a systematic plan. If, however, you have a long history as a nurse or a prior relevant career, your task is more challenging because you have to actively think about what you did in the past and, for a prior career, determine how to translate those experiences into relevance for nursing. The important aspect of this phase is to begin the process and to save it electronically so that you can shape information for specific reasons using a cut-and-paste technique rather than creating an original document each time you need to provide information about yourself.

Compile as many facts as possible for each of the ten categories identified in Table 29-3. Even if you have no entry for a specific category, retain the heading as a reminder and think about what you would like to be able to list there in the future. If you do not have regular access to a computer, at least keep the information on a CD or flash drive so that you do not need to recreate it the next time. This is your private data bank for information to list on a curriculum vitae or to select for a résumé.

TABLE 29-3	DATA COLLECTION

TOPICS	FACTS NEEDED
1. Education	Name of school, address, phone numbers, website address, years of attendance, date of graduation, name of degree(s) received, minor earned, honors received (e.g., Dean's List)
2. Continuing education	Dates attended, places, topics and any special outcomes, type and amount of credit earned
3. Experience	Dates of employment, title of position, name of employing agency, location and phone numbers, website address, name of chief executive officer, chief nursing officer, immediate supervisor, salary range, typical duties (role description)
4. Community/institutional service	Dates of service, name of committee/task force and the parent organization (e.g., name of hospital or professional organization), your role on the committee (e.g., chairperson, secretary, member), general description of committee's functions, any unique accomplishments
5. Publications	Articles: author(s) name(s), year of publication, title, journal, volume, issue, pages; books: author(s), year of publication, title, location and name of publisher
6. Honors	Date, description of award, special factors related to award (e.g., competitive, communitywide, national)
7. Research	Date, title of research, role in research (e.g., principal investigator, co-investigator, team member), funded/unfunded
8. Speeches/presentations given	Date, title of speech presented, place, name of sponsoring organization, nature of the presentation (e.g., keynote, concurrent session), your honorarium
9. Workshops/conferences presented	Date, title of workshop/conference presented, place, name of sponsoring group and nature of the presentation, brief description of the activity, your honorarium
10. Certification	Initial date of certification, expiration date, certifying body, area/type of certification

---

EXERCISE 29-3
Go to the *Evolve* website (http://evolve.elsevier.com/Yoder-Wise/) and draft entries for your data bank. Using that information, draft a curriculum vitae and a résumé for a position you are seeking. As a checkpoint for yourself, make a list of four or five key strengths or facts that you want others to know. Be sure they are listed in your CV and described in your résumé. Save the list for preparing for interviews.

Curriculum Vitae

A curriculum vitae (or CV) is the documentation of one's professional life. It is designed to be all-inclusive of facts but not detailed. A curriculum vitae follows some designated flow of information reflective of the ten categories identified in Table 29-3. However, unlike the data collection stage, in which a category is retained even if no data appear, empty categories are not listed on a CV.

Typically, a CV begins with your name and contact information. Your name should be most prominent (e.g., larger type size, bolded) and should be followed with contact information listed on separate lines. Your contact information should include address with zip code; phone numbers, designated by work, home, and cell; fax number; e-mail address; and, if you have one, a website address. If you include a website address, use an e-mail account with a professional name; avoid usernames that are overly casual such as "*sweetiepie@domain.com*" or those that provide personal information such as "*crabbynurse@domain.com*." Center the contact information on the CV or place a dividing line under it to help a prospective employer quickly locate that information. Information in the body of the CV should be presented in *reverse chronological order*. This approach allows a prospective employer to find the most recent (and theoretically most relevant) information quickly. By drawing attention to your most recent accomplishments, the reader gains a sense of where you are in your career.

Résumé

Résumés are customized documents that relate to the qualifications of a specific organizational position and help create an image of you serving in that position. Unlike the CV, a résumé provides details. It is presented in sentences or phrases (not both) to share the value of the information. For example, rather than listing years of service in a position by title and organization, a résumé might include information that you served as the only nurse to provide some distinctive service. For the experienced nurse, a résumé could be used to reflect increasing skills and abilities; for the new nurse, it could focus on specific "extra" abilities (e.g., competencies) that are not normally expected of a new graduate.

The résumé is a better choice than a CV for advertising your skills and talents to a prospective employer. Because a résumé is brief (typically no more than two pages) and tailored to the position being sought, the information is pointed toward specific position requirements. Details and action words help the reader view you as accomplishing work. Verbs that relate to outcomes (produced, created) are most powerful. Fox (2006) suggested that the purpose of the résumé is to elaborate on what you said during an interview, but often the interviewer will have read your résumé as a basis for scheduling the interview. Either way, it is a good idea to arrive for an interview with a copy of your résumé as a reminder of your capabilities. Bringing a résumé to an interview is especially useful if you were asked previously to provide a CV. This additional work of applying your talents to the specific position in the résumé helps the interviewer see you as fitting in the organization.

Basically, there are two ways to develop a résumé. One is *conventional,* and it provides information by positions and activities. The other approach, called *functional,* may combine multiple positions into role areas you are trying to highlight. So, rather than using experience as a heading (as in a conventional résumé), the functional résumé heading may relate to writing or client education and describe how you achieved results across several positions. A functional approach is best if you are planning a sharp departure from your present position or if you have considerable experience before entering nursing. The focus is on experience in diverse roles/positions rather than the specific positions held.

As with the CV, your résumé should be error-free and grammatically correct, accurate, and logical. Both of these documents should be printed on high-quality paper, preferably 100% cotton bond. Electronic résumés are best sent as a pdf or image file so that no distortion in the design or layout can occur. This is also a universally accepted electronic format, so recipients should have no difficulty opening the attachment.

Professional Letters

During your career, you will need to communicate effectively through letters. Every well-designed letter markets you as a professional. The commonly used letters are a cover letter, a thank-you letter, and a resignation letter. You may also write letters declining positions that you have been offered or recommending others for positions.

All of these types of letters include your name and contact information and should match the comparable contact information on your résumé and CV. This is especially important for the cover letter because it accompanies another document. The same quality paper should be used for letters as is used for the CV and résumé. If any of these documents are sent by e-mail or fax, you may still choose to send a hard copy.

These letters should be no longer than one page. The date and an inside address with the name (and credentials) of the addressee, the person's title, the name of the organization, street address, city, state, and zip code should be included. The next area of the letter is the greeting. The typical salutation (greeting) (e.g., "Dear Ms. Smith") is followed by a colon or comma. The end of the letter (closing) allows several line spaces between the word (e.g., *Sincerely*) and your printed name followed by credentials. If your address did not appear at the top of the letter, it should appear below your typed name. The space between the closing and your name should allow enough room for your signature. Between the greeting and the closing are paragraphs conveying the letter's main message. As with all formal documents, the letters should be proofread for layout, typographical errors, spelling, and content. E-mail communication contains essentially the same information, although no inside address is used. A discussion of each of the major types of letter follows.

Cover Letter

The cover letter is the key to getting your CV read and reiterates or supplements a résumé. A cover letter is a brief and carefully written document that includes why you are writing, why you "fit" the position, and how you will follow up.

Numerous positions may be advertised by an organization simultaneously. In addition, an organization may use a variety of vehicles to issue a call for applicants. Thus immediately stating which position interests you and how you learned of it is helpful. Once you have stated your reason for writing, you should address the issue of "why you."

The second paragraph should indicate why someone should take time to read your attached résumé. This section should state how you see yourself fitting with the organization (by experience, by philosophy, by clinical focus, and so forth). Two or three examples are helpful to provide the details of any general statements. It is also appropriate to refer to the attachment (your CV or résumé, whichever the organization requested).

The final paragraph should convey your optimism—you anticipate being interviewed. If you want to ensure that you have an additional opportunity to market yourself, you should indicate when you will follow up with a phone call.

EXERCISE 29-6

Write a cover letter that highlights information from at least two items from your data bank. Select items that best market you and that will entice the reader to call you for an interview.

Thank-You Letter

The business format described earlier can be used also for a formal thank-you letter, expressing appreciation for the opportunity that you had to interview. A more personal approach is to hand-write a thank-you note. Either way, the thank-you letter is your last chance to provide information about your communication skills and values at this point in the process. A quick e-mail message to acknowledge the interview is not sufficient; if you send an immediate e-mail, a formal note should follow.

The lead paragraph of the thank-you letter may help the interviewer recall your interview. Identify which position you are seeking and perhaps a key statement that you discussed during the interview. If you discussed multiple positions, you should identify which of those positions most interested you. The next paragraph should reiterate one of your strengths and what you found most interesting in the interview. This paragraph could also answer any question that was left unanswered during the interview.

The closing paragraph should reference specific times when you expect to hear about the interview outcomes and when you will follow up. If you decided the position was not a fit, you should thank the person for the time devoted to the interview and wish him or her success in seeking the best candidate. Even the worst interview should be followed by a thank-you letter expressing your appreciation for the interviewer's taking time to talk with you and sending the organization your best wishes for the future. These actions create a positive impression both for the present and for future interactions. Finally, if the position is offered to you, another thank-you letter is appropriate and might include a statement related to your excitement about joining the organization, the date you expect to transition, and any key agreements that were made verbally but that are not yet in writing.

Resignation Letter

When you secure a new position, it is essential to resign effectively from your current position. Occasionally this is not applicable—for example, if you are transitioning from a student or military role or if you were terminated or laid off. Otherwise, being polite and diplomatic in your resignation process keeps communications open with your current agency so that you could return or seek support from the colleagues you left behind. The best approach to resigning is having a personal meeting with your manager and indicating that you will provide a formal letter of resignation. Your resignation should be given with adequate notice, which depends on your conditions of employment. Being flexible in your resignation date and negotiating that date with your manager create a positive exit strategy.

The letter of resignation follows the format guidelines described for other professional letters and begins with an acknowledgment of your intent to resign. Your date of resignation should be stated, and you might include whether this date is negotiable. This paragraph should also reference the oral discussion you had with your manager.

The second paragraph highlights aspects of the employment experience that enhanced your career development. Identifying any major contribution you made to the organization is also appropriate. The worst thing to do would be to offload any negative feelings you have for the organization, manager, or co-workers in writing. Always say something positive about the position you have held.

The closing paragraph concludes by asking for a copy of your exit evaluation. It is important to learn your final standing as you leave an organization, and this appraisal for your own records may be valuable to you in the future.

DATA ASSEMBLY FOR PROFESSIONAL PORTFOLIOS

The checklist in Box 29-1 will help you keep track of your data and assemble the facts attractively. Inclusion of these elements ensures a comprehensive view of your professional contributions and makes up a portfolio. Creating a professional portfolio, the basics of which are found in the citations made in your CV, can help organize one element of your professional life. Keeping notes of recognition, copies of evaluations, and pictures of your successes are examples that help round out the resource documents behind the CV data. Although a portfolio takes time to develop and to maintain, that work pays off at evaluation, promotion, and position-seeking times. The information is always available, and it is easy to expand information in a given area or focus on the most important

or most recent work. In other words, this system of maintaining professional information provides a resource to respond promptly to new or emerging opportunities.

> **EXERCISE 29-7**
>
> Go to the *Evolve* website (http://evolve.elsevier.com/Yoder-Wise) and view the sample portfolio. Based on information in the portfolio, what types of positions in your community would you suggest might be the best fit for this nurse? What information in the portfolio supports your suggestions?

The Interview

After your letters and résumé are effective in career marketing, the next step is participating in an interview. Interviewing is a two-way proposition; the interviewee should be gathering as much information as the interviewer is. Both should be making judgments throughout the process so that if a position is offered, the interviewee will be prepared to accept, decline, or explore further. Interviews may take place with one or more individuals and may include a range of activities. To be at ease, the interviewee should wear professional and comfortable clothing. Rehearse specific questions to ask and points to make so that you can feel more at ease during the interview. Be prepared to cite how you have faced challenges and dilemmas, because those types of questions are likely to be asked.

Even in times of a nursing shortage, employers are using behavioral interviewing techniques to identify the most appropriate applicant for the vacant position. Rather than being asked, "What are your weaknesses?" you may be asked, "Tell me how you handled the last mistake you made" or "How did your educational program prepare you for critical care nursing?" Applicants in some organizations are screened and interviewed by a panel and then asked to participate in a series of interviews to allow fellow employees more say in the hiring process. In business and health-care settings, many prospective employers administer basic skills tests. Researching the organization in advance can help prepare you for the interview. (See the Literature Perspective on p. 584.)

Interview Topics and Questions of Concern

During interviews, employers should ask all applicants for a given position the same questions. In

| BOX 29-1 | CHECKLIST FOR CONSTRUCTING MARKETING DOCUMENTS |

Data Collection
_____ 1. Data sets are used for information development.
_____ 2. Information is assembled in categorical manner.

Data Assembly
_____ 1. Discrete categories are used.
_____ 2. Assembly addresses specific position.
_____ 3. Current name, address, phone numbers, voice mail, e-mail address, and Web address are prominent (use as many as are appropriate for you).
_____ 4. Career summary (if used) (or cover letter) is prominent.
_____ 5. Key points about positions/experiences are evident.
_____ 6. A logical flow is evident.
_____ 7. Grammar, spelling, and syntax are correct.
_____ 8. Writing style is positive and direct, but not terse.
_____ 9. Action verbs are evident.
_____10. If writing in full sentences, third person and passive voice are avoided (i.e., write in the active voice).
_____11. "Canned" résumé language is avoided (e.g., "distinguished" and "all phases of …").
_____12. Emphasis is on competence, not years (cover letter).
_____13. Specific examples of key competencies are cited (cover letter).
_____14. The format is consistent throughout.
_____15. Personal information (e.g., health, marital status) is absent.

Appearance and Format
_____ 1. There are no typographic errors.
_____ 2. The product is "clean" (e.g., no smudges, no discrepant margins).
_____ 3. The product is readable (e.g., layout design is pleasing: white space, capitalization).
_____ 4. The paper is high-quality bond (100% cotton), white or cream.
_____ 5. The type is businesslike (no script); text is at least 10 to 12 point, and fonts are limited to one or two.
_____ 6. Emphasis is evident (e.g., centering and bold print or underlining).
_____ 7. The product is only one or two pages in length (not applicable for a curriculum vitae [CV]).

Overview
_____ 1. It is attractive, interesting, quick-reading, and competency-based.
_____ 2. The package sells you.
_____ 3. You are pleased to have it precede you.
_____ 4. Additional items are enclosed, or they are assembled for personal handling at an interview.
_____ 5. If you were receiving this CV or résumé, you would want to interview this person.

addition to providing comparable information as the basis for a decision, the applicant's expectation for equal treatment is upheld. Only questions related to the position and its description are legitimate. Employers should not ask other questions (Table 29-4), and applicants should express appropriate concern if asked such inappropriate questions.

If the interviewer asks an inappropriate question, the applicant can choose not to answer the direct question by addressing the content area. For example,

if asked about your spouse's employment, you might say, "I believe what you are asking is how long I will be able to be in this position. Let me assure you that I intend to be here for at least 2 years."

Each of the content areas in Table 29-4 may be acceptable, but the question is phrased inappropriately. The second column identifies approaches that are both appropriate and legal. The key to ensuring a fair interviewing process is being prepared, knowing what can be asked legitimately, and knowing how to respond to inappropriate questions.

LITERATURE PERSPECTIVE

Resource: Heath, D., & Heath, C. (2009). *Why it may be wiser to hire people without meeting them.* Mansueto Ventures LLC. Retrieved August 28, 2009, from www.fastcompany.com/magazine/136/made-to-stick-hold-the-interview.html.

Most interviewers believe that they can tell a lot about a prospective employee or student from an interview. However, interviews may tell employers less about a candidate's likely job performance than work samples, job-knowledge tests, and peer ratings of past job performance.

In a study reported by psychologist Robyn Dawes, a unique situation regarding admission interviews for a large medical school class allowed an assessment of the value of interviews. Interview scores were one of the criteria for admission, so most students admitted had earned high scores on their interviews, but some students with the lowest interview scores were also admitted. The faculty was not aware of which students had earned low or high interview scores. At the end of the program, those students who had interviewed poorly and those who had interviewed well graduated and received honors at the same rate.

Implications for Practice
Employers may want to improve the predictive ability of position interviews by including some type of realistic test or description of your performance. Review the job qualifications and responsibilities that are advertised, and then consider what you might be asked to do or think through during an interview related to those qualifications and responsibilities. Some potential interview questions include asking for an example of how you have worked effectively with an anxious or angry patient during his hospitalization or asking you to identify priorities from a given patient situation.

TABLE 29-4   INAPPROPRIATE AND APPROPRIATE QUESTIONS

SAMPLE OF INAPPROPRIATE QUESTIONS	SAMPLE OF APPROPRIATE AND LEGAL QUESTIONS
1. How old are you?	1. Do you know that this position requires someone at least 21 years old?
2. What does your husband (wife) do?	2. This position requires that no one in your immediate family be in the healthcare field or own interests/shares in any healthcare facility. Does this pose a problem?
3. Who takes care of your children?	3. Attendance is important. Are you able to meet this expectation?
4. Are you working "just to help out"?	4. What are your short-term and long-term goals?
5. Do you have any disabilities?	5. Is there anything that would prevent you from performing this work as described?
6. Where were you born?	6. This position requires U.S. citizenship. May I assume you meet this criterion?
7. What are the names of all of the organizations to which you belong?	7. To which professional organizations do you belong?
8. What is your religious preference?	8. As you have read in our philosophy, we subscribe to a Christian philosophy. Do you understand that all employees are expected to promote this philosophy?

EXERCISE 29-8
Select a partner and role-play an interview for a professional nursing position. The potential employer (manager) should focus on competencies of the prospective employee. Include questions and scenarios about common conflicts and challenges seen in the clinical setting. The interviewee (prospective employee) should highlight competencies, decision-making abilities, and critical-thinking abilities when responding to the situation-based questions. Debrief how well you did.

If you have prepared well, you will know what the organization's stated beliefs are and whether they are compatible with yours. The challenge in an interview is to determine whether those stated beliefs are lived or are merely printed words. If numerous people can relate how the mission is translated into a specific role, the beliefs are likely lived ones.

Plank, in a *Wall Street Journal* article, identified the five must-ask questions, and therefore the five must-be-prepared-to-answer questions (2010):

1. In what ways will this role help you stretch your professional capabilities? (This is designed to provide clues about weaknesses.)
2. What have been your greatest areas of improvement in your career? (This identifies weaknesses again and this time identifies what action you took; just knowing one's weaknesses is not good enough.)
3. What's the toughest feedback you've ever received and how did you learn from it? (This question is designed to identify candidates who can be forthright and who are learners.)
4. What are people likely to misunderstand about you? (This question is all about how the candidate "reads" others.)
5. If you were giving your new staff a "user's manual" to you, what would you include in it to accelerate their "getting to know you" process? (This reveals information about how the person will function in the team.)

This chapter includes two tools designed to be used in preparing for an interview: "Checklist for Interviewing" (Box 29-2), and "Interview Goals and Content" (Table 29-5). Using the thank-you letter described earlier in this chapter is an additional opportunity to market yourself, especially if you wish to correct or expand on an answer you provided during the interview.

PROFESSIONAL DEVELOPMENT

Active involvement in education, service, and scholarship opportunities can help prepare you to deal with new roles and challenges in your employment setting and the larger scope of nursing and health care. Engaging in service activities (both community and professional organizations) and sharing your knowledge through research, writing, and speaking (scholarship) allow you to influence others in the profession and through the profession. (See the Research Perspective on p. 586.)

In settings in which positions are scarce or when you are competing for a very desirable position, community/professional service experience and

---

BOX 29-2   **CHECKLIST FOR INTERVIEWING**

1. Check interviewing guides, such as *What Color Is Your Parachute?*
2. Check out the new organization:
   a. Review the organization's mission, vision, and values statements before the interview (via the Web or hard copy).
   b. Obtain statistics and facts.
   c. Ask about new program directions.
3. Recheck your résumé or curriculum vitae for the following:
   a. Emphasis
   b. New information
4. Practice using "action" words.
5. Decide about the following:
   a. Appearance
   b. Key points:
      i. To make
      ii. To learn
   c. Tool for quick check (e.g., a file card with key points)
6. Arrive on time and alone.
7. Make a memorable entrance:
   a. Make eye contact.
   b. Shake hands.
   c. Smile.
   d. Say, "Hello, I'm [name]."
8. Position yourself with the interviewer (e.g., decide to sit at an angle).
9. Keep in mind your key points.
10. Appear interested—project competence, confidence, and energy.
11. Accentuate the positive!
12. Answer questions directly but know when not to.
13. Ask for more information.
14. Say only positive things about your present employer, but do not be untruthful.
15. Secure a time frame for notification of a position offer.
16. Thank interviewer personally.
17. Write a thank-you letter.
18. Let interviewer know your decision.
19. Put commitments in writing.

---

scholarly contributions to nursing may give you the advantage over other candidates.

One of the keys to maintaining competence and versatility is continued learning. "Nursing professional development begins within the basic nursing education program, continues throughout the career of the nurse and encompasses the educational

TABLE 29-5   INTERVIEW GOALS AND CONTENT

INTERVIEW GOALS	CONTENT
1. Personal characteristics	Describe the type of person you are, including personality traits. Be expected to cite examples of when these traits helped or hindered you in previous situations. List situations that characterize your energy, initiative, drive, ambition, and enthusiasm. Clarify your professional values. Have a story ready that illustrates how you see yourself.
2. The work itself	Emphasize what makes you distinctive. Describe how your education and experience prepared you for this position. Describe your skills as a member of a team and a leader of a team. Prepare to address hypothetical situations that display your problem solving, reasoning, self-confidence, knowledge, and critical thinking. (Creates opportunity to evaluate you in action and under some stress.) Ask intelligent questions that suggest you have prepared for this interview and know something about this organization.
3. The organizational fit	Be clear about what you believe to be distinctive about this organization and how it meets your expectations for a position. Articulate your "fit" with the organization's philosophy, mission, and vision.
4. The professional opportunities	Be clear about what you expect to obtain from any position you consider. Include advancement opportunities, educational support, and work/life balance.

 RESEARCH PERSPECTIVE

Resource: Cummings, G., Lee, H., MacGregor, T., Davey, M., Wong, C., Paul, L., & Stafford, E. (2008). Factors contributing to nursing leadership: A systematic review. *Journal of Health Services Research & Policy, 13* (4), 240-248.

Leadership practices contribute to outcomes in health care, so developing strong leaders in healthcare organizations is important to ensure effective health care. Through a systematic review of articles indexed in healthcare databases, authors identified 24 research studies about the development of nursing leaders. Several studies indicated that actively practicing leadership styles, skills, and roles influenced nurses' development of leadership. In addition, after participating in formal leadership educational programs, nurses reported using leadership behaviors more frequently.

Implications for Nursing Practice
Leadership development can be supported through attending educational activities, identifying role models, and practicing leadership behaviors. Look for opportunities to attend workshops, and read articles on leadership. Observe effective leaders in your workplace, and consider whether the ways that those leaders handle challenges might work well for you in similar situations. Volunteer to lead work groups, committees, and community organizations to practice the leadership behaviors that you have read about and observed.

concepts of continuing education, staff development, and academic preparation" (American Nurses Association [ANA], 2000, p. 1). Learning can occur also through informal means: in a conversation with colleagues, by reading an article in the general literature, or sometimes in an "ah ha" reflective thought that provides sudden enlightenment.

ACADEMIC AND CONTINUING EDUCATION

A graduate degree opens the door to numerous career opportunities. Graduate education consists of either master's-level or doctorate-level study in a clinical specialty area, in preparation for a specific role, or a combination of both.

Some employment situations or career specialties require advanced education. For example, nurse practitioner preparation requires graduate-level degree preparation as opposed to the earlier certificate programs. As health care has become more complex, nurses recognized as independent practitioners need more education to meet healthcare demands.

BOX 29-3   FACTORS TO CONSIDER IN SELECTING A GRADUATE PROGRAM

Accreditation	• Does the program have national nursing accreditation (master's/doctoral level)? • Is the institution regionally accredited (e.g., North Central Association of Colleges and Schools)?
Clinical/functional role	• How closely do the descriptions of clinical/functional courses of study meet career goals?
Credits	• How many graduate credits are required to complete the degree? • How many are devoted to clinical or practicum experiences? • How many relate to classroom experiences?
Thesis/research	• Is a thesis/dissertation/capstone project required? • If not, what opportunities exist for research development? • What support is available for graduate students?
Faculty	• What credentials do faculty members hold? • Are they in leadership positions in the state/national/international scenes? • Are they competent in your field of interest? • What is their reputation?
Current research	• What are the current research strengths of the institution?
Flexibility	• Do these strengths fit with your interests, or is there flexibility to create your own direction? • Is flexibility present in scheduling and progress through the program? • Is classroom attendance required or is online attendance an option?
Admission	• What is required? • Is the GRE used? • What is the minimum undergraduate GPA expected? • Is experience required? What kind? How much?
Costs	• What are the total projected costs? • What financial aid is available?

GPA, Grade point average; *GRE*, Graduate Record Examination.

Admission to graduate programs may require taking a test (often the Graduate Record Examination [GRE]), having an above-average grade point average (GPA), and graduating from a professionally accredited school of nursing.

> **EXERCISE 29-9**
> Analyze the academic and clinical preparation you received in your nursing program. Do you feel confident in your knowledge base and clinical skill? Can you effectively manage multiple roles? Based on these answers, determine whether you should pursue graduate education immediately or wait until you have gained additional work experience.

Deciding to pursue graduate education may be very simple. Some applicants to associate degree and baccalaureate programs already have a specific career focus requiring graduate preparation in mind. In the past, new graduates were often encouraged (or even required) to gain work experience before seeking a master's degree or doctorate. Although experience can enrich the learning process, the philosophy of delaying entry into graduate education is changing as nurse leaders have identified the profession's need for nurses who have completed graduate degrees earlier in their careers. Working while attending a graduate program may be difficult, but it is common among graduate students in nursing. Box 29-3 lists some factors to consider in selecting a graduate program.

Consider the following example of seeking out a graduate program that fits:

> You know you want to work with elderly patients. Your library subscribes to the *Journal of Gerontological Nursing* and *Geriatric Nursing*. You review the most recent year's issues of both. You scan the

masthead (i.e., the page with the editors and board members). Where are these individuals affiliated? Now you scan the articles. Are there some that are particularly intriguing? Where are the authors affiliated? Finally, look back over the lists. Are there any places emerging where the leaders in the field may be? What centers of excellence in geriatrics have related graduate programs? This is a good starting place.

Distance education online provides an additional option for earning an advanced degree. Flexible scheduling and the convenience of online courses permit many individuals to participate who would not be able to attend traditional programs because of class times or geographical distance.

EXERCISE 29-10

Assume you are interested in graduate education.
- Use the Internet or the library to locate information about graduate education and financial assistance.
- Determine what specialties exist at the master's/doctoral level.
- Determine the location of programs nearby and access to distance programs.
- Evaluate the clinical interest of the programs of study.
- Decide if the diverse roles of the advanced practice registered nurse appeal.
- Consider doctoral programs, including those permitting entrance from the baccalaureate level.

Continuing education also contributes to professional growth. *Continuing education* is defined as "systematic professional learning experiences designed to augment the knowledge, skill, and attitudes of nurses and therefore enrich the nurses' contributions to quality health care and their pursuit of professional career goals" (ANA, 2000, p. 5).

Numerous opportunities for continuing education exist at local, state, regional, and broader levels. Selecting among the numerous opportunities to pursue may be difficult. Box 29-4 lists factors to consider in selecting any offering, but depending on your particular goal, certain factors may be more influential than others. For example, if cost is a major factor, length and speaker may be less influential factors.

In addition to increasing your knowledge base, continuing education provides professional networking opportunities, contributes to meeting certifica-

tion and licensure requirements, and documents additional pursuits in maintaining or developing clinical expertise. Sponsors of continuing education include employers, professional associations, schools of nursing, and private entrepreneurial groups.

Both types of formal professional development (i.e., graduate education and continuing education) are valuable, and both can contribute to a specific area of career development—certification.

EXERCISE 29-11

Like an organization, you will develop a strategic plan for yourself. Imagine you have decided to earn a master's or doctoral degree in nursing. This decision can be enhanced by a strategic plan.
- What values do you have that influence your plan?
- Are your interests in primary care, administration, or education?
- What is your target date for completion of the program?
- What other factors would interfere with your strategic plan?
- Do you have specific short-term goals or operational plans that must be attained before enrollment?

CERTIFICATION

Certification signifies completion of requirements in a particular field beyond basic nursing educational preparation for licensure. Nurses can be certified in a number of different specialty areas. Certification is an expectation in some employment settings for career advancement; in the field of advanced practice nursing, it is a requirement for practice and reimbursement. In many states, certification in advanced practice is the mechanism to achieve recognition as an advanced practice registered nurse from the board of nursing.

Obtaining certification may require testing, continued education, and documented time in practice in a specific practice area. Recertification is a process of continued recognition of competence within a defined practice area. Many certifications require participation in continuing education, as reported annually in the January issue of *The Journal of Continuing Education in Nursing*.

Certification plays an important part in the advancement of a career and the profession. In some fields, more than one examination exists; in others, there is an examination in the broad field and

BOX 29-4	FACTORS TO CONSIDER IN SELECTING A CONTINUING EDUCATION COURSE
Accreditation/approval	• Is the course accredited/approved? If so, by whom? • Is that recognition accepted by a certification entity and by the board of nursing (if continuing education is required for re-registration of licensure)?
Credit	• Is the amount of credit appropriate in terms of the expected outcomes?
Course title	• Does it suggest the type of learner to be involved (e.g., advanced)? • Does it reflect the expected outcomes?
Speaker(s)	• Is the instructor known as an expert in the field? • Is the instructor experienced in the field?
Objectives	• Are the objectives logical and attainable? • Do they reflect knowledge, skills, attitudes, or a combination of these? • Do they fit a learner's needs?
Content	• Is the content reflective of the objectives? • Is the content at an appropriate level?
Audience	• Is the audience designed as a general or target one (e.g., all registered nurses or experienced nurses in state health positions)?
Cost	• Is the cost equitable with that of similar nursing conferences? • Is travel required? • What is the actual direct expense for an individual to attend? Is it affordable?
Length	• Is the total time frame logical in terms of objectives, personal needs, and time away from work? • Does the time frame permit breaks from intense learning?
Provider	• Does the provider have an established reputation?

numerous options for defined subspecialties. The American Nurses Credentialing Center (ANCC) (www.nursecredentialing.org) offers numerous certification examinations for nurse generalists, nurse practitioners, clinical specialists, nurse administrators, nurse case managers, ambulatory nurses, and informatics nurses. In addition, other certifications are offered by nursing specialty organizations. The websites of these specialty organizations (or their credentialing organizations) provide specific certification requirements.

Certification recognizes competence of the nurse in a specialized area. Nurses, managers, and administrators value certification. The American Board of Nursing Specialties (2006) has identified both intrinsic (internal and defined by personal values) and extrinsic (external and defined by others) types of rewards related to specialty certification. Intrinsic rewards include indicating a level of competence, enhancing professional autonomy, and enhancing personal confidence. Extrinsic rewards include recognition from peers and employers, increased consumer confidence, and in some settings, increased salary.

PROFESSIONAL ASSOCIATIONS

Belonging to a professional association not only demonstrates leadership but also provides numerous opportunities to meet other leaders, participate in policy formation, continue specialized education, and shape the future of the profession. Professional associations (organizations) are groups of people who share a set of professional values and who decide to join their colleagues to effect change. Many nursing associations set standards and objectives to guide the profession and specialty practice. Standards can also serve as critical measurements for the profession and its practitioners. In today's changing healthcare environment, increasing numbers of associations are serving unique healthcare interests in society.

Although associations have very different agendas and goals, many nursing organizations share the same motivation and long-term goal of uniting and advancing the profession.

More than 75 specialty nursing organizations represent nurses in particular areas of the profession. Some are clinically focused, such as the American Association of Critical-Care Nurses, the Oncology Nurses Association, and the American Association of Neuroscience Nurses. Others are role focused, such as the American Organization of Nurse Executives and the National League for Nursing. Still others represent specific groups in nursing, such as the American Assembly for Men in Nursing and the National Black Nurses Association. To attract future members, many specialty organizations offer reduced membership rates to students and new graduates, which include discounted meeting and convention rates, discounts on insurance, networking opportunities, and informative publications and mailings about the association. Go to the *Evolve* website (http://evolve.elsevier.com/Yoder-Wise) to see a listing of nursing specialty organizations.

The "umbrella organization" that represents all nurses is the American Nurses Association (ANA), which comprises registered nurses throughout the United States and its territories and various organizational affiliate members *(www.ana.org)*. The ANA advances the nursing profession by fostering high standards of nursing practice. Some functions of the ANA include promoting the economic and general welfare of nurses in the workplace, projecting a positive and realistic view of nursing, and lobbying Congress and regulatory agencies on healthcare issues affecting nurses and the public (ANA, 2010). When the ANA was formed in 1897 and officially founded in 1901, its purpose was to protect the public from unsafe nursing care and to set standards for practice and education that could be changed and adapted over the years (Joel, 2003). Today, the ANA continues to speak for nursing. Policymakers look to the ANA for guidance on nursing and health policy issues.

EXERCISE 29-12

Research the ANA and your state nursing organization on the Internet *(www.nursingworld.org)*. Find the mission of the organization and the legislative issues of interest. Obtain/download association brochures or further information.

Unlike most professional associations that are open memberships (i.e., if you meet the basic criteria, you are eligible to be a member), Sigma Theta Tau International is an invitational association. Established in 1922, membership is available to nurses enrolled in baccalaureate, master's, and doctoral education programs and community leaders through a nomination process. Its mission is to create a global community of nurses who lead in using scholarship, knowledge, and technology to improve the health of the world's people *(www.nursingsociety.org)*. This organization is one of the primary sources for small grants to aid in beginning research and disseminates research and leadership information through various publications and international meetings.

A MODEL FOR INVOLVEMENT

Few nurses graduate from their basic nursing educational program and then immediately join and become involved in their professional organization. Upon graduation, nurses often are focused on key aspects of professional life, such as learning basic policies and the organizational culture, evaluating peers to determine who to trust and who to avoid, and resolving numerous transitional issues, such as where to live, how to afford housing, how to manage payment of student loans, how to network with old and new friends, and how to be safe practitioners. Few new graduates think about how they can benefit from professional organizational membership, and unfortunately, many nurses never pursue membership in any professional organization. Many others participate only through a financial contribution, by paying the membership dues. Yoder-Wise (2006) describes the common path for development of professional involvement as movement from only a clinical focus (direct patient care) to a broader professional focus (policy-level).

Connecting with an Organization

The size of an organization is not as important as how the group is organized and who is leading it. Therefore it is extremely important to do some online reading about the officers and membership composition of the organization before making a commitment through membership. Most associations have a website that lists information regarding leader contact and biographical information, locations of their next meetings or activities, current policy issues and their positions, election information, and other valuable resource links. Some organizations permit e-mail subscriptions so that you are notified on a regular basis about evolving events.

EXERCISE 29-13
Attend a local meeting of a professional association, observe the dynamics, and network with the members.

Expectations of Membership

Upon joining a nursing organization, you may receive information on the history of the organization, future meetings and current activities, officer contact information, and local contacts. One of the most important things that you can do is connect with your local organization so that you can immediately begin networking. Decide how much time you can allocate to the organization. There are several different ways to be involved, all of which carry different time commitments. Do not assume that a certain role or committee position entails a set amount of time. The fact remains that most associations are composed of volunteers, all of whom have very busy schedules and different motivations for becoming involved. Taking time to talk to an officer or attend a local meeting and observe the group and the dynamics before deciding to make commitments will help ensure that you make an informed decision. Some members enter into the organizational experience with unreal expectations and quickly become disenchanted and disappointed with the organization, which results in completely pulling away from the organization. To maximize your experience, you owe it to yourself to do your homework, research the organization, talk to the members, determine the sense of the group dynamics, and assess what you want to derive from the experience and how you can contribute to the organization. Look at your strengths and talents to determine if there is a need or a fit within the organization. Finally, remember that the organization is composed of humans who are volunteering their time; therefore you should not expect a "perfect" organization. Every organization has its struggles, but you can gain tremendous personal and professional benefits from

your involvement. Examples of tangible benefits of membership can be found in Box 29-5.

BOX 29-5   TANGIBLE BENEFITS FROM ORGANIZATIONAL INVOLVEMENT

- Substantial discounts on continuing education
- Certifications
- Credentialing
- Group insurance plans for professional liability, hospitalization, and disability
- Travel services, such as auto rentals, hotel stays, and restaurant visits
- Quick access to staff experts on practice advocacy
- Legal, legislative, and educational issues
- Professional standards
- Discounts on professional journals

EXERCISE 29-14
While you are at an association meeting, challenge yourself to speak to at least two members to learn about their work setting and their nursing role. Make sure to get contact information or a business card from at least two individuals whom you can call in the near future. On the back of the business card, write something about that person that will help you remember him or her for the future (e.g., long black hair, nurse manager on the neurology unit at General Hospital). It is also helpful to have a date and the name of the meeting so you can "place" the person in your mind. You may use these cards in the future when you are looking for a job or need a specific question answered.

Joining/Reasons for Involvement

Motivation to join an organization can vary a great deal. Organizational membership has become an integral part of one's career development. Nurses may hold membership in a variety of social and professional organizations, devoting more time to one particular area of interest. Nurses who define themselves as leaders and who want to have influence beyond their workplaces should join at least one professional association. Some reasons for joining organizations include feeling a sense of responsibility to the profession, contributing to the greater good of the profession, enhancing résumé and marketability, supporting particular legislative interests, and social networking.

A common belief among nurses is that their organization of choice can help improve conditions and care for their patients. In addition, there are those who choose to be active participants by joining committee work, running for office, or taking on other leadership roles. Organizations need all types of members, both active and passive participants, so that they can carry out their missions and conduct activities and business. Organizational involvement is a socialization process that can improve morale—being around others who take pride in and celebrate the nursing profession is contagious. Whatever your preferred level of involvement, you can contribute greatly to your profession by simply becoming a member of a professional association, and progressing to active involvement guarantees a world of opportunities.

Some nurses choose to belong to their state nurses' association because they want to protect their licensure status and affect health care through influencing legislation. Others choose to belong because of specific benefits such as liability insurance and education. Some individuals belong to professional organizations because they are required to do so; employment contracts can make it mandatory for the nurse to join a union and pay dues in order to receive a paycheck. Many state associations have instituted a workplace advocacy program, which provides the nurse with communication and conflict resolution tools.

EXERCISE 29-15

Think about what motivates you to join the state nurses' organization. Make a list of your strengths (communication, organization, budgeting, legislative interests). Look at positions within the organization that interest you. On a separate list, write out reasons why you would want to be a part of the association.

Personal and Professional Benefits

Some associations offer substantial scholarships for nurses who are pursuing higher education and certifications. They might also offer scholarships to attend policy meetings, such as the Nurse In Washington Internship (organized by the Nursing Organizations Alliance) or the Annual Health Policy Institute, conducted by the Center for Health Policy, Research, and Ethics of George Mason University. These two intern-

ships are examples of opportunities through which nurses can learn about legislative issues, the political process, healthcare advocacy, and how to be more effective on local, state, and national levels. Another potential benefit of membership is the opportunity to travel for conventions and meetings. Most organizations rotate their regular convention meeting sites so that members throughout the country will have an opportunity to attend.

With ever-increasing time demands on individuals, volunteering for activities outside of work and family has become more difficult. Associations are aware that traditional incentives for member participation may not be enough to draw new members; however, additional benefits exist that are not advertised. Networking and exposure to different opportunities within the nursing profession are two of the most valuable benefits of belonging to an organization. Some nurses may stop working for a time because of family or educational priorities. Organizational membership can help these nurses stay connected to professional issues and colleagues through meetings and publications and smooth the transition back into practice.

Membership in nursing organizations can provide a continuous source of professional colleagues for today's nurse to draw upon for advice and support. All nurses encounter ethical dilemmas and professional challenges. Members of a nurses' professional association can be nonbiased, safe colleagues to ask for advice about your situation. They can provide feedback options for your situation, based on their experience, especially when you may not want to discuss it with co-workers who could be directly involved. They also may be connected to the experts in the field and serve as a connection for further dialog.

With abundant opportunities in nursing, chances are that most nurses will work in a variety of settings over the course of their career. Therefore today's nurse needs to socialize with nurses in different professional career paths. This socialization can take place through district meetings or state or national conventions. For example, organizations have conventions at which they might feature a nurse panel representing a variety of innovative positions within the field, which will introduce the member to networking contacts in those emerging fields. In addition

---

BOX 29-6 **SKILLS DEVELOPED THROUGH ORGANIZATIONAL INVOLVEMENT**

- Conflict resolution
- Interpersonal communication
- Public speaking
- Mentoring
- Conducting meetings
- Creating agendas
- Facilitation
- Delegation
- Consensus-building
- Strategic-thinking
- Team-building
- Political advocacy
- Legislative work/lobbying
- Problem solving

to networking, the professional organization can serve as a training ground through which nurses can build skills and gain wonderful experiences. Examples of these skills can be found in Box 29-6. They also provide opportunities for leadership development

through committees or in officer positions, which can provide invaluable skills training.

Professional organization members can influence healthcare policy through opportunities to influence and educate policymakers. Members of nursing associations learn firsthand about diversity among the patient populations and clinical issues of fellow members, as well as diversity within the profession. On the most basic level, nurses can influence legislation for health and the profession by simply becoming a member and adding political strength through numbers. Further, nurses can participate on a legislative committee and become involved in their local grassroots politics. Nurses' ability to advocate for their patients is not confined to the bedside; nurses must learn to use advocacy skills in the political arena as well. By being acquainted with the key political figures in their area, nurses can ensure that they are at the table for discussions on healthcare and policy-making decisions. Consistently, the Harris poll reports that the public trusts information about health care provided by registered nurses. This powerful influence of the nursing profession on public trust reinforces that nurses must be involved in healthcare discussions and decision-making policies.

THE SOLUTION

I started by volunteering in the emergency department (ED) before I graduated, which gave me the firsthand view that this chaotic environment was the right place for me to start. I was confident that I knew myself and my passions, so I was willing to challenge the tradition of working in medical-surgical units before the ED. I had to work hard to convince my friends, my faculty, and myself that I could work in the ED directly out of nursing school. I wrote down the pros and cons, created my résumé, and made phone calls to a nurse I knew who worked at the medical center and could introduce me to the ED manager there. I was hired, so I worked in the ED as a new graduate, and before my first year, I had earned my Certification in Emergency Nursing (CEN).

I thought that creating the non-traditional job that I wanted for myself would be easier if I had the credibility of a graduate degree. I began taking graduate courses one at a time to find a good fit and found that I did not want to obtain the traditional MSN degree, so I applied and was accepted into the new master of healthcare innovation (MHI) degree program. I e-mailed some contacts I had

met while attending conferences, asking them if they had a human patient simulator and if they needed help learning how to use it, all the while staying in contact with the faculty from my undergraduate program. Within 4 years, I had earned my MHI, started my own patient simulation consulting company, published three peer-reviewed articles in national journals, and started coursework in a PhD program.

Navigating the traditions and socialization of nursing is tough, but you should not let other people direct or constrain your dreams. I did not know it at the time, but networking, joining professional organizations, and looking for the right fit in my career goals made a huge difference in how these ventures developed. Connections with mentors, colleagues, and friends who agree with me, as well as those that challenge my views, keep me moving forward.
—*Daniel Weberg*

Would this be a suitable approach for you? Why?

THE EVIDENCE

A wise mentor can provide a safe learning environment for honest reflection and discussion about challenging issues while acting as a sounding board, an advisor, a role model, a bridge to connections with new colleagues, and a support structure for new responsibilities (Boldra, Landin, Repta, Westphal, & Winistorfer (2008). Working with a helpful mentor provides support for career development through facilitating learning new roles and leadership skills. In addition to the benefits for those who work with a mentor, the mentoring relationship can benefit the mentor and the organization in improving organizational commitment. Organizations need to have future leaders prepared at every level to progress into positions of more responsibility as other formal leaders retire or move within the organization. Some organizations offer structured mentoring programs as a path to leadership development.

NEED TO KNOW NOW

- You are responsible for your own career. Make it what you want it to be.
- Identify colleagues who might serve as a mentor for you in considering strategies for career success.
- Keeping track of your professional accomplishments in an organized way will help you prepare position applications efficiently and quickly when opportunities are advertised.
- Networking with colleagues through professional associations or organizations can lead to many career opportunities.

CHAPTER CHECKLIST

Nurses must make decisions about career goals and career development. Managing a career requires a set of planned strategies designed to lead systematically toward the desired goal. The use of each strategy should be geared toward finding a good person-position fit. Career planning and development is a lifelong process focused on continual competence. Continued professional development, whether via graduate education, continuing education, certification, or service in professional associations, is a crucial component of success as a nurse. Involvement in professional associations can open doors to opportunities and skill development that would never have been possible otherwise.

- Career styles contribute to the diversity of the nursing profession and reflect different ways of achieving success.
- The four career styles are as follows:
  - Steady state: characterized by constancy with increasing professional skill
  - Linear: a hierarchical orientation with a steady climb
  - Entrepreneurial/transient: focused on new services and personal priorities
  - Spiral: rational, independent responsibility for shaping the career
- Certain career control strategies are effective with every career style:
  - Selecting professional peers, mentors, and role models helps shape professional development.
  - Designing personal/professional documents that open doors for further action includes the following:
    - The curriculum vitae (a listing of facts) (quantitative)
    - The résumé (a sampling of the most relevant facts, with details) (qualitative)
    - Appropriate business letters that market effectively
- Interviewing at its best is a two-way interaction that enables both people to determine whether there is a good person-position fit.
- Both graduate education and continuing education contribute to a nurse's ability to provide competent care.
- Certification is the designation of special knowledge beyond the basic licensure and is a requirement in some employment settings. Being a

professional carries additional obligations and privileges to ensure that the nurse remains competent, advances the profession, and improves health care.

- Numerous professional associations exist in health care:
  - The American Nurses Association and numerous specialty organizations focus on improving the profession itself and the care patients receive.
  - Most associations have both volunteers and employed staff to accomplish the organizational goals.
- Connecting with an association produces numerous benefits:
  - Involvement levels vary based on personal situations.
  - Strengths and talents should guide selection of involvement.
- Some nurses are covered by employment contracts via union activities.
- Workplace advocacy strategies help nurses interact on an individual or group basis in the employment situation.
- Nurses can make various contributions to the profession through association involvement:
  - Networking is facilitated.
  - Associations provide the input to policymakers who determine policies and legislation affecting the practice of nursing and patient rights and benefits.
  - Attendance at meetings provides valuable contacts and different points of view.
  - Work to reverse the workforce shortage in nursing is being led by the professional associations.

TIPS FOR A SUCCESSFUL CAREER

- Use an expanding file to organize hard copies of your accomplishments, such as continuing education certificates, by year so that you can report accurate data for licensure or certification.
- Update your CV at least once a year (6 months is better, and 3 months is ideal) so that you always have an accurate, current set of data to share with someone should a special opportunity appear. Better yet, make these changes as you complete achievements.
- Keep connected with people.
- Find a mentor; be a mentor; self-mentor.
- Learn from what you do each day: what to do differently, how to preempt errors, who to seek as a supporter.
- Focus on your strengths and build them into spectacular performances; hone the basics so that you are always prepared.
- Create an individual mission statement.
- Think about the future and what you need to be employable.
- Research and create a file of educational programs of interest.
- Join two professional organizations (e.g., the American Nurses Association (broad professional) and the American Association of Critical-Care Nurses (a specialty).
- Read professional journals and, on a regular basis, at least one other journal external to nursing to keep current with the world.
- Attend at least one professional meeting each year, especially outside of your geographic area, to network.
- Volunteer in your profession and your community.

REFERENCES

American Board of Nursing Specialties. (2006). *Specialty nursing certification: Nurses' perceptions, values and behaviors.* Retrieved October 21, 2009, from www.nursingcertification.org/pdf/executive_summary.pdf.

American Nurses Association (ANA). (2000). *Scopes and standards of practice for nursing professional development.* Washington, DC: Author.

American Nurses Association (ANA). (2010). *ANA Nurse's Career Center.* Retrieved April 30, 2010 from www.nursingworld.org/careercenter.

Boldra, J., Landin, C. W., Repta, K. R., Westphal, J., & Winistorfer, W. (2008). The value of leadership development through mentoring: More experienced colleagues can help protégés. *Health Progress, 89*(4), 33-36.

Bolles, R. N. (2009). *What color is your parachute? A practical manual for job-seekers and career-changers.* Berkley, CA: Ten Speed Press.

Buckingham, M. (2008). *The truth about you: Your secret to success.* Nashville, TN: Thomas Nelson.

Citrin, J. M., & Smith, R. A. (2003). *The five patterns of extraordinary careers.* New York: Crown Business Books.

Cummings, G., Lee, H., MacGregor, T., Davey, M., Wong, C., Paul, L., et al. (2008). Factors contributing to nursing leadership: A systematic review. *Journal of Health Services Research & Policy, 13*(4), 240-248.

Deal, J. J. (2007). *Retiring the generation gap: How employees young and old can find common ground.* San Francisco: John Wiley and Sons.

Fox, J. J. (2006). *How to land your dream job: No resume! And other secrets to get you in the door.* New York: Hyperion.

Friss, L. (1989). *Strategic management of nurses: A policy oriented approach.* Owings Mills, MD: AUPHA Press.

Heath, D., & Heath, C. (2009). *Why it may be wiser to hire people without meeting them.* Mansueto Ventures LLC. Retrieved August 28, 2009, from www.fastcompany.com/magazine/136/made-to-stick-hold-the-interview.html.

Joel, L. (2003). *Kelly's dimensions of professional nursing* (9th ed.). New York: McGraw-Hill.

Plank, W. (2010). *Five must-ask questions.* Retrieved May 4, 2010, from online.wsj.com/article/SB10001424052748704302304572 1396.

Yoder-Wise, P. S. (2006). Professional issues: Creating the challenge. *Annual Review of Nursing Education, 4,* 67-83.

SUGGESTED READING

Pagana, K. D. (2008). *The nurse's etiquette advantage: How professional etiquette can advance your nursing career.* Indianapolis, IN: Sigma Theta Tau International.

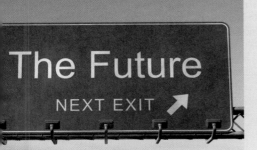

Thriving for the Future

Patricia S. Yoder-Wise

This chapter explores the potential for the future and how the changes we face can be maximized to our benefit—organizationally and personally. The key leadership skills of forecasting and visioning are presented. Projections for the future and their implication for nursing are included.

OBJECTIVES

- Value the need to think about the future while meeting current expectations.
- Ponder two or three projections for the future and what they mean to the practice of nursing.
- Determine three projections for the future that have implications for individual practice.

TERMS TO KNOW

chaos   shared visions   vision
complexity compression

THE CHALLENGE

Sara McCumber, APRN, BC, MSN
Adult/Family Nurse Practitioner, Duluth Clinic, Duluth,
Minnesota

I had been working for several years and had just accepted a position as a correctional nurse working with high-risk adolescents and adults. I pictured my job of completing physical assessments and managing the medication-delivery system. Over time, I learned that I was working with a population who were poor, had high-risk health behaviors, lacked access to health care, and often had physi-

cal and mental health problems. They often were returned to the community with many of the same problems. As the only nurse and health advocate in the facility, I realized that I had to search out and develop innovative solutions to the multitude of unmet health needs. I also knew I didn't have the skills or experiences to develop effective interventions. In addition, I determined that changes in the future that would improve the care for this population were unlikely.

What do you think you would do if you were this nurse?

INTRODUCTION

Leading and managing in nursing constitute a consistent challenge. Even nurses who say they do not want to lead or manage find that new demands call for continuous leadership and increased self-management skills. More important, increased emphasis on teams will continue, and a strong team does not emerge from limited talents. Bringing leadership and management talents to the team strengthens the work of the team. The core point is this: We are all accountable for something, and unless our part in the overall scheme is inconsequential, which it usually is not, we must lead when we have the insight, the ability, or the skill needed to move a situation forward. As stated in Chapter 1, every role has expectations associated with it. Thus every nurse has some leadership role to execute in practice.

Changes affecting healthcare occur at a rapid clip. Just when some stability seems likely, another new project or invention alters the currently established practice. Some years ago, people went to a hospital for invasive surgery and stayed for days. Additionally, many people believed that is where people went to die! Now they go to robotic-equipped surgical centers and stay for hours or maybe a day. The focus is changing from illness to wellness. The implementation of the Affordable Care Act has great potential! Tomorrow people will be rewarded for seeking wellness care and may receive actual physical care in the home, only this time through remote interactive devices. These events illustrate the dichotomous times in which we live and how the future is expected to be.

LEADERSHIP DEMANDS FOR THE FUTURE

Nurse administrators and leaders consistently say that the characteristic they are most seeking in tomorrow's professional nurse is leadership. In probing what that means, we often find themes that relate to our activities that may have serendipitous outcomes. We shape the public's view of the profession, the organization in which we work, and health care in general. We influence interprofessional views of what it is to be a professional, and we create the expectations of the nursing profession's potential. All of those examples form some of the leadership potential that exists for the future.

If we think about the world as a loose web, we know that every element has the potential to influence every other element. This connectivity with each other, whether within our profession or within the team, means that we influence others all of the time, just as others influence us. This influence molds our practices and beliefs as we move health care forward and also changes how we influence others subsequently. Thus even positions without formal leadership titles contain expectations for leadership, and we must all be prepared and willing to lead whenever the need arises. This response is exhibited every time a mass casualty occurs. The ability to be bicultural—both leading and following—is crucial to quality care.

LEADERSHIP STRENGTHS FOR THE FUTURE

Because so much of nursing's work is accomplished in teams, we have considerable strength in inclusivity (the politics of commonalities). This is in contrast to what many of us face in our everyday work of not capitalizing on thinking long-term and acting short-term. Much of the work of the Institute for Healthcare Improvement *(www.ihi.org)*, for example, is built around the fact that change is slow and cumbersome. It has short-circuited that drawn-out process through its program "Transforming Care at the Bedside." Although this rapid change (known as *rapid cycle change*) has produced positive results, nurses' abilities to embrace this intensity of change may be limited. Yet, almost every healthcare organization is actively engaged in determining best practices and finding or validating evidence. This emphasis is critical for safe patient care. However, what we lack by this intense focus is the passion for innovation (see the Literature Perspective at right).

When we are faced with the pressures of providing care to patients versus changing the system, we often remain focused on the patient, thus losing the opportunity to change an issue for many patients. To be effective in the future, we must embrace the opportunities to think longer term and more broadly so that more people are affected by our actions. Perhaps

LITERATURE PERSPECTIVE

Resource: Crenshaw, J. T., & Yoder-Wise, P. S. (2013). Creating an environment for innovation: the risk-taking leadership competency. *Nurse Leader, 11*(1), 24-27.

Most of the efforts of nurses in practice focus on providing evidence-based care and adopting new practices. A relatively small amount of the time (or of the population) is devoted to considered risk-taking. Using Rogers's Theory of Diffusion of Innovation, the authors suggest that little time or talent is spent in being the innovator in the profession. However, being willing to take careful risks (considered risk-taking) leads to innovative approaches of practice. The reason this type of work is not evidence-based is because this work is, in essence, creating the innovation. Innovators are at the cutting edge of change, laggards are at the tail end, and in the middle are the majority of the profession: those who practice based on evidence and who do so in a safe and documented manner. The value of innovation is not only creating the next step for new evidence-based research but also disrupting current thinking and practices.

In order to promote innovation in an organization, the culture has to support the idea of considered risk-taking. Everyone needs to have protected time to reflect on events to consider how a change might have produced even better outcomes.

Implications for Practice
In order to support innovation in the workplace, nurse leaders must support a culture that allows for diverse viewpoints and reflection about events. Providing support for considered risk-taking allows individuals who might not otherwise risk wild thinking to do so in an attempt to find different solutions to ongoing clinical and management concerns.

because of our history of attention to details, we may need to challenge ourselves in developing our ability for leadership. Moving from micromanaging to focusing on setting expectations for those for whom we are accountable may feel uncomfortable. However, that movement reinforces our ability to deal with longer-term issues. In addition, the quest for meaning suggests that our actions today create the foundation on which future leaders will build. Thus if we fail to capitalize on today's opportunities, we are diminishing the place at which future leaders will start their careers. It is incumbent on us to raise expectations about what comprises good, safe, quality care and how nurses contribute to those expectations. This potential is especially critical in times of dramatic changes, such as those that continue to evolve from the Affordable Care Act legislation.

How, then, do today's practitioners know what is expected in the future? The answer may seem trite: Continue to learn and to practice! Our foundation begins with our concern for and advocacy about patient care. That foundation is fairly well engrained in professional nurses' beliefs. The movement from focusing on the nurse-patient relationship to the big picture of nursing (politics and public or health policy activities) may take several years, but the foundation is there. What we do in our professional lives is the legacy we leave for future generations.

EXERCISE 30-3

Think ahead to the time when you might logically die. Rather than being sad that your life has ended, consider all of the good you have done in life and in nursing. Your next of kin is asked to say what he/she believes your nursing legacy to be. What one or two sentences would you want to have said about your contributions to nursing and the patients for whom you provided care?

Nurses who seek leadership opportunities will find that many are available—in the employment setting, in professional organizations, and in voluntary community organizations. Balancing the multiple demands in an era of rapid changes and the resultant new expectations becomes an even greater challenge. Merely being employed is no longer sufficient; we must be *employable*. This suggests that we must constantly be focused on competence, on learning, on what the future holds, and on what patients want and need. Failure to do so will make us unemployable and will make the profession undesirable. To be valued in the future, we need to know what the future might encompass.

VISIONING

Whether you are a leader, a follower, or a manager, being able to visualize in your mind what the ideal future is becomes a critical strategy. A vision can range from that of an individual to that of a group or to a whole organization. No matter how we engage in this visioning activity, we must be open and honest about what we think for the future. Creating our own circle of advisors or brain trusts (those who do not necessarily think as we do, but who are creative thinkers) allows us to test ideas so that we enhance our own thinking and performance to higher levels. (See the

Literature Perspective.) In the classic book, *The Fifth Discipline: The Art and Practice of the Learning Organization* (2006), Senge said that all leadership is really about is people working at their best to create the future. And that, in reality, is what we do everyday.

 LITERATURE PERSPECTIVE

Resource: Batcheller, J. & Yoder-Wise, P. S. (2011). Creating insight when the literature is absent: The circle of advisors. *Nursing Administration Quarterly, 35* (4), 338-343.

Some areas of practice are fairly narrow and few people work in those narrow fields; other areas lag behind the massive push toward safety related issues. Thus, the literature can be limited or absent related to a concern a person might have. Having a circle of advisors is a strategy to overcome lone thinking. This circle of advisors is not restricted by geographic or cultural constraints. Rather, resourceful nurses can find others with similar interests and filter information based on area of the country or world or taking into account various values prevalent in a given field or area. Surrounding yourself with others interested in your specific area provides the opportunity to exchange ideas. The process is somewhat analogous to qualitative research in that little appears in the literature and the task at hand is to gain insight, seek a solution, or propose new ideas. Advisors provide advice and surrounding oneself within a circle of advisors provides for diverse viewpoints to be shared.

Implications for Practice

Although this article was geared toward chief nursing executives, this practice works equally well for nurses in other positions. Careful selection of the advisors is critical to having access to successful advice.

This chapter is designed to share some views about the future so that you can think about them in relation to what it means to lead and manage. This "thinking about" the future, like visions, is further enriched through sharing in open dialogs.

EXERCISE 30-4

Select a group of three or four peers and brainstorm about what you think the future of nursing will be. Consider how technology will affect what we do; consider where our primary place of service will be and how we will deliver care. Think about the changes in society and the political pressures for effective health care and what those might mean for nursing. Think about how you would reform health care. Create a list of ideas to share with others.

Although no one knows the future for certain, many entities engage in formal discussions and predictions. These range from structured groups, such as the World Future Society (*www.wfs.org*), to regular reports and books. Although not everyone is a futurist, each of us needs to be aware of trends. Thinking about the future should be mind-expanding; it is the most non-stereotypical thinking you can do. In everyday practice, you can ask yourself and others "what if" questions. We take for granted that certain practices have remained unchanged. Yet, technology and creative thinkers and investigators prove us wrong on a regular basis. Our challenge is to think about the future in a way that does not necessarily rely on history and yet builds on today.

The Wise Forecast Model©

Yoder-Wise (2011) created The Wise Forecast Model©. Although the model is simplistic (three steps), it is useful in any situation where thinking about the future is important. Box 30-1 portrays the three steps.

This three-step model emphasizes what each of us must do proactively to create our own future rather than to respond to changes as they occur. The first step, learn widely, means that we must extend our sources of knowledge beyond our role and clinical areas of interest. In fact we must extend our learning beyond nursing and health care. Widely might encompass another discipline such as architecture or engineering. This extension doesn't mean that someone has to seek a degree in a new field. Learning about the field and how those professionals think might create new ways to think about issues affecting nursing. Widely might also include works related to the future or general publications, such as FastCompany or Wired. Initially, this kind of learning may be deliberate, in other words, you might need to set aside specified times to make the effort to garner this diverse information. After a few such sessions, however, it is realistic to think that information from other fields will pique your interest to the point that you will create a file of "tidbits" of information.

The second step is to think wildly. In other words, now we are limited only by our imagination. For example, since they were invented, someone wasn't satisfied with what we could do with computers. So computers evolved from one or two room-sized mainframes to something someone could have in a home to something someone could carry in a backpack to something someone could carry in a hand. Step two is designed to create connections among disparate thoughts. This thinking might be seen as the start of innovations. As Crenshaw and Yoder-Wise (2013) identified, risk taking is an important competency to develop. Considered risk taking, that which has the potential to produce innovation without unsafe results, is practiced by a small portion of the population. Yet, others could engage in the practice in order to develop new and improved ways to practice.

Step three, act wisely, is designed to draw us back to the reality of what is possible within the organization in which we work with the funding which we have and with the amount of time we have to vest in an activity. It is, in a sense, a recovery phase to help us balance the wild thinking with reality and provide us with something that will get us to a new way of thinking and practicing without being totally disruptive.

Because the future is about teams and group work, many implications exist for nursing. Skills related to working with others and facilitating their work and ways to reach decisions about practice and the workplace will be crucial. If the work is team-based, how will evaluations and compensation be structured in

---

BOX 30-1	**THE THREE STEPS TO THE WISE FORECAST MODEL ©**

1. Learn widely
2. Think wildly
3. Act wisely

source: Yoder-Wise, P. S. (2011). Creating wise forecasts for nursing: The Wise Forecast Model©. *The Journal of Continuing Education in Nursing: Continuing Competence for the Future, 42*(9), 387.

EXERCISE 30-5

Think about the questions just mentioned and suggest how compensation will be formed in the future. Consider the differences among generations. For example, some generations are interested in being able to see the world. That used to mean travel abroad. A smart, trendy employer might create an international collaborative that allows nurses to retain their home organization benefits while practicing throughout their home country and the world.

the future? Will you receive favorable reviews because the team you work with is productive? Will a team receive a bonus or merit salary increase? If you are not a team player, will you be useful to the organization at all? These are examples of how to rethink the future.

SHARED VISION

The concept of shared vision suggests that several of us buy into a particular view. If we think of a familiar concept, stress, and what Selye (1978) described as *eustress* and *distress,* we have a continuum.

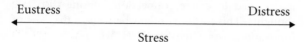

Eustress   Distress

Stress

Again, if you think about stress, you recall that each of us views an event differently and that having no stress results in death. Comparably, we can think about how society is evolving. Stability and total chaos are the ends of a continuum. Moving in some way between those two ends suggests that we live in a constant state of disequilibrium in which we strive toward stability while recognizing we experience chaos. The figure below suggests that in times of great stability, society makes little progress (but life probably seems serene). In times of great chaos, in contrast, society may transform itself (and life may seem uncontrollable). Thus it is even more important to think about the projections for the future. As one example for most of us, think what we were doing, thinking, believing, and valuing on September 10, 2001. Then think about each in relation to September 11, 2001. We moved from some point on that continuum closer to chaos, no matter where we were in the world or what we were doing.

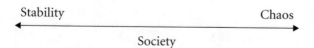

Stability   Chaos

Society

As we continue to move from "traditional" practices to evidence-based ones and from a heavy focus on tertiary care to one that values primary care, we can assume that we might experience more chaos. The comfort of the known is gone; rather, practices are evaluated on a regular basis and changes are incorpo-

rated so that we are all doing the latest "best" for patients. In our efforts to do the best we can as soon as we can, we have experienced the phenomenon complexity compression, a term that means many changes are happening almost simultaneously and before one practice can be firmly implanted in our minds, we are already addressing some other new change. This compression can be distracting or useful. As we increase the educational preparation of nurses worldwide, we will be better able to function in this evolving environment.

It is our ability to retrieve information and analyze and evaluate it that influences our currency with practice expectations. We seem to value the need for shared vision, which include the idea of operating from a rich data-based approach. To be able to do so, however, we also need to hone our skills in projecting for the future so we know where practice is headed, we need to consider how we interact with our patients, and we need to consider how quickly we can elevate all nursing practitioners to a satisfactory level of working with an evidence-based practice approach.

PROJECTIONS FOR THE FUTURE

If you watch future reports on television or read *Trend Letter* or *The Futurist* (The World Society publication) or books such as *The World is Flat: A Brief History of the Twenty-First Century* or *Hot, Flat and Crowded* by Thomas L. Friedman, you will find comparable themes about the future. The following are some forecasts for the future that will affect nursing; it is possible to ask the "what if" questions with each (e.g., What if this happens?):

- Knowledge will change dramatically, requiring that we all be dedicated learners. With or without state law, continuing education will be mandatory.
- Knowledge will evolve from the intensity of the current information evolution so that we will access content with meaning and applicability for our work.
- A power shift will occur toward health care because of the intensity of the developing knowledge and its use in making cost-effective decisions about care.
- As the healthcare system continues to evolve and as employers limit healthcare coverage and

genetics allows us to know more about how an individual would respond to treatment, a shift toward eliminating the current disparities is more likely. Health care may also seem to invade one's rights to privacy and choice because, as an example, everyone will have an electronic health record.

- The world will be seen increasingly as a continuum without borders that prevent trade and inventions, including those related to health care.
- Technology will continue to revolutionize health care.
- Increasing diversity will result in the following:
  - More people who are older
  - More people moving to different parts of the country or the world
  - A greater need for speaking two or three languages
- People will be satisfied with an experience, not simply service.
- There will be increased violence and simultaneously an increased expectation for civility.

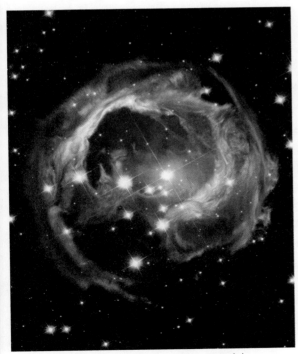

The future explodes with potential.

- Stores will be either very small or huge.
- Macromarketing (targeting masses) will be out; micromarketing (targeting specific populations) will be in.
- We could become narrower in our views of the world because we can be catered to based on our distinctive interests. As an example, think about micro marketing where retailers know what brands and sizes of clothing you prefer and send you information about those products on a regular basis.
- Job security will be out; career options will be in.
- Competition will be out; cooperation will be in.
- Work will be sporadic.
- More people will be living with chronic diseases.
- More people will be overweight and consequently experience various related diseases.
- Robotics will change how chronic diseases can be managed.
- Bioengineering will make possible interventions that currently do not exist.
- Emphasis on prevention will redirect care efforts.
- Work will be accomplished by teams.
- Everyone will need to be a leader.

EXERCISE 30-6

Review the list of projections, and consider how each might affect what you envision as your career. Make a note of one or two phrases that are the top implications. Look at the list again, and evaluate each of the items to determine which ones you believe will be most important to you. Rank in order the top five. Compare your list with two or three colleagues' lists, and offer your rationale for your selection. After you hear other viewpoints, consider if you would change your own rankings.

In nursing, we have issues we can consider in the more narrowed scope of the world, for example:

- How will shared governance continue to enhance the role of direct-care nurses?
- How will Magnet™ designations affect where nurses seek employment?
- Will we have a dramatically richer set of evidence to describe the difference nurses make in patient care and health promotion/disease prevention?

- How will continuing competence be measured in the future?
- How will health care emerge over the next several years as a desirable place to work and as a source of help for health-related needs?
- Will nurses be paid by a classification salary, or will their economic worth be reflected in what they are paid?
- How will the increasing number of men in nursing change the "profile" of the profession?
- What can healthcare organizations learn from business, and vice versa?
- Will increasing concern about terrorism affect the flow of nurses across borders?

IMPLICATIONS

So should we be concerned with these forecasts? Are they likely to come true? Historically, Cornish (1997) analyzed the predictions from the February 1967 issue of *The Futurist*. Of the 34 forecasts that could be judged, 23 were accurate and 11 were not. However, some of the 11 were accurate trends that did not meet the targeted date, often because of shifting national priorities, such as funding. If this is true historically, we might assume that forecasting, which becomes better refined each year, will continue to be a valuable tool for the future. We can see in the economic downturn starting in 2008 that continued movement occurred but most time lines for meeting expectations were altered.

CONCLUSION

Numerous changes will occur throughout our lifetimes. It is only a matter of time before we say (if we haven't already), "When I was young . . . ." Our description might be of something that today is considered fairly advanced. For those who want to thrive, the future forecasts are like the gold ring on the merry-go-round. If you risk and reach far enough, you can grasp it! Lead on … ¡Adelánte!

THE SOLUTION

I joined the professional organization for correctional health professionals and reviewed nursing publications to identify some of the possible options that were viewed as currently successful or likely to happen in the near future. I networked with colleagues at local and state meetings and realized that a graduate degree in public health nursing would help me develop the skills to address the health needs of my population. I also decided to pursue the Clinical Nurse Specialist in Community Health Nursing certification. Clearly, society expected more in the future in both education and credentials. I believed that I had the skills to develop community programs and research studies to help me address the high-risk needs of my client population.

—Sara McCumber

Would this be a suitable approach for you? Why?

NEED TO KNOW NOW

- Ask "what if" when challenged by a problem in your work.
- Use the changes you have seen in health care in the past 6 months as a reminder that the future will be different from the past.

CHAPTER CHECKLIST

This chapter addresses the need to think about the future and what that means for current practice. Involvement by all nurses is needed to keep the profession relevant to the constantly emerging future.

- Leadership demands for the future
- Leadership strengths for the future
- Visioning
- The Wise Forecast Model ©
- Shared Visions
- Projections for the future

■ TIPS FOR THE FUTURE

- Scan literature external to nursing and health care.
- Listen to divergent viewpoints about the economy, federal and state policy, and technology.
- Ask yourself "what if" questions.

- Remember what you find disheartening and use that as a filter for what you learn from numerous fields.

■ WHAT NEW GRADUATES SAY

- Many other disciplines have a very different perspective of life.
- Learning the concepts in nursing really was important because some of the facts already changed.

- Where you work in your first position can shape what you'll be prepared for in the future.

REFERENCES

American Nurses Association (ANA). (2010). *Nursing administration: Scope and standards for practice.* (3rd ed.). Washington, DC: Author.

Batcheller, J. & Yoder-Wise, P. S. (2011). Creating insight when the literature is absent: The circle of advisors. *Nursing Administration Quarterly, 35*(4), 338-343.

Cornish, E. (1997). The Futurist forecasts 30 years later. *The Futurist, 31*(January/February), 45-48.

Crenshaw, J. T. & Yoder-Wise, P. S. (2013). Creating an environment for innovation: the risk- taking leadership. competency. *Nurse Leader, 11*(1), 24-27.

Saffo, P. (2009). A looming American diaspora. *Harvard Business Review,* (February), 27.

Selye, H. (1978). *The stress of life.* New York: McGraw-Hill.

Senge, P. (2006). *The fifth discipline: The art and practice of the learning organization.* New York: Doubleday Currency.

Yoder-Wise, P. S. (2011). Creating wise forecasts for nursing: The Wise Forecast Model©. *The Journal of Continuing Education in Nursing: Continuing Competence for the Future, 42*(9), 387.

SUGGESTED READINGS

Auerbach, D. I. (2012). Will the NP workforce grow in the future? New forecasts and implications for healthcare delivery. *Medical Care, 50*(7), 606-610.

Begun, J. W., & White, K. R. (1995). Altering nursing's dominant logic: Guidelines from complex adaptive systems theory. *Complexity and Chaos in Nursing, 2*(1), 5-15.

Dennison Himmelfarb, C. R. & Hayman, L. L. (2012). Heads up: The forecast for cardiovascular health and disease is formidable. *Journal of Cardiovascular Nursing, 27*(6), 461-463.

Institute for Alternative Futures. (2013). What will chiropractic in the US look like in 2025? *Futurist.* http://www.altfutures.org/chiropracticfutures.

Kowalski, K., Cherry, B., & Yoder-Wise, P. S. (2012). A conversation with Peter Buerhaus: Crucial ideas for the next decade of leadership and administrative research. *Journal of Nursing Administration, 43*(3), 127-129.

Porter-O'Grady, T., Igein, G., Alexander, D., Blaylock, J., McComb, D., & Williams, S. (2005). Critical thinking for nursing leadership. *Nurse Leader, 3*(4), 28-31.

Scott, E. S. & Yoder-Wise, P. S. (2013). Increasing the intensity of nursing leadership: Graduate preparation for nurse leaders. *Journal of Nursing Administration, 43*(1), 1-3.

Yoder-Wise, P. S. (2012). Preparing tomorrow's service leaders: An educational challenge. *Nursing Administration Quarterly, 36*(2), 169-178.

Yoder-Wise, P. S. (2012). The complex challenges of administrative research for the future. *Journal of Nursing Administration, 42*(5), 239-241.

ILLUSTRATION CREDITS

Chapter 2

Unnumbered Figure 2-1: From Lewis, S., Heitkemper, M., Dirksen, S., O'Brien, P., & Bucher, L. (2007). *Medical-surgical nursing* (7th ed.). St. Louis: Mosby.

Unnumbered Figure 2-2: Courtesy Institute of Medicine.

Chapter 3

Figure 3-1: From Fagin, C. (2000). *Essays on nursing leadership.* New York: Springer Publishing.

Unnumbered Figure 3-2: ©2010 Photos. com, a division of Getty Images. All rights reserved.

Chapter 4

Unnumbered Figure 4-2: ©Getty Images, Ablestock.com.

Chapter 5

Unnumbered Figure 5-2: From Leake, P. (2010). *Community/public health nursing online for Stanhope and Lancaster, foundations of nursing in the community* (3rd ed.). St. Louis: Mosby.

Chapter 6

Figure 6-1: Modified from Sullivan, E.J., & Decker, P.J. (1992). *Effective management in nursing.* Menlo Park, CA: Addison-Wesley.

Chapter 7

Unnumbered Figure 7-1: From Leake, P. (2010). *Community/public health nursing online for Stanhope and Lancaster, foundations of nursing in the community* (3rd ed.). St. Louis: Mosby.

Unnumbered Figure 7-2: From Leake, P. (2010). *Community/public health nursing online for Stanhope and Lancaster, foundations of nursing in the community* (3rd ed.). St. Louis: Mosby.

Chapter 11

Figure 11-1: From Graves, J.R., Amos, L.K., Huether, S., Lange, L.L., & Thompson, C.B. (1995). Description of a graduate program in clinical nursing informatics. *Computers in Nursing,* 13(2), 60-70.

Chapter 12

Figure 12-2: Modified from Ward, W. (1988). *An introduction to health care financial management.* Owings Mills, MD: National Health Publishing.

Chapter 14

Figure 14-1: From Kane, R.L., Shamliyan, T.C., Duval, S., & Wilt, T. (March 2007). *Nursing staffing and quality of patient care: Evidence Report/Technology Assessment No. 151.* (Prepared by the Minnesota Evidence-based Practice Center under Contract N. 290-02-0009.) AHRQ Publication N. 07-E00005. Rockville, MD: Agency for Healthcare Research and Quality.

Chapter 18

Figure 18-1: Adapted from Satir, V. (1988). *The new peoplemaking.* Mountain View, CA: Science & Behavior Books; and Olen, D. (1993). *Communicating: Speaking and listening to end misunderstanding and promote friendship.* Germantown, WI: JODA Communications.

Figure 18-2: Adapted from St. Charles Medical Center. (1993). *People centered teams.* Bend, OR: Author.

Chapter 21

Figure 21-1: From Stetler, C.B. (2001). Updating the Stetler model of research utilization to facilitate evidence-based practice. *Nursing Outlook,* 49(6), 272-279, Figure 3A, p. 276.

Figure 21-2: Adapted from Collins, S., Voth, T., DiCenso, A., & Guyatt, G. (2005). Finding the evidence. In A. DiCenso, G. Guyatt, & D. Ciliska (Eds.), *Evidence-based nursing: A guide to clinical practice* (pp. 20-43). St. Louis: Mosby.

Unnumbered Figure 21-2: From Lowdermilk, D., & Perry, S. (2007). *Maternity and women's health care* (9th ed.). St. Louis: Mosby. Courtesy Cheryl Briggs, RN, Annapolis, MD.

Chapter 22

Unnumbered Figure 22-2: From Leake, P. (2010). *Community/public health nursing online for Stanhope and Lancaster, foundations of nursing in the community* (3rd ed.). St. Louis: Mosby.

Chapter 23

Figure 23-2: Almost, J. (2006). Conflict within nursing work environments: Concept analysis. *Journal of Advanced Nursing,* 53(4), 444-453, Blackwell Publishing.

Chapter 25

Figure 25-1: From *2006 Survey of occupational injuries and illnesses.* (October 2007). Bureau of Labor Statistics, U.S. Department of Labor.

Figure 25-2: From *Workplace injuries and illnesses in 2007.* (October 2008). Bureau of Labor Statistics, U.S. Department of Labor.

Figure 25-3: © 2009 by the American Nurses Association. Reprinted with permission. All rights reserved.

Chapter 28

Figure 28-1: Adapted from Selye, H. (1991). History and present status of the stress concept. In A. Monat & R. Lazarus (Eds.), *Stress and coping: An anthology* (pp. 21-36). New York: Columbia University Press.

Figure 28-2: Adapted from Covey, S.R., Merrill, A.R., & Merrill, R.R. (1994). *First things first: To love, to learn, to leave a legacy.* New York: Simon & Schuster.

Chapter 29

Unnumbered Figure 29-1: ©José Luis Gutiérrez, iStock Photo.

Chapter 30

Unnumbered Figure 30-1: ©Geoffrey Holman, Zargon Studios Corp.

Unnumbered Figure 30-2: NASA and The Hubble Heritage Team (STScI/AURA), Hubble Space Telescope ACS, STScI-PRC04-10.

GLOSSARY

Absenteeism The rate at which an individual misses work on an unplanned basis. (Ch. 24)

Accommodating An unassertive, cooperative approach to conflict in which the individual neglects personal needs, goals, and concerns in favor of satisfying those of others. (Ch. 23)

Accountability The expectation of explaining actions and results. (Ch. 26)

Accreditation Process by which an authoritative body determines that an organization meets certain standards to such a degree that the organization is able to meet the standards as a whole and without ongoing monitoring of each aspect of performance. (Ch. 7)

Acculturation Process by which a person becomes a competent participant in the dominant culture. (Ch. 9)

Acknowledgment Recognition that an employee is valued and respected for what he or she has to offer to the workplace, team, or group; acknowledgments may be verbal or written, public or private. (Ch. 18)

Active listening Focusing completely on the speaker and listening without judgment to the essence of the conversation; an active listener should be able to repeat accurately at least 95% of the speaker's intended meaning. (Ch. 18)

Advanced generalist Clinical nurse leader, which is a protected title for those who successfully complete the CNL certification examination. (Ch. 13)

Advocate One who proactively speaks for another to ensure certain needs or wishes are met. (Ch. 22)

Agency for Healthcare Research and Quality (AHRQ) The primary federal agency devoted to improving quality, safety, efficiency, and effectiveness of health care. (Ch. 2)

Agenda A written list of items to be covered in a meeting and the related materials that meeting participants should read beforehand or bring along. Types of agendas include structured agendas, timed agendas, and action agendas. (Ch. 28)

Apparent agency Doctrine whereby a principal becomes accountable for the actions of his or her agent; created when a person holds himself or herself out as acting on behalf of the principal; also known as *apparent authority*. (Ch. 5)

Associate nurse A licensed nurse in the primary care model who provides care to the patient according to the primary nurse's specification when the primary nurse is not working. (Ch. 13)

At-will employee An individual who works without a contract. (Ch. 19)

Autocratic An authoritarian style that places control within one person's position. (Ch. 6)

Autonomy Personal freedom and the right to choose what will happen to one's own person. (Ch. 5)

Average daily census (ADC) Average number of patients cared for per day for a reporting period. (Ch. 14)

Average length of stay (ALOS) The number of patient days in a specific time period divided by the number of discharges in that same period. (Ch. 14)

Avoiding An unassertive, uncooperative approach to conflict in which the avoider neither pursues his or her own needs, goals, and concerns nor helps others to do so. (Ch. 23)

Bar code technology Systems that encode data electronically into a format of bars and spaces that represents letters or numbers. (Ch. 11)

Barriers Factors, internal or external to the change situation, that interfere with movement toward a desirable outcome. (Ch. 17)

Benchmarking Best practices, processes, or systems identified by a quality improvement team to be compared with the practice, process, or system under review. (Ch. 20)

Beneficence Principle that states that the actions one takes should promote good. (Ch. 5)

Biomedical technology The technological devices and systems that relate to biologic and medical sciences. (Ch. 11)

Blog An electronic communication resembling a journal. (Ch. 11)

Budget A detailed financial plan, stated in dollars, for carrying out the activities an organization wants to accomplish within a specific period. (Ch. 12)

Budgeting process An ongoing activity of planning and managing revenues and expenses to meet the goals of the organization. (Ch. 12)

Bullying A practice closely related to lateral or horizontal violence, but a real or perceived power differential between the instigator and recipient must be present in bullying. (Chs. 23, 25)

Bureaucracy Characterized by formality, low autonomy, a hierarchy of authority, an environment of rules, division of labor, specialization, centralization, and control. (Ch. 8)

Burnout Disengagement from work characterized by emotional exhaustion, depersonalization, and decreased effectiveness. (Ch. 28)

Capital expenditure budget A plan for purchasing major capital items, such as equipment or a physical plant, with a useful life greater than 1 year and exceeding a minimum cost set by the organization. (Ch. 12)

Capitation A reimbursement method in which healthcare providers are paid a per-person-per-year (or per-month) fee for providing specified services over a period of time. (Ch. 12)

Career Progressive achievement throughout a person's professional life. (Ch. 29)

Case management A person-oriented service that reflects multidisciplinary cooperation and coordination. (Ch. 4)

Case-management model A model of delivering patient care based on patient outcomes and cost containment. Components of case management are a case manager, critical paths/critical pathways, and unit-based managed care. (Ch. 13)

Case manager A baccalaureate degree– or master's degree–prepared clinical nurse who coordinates patient care from preadmission through discharge. (Ch. 13)

Case method A model of care delivery in which one nurse provides total care for a patient during an entire work period. (Ch. 13)

Case mix The volume and type of patients served by a healthcare provider. (Ch. 12)

Cash budget A plan for an organization's cash receipts and disbursements. (Ch. 12)

Centers for Disease Control and Prevention (CDC) The main federal agency protecting the health and safety of people in the United States. (Ch. 19)

Certification Designation of special knowledge beyond basic licensure. (Ch. 29)

Chain of command The hierarchy depicted in vertical dimensions of organizational charts. (Ch. 8)

Change agents Individuals with formal or informal legitimate power whose purpose is to initiate, champion, and direct or guide change. (Ch. 17)

Change management The overall processes and strategies used to moderate and manage the preparation for, effect of, responses to, and outcomes of any condition or circumstance that is new or different from what existed previously. (Ch. 17)

Change outcome The end product of a change process. (Ch. 17)

Change process The series of ongoing efforts applied to managing a change. (Ch. 17)

Change situations The field comprising various factors and dynamics within which change is occurring. (Ch. 17)

Chaos A condition of disorder or confusion. (Ch. 30)

Chaos theory Theoretical construct defining the random-appearing yet deterministic characteristics of complex organizations (see *Nonlinear change*). (Ch. 17)

Charge nurse A registered nurse responsible for delegating and coordinating patient care and staff on a specific unit. A resource person for all staff; there is usually one charge nurse each shift per unit. (Ch. 13)

Charges The cost of providing a service plus a markup for profit. (Ch. 12)

Chemically dependent A psychophysiological state in which an individual requires a substance, such as drugs or alcohol, to prevent the onset of symptoms of abstinence. (Ch. 24)

Clinical decision support/clinical decision support systems Defined broadly, CDS is a clinical computer system, computer application, or process that helps health professionals make clinical decisions to enhance patient care. (Ch. 11)

Clinical guidelines Statements of practice expectations developed by a group of healthcare practitioners to guide the clinical management of patients. (Ch. 21)

Clinical nurse leader An evolving role of the professional nurse being developed by the American Association of Colleges of Nursing (AACN). (Ch. 13)

Coaching The strategy a manager uses to help others learn, think critically, and grow through communications about performance. (Ch. 15)

Coalitions Groups of individuals or organizations that join together temporarily around a common goal. This goal often focuses on an effort to effect change. (Ch. 10)

Collaborating Involves a group of people working together to achieve a common goal. (Ch. 23)

Collective action A mechanism for achieving professional practice through group decision making. (Ch. 19)

Collective bargaining Mechanism for settling labor disputes by negotiation between the employer and representatives of the employees. (Chs. 5, 19)

Commitment A state of being emotionally impelled; feeling passionate about and dedicated to a project or event. (Ch. 18)

Communication technology An extension of wireless (WL) technology that enables hands-free communication among mobile hospital workers. (Ch. 11)

Competing Assertive, uncooperative approach to conflict in which the individual pursues own needs at the expense of others. (Ch. 23)

Complexity compression The intensity of increasing functions and expectations without a change in resources, including time. (Ch. 30)

Complexity theory Requires leaders to expand and respond to engaging dynamic change and focus on relationships rather than on prescribing and approaching change as a lock-step, preprescribed method. Traditional organizational hierarchy plays a less significant role as the "keeper of high level knowledge" and replaces it with the idea that knowledge applied to complex problems is better distributed among the human assets within an organization, without regard to hierarchy. Leaders try less to control the future and spend more time influencing, innovating, and responding to the many factors that influence health care. (Ch. 1)

Compromising Moderately assertive, cooperative approach to conflict in which the individual's ability to negotiate and willingness to give and take result in conflict resolution and fulfillment of priorities for all involved. (Ch. 23)

Computerized provider order entry (CPOE) System that uses computers for creating orders for care to be made electronically and to coordinate with other elements of an individual's care and record so that one entry performs multiple functions. (Ch. 11)

Confidentiality Right of privacy to the medical record of a patient; also, a respect for the privacy of information and the ethical use of information for its original purpose. (Ch. 5)

Conflict A perceived difference among people and a four-stage process including frustration, conceptualization, action, and outcomes. (Ch. 23)

Consolidated systems A group of healthcare organizations that are united based on common characteristics of ownership, regional location, or mutual performance objectives for the purpose of optimizing utilization of their resources in achieving their missions. (Ch. 7)

Consumer focus Centering of action or attention on the participant or user as a whole. (Ch. 22)

Continuing education Learning that builds on prior knowledge and experience with the goal of being a more competent professional. (Ch. 29)

Continuous quality improvement (CQI) A comprehensive program designed to continually improve the quality of care. Often used interchangeably with *total quality management, quality management, quality improvement,* and *performance improvement.* (Ch. 20)

Contractual allowance A discount from full charges. (Ch. 12)

Coping The immediate response of a person to a threatening situation. (Ch. 28)

Corporate liability The condition of being responsible for corporate loss related to acts performed and not performed in meeting obligations to operate legally and judiciously. (Ch. 5)

Cost The amount spent on something. The national healthcare costs are a function of the price and utilization of healthcare services; a healthcare provider's costs are the expenses involved in providing goods or services. (Ch. 12)

Cost-based reimbursement A retrospective payment method in which all allowable costs are used as the basis for payment. (Ch. 12)

Cost center An organizational unit for which costs can be identified and managed. (Chs. 12, 14)

Creativity Conceptualizing new and innovative approaches to solving problems or making decisions. (Ch. 6)

Critical path/critical pathway A component of a care MAP that is specific to diagnosis-related group reimbursement. The purpose is to ensure patients are discharged before insurance reimbursement is eliminated. (Ch. 13)

Critical thinking A composite of knowledge, attitudes, and skills; an intellectually disciplined process. Also, the ability to assess a situation by asking open-ended questions about the facts and assumptions that underlie it and to use personal judgment and problem-solving ability in deciding how to deal with it. (Ch. 6)

Cross-culturalism Mediating between and among cultures. (Ch. 9)

Cultural competence The process of integrating values, beliefs, and attitudes different from one's own perspective in order to render effective nursing care. (Chs. 9, 22)

Cultural diversity The differences that exist between multiple viewpoints based on ethnicity, gender, religion, socioeconomic status, and other variables. (Ch. 9)

Cultural imposition The condition that exists when one individual or organization attempts to require another individual or group to accept the values, attitudes, and beliefs of the first. (Ch. 9)

Cultural marginality A condition of bordering on one or more cultures and perceiving no membership or affiliation with either. (Ch. 9)

Cultural sensitivity Capacity to feel, convey, and react to ideas, habits, customs, or traditions unique to a group of people. (Ch. 9)

Culture A way of life conveyed strongly enough for a group of people to describe its meaning. It consists of values, beliefs, attitudes, practices, rituals, and traditions. (Chs. 9, 19)

Curriculum vitae A listing of professional life activities. (Ch. 29)

Cybernetic theory Regulation of systems by managing communication and feedback mechanisms. (Ch. 17)

Data Discrete entities that describe or measure something without interpretation. (Ch. 11)

Database A collection of data elements organized and stored together. (Ch. 11)

Decision making Purposeful and goal-directed effort using a systematic process to choose among options. (Ch. 6)

Deeming authority A power granted by one with power so that the recipient acts in his or her place. (Ch. 7)

Delegatee The individual who becomes accountable for performing delegated activities. (Ch. 26)

Delegation Achieving performance of care outcomes for which an individual is accountable and responsible by sharing activities with other individuals who have the appropriate authority to accomplish the work. (Chs. 26, 28)

Delegator The individual with authority to share activities with another. (Ch. 26)

Democratic A leadership style that places control within the group at large where shared authority leads to decisions. (Ch. 6)

Depersonalization Inability to become involved in human relationships and interactions. (Ch. 28)

Differentiated nursing practice A model of care that recognizes the difference in the level of education and competency of each registered nurse. The differentiation is based on education, position, and clinical expertise. (Ch. 13)

Diffusion of innovation Process by which ideas spread through a culture. (Ch. 21)

Direct care hours The amount of time spent in providing care to patients. (Ch. 14)

Disease management Continuous, coordinated processes to manage the progression of care over the course of a disease. (Ch. 13)

DNV (Det Norske Veritas) A new deeming organization as of 2008 to accredit healthcare organizations. (Ch. 2)

Dualism An "either/or" way of conceptualizing reality in terms of two opposing sides or parts (right or wrong, yes or no), limiting the broad spectrum of possibilities that exists between. (Ch. 18)

Effective communication A process that leads to positive outcomes for senders and receivers in terms of clarity, usefulness, and efficiency. (Ch. 18)

Electronic health record (EHR)/ electronic medical record (EMR) Computer-based patient record that capitalizes on the features of electronic processes. (Ch. 11)

Emancipated minor Person younger than adulthood who is no longer under the control and regulation of parents and who may give valid consent for medical procedures; examples include married teens, underage parents, and teens in the armed services. (Ch. 5)

Emerging workforce The so-called *20-something generation,* who were born between the years of 1965 and 1985. (Ch. 3)

Emotional intelligence Monitoring emotions in a situation to guide actions and inform thought processes. (Ch. 1)

Employee assistance program Program designed to provide counseling and other services for employees through either in-house staff or a contracted mental health agency. (Ch. 28)

Empowerment A sharing of power and control with the expectation that people are responsible for themselves; also, the process by which we facilitate the participation of others in decision making within an environment in which power is equally distributed. (Chs. 10, 15, 19)

Entrenched workforce Employed persons older than 35 years who are thought of as the *Baby Boomer genera-tion*. (Ch. 3)

Ethics   Science relating to moral actions and moral values; rules of conduct recognized in respect to a particular class of human actions. (Ch. 5)

Ethics committee   Group of persons who provide structure and guidelines for potential healthcare problems, serve as an open forum for discussion, and function as patient advocates. (Ch. 5)

Ethnicity   An affiliation with a group often based on race or language. (Ch. 9)

Ethnocentrism   Viewing the world based on one's own reference group. (Ch. 9)

Evidence-based practice (EBP)   The integration of individual clinical expertise, built from practice, with the best available clinical evidence from systematic research applied to practice. (Chs. 11, 21)

Expected outcomes   The result of patient goals that are achieved through a combination of medical and nursing interventions with patient participation. (Ch. 13)

Facilitators   Factors, internal or external to the change situation, that promote movement toward a desired outcome. (Ch. 17)

Factor evaluation system   A patient classification system that incorporates specific elements or critical indicators and rates patients on each of these elements. Each indicator is assigned a weight or numerical value. (Ch. 14)

Failure mode and effects analysis (FMEA)   A method to analyze reliability problems proactively to avoid negative outcomes. (Ch. 20)

Failure to warn   Newer area of potential liability for nurse managers that involves the responsibility to warn subsequent or potential employers of nurses' incompetence or impairment. (Ch. 5)

Fee-for-service   A system in which patients have the option of consulting any healthcare provider, subject to reasonable requirements that may include utilization review and prior approval for certain services but does not include a requirement to seek approval through a gatekeeper. (Ch. 7)

Fidelity   Keeping one's promises or commitments. (Ch. 5)

Fixed costs   Costs that do not change in total as the volume of patients changes. (Ch. 12)

Fixed FTEs   Full-time equivalent roles that do not fluctuate based on patient care demands. (Ch. 14)

Flat organizational structure   Characterized by decentralization of decision making to the level of personnel carrying out the work. (Ch. 8)

Follower   Person who contributes to a group's outcomes by implementing activities and providing appropriate feedback. (Ch. 4)

Followership   Those with whom a leader interacts; involves assertive use of personal behaviors in contributing toward organizational outcomes while still acquiescing certain tasks to the leader or other team members. (Chs. 1, 19)

Forecast   The process of making decisions about the future based on multiple sources of data. (Ch. 14)

Foreseeability   Concept that certain events may reasonably be expected to cause specific consequences; third element of negligence/malpractice. (Ch. 5)

For-profit organization   An organization, such as a hospital, that is operated to create excess income (profit) for the benefit of owners or stockholders. (Ch. 7)

Full-time equivalent (FTE)   An employee who works fulltime, 40 hours per week, 2080 hours per year. (Chs. 12, 14)

Functional model of nursing   A method of providing patient care by which each licensed and unlicensed staff member performs specific tasks for a large group of patients. (Ch. 13)

Functional structure   Arrangement of departments and services by specialties. (Ch. 8)

Gatekeeper   Liaison between the consumer and the healthcare market. (Ch. 22)

General adaptation syndrome (GAS)   A set of characteristics first described by Hans Seyle that are identifiable when people experience stress. (Ch. 28)

Governance   System by which an organization controls and directs formulation and administration of policy. (Ch. 19)

Group   A number of individuals assembled together or having a unifying relationship. (Ch. 18)

Halo effect   Only positive (halo) or recent (recency) performances are acknowledged. (Ch. 15)

Healthcare consumer   Patient/customer who uses healthcare provider resources. (Ch. 22)

Healthcare providers   Agencies, insurers, physicians, nurses, and allied health people providing health-related business to consumers. (Ch. 22)

Health literacy   An individual's capacity to obtain, process, and understand health information needed to make appropriate health decisions. (Chs. 5, 22)

Hierarchy   Chain of command that connotes authority and responsibility. (Ch. 8)

High-complexity change   A complicated change situation characterized by the interactions of multiple variables of people, technology, and systems. (Ch. 17)

High tech   Mechanistic perspective that relates to the use of technology in the diagnosis and treatment of disease. (Ch. 22)

High touch   Caring, humanistic perspective that relates to the use of human skills in the care and treatment of patients. (Ch. 22)

Horizontal integration   The condition that results when two (or more) organizations with similar services come together. (Ch. 7)

Horizontal violence   Involves conflictual behaviors among individuals who consider themselves peers with equal power but with little power within the system (Ch. 23). Describes aggressive and destructive behavior of co-workers against each other (Ch. 25).

Horn effect   Only negative performances being acknowledged. (Ch. 15)

Hybrid   Possessing characteristics from several types of organizational structures. (Ch. 8)

Incivility   The condition of acting in a rude or disruptive manner. (Ch. 25)

Indemnification   Obligation resting on one person to make good any loss or damages another has incurred because of the person's actions or inactions; refers to the total shifting of the economic loss to the party chiefly responsible for that loss. (Ch. 5)

Independent contractor One who makes an agreement with another to perform a service or piece of work and retains in himself or herself control of the means, method, and manner of producing the result to be accomplished; sometimes called an *independent practitioner*. (Ch. 5)

Indirect care hours The amount of time spent in activities that support the care of patients but do not involve direct provision of care. (Ch. 14)

Influence The process of using power; may range from the punitive power of coercion to the interactive power of collaboration. (Ch. 10)

Informal change agent Person without designated authority who advances the change among a group of people. (Ch. 17)

Informatics The use of knowledge technology. (Ch. 11)

Information Communication of reception of knowledge, consisting of interpreted, organized, or structured data. (Ch. 11)

Information overload A state of stress brought about by a lack of information-processing skills. (Ch. 28)

Information technology The use of computer hardware and software to process data into information to solve problems. (Ch. 11)

Informed consent Authorization by patient or patient's legal representative to do something to the patient. (Ch. 5)

Institute for Healthcare Improvement (IHI) An independent organization devoted to improving patient safety and health care globally. (Ch. 2)

Institute of Medicine (IOM) An organization that works outside of the federal government to provide independent, scientific advice. (Ch. 2)

Interpersonal conflict Conflict that occurs between or among people. (Chs. 23, 25)

Intrapersonal conflict Conflict that occurs within an individual. (Ch. 23)

Justice Principle that persons should be treated equally and fairly. (Ch. 5)

Knowledge technology The use of expert and decision support systems to assist in making decisions about patient care delivery. (Ch. 11)

Knowledge worker An individual who performs nonrepetitive, nonroutine work consuming considerable levels of cognitive activity and judgment. (Ch. 11)

Labor cost per unit of service A comparison of budgeted salary costs per budgeted volume of service with actual salary costs per actual volume of service. (Ch. 14)

Lateral aggression Aggressive and destructive behavior of co-workers against each other. (Ch. 25)

Lateral violence Aggressive and destructive behavior or psychological harassment of nurses against each other. (Ch. 23)

Law Sum total of rules and regulations by which a society is governed; rules and regulations established and enforced by authority or custom within a given community, state, or nation. (Ch. 5)

Leader Person who demonstrates and exercises influence and power over others. (Ch. 4)

Leadership The use of personal traits to constructively and ethically influence patients, families, and staff through a process in which clinical and organizational outcomes are achieved through collective efforts. (Chs. 1, 3)

Learning organization The designation of a type of organization in which continual learning as an expectation permeates all levels to promote adequate responses required by dynamic, accelerated change. (Ch. 17)

Liability Refers to one's responsibility for his or her own conduct; an obligation or duty to be performed; responsibility for an action or outcome. (Ch. 5)

Liable Refers to one's responsibility for his or her actions or inactions. (Ch. 5)

Licensure A right granted that gives the licensee permission to do something that he or she could not legally do absent such permission; the minimum form of credentialing, providing baseline expectations for those in a particular field without identifying or obligating the practitioner to function in a professional manner as defined by the profession itself. (Chs. 5, 29)

Line function A function that involves direct responsibility for accomplishing

the objectives of a nursing department, service, or unit. (Ch. 8)

Low-complexity change An uncomplicated change situation characterized by the interactions of the limited influences of people, technology, and systems. (Ch. 17)

Magnet™ recognition A distinction granted by the American Nurses Credentialing Center for quality nursing services. (Ch. 1)

Magnet Recognition Program® The only national designation built on and evolving through research. This program is designed to acknowledge nursing excellence. (Ch. 2) Designed for healthcare organizations to achieve recognition of excellent nursing care through a self-nominating, self-appraisal process. (Ch. 13)

Malpractice Failure of a professional person to act in accordance with the prevalent professional standards or failure to foresee potential consequences that a professional person, having the necessary skills and expertise to act in a professional manner, should foresee. (Ch. 5)

Managed care Care purchased through a public or private healthcare organization whose goal is to promote quality healthcare outcomes for patients at the lowest cost possible through planning, directing, and coordinating care delivered by healthcare organizations that it may own, have contractual agreements with, or have authority over by virtue of the fact that it reimburses the organization for services provided its patients. This model rewards providers for low utilization of care that is relatively low in cost; also, a system of care in which a designated person determines the services the patient uses. (Chs. 4, 7, 12)

Management The activities needed to plan, organize, motivate, and control the human and material resources needed to achieve outcomes consistent with the organization's mission and purpose. (Chs. 1, 3)

Management theory The theory related to the activities described in *Management*. (Ch. 1)

Manager The person with accountability for a group of people. (Ch. 4)

Mandatory overtime The expectation that staff will work beyond the hours assigned, often accompanied by a real or perceived threat. (Ch. 14)

Marketing Analysis, planning, implementation, and control of programs for meeting organizational objectives. (Ch. 16)

Matrix structure An organizational structure influenced by dual authority, such as product line and discipline. (Ch. 8)

Mediation A process using a trained third party to assist with conflict resolution. (Ch. 23)

Medical home Patient-centered, multifaceted source of personal primary health care. (Ch. 22)

Mentor An experienced person who helps a less experienced person navigate into expertise. (Chs. 3, 19, 27)

Meta-analysis Statistically combines similar studies on a particular issue to determine if the findings are significant across settings. (Ch. 21)

Mission Statement of an organization's reason for being. (Ch. 8)

Moral distress A type of distress that occurs when faced with situations in which two ethical principles compete, such as when the nurse is balancing the patient's autonomy issues with attempting to do what the nurse knows is in the patient's best interest. Moral distress may occur also when the nurse manager is balancing a staff nurse's autonomy with what the nurse manager perceives to be a better solution to an ethical dilemma. (Ch. 5)

Motivation The instigation of action based on various factors, both intrinsic and extrinsic. (Ch. 1)

Multiculturalism Maintaining several different cultures. (Ch. 9)

National Quality Forum (NQF) A membership-based organization that sets priorities and goals for performance improvement and endorses standards for measurement. (Ch. 2)

Near miss A clinical situation that resulted in no injury but that highlights the need for action (e.g., attempted suicide, last minute cancellation of surgery on wrong patient). (Ch. 20)

Negative feedback Information indicating a correction is needed. (Ch. 17)

Negligence Failure to exercise the degree of care that a person of ordinary prudence, based on the reasonable person standard, would exercise under the same or similar circumstances; also known as *ordinary negligence*. (Ch. 5)

Negotiating Conferring with others to bring about a settlement of differences. (Chs. 10, 23)

Networks Resources of colleagues upon whom you can draw for advice; formal systems to provide services. (Ch. 7)

Never event Error in medical care that is clearly identifiable, preventable, and serious in its consequences for the patient and that indicates a real problem in the safety and credibility of a health care facility. These errors should never occur. Examples of never events include surgery on the wrong body part, foreign body left in a patient after surgery, mismatched blood transfusion, major medication error, severe pressure ulcer acquired in the hospital, and preventable postoperative death. (Ch. 20)

Nonlinear change Change occurring from self-organizing patterns, not human-induced ones, in complex, open-system organizations. (Ch. 17)

Nonmaleficence Principle that states that one should do no harm. (Ch. 5)

Nonproductive hours See *Nonproductive time.* (Ch. 12)

Nonproductive time Benefit time such as vacation or sick time. (Ch. 14)

Nonpunitive discipline A disciplinary measure, usually verbal, describing existing standards and goals to which the parties agreed; pay is not withheld; employee agrees either to adhere to the standards in the future or to be terminated. (Ch. 24)

Nurse outcomes Typically, a system of classification to evaluate nursing care. (Ch. 14)

Nurse practice act Legal scope of practice allowed by state legislation and authority. (Ch. 5)

Nurse-sensitive data The actual data elements collected that relate to nursing-sensitive outcomes. (Ch. 14)

Nursing care delivery model The method used to provide care to patients. (Ch. 13)

Nursing case management The process of a nurse coordinating health care by planning, facilitating, and evaluating interventions across levels of care

to achieve measurable cost and quality outcomes. (Ch. 13)

Nursing Minimum Data Set (NMDS) A specific system to collect essential data using a standardized effort. (Ch. 11)

Nursing productivity The ratio of required staff hours to actual provided staff hours. (Ch. 14)

Nursing-sensitive outcome Patient outcomes that relate to the quality of nursing care provided. (Ch. 20)

Operating budget A financial plan for day-to-day activities of an organization. (Ch. 12)

Optimizing decision Selecting the ideal solution or option to achieve goals. (Ch. 6)

Organization A business structure designed to support specific business goals and processes; or a group of individuals working together to achieve a common purpose. (Ch 8)

Organizational chart A chart that defines organizational positions' responsibility for specific functions. (Ch. 8)

Organizational conflict Conflict that occurs when a person confronts an organization's policies and procedures for patient care and personnel and its accepted norms of behavior and communication. (Ch. 23)

Organizational culture The attitudes, behaviors, and policies evident in an organization that create the ambiance and operation of the workplace. (Chs. 4, 8)

Organizational structure A framework that divides work within an organization and delineates points of authority, responsibility, accountability, and non–decision-making support. (Ch. 8)

Organizational theory The systematic analysis of how organizations and their component parts act and interact. (Ch. 8)

Organized delivery system (ODS) Network of healthcare organizations, providers, and payers who provide a comprehensive package of healthcare services at a competitive price. (Ch. 12)

Outcome criteria The result of patient goals that are expected to be achieved through a combination of nursing and medical interventions. (Ch. 13)

Outcomes Anticipated or actual effects of program activities and outputs. (Ch. 21)

Overtime Time in excess of the standard amount per day; often based on an 8-, 10-, or 12-hour shift. (Ch. 14)

Overwork A situation in which employees are expected to become more productive without additional resources. (Ch. 28)

Participative Comparable to democratic style; involves others in making decisions. (Ch. 6)

Partnership model A method of providing patient care when an RN is paired with an LPN/LVN or an unlicensed assistive person to provide total care to a number of patients. (Ch. 13)

Paternalism Principle that allows one to make decisions for another; often called *parentalism*. (Ch. 5)

Patient-care outcome A measurable end result of patient care. (Ch. 20)

Patient-focused care A model in which staff functions become centralized on a unit to reduce the number of staff required; emphasizes quality, cost, and value. (Ch. 13)

Patient outcomes See *Expected outcomes*. (Chs. 13, 14)

Patient satisfaction Measurement, frequently by an external service, of patient perception about care and services; frequently presented in reports or ratings and often compared with a prior time period and comparable service. (Ch. 22)

Payer mix The volume and type of reimbursement sources for a healthcare provider. (Ch. 12)

Payers Sources of healthcare financing or payment for health services; includes government, private insurance, and individuals (self-pay). (Ch. 12)

Percentage of occupancy The patient census divided by the number of beds on the unit. (Ch. 14)

Perfectionism The tendency to never finish anything because it is not quite perfect. (Ch. 28)

Performance appraisal Individual evaluation of work performance. (Ch. 15)

Performance improvement (PI) The application of quality improvement principles on an ongoing basis. Often used interchangeably with *total quality management, continuous quality management, quality improvement,* and *quality management.* (Ch. 20)

Personal liability Serves to make each person responsible at law for his or her own actions. (Ch. 5)

Philosophy Values and beliefs regarding nature of work derived from a mission and the rights/responsibilities of people involved. (Ch. 8)

Planned change Change expected and deliberately prepared beforehand by using systematic directional processes to develop and carry out activities to accomplish a desired outcome. (Ch. 17)

Policy A specifically designated statement to guide decisions and actions. (Ch. 10)

Politics A process of human interaction within organizations. (Ch. 10)

Portfolio A professional assemblage of materials that represent the work of the professional. These materials include such elements as evaluations, letters of recommendation or appreciation, certificates of accomplishment, copies of articles, documentation of projects (e.g., research, clinical changes, management projects), and additional educational achievements (continuing education and degree achievement). (Ch. 29)

Position description A general overall description of the duties and responsibilities of the employee. (Ch. 15)

Power The ability to influence others in the effort to achieve goals. (Ch. 10)

Practice-based evidence A research methodology that helps inform practice decisions by examining outcomes in the real world where patients may not be similar and the actual application of an intervention may have multiple variations. (Ch. 21)

Practice-based research network (PBRN) Originally formed to address research issues in primary care, PBRNs are increasingly being used in large healthcare organizations having the capability of integrating systems across multiple practice sites. Practice-based research networks in nursing exist for primary care, community nursing centers, and school nursing. (Ch. 21)

Price See *Charges*. (Ch. 12)

Primary care First access to care. (Ch. 7)

Primary nurse One who delivers autonomous care. (Ch. 13)

Primary nursing A model of patient care delivery whereby one registered nurse functions autonomously as the patient's main nurse throughout the entire hospital stay. (Ch. 13)

Privacy The right to protection against unreasonable and unwarranted interference with one's solitude; the right of an individual to be left alone. (Ch. 5)

Private non-profit (or not-for-profit) organization Organization that has funds redirected to maintenance and growth rather than as dividends to stockholders. (Ch. 7)

Problem solving Using a systematic process to solve a problem. (Ch. 6)

Process of care The desired sequence of steps that have been designed to achieve clinical standardization. (Ch. 1)

Procrastination Doing one thing when one should be doing something else. (Ch. 28)

Productive hours Paid time that is worked. (Ch. 12)

Productive time Time an employee actually works. (Ch. 14)

Productivity The ratio of outputs to inputs or, in nursing terms, of services to resources used to provide services. (Ch. 12)

Productivity report Documentation of the volume of efforts consumed. (Ch. 14)

Professional association (organization) An alliance of practitioners within a profession that provides opportunities for its members to meet leaders in the field, hone their own leadership skills, participate in policy formation, continue specialized education, and shape the future of the profession. (Ch. 29)

Profit An excess of revenues over expenses. (Ch. 12)

Progressive discipline A step-by-step process of increasing disciplinary measures, usually beginning with an oral warning, followed by a written warning, suspension, and termination, if necessary. (Ch. 24)

Prospective reimbursement A method of payment in which the third-party payer decides in advance the flat rate that will be paid for a service or episode of care. (Ch. 12)

Prototype evaluation system System of classifying in broad categories. (Ch. 14)

Providers See *Healthcare provider.* (Ch. 12)

Public institution Providing health services under the support and direction of local, state, or federal government. (Ch. 7)

Quality assurance (QA) A process that focuses on the clinical aspects of a provider's care, often in response to an identified problem. (Ch. 20)

Quality improvement (QI) An ongoing process of innovation, prevention of error, and staff development used by an organization that has adopted a quality management philosophy. Often used interchangeably with *total quality management, continuous quality management, quality improvement,* and *quality management.* (Ch. 20)

Quality indicators Measurable elements of quality that specify the focus of evaluation and documentation. (Chs. 4, 22)

Quality management (QM) A corporate culture emphasizing customer satisfaction, innovation, and employee involvement in quality improvement activities. Often used interchangeably with *total quality management, continuous quality management, quality improvement,* and *performance improvement.* (Ch. 20)

Quantum theory A physics theory stating that energy is not a smooth-flowing continuum but, rather, bursts of energy that are related. (Ch. 4)

Randomized controlled trial (RCT) Study in which patients are assigned by chance to one of the groups defined in the study. (Ch. 21)

Redesign Technique to analyze tasks to improve efficiency. (Ch. 8)

Reengineering A total reorganization of how an organization will function, with the goal of increased efficiency. (Ch. 8)

Research A systematic investigation to determine the truth or falsehood of a hypothesis. (Ch. 21)

Research utilization Process of synthesizing, discriminating, and using research-generated knowledge to make an impact or change in existing practices. (Ch. 21)

Respect for others The highest ethical principle, respect for others acknowledges the right of individuals to make decisions and to live by those decisions. (Ch. 5)

Respondeat superior A doctrine by which the employer is given accountability and responsibility for an employee's negligent actions incurred during the course and scope of employment. (Ch. 5)

Responsibility The condition of being reliable and dependable and being obligated to accomplish work. (Ch. 26)

Restructuring Technique to enhance organizational productivity. (Ch. 8)

Résumé A summary of professional abilities and facts designed for specific opportunities. (Ch. 29)

Revenue Money earned by an organization for providing goods or services. (Ch. 12)

Risk management Integrated into a quality management program as a process of developing and implementing strategies that will minimize risks and mitigate the impact of adverse effects. This includes preventing patient injury, minimizing financial loss after a problem/error occurs, and preserving agency reputation. (Ch. 20)

Role Expected or actual behavior, determined by a person's position or status in a group. (Ch. 4)

Role ambiguity A condition in which individuals do not have a clear understanding about performance and evaluation. (Ch. 15)

Role conflict A condition in which individuals understand the role but are unwilling or unable to meet the requirements. (Ch. 15)

Role development Choosing to change role expectations and/or role performance. (Ch. 27)

Role discrepancy A gap between role expectations and role performance. (Ch. 27)

Role expectations The attitudes and behaviors another anticipates a person in the role will possess or demonstrate. (Ch. 27)

Role internalization Stage at which a person has learned behaviors that maintain a role so thoroughly that the person performs them without consciously considering them; energy once spent on establishing these behaviors can be redirected to other goals. (Ch. 27)

Role model A person who enacts a role, typically in a positive way, so that others can follow the example. (Ch. 19)

Role negotiation Resolving conflicting expectations about personal management performance through communication. (Ch. 27)

Role strain The subjective feeling of discomfort experienced as a result of role stress; may manifest through increased frustration, heightened emotional awareness, or emotional fragility to situations. (Chs. 24, 27)

Role stress A social condition in which role demands are conflicting, irritating, or impossible to fulfill. (Chs. 24, 27, 28)

Role theory A framework used to understand how individuals perform within organizations. (Chs. 4, 15)

Role transition The process of unlearning an old role and learning a new role. Transforming one's identity from being an individual contributor as a staff nurse to being a leader as a nurse manager. (Ch. 27)

ROLES An acronym used to identify the components of a role: **r**esponsibilities, **o**pportunities, **l**ines of communication, **e**xpectations, and **s**upport. (Ch. 27)

Root-cause analysis The process used to identify all possible causes of a sentinel event and all appropriate risk-reduction strategies. (Ch. 20)

Satisficing decision Selecting an option that is acceptable but not necessarily the best option. (Satisfy + suffice = satisfice.) (Ch. 6)

Scheduling The implementation of the staffing plan by assigning unit personnel to work specific hours and days. (Ch. 14)

Secondary care Disease restorative care. (Ch. 7)

Self-management The ability of individuals to actively gain control of their lives; components include stress management, time management, meeting management, and the ability to delegate. (Ch. 28)

Sentinel event A serious, unexpected occurrence involving death or injury, such as suicide, infant abduction, or wrong-site surgery. (Ch. 20)

Service In a healthcare context, the interaction between a consumer and the system to the extent needs are addressed. (Ch. 22)

Service-line structures A type of structure in which the functions necessary to produce a specific service or product are brought together into an integrated organizational unit under the control of a single manager or executive. (Ch. 8)

Service recovery A strategy for identifying complaints and rectifying service failures to retain or "recover" dissatisfied customers. (Ch. 22)

Shared governance A flat type of organizational structure with decision making decentralized. (Chs. 8, 19)

Shared vision Agreement among a team of people working toward a common end; concurrence on what the desired state in the future will be. (Ch. 30)

Smart card Credit card–like device that stores data. (Ch. 11)

Social networking The use of technology and other mechanisms to create a web of relationships with common involvement in an area of focus or concern. (Ch. 1)

Span of control The number of individuals a supervisor manages. For budgetary reasons, span of control is often a major focus for organizational restructuring. (Ch. 8)

Speech recognition (SR) Electronic devices and programs that permit data entry via oral entry methods. (Ch. 11)

Staff function Function that assists those in line positions in accomplishing primary objectives. (Ch. 8)

Staff mix The proportion of RNs to LPNs/LVNs to UAPs in a specific setting. (Ch. 13)

Staffing The function of planning for hiring and deploying qualified personnel to meet the needs of patients for care and services. (Ch. 14)

Staffing plan The conceptual approach of accomplishing the work to be done on a given unit. (Ch. 14)

Staffing regulations Licensing regulations required by the state department of health, usually related to the minimum number of professional nurses on a unit at a given time. (Ch. 14)

Standard of care Level of quality considered adequate by a profession; skills and learning commonly possessed by members of a profession; also written at a minimum level. (Ch. 5)

Statute Rule/regulation created by elected legislative bodies; also known as *statutory law.* (Ch. 5)

Strategic planning A process designed to achieve goals through allocation of resources. (Ch. 16)

Strategies Approaches designed to achieve a specific purpose. (Ch. 17)

Structured nursing terminology A specific approach to create a common understanding of words, especially for the purpose of data entry. (Ch. 11)

Subculture Element of a main culture that has formed its own culture that differs in some way. (Ch. 19)

Synergy A phenomenon in which teamwork produces extraordinary results that could not have been achieved by any one individual. (Ch. 18)

Synergy Model A model of care delivery adopted by the American Association of Critical-Care Nurses that matches the needs and characteristics of the patient with the competencies of the nurse. Seven characteristics are unique to every patient, and each nurse has varying levels of ability, which are categorized into eight competencies. When the knowledge, skills, and competencies of the nurse are utilized to meet the complex needs of the patient and family, the care is optimal. (Ch. 13)

System A group or organization working together as a unified whole. (Ch. 8)

Systems theory An approach to consider how various independent parts interact to form a unified whole or to disrupt a unified whole; the construct related to the operation of the whole process or entity. (Ch. 8)

Tacit knowledge An implied, unspoken knowledge (Ch. 1)

Teaching institution An academic health center and affiliated hospital. (Ch. 7)

Team A number of people associated together in specific work or activities. (Ch. 18)

Team nursing A small group of licensed and unlicensed personnel, with a team leader, responsible for providing patient care to a group of patients. (Ch. 13)

Telehealth Use of modern telecommunications and information technologies for provision of health care to individuals at a distance and transmission of information to provide that care; involves use of two-way interactive video-conferencing, high-speed phone lines, fiberoptic cable, and satellite transmissions. (Ch. 11)

Tertiary care Rehabilitative or long-term care. (Ch. 7)

The Joint Commission An organization that accredits healthcare organizations and is deemed by the Center for Medicare & Medicaid Services (CMS) as holding healthcare facilities to CMS standards. (Ch. 2)

Third-party payers Private and public agencies that contract with an individual to assume responsibility to pay under defined conditions for specified healthcare services. (Ch. 7)

Time management The use of tools, techniques, strategies, and follow-up systems to control wasted time and to ensure that the time invested in activities leads toward achieving a desired, high-priority goal. (Ch. 28)

Total patient care See *Case method.* (Ch. 13)

Total quality management (TQM) A comprehensive program designed to achieve perfection in quality of care. Often used interchangeably with *continuous quality management, quality management, quality improvement,* and *performance improvement.* (Ch. 20)

Toxic workplace An organization in which people feel devalued or dehumanized and in which disruptive behavior often flourishes. (Ch. 25)

Transactional leadership The act of using rewards and punishments as part of daily oversight of employees in seeking to get the group to accomplish a task. (Ch. 3)

Transculturalism Bridging significant differences in cultural practices. (Ch. 9)

Transformational leadership An act of encouraging followers to follow the leader's style and change their interests into a group interest with concern for a broader goal. (Ch. 3)

Transforming Care at the Bedside (TCAB) A program of the Institute for

Healthcare Improvement designed to improve care of patients. (Ch. 13)

Translating research into practice (TRIP) Approaches that integrate the use of evidence into patient care. (Ch. 21)

Unit of service A measure of the work being produced by the organization, such as patient days, patient or home visits, or procedures. (Chs. 12, 14)

Unlicensed assistive personnel Healthcare workers who are not licensed and who are prepared to provide certain elements of care under the supervision of a registered nurse (e.g., technicians, nurse aides, certified nursing assistants). (Ch. 13)

Unlicensed nursing personnel A term used to distinguish those for whom nurses are accountable as opposed to the numerous unlicensed assistive personnel providing aid in other clinical disciplines. (Ch. 26)

Utilization The quantity or volume of services provided. (Ch. 12)

Values Inner forces that influence decision making and priority setting. (Ch. 1)

Variable costs Costs that vary in direct proportion to patient volume or acuity. (Ch. 12)

Variable FTEs Those full-time equivalent positions that depend on the demand for care, typically staff positions. (Ch. 14)

Variance Anything that alters a patient's progress through a normal care path. (Chs. 12, 13)

Variance analysis Budget-control process to determine differences between income and expense, projected and actual costs. (Ch. 12)

Variance report A report defining the difference between the actual and projected staffing or budgeting. (Ch. 14)

Veracity Principle that compels the truth be told completely. (Ch. 5)

Vertical integration Alignment of organizations to provide a full array or continuum of services. (Ch. 7)

Vicarious liability Imputation of accountability upon one person or entity for the actions of another person; substituted liability or imputed liability. (Ch. 5)

Vision The desired future state. (Chs. 1, 8, 30)

Weblog *See* Blog. (Ch. 11)

Whistleblower A person who makes public a serious wrongdoing or danger concealed within an organization when internal actions have failed to correct or make public a situation. (Ch. 19)

Workload The amount of work distributed to a person or unit for a given time period. (Ch. 14)

Workplace advocacy Refers to acting on or in behalf of another who is unable to act for himself or herself to effect change about workplace conditions. (Ch. 19)